Applied Neuromuscular Pharmacology

Edited by

B. J. POLLARD

Oxford   New York   Tokyo

OXFORD UNIVERSITY PRESS

1994

Oxford University Press, Walton Street, Oxford OX2 6DP

Athens Auckland Bangkok Bombay
Calcutta Cape Town Dar es Salaam Delhi
Florence Hong Kong Istanbul Karachi
Kuala Lumpur Madras Madrid Melbourne
Mexico City Nairobi Paris Singapore
Taipei Tokyo Toronto
Oxford is a trade mark of Oxford University Press

Published in the United States
by Oxford University Press Inc., New York

A catalogue record for this book is available from the British Library

Library of Congress Cataloging in Publication Data

Applied neuromuscular pharmacology / edited by B. J. Pollard
Includes bibliographical references.
1. Neuromuscular blocking agents. I. Pollard, B. J.
[DNLM: 1. Neuromuscular Blocking agents — pharmacology. 2. Muscle
Relaxants, Central — pharmacology. 3. Drug Interactions — physiology.
4. Muscles — drug effects. QV 140 1994]
RM312.A66   1994   615'.773 — dc20   94–14338

ISBN 0 19 262148 3

Typeset by EXPO Holdings, Malaysia
Printed and bound in Great Britain by
Bookcraft (Bath) Ltd, Midsomer Norton, Avon

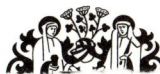

Applied Neuromuscular Pharmacology

Preface

There can be few families of drugs which have been so extensively investigated as the neuromuscular blocking agents. Indeed, the neuromuscular junction is the most comprehensively investigated synapse in existence. Despite all of this attention, we still do not know everything that there is to know about this structure and the drugs which affect it.

The muscle relaxants are central to the practice of modern anaesthesia and the 50th anniversary of their introduction into clinical anaesthetic practice was celebrated only 2 years ago. In 1942, there was only one neuromuscular blocking agent, Intocostrin. Continued research has given us a wide range of these agents, many of which have only appeared in the last 10–12 years. It is certain that more will appear in the future.

As well as new drugs, new techniques of research into neuromuscular transmission continue to be developed. There are better techniques of monitoring and it is presently possible to measure minute plasma levels with sensitive assays. We thus have an ever-increasing level of information concerning the pharmacokinetics and pharmacodynamics in normal patients and also in those with a range of pathological processes.

This book is designed to look at the subject of neuromuscular pharmacology in a different way to many of the established texts. It is not a compilation of monographs on the individual drugs and families of drugs. Instead, it is subdivided in a way which examines the characteristics and application of the drugs, for example, onset, recovery, species differences — hence the title *Applied Neuromuscular Pharmacology*. I believe that both the trainee and specialist anaesthetist, as well as scientists engaged in basic or applied research will find this book to be a valuable addition to their library.

In a multi-author book, there are inevitably differences in style between the chapters. No attempts have been made to move to a unified style and I hope that these differences in style will better hold the reader's interest. Likewise, in a multi-author book there are repetitions. No attempt has been made to remove these because when the same fact is described in two different ways in two different contexts, the reader is more likely to understand and remember it.

I have been able to assemble a group of authors with a widespread knowledge in neuromuscular pharmacology and the clinical applications of these drugs. I am grateful to all of the authors of the individual chapters for their excellent contributions.

Finally, thanks must go to my personal secretary, Mrs K. Dimelow, without whose organizational and word-processing skills much would not be possible.

Manchester   B.J.P.
May 1994

Contents

Contributors

Hassan H. Ali Department of Anesthesia, Massachusetts General Hospital, Boston, MA 02114, USA.

J. R. Barrie University Department of Anaesthesia, Withington Hospital, Nell Lane, West Didsbury, Manchester M20 8LR, UK.

E. Baubillier Service d'anesthesie reanimation, Hospital Henri Mondor, 94010, Creteil, Cedex, France.

David R. Bevan Department of Anaesthesia, University of British Columbia, Vancouver, BC, Canada.

Jan Bonde Department of Anaesthesia, Herlev Hospital, University of Copenhagen, Herlev Ringvej, DK-2730, Denmark.

L. H. D. J. Booij Department of Anaesthesiology, University of Nijmegen, Nijmegen, Netherlands.

François Donati Department of Anaesthesia, Royal Victoria Hospital, 687 Pine Avenue W., Montreal, Quebec, Canada, H3A 1A1.

P. Duvaldestin Service d'anesthesie reanimation, Hospital Henri Mondor, 94010, Creteil, Cedex, France.

N. Fauvel Magill Department of Anaesthetics, Charing Cross and Westminster Hospitals, Fulham Road, London, SW10 9NH, UK.

S. A. Feldman Magill Department of Anaesthetics, Charing Cross and Westminster Hospitals, Fulham Road, London, SW10 9NH, UK.

Francis F. Foldes Department of Anesthesiology, University of Miami School of Medicine, PO Box 016370, Miami, Florida, 33101, USA.

Nishan G. Goudsouzian Department of Anesthesia, Massachusetts General Hospital, Boston, MA 02114, USA.

N. J. N. Harper Department of Anaesthesia, Manchester Royal Infirmary, Oxford Road, Manchester M13 9WL, UK.

T. E. J. Healy University Department of Anaesthesia, Withington Hospital, Nell Lane, West Didsbury, Manchester M20 8LR, UK.

Jennifer M. Hunter University Department of Anaesthesia, Royal Liverpool University Hospital, Prescot Street, PO Box 147, Liverpool L69 3BX, UK.

R. S. Jones University Department of Anaesthesia, Royal Liverpool University Hospital, Prescot Street, PO Box 147, Liverpool L69 3BX, UK.

G. J. McCarthy Department of Anaesthetics, The Queen's University of Belfast, Whitla Medical Building, Lisburn Road, Belfast, UK.

I. G. Marshall Department of Physiology and Pharmacology, University of Strathclyde, George Street, Glasgow G1 1XW, UK.

Claude Meistelman Department of Anaesthesia, Institut Gustave Roussy, Rue Camille Desmoulins, 94805, Villejuif, Cedex, France.

R. K. Mirakhur Department of Anaesthetics, The Queen's University of Belfast, Whitla Medical Building, Lisburn Road, Belfast, UK.

B. J. Pollard University Department of Anaesthesia, Manchester Royal Infirmary, Oxford Road, Manchester M13 9WL, UK.

George D. Shorten Department of Anesthesia, Massachusetts General Hospital, Boston, MA 02114, USA.

Jorgen Viby-Mogensen Department of Anaesthesia, Rigshospitalet, University of Copenhagen, 9 Blegdamsvej, DK-2100, Copenhagen, Denmark.

R. D. Waigh Department of Pharmaceutical Sciences, University of Strathclyde, George Street, Glasgow G1 1XW, UK.

1

Introduction and historical perspectives

Francis F. Foldes

There can be little doubt that the introduction of neuromuscular blocking agents (muscle relaxants) into anaesthetic practice heralded the start of the modern era of anaesthesiology. It made possible the performance of major intraperitoneal operations requiring muscular relaxation in light planes of general anaesthesia, all but eliminated the concept of inoperability due to advanced pathophysiological changes or extremes of age, and made possible the development of open heart and organ transplant surgery. Only those anaesthetists who, before the advent of curare, had to provide adequate operating conditions for intraperitoneal, intrathoracic and intracranial surgery with ether or cyclopropane anaesthesia can really appreciate the significance of muscle relaxants.

The then prevailing conditions were eloquently depicted by Gillies (1952) who stated:

In many clinics uncompensated depression of respiratory and circulatory functions, seen at its worse in third and fourth plane ether anaesthesia and regarded as ideal for abdominal surgery became routine. In submitting to operations involving vital functions directly or indirectly to an extent never before known, patients had enough to overcome on their way to recovery without the extra burden of the metabolic, respiratory and cardiovascular disturbances added by prolonged general anaesthesia.

The availability of muscle relaxants made possible the development of balanced anaesthesia (Gray and Halton 1946), a concept advocated earlier by Lundy (1942), in the true sense of the word, and facilitated the revolutionary advances in open-heart, organ transplant, and intracranial surgery.

More than four centuries elapsed between the time that the news of a mysterious arrow poison, used by the Indians of South America reached Europe, and the first use of a standardized extract of *Chondodendron tomentosum*, Intocostrin, by Griffith and Johnson (1942) for the production of muscular relaxation in anaesthetized patients. The fiftieth anniversary of this momentous event having recently taken place, it might be of interest to anaesthesiologists to retrace the slow and tortuous progress that changed the lethal arrow poison of Indians to one of the most frequently used drugs, and which contributed so significantly to the reduction of operative and postoperative morbidity and mortality of surgical patients.

EARLY HISTORY

The first news of the existence of deadly arrow poisons reached Europe soon after the discovery of the 'New World' by Columbus in 1492. Peter Martyr d'Anghera (1516), an Italian friar, who lived in the Court of Ferdinand and Elizabeth in Madrid, described in his book several incidents in which Spanish sailors and soldiers, who accompanied the conquistadors in the early explorations of Central and South America, were killed by poisoned arrows. On one occasion, described by d'Anghera (1516) (Thomas 1963, p. 14), 700 warriors of an 'Indian King' attacked a group of sailors who landed to replenish their water supplies and killed 47 of them. In the course of the next two centuries numerous accounts were published on the geographic distribution of the use, botanical origin, and modes of preparation of these mysterious arrow poisons, referred to as urari, wourari, curara, and many other names (Thomas 1963, p. 22). These accounts consist of variable mixtures of fact and fancy. I would like to refer those interested in these fascinating stories to the detailed, absorbing monographs of Gill (1940), McIntyre (1947), Thomas (1963), and Smith (1969).

GEOGRAPHIC DISTRIBUTION OF ARROW POISONS

Arrow poisons had been used primarily by natives of the northern part of South America, in an area located between 10 degrees north and 10 degrees south of the equator, encompassing the Guyanas, the northern part of Brazil, Venezuela, Columbia, Ecuador, and Peru (Thomas 1963, pp. 16–18). It appears that the main ingredient of curares produced in the western part of this area was *Chondodendron tomentosum*, later shown to contain *d*-tubocurarine (Wintersteiner and Dutcher 1943). In most other areas curares were produced from *Strychnos toxifera* and other varieties of *Strychnos*. The main ingredients of these poisons were probably toxiferines (Karrer and Schmidt 1946). It is possible, however, that poisoned narrows have also been used much further south. One of Magellan's sailors was killed by a poisoned arrow, when in 1520 during an expedition searching for the westward passage to India, he wintered in Patagonia (Karrer 1967). It is not at all sure, however, that the arrow poison used by the Patagonian natives contained any neuromuscular blocking agent. In the rest of this chapter, chemically unidentified arrow poisons will occasionally be referred to as curare(s).

CHEMISTRY OF ARROW POISONS

In all probability the first European witnesses of the preparation of curares were Bancroft (1769) (see Thomas 1963, pp. 27–28), Von Humboldt and Bonland (1807) (see McIntyre 1947, pp. 28–30), Schomburgk (1841) (see McIntyre 1947, pp. 30–35). They all reported that the main ingredient of the toxin prepared in Guyana was the extract of the bark of *Strychnos toxifera*. Boehm (1897), the famous German chemist, based on the chemical analysis of samples available in different types of containers, distinguished tube-, pot-, and calabash-curares. Gill (1946), however, was of the opinion, that the chemical characteristics of various arrow poisons could not be based on the type of container. In his experience the natives who prepared these poisons used whatever container was handy. Thanks to the pioneering work of King (1935), it was definitely established that the main active ingredient of tube-curare is *d*-tubocurarine, later extracted from *Chondodendron tomentosum* by Winterseteiner and Dutcher (1943). Pot-curare and gourd-curare contain alkaloids extracted from *Strychnos toxifera* and other *Strychnos* varieties, referred to by Wieland and Pistor (1938) as curarines. Some of these were shown to be tertiary and others quaternary alkaloids (Karrer 1967) and were collectively name toxiferines. The tertiary alkaloids were the starting materials for the synthesis of toxiferine I and the closely related diallylnortoxiferine (alcuronium) (Schmidt 1967). Toxiferine I is the most potent nondepolarizing muscle relaxant ever used in clinical practice (Foldes *et al.* 1961*a*).

EARLY EXPERIMENTAL USE OF CURARES

Early animal experiments with curares had been conducted since the 1730s by de la Condamine, Ulloa, Herrisant, Brocklesby, Bancroft, Fontana, Von Humboldt, and others (for details see Thomas 1963, pp. 24–43). In the early 19th century, the famous British surgeon Brodie (1812) was the first to show that rabbits paralysed with curare could be kept alive with artificial respiration, administered through an opening in the trachea. This was probably the first time that artificial respiration was administered through a tracheostomy opening (Thomas 1963, p. 33). His most famous experiment in 1814 was carried out on an ass, appropriately named Wouralia. In this experiment, described by him much later in 1851 (see Thomas 1963, p. 34) he was assisted by the veterinarian Sewel. The explorer Charles Waterton, who supplied the curare and the ass, was also present. The poison, wouraly, was administered to the ass through a shoulder wound and complete paralysis ensued in 10 minutes. Subsequently the animal was tracheotomized, ventilated with a pair of bellows for two hours, survived the experiment and lived for another 25 years. Both Brodie and Waterton (see Thomas 1963, p. 34) independently described the experiment. It appears that the quest for priority was not much different in the early 19th century from what it is today: Brodie credited Waterton with supplying the ass and the arrow poison and Waterton does not even mention that Brodie participated in the experiment.

EARLY CLINICAL USE OF CURARE

Early clinical uses of curare, from the beginning of the 19th century up to 1938 are described in detail by McIntyre (1947, pp. 85–88) and by Thomas (1963, pp. 85–104). The first clinical use of curare can also be traced back to Brodie (1812) who in 1811 suggested its use in tetanus. During the 19th century numerous attempts were made to use carare for the treatment of tetanus, hydrophobia, epilepsy, and chorea. Considering the variable potency of the available curare preparations and the unscientific methods of its administration, e.g. topical application (Sayres 1858), it is no wonder that these attempts were usually unsuccessful. In 1938 Bennett, on the suggestion of McIntyre, used a standardized curare preparation, Intocostrin, for the prevention of trauma in convulsive therapy (Bennett 1941).

CLARIFICATION OF THE MODE OF ACTION OF MUSCLE RELAXANTS

Until the classical experiments of Claude Bernard (1850) on the frog nerve–muscle preparation there was considerable disagreement on the site of action of curare. The nerve, the muscle, and the brain were all proposed as sites of the paralysing effect of curare. The work of Bernard, confirmed by the Swiss physiologist Kollicke (1858), definitely established the neuromuscular junction as the site of the paralysing effect of curare.

It was suggested by Lapicque and his wife Marcelle (1913) that the nerve impulse is transmitted to the muscle by an electrical current and that curare inhibits the sensitivity of the muscle to this electrical stimulus. This theory was supported by other investigators (Thomas 1963, pp. 69). A modified form of the electrical transmission theory was proposed by Nachmansohn (1959) who suggested that intraneurally released acetylcholine (ACh) initiated an electrical current which traversed the synaptic cleft, depolarized the postjunctional membrane, and initiated the endplate action potential that ultimately elicits contraction of the muscle fibre. These theories of 'electrical transmission' of the nerve impluse have been discredited. It is now universally accepted that ACh is stored in the motor nerve terminal in synaptic vesicles which contain several thousand molecules of ACh, and is released from the vesicles by the nerve impulse (quantal release). ACh diffuses through the synaptic cleft, and interacts with specific nicotinic receptors (cholinoceptors) of the postjunctional membrane (endplate). This interaction depolarizes the endplate and initiates the electrical current responsible for the contraction of the muscle fibre. Within a few milliseconds ACh is hydrolysed by acetylcholinesterase, the endplate becomes repolarized and the muscle relaxes (for further details see Chapters 2 and 3; Foldes 1957; Bowman 1990; I. G. Marshall, 1991). This depolarization–repolarization sequence is essential for physiological neuromuscular transmission.

At first it was generally accepted that both depolarizing and nondepolarizing neuromuscular blocking agents act postjunctionally and produce neuromuscular block by preventing the repolarization or depolarization of the endplate (Foldes 1957). Subsequently it became evident that neuromuscular blocking agents also interact with presynaptic nicotinic receptors and thereby inhibit the positive feedback mechanism of ACh mobilization from reserve stores to release sites (Glavinovic 1979; Foldes *et al.* 1989; Bowman *et al.* 1990). The amount of ACh available for release by the nerve impulse is thereby inhibited. This has been demonstrated by direct measurement of the ACh released by the nerve impulse in the absence or presence of muscle relaxants (Foldes *et al.* 1984; Foldes and Vizi 1985; Vizi *et al.* 1985). When used in large doses, neuromuscular blocking agents may obstruct the ion channels of the postjunctional membrane and thereby contribute to the intensity of the neuromuscular block (Katz and Miledi 1978; Standaert 1986; Bowman 1990, pp. 145–149).

DEVELOPMENTS LEADING TO THE INTRODUCTION OF MUSCLE RELAXANTS INTO ANAESTHETIC PRACTICE

The first steps toward the introduction of muscle relaxants into clinical practice had to await two important developments in the chemistry of these compounds. The first of these was the extraction of curarine from calabash curare (Boehm 1897). In retrospect, based on the botanical origin of calabash curare (*Strychnos toxifera* and other varieties of *Strychnos*) and the high potency of curarine, it may be assumed that it consisted mostly of c-toxiferine I isolated a half century later from the bark of *Strychnos toxifera* by Karrer and Schmidt (1946). On the instigation of Boehm, A. Läwen (1912), a German surgeon, administered 0.8 mg curarine intramuscularly to surgical patients anaesthetized with ether. In his paper he points out the dangers of deep ether or chloroform anaesthesia required for the provision of adequate muscular relaxation for the then developing intraperitoneal surgery. He attempted to produce surgical relaxation under light general anaesthesia by the concomitant use of high extradural (paravertebral) anaesthesia. It is not surprising that with the 0.5–2.0 per cent procaine solution used, the relaxation obtained with combined regional and general anaesthesia was often unsatisfactory. This prompted him to attempt the use of curarine. He pointed out that:

1. Curarine, in contrast to other curare preparations, has uniform potency and its neuromuscular effect is reproducible.

2. With the appropriate dose of curarine it is possible to paralyse the skeletal muscles of mice and guinea pigs, without paralysing the diaphragm.

3. When, with higher doses of curarine, the respiratory muscles are also paralysed the animals can be kept alive by artificial ventilation.

He further observed that to produce relaxation of abdominal muscles it is not necessary to produce complete paralysis, and that this goal can be achieved by the combination of regional and/or general anaesthesia, with moderate doses of curarine. Lawen pointed out that although he never administered more than 0.8 mg curarine intramuscularly or subcutaneously it would be permissible to increase the dose or to administer smaller doses i.v. He stated that because of the unavailability of adequate supplies of curarine he was unable to further explore the clinical usefulness of curarine.

This remarkably intuitive surgeon described in one publication the use of high epidural block, the clinical use of which is generally attributed to Paget (1921), and the first anaesthetic use of muscle relaxants 30 years before Harold Griffith and Enid Johnson (1942) administered curare to their patients. It is interesting to speculate how the course of the development of anaesthesia and surgery would have changed if the First World War and its aftermath had not interfered with the progress of German science and medicine.

The second important development occurred more than 20 years later when, in England, H. King (1935) extracted crystalline *d*-tubocurarine from a museum sample of tube-curare. This preparation was used by West (1936) in continuous intravenous infusion for the treatment of tetanus in three patients. No attempt was made, again perhaps because of the paucity of supplies, to use crystalline *d*-tubocurarine for the production of muscular relaxation during surgery. Just as World War I interrupted the work of Lawen in Germany, the impending World War II might have disrupted progress in the clinical use of curare in England.

THE FINAL STEPS LEADING TO THE INTRODUCTION OF MUSCLE RELAXANTS INTO ANAESTHETIC PRACTICE

At about the same time that King (1935) isolated and determined the chemical structure of *d*-tubocurarine, Gill (1940) brought from Ecuador to the USA substantial quantities of crude curare and also vines and bark of *Chondodendron tomentosum*, which he believed to contain the active ingredient of curare. A. R. McIntyre (1947) prepared a standardized extract of Gill's crude curare. Starting in 1938 at his suggestion, it was used first by Bennett (1941), and subsequently by many other psychiatrists, for the prevention of trauma in psychiatric patients receiving electroconvulsive or metrazol-shock therapy. Soon afterwards Intocostrin, an extract of 'unauthenticated curare', was prepared in the laboratories of E.R. Squibb and Sons from the vines of *Chondodendron tomentosum*. This extract was standardized with the rabbit 'head drop' test of H. A. Holaday (1947). By the end of 1941 Intocostrin had been used by psychiatrists on thousands of occasions and several publications appeared on its use in conjunction with shock therapy and for the treatment of spastic conditions (for references see McIntyre 1947, pp. 190–193). For some reason these developments failed to arouse the interest of anaesthesiologists, who continued to administer dangerously deep levels of anaesthesia for the provision of muscular relaxation for intraperitoneal and the then developing intrapleural surgery.

Much of the credit for the introduction of curare (Intocostrin) into anaesthetic practice is due to Lewis H. Wright who, at the time of the development of Intocostrin, was affiliated to the medical department of E. R. Squibb and Sons. Wright was originally trained as an obstetrician, but between February 1938 and October 1939 he also received training in anaesthesiology in Professor Rovenstine's department at Bellevue Hospital in New York (Professor H. Turndorf, personal communication). As an anaesthesiologist, Wright was undoubtedly cognizant of the difficulties associated with the production of adequate muscular relaxation for abdominal surgery with ether, and even more so with cyclopropane, frequently used at Bellevue Hospital. Because of his connections with E. R. Squibb and Sons, he had the opportunity to observe the prevention of the traumatic effects of shock therapy by Intocostrin. It occurred to him that, when combined with general anaesthesia, it would provide excellent operating conditions for abdominal surgery. At first he had no success in selling his idea to anaesthesiologists. In retrospect it should not be surprising that the concept of using a drug that could paralyse the respiratory muscles was abhorrent to anaesthesiologists, whose motto was *'dum spiro speroll'* (as long as there is breath there is hope). It should be remembered that at that time tracheal intubation was seldom practised and controlled ventilation was only used as an emergency measure. Finally in 1941 it seemed that Wright's efforts were not in vain. Two prominent anaesthesiologists, E. A. Rovenstine of New York and S. C. Cullen of Iowa City, agreed to give Intocostrin a try. His expectations, however, were not to be fulfilled. Professor Rovenstine asked his assistant E. M. Papper to test Intocostrin in anaesthetized surgical patients. Papper, who throughout his illustrious career did so much for the development of anaesthesiology, missed the chance of a lifetime on this occasion. He probably administered a large dose or an exceptionally potent sample of Intocostrin to his two patients, anaesthetized with ether, and had to administer artificial respiration to both for several hours to keep them alive. The standardized curare preparation, Intocostrin, of the early 1940s did not have uniform potency. According to Thomas (1963, p. 105) the *d*-tubocurarine content of 1 unit of Intocostrin varied between 0.15 and 3.3 mg. Papper told Rovenstine that curare was far too dangerous for clinical use.

Cullen got even less far. Based on his dog experiments he also considered curare too dangerous for clinical use. However, after learning of Griffith's excellent results (Griffith and Johnson 1942), he became the foremost advocate of the clinical use of curare in the USA (Cullen 1943).

The disappointed Wright met Griffith at a medical meeting in Montreal in 1941. Griffith asked Wright whatever happened to his hopes of using curare for the provision of relaxation during surgery. In spite of Wright's disappointing story he made up his mind to try curare. On 23 January 1942, Harold Griffith and Enid Johnson took the giant step that changed the course of anaesthesiology and made possible the dramatic advances of modern surgery.

It is interesting to speculate why Harold Griffith was willing to test curare in anaesthetized patients and why he succeeded in administering it safely and effectively. He was well aware of the fact that it was more difficult to produce good surgical relaxation with cyclopropane, his favourite inhalation anaesthetic agent, than with ether, used by most contemporary anaesthesiologists. Curare promised a solution to this problem, that caused him much concern. After he studied the reports on the experimental results obtained with curare and on its use in electroshock therapy he became convinced that, applied cautiously, it could become a valuable adjunct to general anaesthesia. He was confident that he could manage the paralysis of the respiratory muscles, that may be encountered with curare. He also realized that curare should be used to produce good muscular relaxation in lightly anaesthetized patients and not complete paralysis in insufficiently anaesthetized patients. His first attempts with the use of curare in anaesthetised patients were uniformly successful and the publication of his classical succint report, later in 1942, heralded the start of the modern era of anaesthesiology.

THE SPREAD OF THE USE OF CURARE IN ANAESTHETIC PRACTICE

In spite of its obvious advantages, the use of curare in anaesthesiology was slow to take hold. Two unrelated factors may have been responsible for this. The first of these was that deliberate depression of respiration was considered a heresy. Gray and Halton (1946) were the first to meet this challenge head-on. They pointed out that when muscle relaxants are used, it may be necessary to paralyse spontaneous breathing deliberately and to control the patient's ventilation. The second factor that inhibited the rapid spread of the use of curare was the fact that most of the younger generation of anaesthetists, who perhaps would have been more receptive to this new, revolutionary concept, were serving in the armed forces. It is interesting that Adriani (1945) did not consider curare important enough to include a reference to it in the third printing of the second edition of his *Pharmacology of Anaesthetic Drugs*.

In the first decade after its introduction there was considerable criticism of the use of muscle relaxants. Beecher and Todd (1954), in a detailed analysis of 600 000 surgical cases in 10 university hospitals, concluded that the use of muscle relaxants caused a six-fold increase of anaesthesia related deaths. This report caused much concern among anaesthesiologists who by then were using not only curare but also the new synthetic muscle relaxants with increasing frequency. The widespread discussion of this report helped to clarify many aspects of the use of muscle relaxants. It became evident that muscle relaxants, despite their advantages, are potentially dangerous drugs which have to be administered with extreme care. It was pointed out in a joint publication by 16 of the leading exponents of the use of muscle relaxants (Abajian *et al.* 1955) that, whenever they are used, the patient's ventilation should be adequately assisted or controlled, the residual curarization at the end of anaesthesia should be antagonized, and that hypokalaemia, dehydration, and respiratory and circulatory acidosis should be avoided. Attention was drawn to the potentiation of the effect of muscle relaxants by magnesium, certain antibiotics and other drugs that may be used in the perioperative period (Foldes 1959). The increased sensitivity to nondepolarizing muscle relaxants in certain pathological conditions (e.g. myasthenia gravis, carcinomatous neuropathy) (Foldes and McNall 1962) and to suxamethonium in genetically determined anomalies of plasma cholinesterase (Kalow 1956; Foldes *et al.* 1963*a*) became recognized. It became evident that, when used properly, the advantages of muscle relaxants far outweigh their disadvantages and that competent anaesthesiologists deserve muscle relaxants and incompetent anaesthesiologists need them.

SEARCH FOR NEW MUSCLE RELAXANTS

As more experience had been gathered with curare it was pointed out by Landmesser (1947), that even when used correctly tubocurarine may cause hypotension and/or bronchiolar constriction in certain patients. These complications are caused

Table 1.1 Muscle relaxants in clinical use or investigated in humans

Gallamine	Huguenard and Boue (1950)
	Mushin *et al.* (1949)
Dimethyltubocurarine	Stoelting *et al.* (1948)
Decamethonium	Organe (1949)
Suxethonium	Valdoni (1949)
Benzoquinonium	Arrowood (1951)
	Foldes *et al.* (1952)
Suxamethonium	Brucke *et al.* (1951)
	von Dardel and Thesleff (1951)
	Mayrhofer and Hassfurther (1951)
Laudolissin	Bodman *et al.* (1952)
Imbretil	Holzer *et al.* (1954)
	Mayrhofer *et al.* (1955)
Prestonal	Frey (1955)
	Rendell-Baker *et al.* (1957)
Toxiferine	Waser and Harbeck (1959)
	Foldes *et al.* (1961*a*)
Alcuronium	Hügin and Kissling (1961)
	Foldes *et al.* (1963*b*)
Pancuronium	Baird and Reid (1967)
	Foldes *et al.* (1971)
	Katz (1971)
Fazadinium	Simpson *et al.* (1972)
Vecuronium	Agoston *et al.* (1980)
	Booij *et al.* (1980)
Atracurium	Hunt *et al.* (1980)
	Payne and Hughes (1981)
Pipecuronium	Boros *et al.* (1980)
	Tassonyi (1981)
Mivacurium	Savarese *et al.* (1985)
	Savarese *et al.* (1988)
Doxacurium	Basta *et al.* (1988)
	Murray *et al.* (1988)
Rocuronium	Wierda *et al.* (1990)
(ORG 9426)	Foldes *et al.* (1990)
	Foldes *et al.* (1991)

Modified from Foldes (1990)

by inhibition of synaptic transmission in the sympathetic nervous system and/or histamine release. These side effects of *d*-tubocurarine prompted the search for muscle relaxants that would retain the desirable neuromuscular blocking activity, but would be free of the unwanted side-effects of curare.

In the 50 years that have elapsed since the introduction of curare into anaesthetic practice by Griffith and Johnson (1942), numerous compounds have been synthesized and tested in clinical practice (Table 1.1). In some respects, however, the pharmacodynamic and pharmacokinetic profiles of all of these compounds differ from those of the hypothetical ideal muscle relaxant (Foldes 1990) (Table 1.2). Vecuronium, pipecuronium, rocuronium (ORG 9426), and doxacurium (R. J. Marshall 1991) appear to be free of significant cardiovascular or other unwanted side effects.

Atracurium breaks down by the processes of Hofmann elimination, nucleophilic substitution, and hydrolysis, and is probably also attacked by carboxylesterase (Nigrovic 1991). The duration of action of its neuromuscular effect is not significantly affected by kidney or liver failure. Mivacurium is metabolized by plasma cholinesterase, but at a slower rate than suxamethonium (Brandom *et al.* 1989). With the exception of suxamethonium and rocuronium (Foldes *et al.* 1991), the onset of action of all the presently available muscle relaxants is too slow to provide acceptable conditions for rapid sequence intubation. Their onset time, however, can be increased by 'priming' (Foldes 1984; Schwartz *et al.* 1985).

Some of the synthetic muscle relaxants are unstable in solution and either must be dissolved immediately before use (e.g. suxamethonium, vecuronium, pipecuronium, rocuronium) or must be stored in the refrigerator (e.g. atracurium).

Because of the shortcomings of the presently available compounds, the search for the ideal muscle relaxant will continue. This search will be both time-consuming

Table 1.2 Properties of the ideal muscle relaxant

Nondepolarizing agent

Rapid onset and short duration of action

Non cumulative effect

Easily antagonized

No side-effect liability due to:
  ganglionic blockade
  inhibition of muscarinic receptors
  increased release (or inhibition of reuptake) of endogenous catecholamines
  histamine release
  significant inhibition of muscle cholinesterase

It should:
  break down spontaneously at physiological pH to inactive components
  be excreted by both kidney and liver
  have long shelf life in solution

Foldes (1990)

and expensive. The reason for this is that there is a wide variation in potency of the same muscle relaxant in different species and that the relative potencies of various muscle relaxants may change in the opposite direction in different species. As suggested earlier by Waud (1977), the effects of muscle relaxants on the skeletal muscles of humans and guinea-pigs are similar. This has been confirmed (Foldes 1991, unpublished) by comparing the potencies of tubocurarine, pancuronium, vecuronium, pipecuronium, rocuronium, and atracurium in humans, guinea-pigs, and rats. The ED_{90} values of all these compounds are closer in humans and guinea-pigs than in humans and rats. Furthermore, the five newer muscle relaxants are more potent than tubocurarine in humans and guinea-pigs and are less potent than tubocurarine in the rat. The onset time, duration of action, and recovery rate of the various muscle relaxants are also more similar in humans and guinea-pigs than in humans and rats. Consequently, the guinea-pig appears to be more suitable for the preliminary screening of muscle relaxants than the more frequently employed rat.

It is evident from the above discussion that the suitability of any new muscle relaxant for clinical use must be determined in clinical pharmacological studies in humans. The present monograph is dedicated to this concept. Because of the requirements of drug regulatory authorities, large scale clinical pharmacological studies with muscle relaxants must be preceded by extensive toxicity studies in several species.

It can occur, however, that in subsequent clinical pharmacological studies, a compound found to be safe from the point of view of organ toxicity may prove to be no better than or inferior to already available muscle relaxants. It is suggested that, before time-consuming and expensive toxicity studies are planned, promising compounds could be tested in a small number of unanaesthetized volunteers. Because of the resistance of the diaphragm to nondepolarizing muscle relaxants, considerable information can be obtained on the potency and time course of the compounds tested, with little or no discomfort to the volunteer. Repeated administration of all the muscle relaxants in clinical use revealed no significant organ toxicity. Therefore it is highly unlikely that the administration of a single, moderate dose of a new muscle relaxant, structurally similar to compounds in clinical use, should have any toxic effect. If the information obtained in these preliminary studies is favourable it is justifiable to subject the new muscle relaxant to extensive pharmacodynamic and pharmacokinetic studies in anaesthetized subjects before the required toxicity studies in several species. The feasibility of this approach has been demonstrated with tubocurarine, gallamine, toxiferine, decamethonium, and suxamethonium (Foldes *et al.* 1961*b*), pancuronium (Foldes *et al.* 1971), alcuronium (Foldes *et al.* 1963*b*), and pipecuronium (Foldes and Nagashima 1983 unpublished).

CONCLUSIONS

Anaesthetists and surgeons should be ever grateful to the dedication, persistence and courage of C. H. Gill, A. R. McIntyre, L. H. Wright, H. R. Griffith, and G. E. Johnson. Gill, in spite of his physical handicaps and in the face of great hardships, traced the source of curare to *Chondodenron tomentosum* (Gill 1940). He brought to the USA significant quantities of the bark and vines of this plant. This enabled McIntyre to prepare a clinically usable extract, Intocostrin, standardized with the rabbit head-drop test of Holaday (1947). The vision and persistence of Wright, and the support of E. R. Squibb and Sons, enabled Griffith and Johnson (1942) to take the final, courageous step that revolutionized anaesthesia and made possible the explosive development of surgery. Since the introduction of curare many new muscle relaxants have been introduced into clinical practice. Several of these have major advantages over tubocurarine. The search for even better compounds continues and there is hope that the ideal muscle relaxant will become available for clinical use in the not too distant future.

ACKNOWLEDGEMENTS

Some of the material used in this chapter was previously presented in Chapter 1 of *Muscle relaxants* (1990), A. Agoston and W. C. Bowman (ed.), Elsevier, Amsterdam. I would like to thank the editors and the publisher for their permission to use this material.

REFERENCES

Abajian, J., Jr, Arrowood, J. G., Barrett, R. H., Dwyer, C. S., Eversole, U. H., Fine, J. H., *et al.* (1955). Critique of study of the deaths associated with anesthesia and surgery. *Annals of Surgery*, **142**, 138–41.

Adriani, J. (ed.) (1945). *Pharmacology of anesthetic drugs*. Thomas, Springfield.

Agoston, S., Newton, D., Bencini, A., Boomsma, P., and Erdmann, P. (1980). The neuromuscular blocking action of ORG NC45, a new pancuronium derivative, in anaesthetized patients. *British Journal of Anaesthesia*, **52**, 53S–60S.

Arrowood, J. G. (1951). Mytolon chloride: a new agent for producing muscular relaxation. *Anesthesiology*, **12**, 754–61.

Baird, W. L. M., and Reid, A. M. (1967). The neuromuscular blocking properties of a new steroid compound, pancuronium bromide. *British Journal of Anaesthesia*, **39**, 775–80.

Bancroft, E. (1769). *Essay on the natural history of Guiana and South America*. p. 281 et seq.

Basta, S. J., Savarese, J. J., Ali, H. H., Embree, P. B., Schwartz, A. F., Rudd, G. D., *et al.* (1988). Clinical pharmacology of doxacurium chloride. A new long-acting nondepolarizing muscle relaxant. *Anesthesiology*, **69**, 478–86.

Beecher, H. K. and Todd, D. P. (1954). A study of the deaths associated with anesthesia and surgery. *Annals of Surgery*, **140**, 2–34.

Bennett, A. E. (1941). Curare: a preventive of traumatic complications in convulsive shock therapy. *American Journal of Psychiatry*, **97**, 1040–60.

Bernard, C. (1850). Action de curare et de la nicotine sur le système nerveux et sur le systèmes musculaire. *Compte Rendu de la Société de Biologie*, **2**, 195.

Bodman, R. I., Morton, H. J. V., and Wylie, W. D. (1952). A new synthetic curarising agent: clinical trial of compound 20 (Laudolissin). *Lancet*, **263**, 517–8.

Boehm, R. (1897). Ueber Curare und Curarealkaloide. *Archive Pharmakologie Berlin*, **235**, 660–84.

Booij, L. H. D. J., Edwards, R. P., Sohn, Y. J., and Miller, R. D. (1980). Cardiovascular and neuromuscular effects of ORG NC45 pancuronium, metocurine and *d*-tubocurarine in dogs. *Anesthesia and Analgesia*, **59**, 26–31.

Boros, M., Szenohradszky, J., Marosi, G. Y., and Toth, J. (1980). Comparative clinical study of pipecuronium bromide and pancuronium bromide. *Arzneimittel Forschung*, **30**, 389–93.

Bowman, W. C. (ed.) (1990). *Pharmacology of neuromuscular function*, (2nd edn). Wright, London.

Bowman, W. C., Prior, C., and Marshall, I. G. (1990). Presynaptic receptors in the neuromuscular junction. *Annals of the New York Academy of Science*, **604**, 69–81.

Brandom, B. W., Woelfel, S. K., Cook, D. R., Weber, S., Powers, D. M., and Weakly, J. N. (1989). Comparison of mivacurium and suxamethonium administered by bolus and infusion. *British Journal of Anaesthesia*, **62**, 488–93.

Brodie, B. (1812). Further experiments and observations on the action of poisons on the animal system. *Philosophical Transactions of the Royal Society of London*, **1**, 205–27.

Brucke, H., Ginzel, K. H., Klupp, H., Pfaffenschlager, F., and Werner, G. (1951). Bischolinester von Dicarbonsäuren als Muskelrelaxatien in der Narkose. *Wiener Klinische Wochenschrift* **63**, 464–6.

Cullen, S. C. (1943). The use of curare for the improvement of abdominal muscle relaxation during inhalation anesthesia. *Surgery*, **14**, 261–6.

d'Anghera, P. M. (1516). *De orbe novo*, Vol.1, p.75, (trans. F.A. Macnutt). Putnam, New York (1912).

Foldes, F. F. (1957). *Muscle relaxants in anesthesiology*. Thomas, Springfield.

Foldes, F. F. (1959). Factors which alter the effects ofmuscle relaxants. *Anesthesiology*, **20**, 464–504.

Foldes, F. F. (1984). Rapid tracheal intubation with non-depolarizing neuromuscular blocking drugs: the priming principle. *British Journal of Anaesthesia*, **56**, 663.

Foldes, F. F. (1990). The impact of neuromuscular blocking agents on the development of anaesthesia and surgery. In *Monographs in anaesthesiology*, Vol. 19 (ed. S. Agoston and W. C. Bowman), pp. 1–17. Elsevier, Amsterdam.

Foldes, F. F. and McNall, P. (1962). Myasthenia gravis: a guide for anaesthesiologists. *Anesthesiology*, **23**, 837–72.

Foldes, F. F. and Vizi, E. S. (1985). The effect of nondepolarizing muscle relaxants on transmitter release at peripheral cholinergic receptor sites. In *Proceedings of the 4th Congress of the Hungarian Pharmacological Society*, (ed. E. S. Vizi, S. Furst, and G. Zsilla) Vol. 2, pp. 3–46 Akademiai Kiado, Budapest.

Foldes, F. F., Hunt, R. D., and Ceravolo, A. J. (1952). Use of mytolon chloride with pentothal sodium and nitrous oxide-oxygen for abdominal surgery. *Anesthesia and Analgesia*, **30**, 185–92.

Foldes, F. F., Wolfson, B., and Sokoll, M.(1961*a*). The use of toxiferine for the production of surgical relaxation. *Anesthesiology*, **22**, 93–9.

Foldes, F. F., Monte, A. P., Brunn H. M., and Wolfson, B. (1961*b*). Studies with muscle relaxants in unanesthetized subjects. *Anesthesiology*, **22**, 230–6.

Foldes, F. F., Foldes, V. M., Smith, J. C., and Zsigmond, E. K. (1963*a*). The relation between plasma cholinesterase and prolonged apnea caused by succinylcholine. *Anesthesiology*, **24**, 208–16.

Foldes, F. F., Brown, I. M., Lunn, J. M., Moore, J., and Duncalf, D. (1963*b*). The neuromuscular effects of diallylnortoxiferine in anesthetized subjects. *Anesthesia and Analgesia*, **42**, 177–87.

Foldes, F. F., Klonymus, D. H., Maisel, W., Sciammas, F., and Pan, T. (1971). Studies of pancuronium in conscious and anesthetized man. *Anesthesiology*, **35**, 496–503.

Foldes, F. F., Somogyi, G. T., Chaudhry, I. A., Nagashima, H., and Duncalf, D. (1984). Assay of 3H acetylcholine release from mouse diaphragm without cholinesterase inhibition. *Anesthesiology*, **61**, A395.

Foldes, F. F., Chaudhry, I. A., Kinjo, M., and Nagashima, H. (1989). Inhibition of mobilization of acetylcholine: the weak link in neuromuscular transmission during partial neuromuscular block with *d*-tubocurarine. *Anesthesiology*, **71**, 218–23.

Foldes, F. F., Nagashima, H., Nguyen, H., and Ohta, Y. (1990). The clinical pharmacology of Org 9426. In *Neuromuscular blocking agents: past, present and future.* Proceedings of the David Savage Memorial Interface Symposium, London, (ed. W. C. Bowman, P. A. F. Denissen, and S. Feldman), pp. 171–81. Excerpta Medica, Amsterdam.

Foldes, F. F., Nagashima, H., Nguyen, H. D., Schiller, W. S., Mason, M. M., and Ohta, Y. (1991). The neuromuscular effects of ORG9426 in patients receiving balanced anesthesia. *Anesthesiology*, **75**, 191–6.

Frey, R. (1955). A short acting muscle relaxant: Prestonal (G. 25178) preliminary report. In *Proceedings of the World Congress on Anesthesiology*, p. 262.

Gill, R. C. (1940). *White water and black magic*, pp. 242–360. Holt, New York.

Gill, R. C. (1946). Published misconceptions regarding the new clinically adequate curare. *Science*, **103**, 147.

Gillies, J. (1952). Physiological trespass in anaesthesia. *Proceedings of the Royal Society of Medicine*, **45**, 1–6.

Glavinovic, M. I. (1979). Presynaptic action of curare. *Journal of Physiology*, **290**, 499–506.

Gray, T. C. and Halton, J. (1946). Technique for the use of *d*-tubocurarine chloride with balanced anaesthesia. *British Medical Journal*, **2**, 293–5.

Griffith, H. R. and Johnson, G. E. (1942). The use of curare in general anesthesia. *Anesthesiology*, **3**, 418–20.

Holaday, H. A. (1947). Report of the committee on pharmacological assays. *Proceedings of the American Drug Manufacturing Association Meeting*, pp. 143–5.

Holzer, H., Waltner, H., and Willomitzer, E. (1954). Klinische Erprobung eines neuen Muskelrelaxans (Hexamethyl-bis-carbaminoyl-cholinbromid). *Wiener Medizinische Wochenschrift*. **104**, 637–8.

Huguenard, P. and Boue, A. (1950). Un nouveau curarisant francais de synthese, le 3697 R.P. *Anesthesie et Analgesie (Paris)*, **7**, 55–72.

Hügin, W. and Kissling, P. (1961). Vorläufige Mitteilungen über ein neues kurzwirkendes Relaxans vom depolarisationshindernen Typus, das Ro4-3816. *Schweizerische Medizinische Wochenschrift*, **91**, 455–7.

Hunt, T. M., Hughes, R., and Payne, J. P. (1980). Preliminary studies with atracurium in anaesthetised man. *British Journal of Anaesthesia*, **52**, S238–9.

Kalow, W. (1956). Relationship of plasma cholinesterase to response to clinical doses of succinylcholine. *Canadian Anaesthetists Society Journal*, **3**, 22–30.

Karrer, P. (1967). Geschichte der Curareforschung. In *Curare*, Symposium der Schweizerischen Akademie der Medizinischen Wissenschaften, pp. 391–8. Schwabe, Basel.

Karrer, P. and Schmidt, H. (1946). Über Curare-Alkaloide aus Calebassen. *Helvetica Chirurgica Acta*, **29**, 1853–70.

Katz, R. L. (1971). Clinical neuromuscular pharmacology of pancuronium. *Anesthesiology*, **34**, 550–6.

Katz, B. and Miledi, R. (1978). A re-examination of curare action at the motor and endplate. *Proceedings of the Royal Society* (Series B), **196**, 59–72.

King, H. (1935). Curare alkaloids, I. Tubocurarine. *Journal of the Chemical Society*, **57**, 1381–9.

Kollicke, A. (1858). Die Lähmung der Herzaste des Vagus durch das amerikanische Pfeilgift. *Allgemeine Medizinische Zeitschrift*, **27**, 457.

Landmesser, C. N. (1947). A study of the bronchoconstrictor and hypotensive actions of curarizing drugs. *Anesthesiology*, **8**, 506–23.

Lapicque, L. and Lapicque, M. (1913). Quelques points de l'action du curare. *Compte Rendu de la Société Biologique de Paris*, **74**, 1392–5.

Läwen, A. (1912). Über die Verbindung der Lokalanaesthesie mit der Narkose, über hohe Extraduralanaesthesia und epidurale Injektionen anaesthesierender Lösungen bei tabischen Magenkrisen. *Beiträge zur Klinischen Chirurgie*, **80**, 168–89.

Lundy, J. S. (1942). *Clinical anesthesia*. Saunders, Philadelphia.

Marshall, I. G. (1991). Prejunctional aspects of neuromuscular transmission: physiology, biochemistry and pharmacology. *Current Opinion in Anaesthesiology*, **4**, 577–82.

Marshall, R. J. (1991). Cardiovascular effects of neuromuscular blocking drugs. *Current Opinion in Anaesthesiology*, **4**, 599–602.

McIntyre, A. R. (1947). *Curare, its history, nature and clinical use*. University of Chicago Press.

Mayrhofer, O. K. and Hassfurther, M. (1951). Kurzwirkende Muskelerschlaffungsmittel. *Wiener Klinische Wochenschrift*, **47**, 885–9.

Mayrhofer, O., Remes, I., and Schuster, H. (1955). Zur Frage der Antagonisierbarkeit des langwirkenden, depolarisierenden Muskelrelaxans Imbretil. *Anaesthesist*, **4**, 174–5.

Murray, D. J., Mehta, M. P., Choi, W. W., Sokoll, M. D., Gergis, S. D., *et al.* (1988). The neuromuscular blocking and cardiovascular effects of doxacurium chloride in patients receiving nitrous oxide narcotic anesthesia. *Anesthesiology*, **69**, 472–7.

Mushin, W. W., Wien, R., Mason, D. F. J., and Langston, G. T. (1949). Curare-like actions of tri (diethylamino-ethoxy) benzene triethyliodide. *Lancet*, **i**, 726–8.

Nachmansohn, D. (1959). *Chemical and molecular basis of nerve activity*. Academic Press, New York.

Nigrovic, V. (1991). New insights into the toxicity of neuromuscular-blocking drugs and their metabolites. *Current Opinion in Anaesthesiology*, **4**, 603–7.

Organe, G. (1949). Decamethonium iodide (bis-trimethyl ammonium decane diiodide) in anaesthesia. *Lancet*, **256**, 773–4.

Paget, F. (1921). Anesthesia metamerica. *Revista Sanitario Militar*, **11**, 315.

Payne, J. P. and Hughes, R. (1980). Evaluation of atracurium in anaesthetized man. *British Journal of Anaesthesia*, **53**, 45–54.

Rendell-Baker L., Foldes F. F., Birch J. H., and D'Souza, P. (1957). Experimental studies with prestonal, a new short-acting muscle relaxant. *British Journal of Anaesthesia*, **29**, 303–10.

Savarese, J. J., Basta, S. J., Ali, H. H., Scott, R. F. P, Sunder, N., Gargarian, M., *et al.* (1985). Cardiovascular effects of BW B109OU in patients under nitrous oxide-oxygen-thiopentone-fentanyl anesthesia. *Anesthesiology*, **63**, A319.

Savarese, J. J., Ali, H. H., Basta, S. J., Embree, P. B., Scott, R. P. F., Sunder, N., *et al.* (1988). The clinical neuromuscular pharmacology of mivacurium chloride (BW B109OU). A short-acting nondepolarizing ester neuromuscular blocking drug. *Anesthesiology*, **68**, 723–32.

Sayres, L. A. (1858). Two cases of traumatic tetanus. *New York Journal of Medicine*, **4**, 250.

Schmid, H. (1967). Chemie des Calebassencurare. In *Curare*, Symposium der Schweizerischen Akademie der Medizinischen Wissenschaften, pp. 415–31. Schwabe, Basel.

Schomburgk, R. (1841). On the Urari. *Annals and Magazine of Natural History*, **7**, 409.

Schwartz, S., Ilias, W., Lackner, F., Mayrhofer, O. and Foldes, F. F. (1985). Rapid tracheal intubation with vecuronium: the priming principle. *Anesthesiology*, **62**, 388–91.

Simpson, B. R., Savage, T. M., Foley, E. I., Ross, L. A. Strunin, L., Walton, B., *et al.* (1972). An azobisarylimidazo-pyridinium derivative: a rapidly acting, nondepolarizing muscle-relaxant. *Lancet*, **i**, 516–9.

Smith, P. (1969). *Arrows of mercy*. Doubleday, New York.

Standaert, F. G. (1986). Basic physiology and pharmacology of the neuromuscular junction. In *Anesthesia* (2nd edn) (ed. R. D. Miller), pp. 835–70. Churchill-Livingstone, New York.

Stoelting, V. K., Graf, J. P., and Vieira, Z. (1948). Use of a new curarising drug. Dimethyl ether of *d*-tubocurarine iodide as an adjunct to anesthesia. *Anesthesia and Analgesia*, **28**, 130–43.

Tassonyi, E., Szabo, G., and Vereckey, L. (1981). Pharmacokinetics of pipecuronium bromide, a new non-depolarizing neuromuscular blocking agent, in humans. *Arzneimittel Forschung*, **31**, 1754–6.

Thomas, K. B. (1963). *Curare, its history and usage*. Lippincott, Philadelphia.

Valdoni, P. (1949). Osservazioni cliniche sull'impiego del curarizzante 362 I. S. *Rendiconti Instituto Superiore di Sanita (Roma)* **12**, 255–62.

Vizi, E. S., Harsing, L. G., Jr, Duncalf, D., Nagashima, H., Potter, P., and Foldes, F. F. (1985). A simple and sensitive method of acetyl-choline identification and assay. *Journal of Pharmacological Methods*, **13**, 201–11.

Von Dardel, O., and Theslef F. S. (1951). Kliniska erf arenheter med succinylkolinjodid ett mytt medel som ger muskelavslapping. *Nordisk Medicinsk Tidskrift*, **46**, 1308–11.

Von Humboldt, A. and Bonland, A. (1807). *Voyage aux régions équinoxiales du nouveau continent*, Paris.

Waser, P. and Harbeck, P. (1959). Erste klinische Anwendung der Calebassenalkaloide Toxiferin I and Curarin I. *Anaesthetist*, **8**, 193.

Waud, B. E. (1977). Neuromuscular blocking agents. *Current Problems in Anesthesia and Critical Care Medicine*, **1**, 3–47.

West. R. (1936). Intravenous curarine in the treatment of tetanus. *Lancet*, **ii**, 12–6.

Wieland, H., and Pistor, H. (1938). Curarin from calabash-curare. *Annals of Chemistry*, **527**, 160.

Wintersteiner, D. and Dutcher, J. D. (1943). Curare alkoloids from Chondrodendron tomentosum. *Science*, **97**, 467–70.

Wierda, J. M. K. H., De Wit, A. P. M., Kuizenga, K., Agoston, S. (1990). Clinical observations on the neuromuscular blocking agent (Org 9426) in anaesthetized cats and pigs and in isolated nerve–muscle preparations. *British Journal of Anaesthesia*, **64**, 521–3.

2

Components of the neuromuscular junction

B. J. Pollard

Sir Walter Raleigh is credited with the introduction of tobacco into the western world. It is possible that he was also the first with a muscle relaxant (Sykes 1982). Among his expeditions he visited Guiana and South America and described an unusual arrow poison used by the natives. It seems likely that this was a preparation of curare, though the details are not well reported. It is likely that a few cursory investigations were undertaken using the sample which Sir Walter Raleigh brought home, but the matter was not followed up.

Approximately 300 years later, in the early 19th century (Sykes 1982), Charles Waterton, during his wanderings in South America, made an observation similar to that of Raleigh. He made a number of observations concerning the preparation and use of the arrow poison. The preparation was surrounded by ritual and included many ingredients, although Waterton suspected the principal active ingredient to be the bark from the wourali plant. He and Brodie are credited with the first scientific experiments on the substance when they showed that the substance was inactive by mouth, but rapidly fatal when injected parenterally. Waterton postulated that the substance affected the muscles of respiration, a view which was supported in 1850 by Claude Bernard, who showed that the site of action was the junction between nerve and muscle (Bernard 1856).

For nearly 100 years curare was used empirically in medicine for the treatment of conditions including hydrophobia and tetanus (Bennett 1968). In 1939, Bennett reported the introduction of the drug into psychiatry as an adjuvant to lessen the side-effects of pentylenetetrazol shock therapy (see Bennett 1968). It is likely that the first use in anaesthesia was by Lawen (1912), although it is Harold Griffiths of Montreal who is credited with the introduction of curare into clinical practice (Griffiths and Johnson 1942).

Under the umbrella term of 'curare' (synonyms include wourali, ourari, urari), come several varieties of plant extract (Wallis 1967). These are all prepared by the Indians of the Amazonian and Orinoco basins from the bark of certain plants, in particular *Strychnos toxifera, S. castenoei, S. gubleri,* and *S. crevauxii.* The extract is dark brown or black in colour, of a thick, viscid constituency, odourless, and bitter tasting. For a time it was imported into England in three different types of containers – gourds, bamboo tubes or earthenware pots depending upon the source. This gave rise to the eponymous names 'calabash-curare', 'tube-curare' and 'pot-curare' respectively. The different types contain varying ratios of alkaloids which include curarine, calabashcurarine I, calabashcurarine II, protocurine, protocurarine, protocuridine, and neoprotocuridine. Strychnine was not present because of this alkaloid is derived from the related plant *Strychnos nux-vomica*. As it is an extract of naturally occurring alkaloids, standardization was initially performed by biological assay and an extract of the crude drug was used clinically until the active ingredient, tubocurarine, was isolated and purified. It was subsequently shown that tubocurarine could be more easily obtained from the plant *Chondrodendron tomentosum* which is presently the main source of the drug.

CHEMISTRY

The active ingredient of curare was identified by King (1935) as a quaternary ammonium compound which he named *d*-tubocurarine (Fig. 2.1). He believed that both nitrogen atoms were in the quaternary state, a view which remained until evidence showed that only one nitrogen was positively charged, although the second may become protonated at body pH (Everett *et al*. 1970).

The introduction of tubocurarine into clinical practice stimulated the search for other compounds which also possessed neuromuscular blocking activity and which might be superior to tubocurarine. The belief in the need for two quaternary nitrogens atoms in the molecule which were separated by a fixed distance governed much of the early work. A number of compounds containing two such quaternary nitrogen atoms separated by variable distances were synthesized. Two groups, Barlow and Ing (1948) and Paton and Zaimis (1948), independently examined two very similar series of compounds where two quaternary nitrogens were separated by a simple carbon chain of varying length. Their conclusions were that as the length of the carbon chain rose, neuromuscular blocking activity increased, reaching a peak at a 10 carbon chain and subsequently declining again. It was also

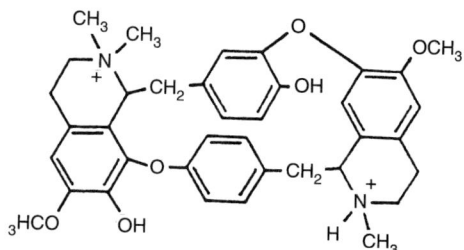

Fig. 2.1 The structural formula of tubocurarine as described by King (1935). Both nitrogens are shown in the quaternary state although this only applies at body pH by protonation of the second (right hand) nitrogen.

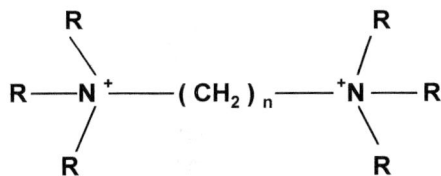

Fig. 2.2 The generic structural formula of the methonium series. In hexamethonium ($n = 6$), and decamethonium ($n = 10$), the R groups are all methyl groups (CH_3).

observed that ganglionic blocking activity exhibited a similar peak, but at a chain length of six carbon atoms. Two compounds were then examined more carefully — decamethonium and hexamethonium (Paton and Zaimis 1952) (Fig. 2.2) — both of which subsequently entered clinical usage. From these studies and others, it was calculated that the distance between the two quaternary nitrogen centres should be approximately 1 nm for optimum neuromuscular activity. This led to the synthesis of many more substances, some of which were based on a rigid hydrocarbon ring structure in an attempt to hold the quaternary nitrogen groups at the desired fixed distance with respect to each other. It also became evident at the time that drugs which have a depolarizing action tended to be smaller, more flexible molecules, while those which had a competitive (nondepolarizing) character were larger, bulkier, less flexible molecules. It is interesting to note that when the crystal structure of tubocurarine was finally delineated by Sobell *et al.* (1972) the inter-nitrogen distance was measured to be 1.07 nm.

Table 2.1 Neuromuscular blocking agents which have been introduced into clinical practice

Neuromuscular blocking agent	Year of first clinical use
d-tubocurarine	1942
Gallamine	1947
Decamethonium	1948
Metocurine (dimethyltubocurarine)	1948
Suxethonium	1949
Suxamethonium (succinylcholine)	1951
Alcuronium (diallylnortoxiferine)	1961
Pancuronium	1967
Fazadinium	1972
Pipecuronium	1980
Atracurium	1982
Vecuronium	1982

It is impossible to list all of the substances which have been investigated with respect to their neuromuscular blocking activity, but there are a number which have found clinical use. Not every drug is universally available, different countries having different agents in regular use. The reader is referred to Chapter 1, page 9 for a complete list. Those in regular clinical use are listed in Table 2.1. Decamethonium, suxethonium, and fazadinium have been withdrawn from clinical use. Metocurine is only available in the USA and pipecuronium in some European countries, although it is likely soon to be marketed in the UK and the USA. Doxacurium, rocuronium, and mivacurium are new neuromuscular blocking agents, the first long acting, the second intermediate acting with a rapid onset, and the third short acting.

THE NEUROMUSCULAR JUNCTION

Nerve supply

The motor nerves to striated muscle in mammals are large myelinated fibres of the 'A alpha' type (Guyton 1976). The cell body is in the brain or spinal cord and there is one single long axon which enters the muscle at the motor point. This point is usually towards the centre of the belly of the muscle. The nerve fibre then branches repeatedly. In muscles that perform fine movements, one nerve fibre will supply relatively few muscle fibres (low innervation ratio) whereas those muscles which perform relatively crude movements, e.g. the muscles of posture, have a high innervation ratio – one nerve fibre supplies a large number of muscle fibres (Guyton 1976). Each nerve cell, together with the muscle fibres which it supplies, is one motor unit. As the axon comes into contact with the muscle fibre, it loses its myelin sheath and enters a shallow trough, in which it may subdivide further before ending. The nerve at its terminal is therefore in intimate contact with the muscle fibre, separated by a space, the synaptic cleft. This cleft is filled with a basement membrane material and is about 50–100 nm across (Katz 1966). Neuromuscular transmission consists of the events which lead to a transfer of the electrical impulse from the nerve to the muscle fibre.

Identification of the transmitter

The neuromuscular junction of striated muscle is probably the most extensively studied of all synapses. The concept of a distinct junction between nerve and muscle probably began with Claude Bernard's work in the mid-19th century (Bernard 1856), although it was not until 50 years later that the principle of chemical transmission began to be properly established.

This initial pioneering work which established the concept of chemical transmission was centred on the adrenergic system. Lewandowsky (1898) and Langley (1901) independently observed that when an extract of the adrenal gland was injected into an animal, the effect was similar to that of stimulating the sympathetic nervous system. Adrenalin also had the same effect (Elliot 1905). This clearly led to the suggestion that sympathetic nerve impulses might release minute amounts of a substance which was very similar to adrenalin (Elliot 1905) with respect to the cholinergic system. Thirty years earlier, Schmeideberg had shown that the administration of the alkaloid muscarine mimicked the action of vagus nerve stimulation (Schmiedeberg and Harnack 1877). It was therefore logical for the existence of a second, non-adrenergic system to be proposed by Dixon from his own observations of the similarity of effect between the administration of muscarine and the responses to vagal stimulation (Dixon 1909). Both had also been shown to be affected in a similar way by atropine (Dixon 1906), leading to the suggestion that the vagus nerve liberated a substance similar to muscarine, which functioned as a chemical transmitter across the synapse. In 1914, Dale examined the pharmacological properties of the chemical compound acetylcholine and its similarity to muscarine (Dale 1914). Seven years later, Otto Loewi (1921) provided the first conclusive proof of chemical transmission of nerve impulses and it is to Loewi that credit must be given for the first use of the term 'neurohumoral transmission' (Loewi and Navratil 1926). While stimulating the vagus nerve of one frog's heart, he allowed the perfusate to bathe a second heart which also slowed in tandem with the first (Loewi 1921). The mediator he called 'Vagusstoff'. Vagusstoff and acetylcholine had the same effect and he concluded that they were probably the same substance (Loewi and Navratil 1926). His evidence for this included the following: atropine inhibited the action of both; both were rapidly destroyed by an esterase present in heart muscle; activity could then be restored by acetylating the residue; eserine inhibited the breakdown of both; eserine resulted in a potentiation of the actions of both. All of Loewi's work had been performed in frogs but subsequent work established the same to be true in mammals (Dale and Feldberg 1933; Feldberg and Krayer 1933; Dale 1934; Dale *et al.* 1936). Furthermore, acetylcholine is the only ester of choline known to occur naturally in the body (Dale 1934).

Previous work (Dale 1934) had shown that when atropine was given to an animal, muscarine had no effect, but a larger dose of acetylcholine would then produce a different action, which was mimicked by nicotine. Thus the concept of two receptor subtypes, 'nicotinic' and 'muscarinic', was introduced. The action of nicotine (as opposed to muscarine) in mimicking the action of acetylcholine on the neuromuscular junction, and its block by curare and not by atropine, helped to confirm suspicions that neurohumoral transmission is also present at the skeletal nerve–muscle junction, that acetylcholine is the transmitter, and that those acetylcholine receptors on the neuromuscular junction are of the nicotinic type (Dale 1934).

The prejunctional nerve terminal

Intracellular structures, including endoplasmic reticulum, Golgi apparatus, microtubules, and lysosomes, are all present throughout the nerve, including the nerve terminal. Within the nerve terminal there are many mitochondria and also a large number of vesicles of approximately 30–50 nm diameter (Palay 1954; Robertson 1956; Bowden and Duchen 1976). Although present throughout the axoplasm of the nerve terminal, the vesicles are principally located in the vicinity of the junction and grouped more densely behind thickened bands, each about 50 nm wide. These run transversely across the synaptic surface of the cell membrane. There are up to 1000 of these thickened areas, or 'active zones', in each nerve ending and they are thought to represent the sites of acetylcholine release (Peper *et al.* 1974; Ceccarelli and Hurlbut 1980).

The transmitter acetylcholine is synthesized in the nerve ending from choline, which is acetylated in an energy dependent process. The acetyl group is supplied bound to coenzyme A (CoA) (Tucek and Cheng 1974) and the process is catalysed by choline-*O*-acetyltransferase (choline acetylase). This enzyme is manufactured within the cell body and transported down the axon to the nerve ending (Ekstrom and Emmelin 1971; Droz *et al.* 1979). It exists both free in the cytoplasm and also bound to membrane structures (Hebb 1972; Fonnum 1973). The acetyl-CoA is supplied by intracellular metabolic processes (Tucek and Cheng 1974) and choline is supplied by active transport into the cell from the surrounding extracellular fluid (Haga and Noda 1973; Vaca and Pilar 1979). It has been estimated that about 50% of this choline comes from that liberated by the breakdown of previously released acetylcholine (Potter 1970) and the remainder from what is freely available in the extracellular fluid. Sodium flux seems to be an important factor and both the uptake of choline and the activity of choline-*O*-acetyltransferase are linked to the entry of sodium into the nerve ending (Birks 1963; Beach *et al.* 1980).

There are three sites within the nerve terminal where acetylcholine may be found. Approximately half is present in neural tissues and half in non-neural tissues (e.g. Schwann cells) (Marchbanks and Israel, 1972; Israel *et al.*; Miledi *et al.* 1980). That acetylcholine in the neural tissues, is mainly in the vesicles (about 60%) with the remainder dissolved in the cytoplasm.

The storage and release of acetylcholine

It is appropriate to consider the storage and release of acetylcholine at the same time. When an action potential reaches the nerve endings, acetylcholine is released. This causes a transient change in the potential difference across the membrane which rapidly returns to the previously polarized state. This change is referred to as the endplate potential (e.p.p.). These electrical changes in the postjunctional membrane can be observed by the use of microelectrodes. Whilst conducting such studies using intracellular microelectrodes, Fatt and Katz (1950, 1952) observed that small spontaneous depolarizations were also present at the neuromuscular junction. These potentials were each about 0.5–1.0 mV in amplitude, whereas the e.p.p. was about 50–100 mV in amplitude. These small depolarizations occurred randomly in time, but were constant in amplitude. They resembled the e.p.p. in time course and in the effect of drugs, being depressed or abolished by tubocurarine, increased by anticholinesterase, and reduced in frequency by botulinum toxin (Brooks 1956; Hubbard *et al.* 1968; Llinas and Heuser 1977). The term 'miniature endplate potentials' (m.e.p.p.) was therefore used to describe them. One m.e.p.p. will not produce a contraction of the muscle because the potential change does not exceed the threshold required to generate an action potential. If the calcium concentration in the extracellular fluid is reduced or the magnesium concentration is raised, then the amount of acetylcholine released and also the size of the e.p.p. resulting from stimulation of the motor nerve falls (Hubbard *et al.* 1968). Careful control of the ratio of calcium and magnesium allowed these changes in the size of the e.p.p. to be examined more closely. It was observed that the size of the e.p.p. changed in a stepwise fashion and that when the e.p.p. was very small, the size of each step was equal to the size of a m.e.p.p. (Del Castillo and Katz 1954; Boyd and Martin 1956; Katz 1966). One m.e.p.p. is thus the lowest common denominator of transmitter release and every e.p.p. is made up of a large number of m.e.p.p.s combined together.

The next question to arise related to the origin of the m.e.p.p.s. It appeared likely that they were the result of the spontaneous release of acetylcholine from the nerve ending. When the effect of acetylcholine which had been applied directly to the region of the endplate by iontophoresis was examined it was seen that the potential change evoked by just a few molecules of acetylcholine could not be detected and it required several thousand molecules of acetylcholine to produce a depolarization the size of a m.e.p.p. Furthermore, varying the amount of acetylcholine produced a continuously variable change in the size of the e.p.p. and not a stepwise change. Thus it became clear that m.e.p.p.s were not the result of the spontaneous discharge of individual molecules of acetylcholine but rather the result of spontaneous discharge of discrete packets or 'quanta', each containing several thousand molecules of acetylcholine. The e.p.p. is then produced by many quanta being released simultaneously (Boyd and Martin 1956); estimates range from about 200 to 400 (Hubbard and Wilson 1973; Katz and Miledi 1979).

Simultaneously, attention had been directed to the prejunctional vesicles which had also been described at around the same time (Robertson 1956). It was logical to postulate that these vesicles were the source of the transmitter, each holding one 'quantum' of acetylcholine (Del Castillo and Katz 1955; Martin 1966). The vesicular hypothesis of transmitter release was born and has been central to all subsequent studies of the neuromuscular junction. This hypothesis states that each vesicle holds a certain amount of acetylcholine, and it is the acetylcholine within the vesicles which is available for release, all other sources being simply stores. One m.e.p.p. is produced by random fusion of one vesicle with the cell membrane and extrusion of its contents into the junctional cleft. An e.p.p. is produced by the synchronized fusion of a large number of vesicles with the cell membrane following the arrival of an action potential along the axon of the motor nerve.

Returning to the structure of the neuromuscular junction, can further proof be obtained to confirm that the vesicular hypothesis is correct? Electron microscopy has demonstrated the presence of rows of pits of approximately uniform size alongside the 'active zone' bands. The number of pits increases with time after nerve stimulation (Peper *et al.* 1974; Heuser and Reese 1973; Heuser *et al.* 1979). The active zones are directly above the shoulders of the folds in the postjunctional membrane, which is the site of the greatest density of receptors (Land *et al.* 1980). The administration of drugs which prevent the loading of acetylcholine into the vesicles results in a block of neuromuscular transmission (Marshall 1970; Gandiha and Marshall 1973; Anderson *et al.* 1983). Black widow spider venom, which results in a disappearance of the vesicles and prevents them from reforming, causes the disappearance of both m.e.p.p.s and e.p.p.s. There is also an initial large increase in acetylcholine output following treatment with black widow spider venom and the area of the cell membrane is found to have increased (Hurlbut and Ceccarelli 1979). If the synthesis of acetylcholine is inhibited using hemicholinium, there is a reduction in the size and acetylcholine content of the vesicles together with a reduction in m.e.p.p. amplitude (Elmqvist and Quastel 1965*a*; Jones and Kwanbunbumpen 1970).

The fate of the vesicles is a matter of interest. The cell membrane area does not usually change with stimulation and so it is likely that vesicles can be reformed and recycled (Bittner and Kennedy 1970). Furthermore, the vesicular membrane can only be synthesized in the nerve cell body (Bowman 1985) and it is hard to imagine that it could be transported along the axon fast enough to keep pace with the needs of an active nerve. In order to try and address this point, electron micrographs of neuromuscular junctions flash frozen at predetermined intervals following stimulation were taken (Heuser *et al.* 1979; Heuser and Reese 1981). These images appeared to show vesicles fusing with the membrane and flattening out to blend in with the cell membrane. The vesicles are then thought to be recycled by invaginating the membrane at a site adjacent to the active zone (Heuser and Reese 1973). The question then arises as to how the cell recognizes the correct section of membrane for this to take place. The membrane in the region of the active zones appears on electron microscopy to be studded with large protein particles, the number of which increase when the nerve is stimulated. It is possible that these may be markers involved in the recognition of a vesicle (Heuser and Reese 1981).

Established theories are continually being re-examined, and the vesicular theory of acetylcholine release is no exception (Marchbanks 1979). Of the total acetylcholine present within the nerve terminal, a substantial part is not within the vesicles; estimates range from 20% (Israel *et al.* 1968) to 50% (Miledi *et al.* 1980). The site of manufacture of acetylcholine is probably the cytoplasm, choline-*O*-acetyltransferase being a soluble enzyme. That free in the cytoplasm may then represent newly synthesized acetylcholine, before it has been loaded into the vesicles. There are, however, other considerations. The acetylcholine released spontaneously (that accounting for the m.e.p.p.s), has been reported to be only about 2% of the total acetylcholine spontaneously released from the nerve ending (Mitchell and Silver 1963; Katz and Miledi 1977). There would appear to be a continual leakage or secretion of acetylcholine from the nerve ending which gives rise to a small persistent depolarization of the postjunctional membrane (Bittner and Kennedy 1970). There is an increased release of non-vesicular acetylcholine during motor nerve stimulation (Vizi and Viskocil 1979), although its contribution (if any) to stimulus evoked transmission is unclear (Katz and Miledi 1981). Furthermore, acetylcholine is known to be synthesized and released from Schwann cells (Ito and Miledi, 1977), axons (Nachmansohn 1975), and other non-neural tissues (Rama Sastry and Sadavongvivad 1979) but the function of this is unknown. It is possible that non-vesicular release of transmitter has a tonic or trophic function.

The total pool of acetylcholine is dynamic in nature, as freshly synthesized acetylcholine mixes freely with older acetylcholine in the vesicles and in the cyto-plasm (Whittaker and Luqmani 1980). That which is released also constitutes a mixture of old and new and has even been suggested to favour the more recently synthesized transmitter (Potter 1970). This, although not incompatible with the vesicular theory, is difficult to understand. Newly formed acetylcholine would be expected to be in some vesicles and older acetylcholine in others, with the latter closer to the sites of release. Inhibition of synthesis by hemicholinium results in a uniform reduction in size of all vesicles throughout the nerve ending and not just those which have been recently synthesized or filled (Elmqvist and Quastel 1965*a*; Jones and Kwanbunbumpen 1970).

The assumption that acetylcholine molecules are released in quanta does not require that the molecules must come directly from vesicles (Israel and Dunant 1979; Israel *et al.* 1979; Marchbanks 1979; Tauc 1979). An alternative theory could be advanced where ion 'gates' may exist which open and close allowing a discrete amount of non-vesicular acetylcholine into the junctional cleft on each occasion. This might also result in another form of quantal release (Van der Kloot 1977; Marchbanks 1979; Thesleff and Molgo 1983). Random opening of the channels might give rise to m.e.p.p.s and coordinated opening to an e.p.p. The outflow of acetylcholine from the nerve ending could be readily explained by the concentra-tion gradient from nerve cell to synaptic cleft. There are specific channels for sodium, potassium, and calcium, so why not one for acetylcholine?

Taking into account all of these arguments, it seems that the weight of evidence is at present heavily in favour of the vesicular hypothesis of acetylcholine release (Heuser *et al.* 1979; Pecot-Dechavassine 1982). The available evidence, however, does not allow the total exclusion of other forms of acetylcholine release. The ves-icles certainly do contain acetylcholine and they lie close to the cell membrane directly above the receptors on the postjunctional membrane. They do appear to fuse with the cell membrane after stimulation in numbers proportional to the amount of transmitter released (Pecot-Dechavassine 1982). Although the time-course does relate the fusion of the vesicles with the release of acetylcholine (Heuser and Reese 1981), the appearance of the pits on electron microscopy is slower than the time course of transmitter release as evidenced by studies of endplate currents.

The breakdown of acetylcholine

In order to reset the mechanism rapidly and to allow repeated stimuli to pass, the transmitter must be removed from the vicinity of the receptors very rapidly. Diffusion away from the active sites will help to accomplish this reduction, but the most impor-tant mechanism is the destruction of the acetylcholine by the enzyme acetyl-cholinesterase. This enzyme is present within the junction in the basement membrane and within the depths of the junctional folds (Davis and Koelle 1967; Koelle *et al.* 1967; Salpeter 1967; Dreyer 1982). The enzyme possesses two active sites — an anionic site and an esteratic site. The former binds the quaternary ammonium moiety of the acetylcholine molecule and the latter binds the opposite end of the molecule before attacking it to split the ester linkage separating the molecule into its two component parts, choline and acetate. The efficiency of the enzyme is so great that it takes only 0.1 ms to destroy a molecule of acetylcholine (Lawler 1961) and most of the acetylcholine released from one nerve impulse will be destroyed within 1 ms (Hobbiger 1976). It is likely therefore that under normal conditions, an acetylcholine molecule only lasts long enough to combine with one receptor site (Hobbiger 1976).

THE ACETYLCHOLINE RECEPTORS

At the end of the 19th century, one of the topical questions under discussion regarded the nature of the action of drugs: was it physical or chemical in nature? Supporters of the former hypothesis held the view that drugs exerted their effects by altering certain physical properties of cells, e.g. surface tension or osmotic pressure; supporters of the latter hypothesis regarded the action of a drug as being mediated by the formation of a chemical union with some constituent of a cell. The answer to the questioning came from the pioneering work of Langley and Ehrlich (Langley 1878, 1906, 1909; Ehrlich 1900) which subsequently gave rise to the concept of receptors.

Langley was involved in studies of the nervous system, particularly concerning the effect of cholinomimetic compounds on the stimulation of secretion and their antagonism by atropine. Those studies led him to suggest that 'there is some substance or substances in the nerve endings or gland cells with which both atropine and pilocarpine are capable of forming compounds' (Langley 1878). These he called 'specific receptive substances', and he advanced the hypothesis that such substances were present at the nerve ending and were capable of receiving or transmitting stimuli (Langley 1906). Interestingly enough, during the course of his studies, he suggested that the alkaloid nicotine could form a dissociable complex with these specific receptive substances upon skeletal muscle (Langley 1909), a theory which was later shown to be true.

Ehrlich was working with stains and dyes on biological tissues and also conducting early investigations into immunological mechanisms (Ehrlich 1900). His work led him to formulate the concept of the existence of surface groups on cells which showed specific binding properties with toxin molecules; these groups he called 'receptors'. It was through the work of A. J. Clarke, however, that the drug receptor theory became fully established in pharmacology.

His early work concerned the glycoside strophanthin and led him to the conclusion that strophanthin acted on heart cells without entering them. He initially thought that this effect was likely to be of a physical nature (Clarke 1913). Subsequent work, which centred around the quantitative relation between concentration and action of acetylcholine, however, led him to reconsider this position. He measured the existence of a graded response to increasing concentrations of acetylcholine. The concentration of acetylcholine and the effect produced by that concentration when plotted in the form of a graph produced a sigmoid curve which could be expressed mathematically in the following way:

$$x = k \frac{y}{(100 - y)}$$

where x is the concentration of acetylcholine, y is the effect expressed as % of maximum possible effect, and k is a constant.

The simplest explanation for this relationship would be a reversible monomolecular reaction between two entities, in this case the drug and a binding site on the cell. Clarke also observed that there appeared to be no relation between the amount of drug entering a cell and the effect produced. Clarke then calculated the number of molecules which became attached to each cell. This led him to conclude that they could only occupy a very small area of the cell surface, insufficient to exert any significant physical effect (Clarke 1926, 1927). Clarke therefore revised his previous views and concluded that the drugs were acting upon a small number of sites on the surface of the cells.

Even though the concept of surface receptors were soon established, they remained a conceptual entity until the 1970s when advanced techniques of electron microscopy first allowed the receptors to be visualized. Simultaneous advances in biochemistry allowed receptors to be isolated and purified and then to be re-inserted into artificial lipid membranes for further electrophysiological examination (Boheim *et al.* 1981). Of possibly greater importance at that time was the development of immunological binding techniques. It became possible to raise antibodies to receptors in small animals, usually rabbits (James *et al.* 1980; Conti-Tronconi *et al.* 1981). In addition, toxins from the Taiwanese banded krait, *Bungarus multicinctus* (alpha-bungarotoxin and beta-bungarotoxin) were discovered. Alpha-bungarotoxin blocks neuromuscular transmission by binding specifically and irreversibly to acetylcholine receptors (C. Y. Lee 1972). The application of radiolabelled alpha-bungarotoxin to the neuromuscular junction results in it being localized almost exclusively to the crests of the folds in the postjunctional membrane (Fertuk and Salpeter 1974, 1976; Daniels and Vogel 1975). Using freeze etching methods, particles of about 7–10 nm diameter, which had the appearance from above of rosettes with a central pit, were found at this location (Dreyer *et al.* 1973; Peper *et al.* 1974; Groharaz *et al.* 1982; Hirokawa and Heuser, 1982). The immediate assumption was that these were probably the receptor structures. Close examination revealed the particles to be in double rows (Hirokawa and Heuser 1982; Ellisman *et al.* 1976) with an overall density of 10 000–20 000 μm^{-2} on the cell surface (Dreyer *et al.* 1973; Peper *et al.* 1974; Heuser and Salpeter 1979; Hirokawa and Heuser 1982).

The greatest concentrations of acetylcholine receptors are found on the postjunctional membranes of the electric organs of *Electrophorus* and *Torpedo* species (electric eels) and much of the research into the structure and function of the receptors has been undertaken using material from these sources. Antibodies against *Torpedo* receptors were observed to cross-react with mammalian receptors, implying that the structure was likely to be similar (Conti-Tronconi *et al.* 1981). This observation does not, of course, prove that they are identical, because the antibody could simply be reacting with one protein component which happens to be common to both.

The *Torpedo* receptors, which appear to be large protein macromolecules, span the cell membrane, which is about 5 nm across. The receptors protrude about 5 nm into the extracellular space and 1.5 nm into the intracellular space (Ross *et al.* 1977; Strader and Raftery 1980; Stroud 1983). The molecular weight of this receptor macromolecule is about 250 000 and as it exists as a dimer the total molecular weight is approximately 500 000 (Reynolds and Karlin 1978; Lindstrom *et al.* 1980). Each receptor molecule consists of five subunits as follows (Lindstrom *et al.* 1980; Raftery *et al.* 1980; Raftery *et al.* 1983):

two with a molecular weight of 40 000 (alpha subunits);

one with a molecular weight of 49 000 (beta subunits);

one with a molecular weight of 60 000 (gamma subunits);

one with a molecular weight of 67 000 (delta subunits).

The five subunits are arranged longitudinally, parallel to one another to form a cylinder with a channel down the middle (Guy 1984; Sargent *et al.* 1984) (Fig. 2.3). The amino acid sequence of the receptor macromolecule and its component parts has now been elucidated (see Chapter 3).

The central channel which is formed by the components of the receptor structure allows cations to pass when activated (Dwyer *et al.* 1980). This would explain the surface views of the receptors because the microscope is looking end-on into a

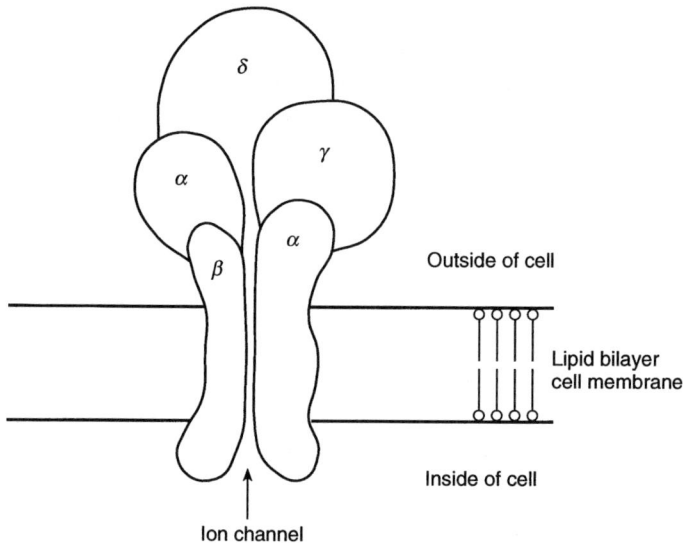

Fig. 2.3 Diagrammatic representation of the structure of the acetylcholine receptor at the neuromuscular junction. It comprises five macromolecules arranged longitudinally to form a cylinder with an ion channel down the centre. As the broad heads lie together on the outside of the cell, the channel has a funnelled entrance on the exterior of the cell. Two of the subunits are identical (alpha). The acetylcholine binding sites are situated one on each alpha subunit.

cylindrical structure (Stroud 1983). The binding sites for acetylcholine and alpha-bungarotoxin are on the alpha subunits (Heidmann and Changeux 1978; Peper *et al.* 1982; Guy 1984) on the extracellular part. Acetylcholine will therefore only activate the receptor when applied to the outside of a cell. The human acetylcholine receptor appears to be similar in structure, with corresponding subunits which have molecular weights of approximately 42 000, 56 000, 66 000, and 85 000 (Raftery *et al.* 1975; Reynolds and Karlin 1978; Linstrom *et al.* 1980).

Chemical analysis has indicated that the receptor system binds the cationic moiety of agonists and antagonists (all have at least one positively charged nitrogen atom) and that they attach to a previously orientated anionic site (Eldefrawi *et al.* 1975). These are closely associated with disulphide bonds which can be readily reduced. It is probably a stereochemical change which is, at least partly, responsible for the opening of the ion channel (Karlin 1969).

The receptors at the neuromuscular junction seem to be in a constant state of flux. There is a continual turnover of receptors, older ones being constantly removed and new ones being manufactured. The site of manufacture is likely to be the Golgi apparatus, from where the receptors are inserted into the membrane of the cell in an energy dependent process. This process probably involves microtubules (it is retarded by colchicine), but not microfilaments. In denervated or embryonic muscle the receptors are not restricted to the endplate but are spread over the entire surface of the muscle membrane (Fambrough 1979). Once a muscle is innervated, however, receptors become concentrated at the neuromuscular junction and extrajunctional ones almost totally disappear (Fambrough 1979).

There are fundamental differences between the receptors at the neuromuscular junction and those on extrajunctional sites, other than the part of the membrane in which they are inserted (Steinbach 1981). Amongst these difference are the following:

1. The rate at which they are synthesized and degraded differs — Their lifetime is about 17–20 hours for extrajunctional receptors and 7–14 days or longer for junctional receptors (Edwards 1979; Pumplin and Fambrough 1982; Bowman 1985).

2. There are different stimuli for their formation (Edwards 1979).

3. The extrajunctional receptors have longer channel open times and lower single channel conductances (Gage and Hamill 1980; Brenner and Sakmann 1983);

4. Extrajunctional receptors are more sensitive to depolarizing agents and less sensitive to nondepolarizing agents than junctional receptors (McIntyre *et al.* 1945; Beranek and Vyskocil 1967).

Upon activation by an agonist, a receptor macromolecule changes its structural conformation. This has been determined by binding a fluorescent marker to the receptor. Activation by an agonist changes the spectrum of light emitted, an effect which was prevented by the prior addition of an antagonist which itself had no effect (Changeux *et al.* 1976). Activation opens an ion channel allowing Na^+ and K^+ (and possibly Ca^{2+}) to cross (Boheim *et al.* 1981). The synchronous opening of

a large number of channels results in an endplate potential followed by the generation of an action potential across the surface of the muscle (Fatt and Katz 1951).

Using microelectrode techniques, it was determined that two molecules of acetylcholine must combine simultaneously with the receptor system for activation
(Trautmann and Feltz 1980; Dreyer 1982; Feltz and Trautmann 1982; Neubig *et al.*
1982) and that the binding of the first affects the affinity for the second (Dreyer *et al.*
1978). This may explain the non-linearity of the relationship between concentration of
acetylcholine and endplate current (Magelby and Terrar 1975; Dreyer *et al.* 1978;
Neubig *et al.* 1982; Peper *et al.* 1982). An additional consideration is that the two
alpha subunits do have a different environment, each being flanked by a different pair
of the other subunits. The receptor macromolecules are arranged in pairs on the
postjunctional membrane and, although they function independently, it is possible that
there is some cooperation between the two receptors in a pair (Raftery *et al.* 1983). A
number of the characteristics of the channels have been identified (Ginsborg and
Jenkinson 1976; Rang 1981; Dreyer 1982; Peper *et al.* 1982; Lambert *et al.* 1983):

1. At a normal resting membrane potential, the opening of one channel results in
    the passage of a current of about 2 pA, which is capable of producing a depo-
    larization of about 2 μV on the postjunctional membrane.

2. The single channel conductance is approximately $25–40 \times 10^{-12}$ ohms^{-1}). This
    is not the same for all nicotinic agonists (Colquhoun *et al.* 1975; Sachs and
    Lechar 1977).

3. The time constant of a channel can be calculated from power spectrum analy-
    sis. The time constant is approximately 3 ms for acetylcholine at a resting
    membrane potential of –80 mV and a temperature of 15°C (Colquhoun *et al.*
    1975; Lehter 1977).

4. The mean channel open time decreases if the resting membrane potential is
    increased (Lehter 1977).

5. Channels close faster when the membrane is depolarized than when it is
    polarized (Magelby and Stevens 1972; Lehter 1977; Sachs and Lechar 1977).
    The triggered action potential will therefore accelerate channel closing. This
    would be compatible with the suggestion that an integral part of the operation
    of the channel is a moving dipole. The ease with which it opens and closes
    would then depend upon the magnitude of the surrounding electrical field.

6. An increase in the concentration of acetylcholine, or other agonist, increases
    the frequency of channel opening but does not change the amount of current
    flow per event.

7. The mean channel open time is approximately 1 ms at 20°C but only 0.3 ms at
    37°C.

8. The mean channel open time is not the same for different agonists; e.g. for
    acetylcholine it is 1 ms, nicotine 0.22 ms, suxamethonium 0.25 ms, carbachol
    0.35 ms (all measured at 20°C) (Wray 1980; Dreyer 1982).

9. The mean channel open time is different in different muscle types (Anderson and Stevens 1973).

10. During 1 ms of open time approximately 1000 ions, principally sodium and potassium, pass through.

11. Only small diameter positively charged ions can pass through the channel. Larger positively charged ions can enter the channel but may not pass right through. From observations of the molecules that can cross, it appears that the channel is approximately 0.65 nm in diameter at its narrowest point (Dwyer *et al.* 1980).

As the ion channels close, acetylcholine dissociates from the receptor sites and is destroyed by acetylcholinesterase. It is probable that one molecule of acetylcholine lasts long enough to only open one channel. It is important to note that each channel opening event produces a pulse of current which is of a square wave nature. Channel openings are 'all-or-none' events and changes in the concentration of acetylcholine alter the frequency of channel opening and not the individual elementary events. The increase in endplate current gives rise to an endplate potential which, if it reaches a certain threshold, triggers an action potential which spreads across the muscle membrane to result in activation of the contractile mechanism.

The prejunctional nerve ending — prejunctional receptors

A nerve possesses receptors along its entire length. It is likely, however, that only those receptors at the cell body and at the nerve terminals have physiological importance (Starke 1981).

The presence of receptors on the nerve endings at the neuromuscular junction was recognized following the observation that adrenalin and noradrenalin increased the endplate potentials resulting from motor nerve stimulation but not those produced by iontophoretically applied acetylcholine (Krnjevic and Miledi 1958). (An anticurare action of adrenalin was in fact first reported by Panella (1907).) Since that time, the existence of prejunctional receptors for many other humoral mediators have been reported. It is possible that receptors for the following mediators exist on the presynaptic nerve terminal at cholinergic nerve endings: acetylcholine (nicotinic and muscarinic), noradrenalin (alpha- and beta-adrenergic), dopamine, gamma-amino butyric acid (GABA), opioids, substance P, adenosine, 5-hydroxytryptamine, prostaglandins, glutamate, benzodiazepines, and angiotensin-2 (Starke 1981). The physiological function of the majority of these receptors is presently unclear. It is possible that their function is to allow modulation of transmission by physiological mediators either released from neighbouring cells, or blood-borne.

The prejunctional nicotinic acetylcholine receptor

This receptor has probably attracted the most attention of all of the prejunctional receptors. Acetylcholine depolarizes the nerve endings, an effect which is antagonized by tubocurarine. It was postulated therefore that the prejunctional receptor might control acetylcholine release: a small amount of acetylcholine released by the motor nerve action potential might act upon the prejunctional receptors to stimulate the main release (Koelle 1962). However, although acetylcholine depolarizes the nerve ending, such a depolarization causes little or no increase in either m.e.p.p. frequency or quantal content (Ciani and Edwards 1963; Hubbard *et al.* 1965). Nor does tubocurarine, in a dose sufficient to abolish the action of acetylcholine on nerve ending, affect m.e.p.p. frequency or quantal content. The prejunctional acetylcholine receptors must therefore subserve some function other than simply an amplification system.

The application of acetylcholine to a nerve–muscle preparation produces three detectable actions: fasciculation; potentiation of any simultaneous contractors induced by stimulation of the motor nerve; and neuromuscular blockade. The first and second of these appear to be prejunctional in origin, and the third, postjunctional (Riker 1966). The synthesis of acetylcholine in nerve endings is known to be enhanced by nerve stimulation (Potter 1970) and this may be linked to intracellular sodium changes (Grewaal and Quastel 1973). Acetylcholine-sensitive sodium channels exist on the axon and it was suggested that these may be involved in the generation or maintenance of the action potential (Nachmansohn 1975) although this theory is not presently upheld. The release of acetylcholine does appear to be affected by the concentration of sodium in the cytoplasm which might give these prejunctional acetylcholine activated sodium channels a possible role in the mobilization of acetylcholine. Choline transport into cells also rises immediately following a nerve impulse (Collier and MacIntosh 1969; Yamamura and Snyder, 1973; Bowman 1985).

In the presence of rapid rates of firing of the motor nerve, tubocurarine has a marked effect resulting in a failure of transmission. There is a reducing amplitude of successive stimuli from the first, which is the largest, until a constant lower amplitude is reached (tetanic fade) (Lilleheil and Naess 1961; Standaert, 1964). The more rapid is the rate of firing, the more rapid is this fade. Under normal circumstances, the amount of acetylcholine released by a nerve impulse is considerably in excess of that required to just evoke depolarization of the endplate (Paton and Waud 1967). The rate of output of acetylcholine declines over the duration of a stimulus train ultimately to reach a constant level lower than at the beginning of the train. The higher the rate of stimulation, the higher the rate of acetylcholine output, although the output per impulse is less (Elmqvist and Quastel 1965*b*). In order to sustain acetylcholine release at the high rate caused by rapid stimulation, the nerve terminal must be capable of rapidly mobilizing transmitter. It is tempting therefore to speculate that acetylcholine released from the nerve ending acts upon prejunctional receptors to increase its own mobilization at higher rates of stimulation — a positive feedback system. If these receptors are blocked by the presence of tubocurarine, mobilization decreases, resulting in fade at higher rates of stimulation (Hubbard and Wilson 1973; Glavinovic 1979). Decamethonium, a substance with cholinomimetic properties increases acetylcholine mobilization, an effect which is blocked by tubourarine (Blaber 1970).

It was reported by Bowman (1980) that the pharmacological profile of the pre-junctional nicotinic receptors differed from the postjunctional ones. Having con-sidered the relative effects of hexamethonium (a potent ganglion blocker) and pancuronium (a weak ganglion blocker and potent neuromuscular blocker), upon this system, Bowman reached the conclusion that the prejunctional receptors resemble nicotinic acetylcholine receptors in autonomic ganglia more than they do the postjunctional receptors. This conclusion is supported by the observation that alpha-bungarotoxin, which binds selectively and irreversibly to the acetylcholine recognition sites on the postjunctional membrane (Chang and Lee 1963), neither binds to the nerve endings nor produces fade (Jones and Salpeter 1983).

Bowman and colleagues made an additional observation concerning the nature of the block at the prejunctional receptors, namely that it is rate-dependent (Bowman and Webb 1976; Bowman 1980). The degree of tetanic fade increased with the rate of stimulation. This pattern of effect might suggest an action by blockade of open ion channels rather than by occlusion of a receptor recognition site (Strichartz 1976). Furthermore, it had been reported that hexamethonium may not compete with acetylcholine at receptors in ganglia, but may exert its effect by open channel blockade (Ascher *et al.* 1979). If the tetanic fade resulting from the action of tubocurarine was due to open channel blockade the administration of neostigmine, which increases channel open time, should have accentuated the block. The admin-istration of neostigmine reduced tetanic fade produced by tubocurarine (C-M. Lee 1975). Channel blockade should only be seen with higher concentrations of a drug. Fade was produced by very small doses of tubocurarine. Channel blockade is dependent on the membrane potential (Colquhoun *et al.* 1979; Gibb and Marshall 1984), yet tetanic fade with tubocurarine (measured by run down of endplate current) was unaffected by any change in the membrane potential (Magleby *et al.* 1981). It seems unlikely therefore that channel block was the principal mechanism.

The exact function of the prejunctional nicotinic receptors and the effect of drugs on those receptors has not yet been fully explained. It is likely that they play a role in the production of tetanic fade but it cannot be concluded with certainty that block of prejunctional receptors is the only mechanism underlying tetanic fade.

Prejunctional muscarinic receptors

In 1980, it was reported that neuromuscular junctions in the electric organs of *Torpedo occellata* contain presynaptic muscarinic receptors (Kloog *et al.* 1980). Stimulation of these receptors was shown to inhibit the release of acetylcholine from nerve endings (Michaelson *et al.* 1979; Michaelson *et al.* 1980) and also to lead to a reduction in m.e.p.p. frequency (Duncan and Publicover 1979). There is no general agreement on these muscarinic actions, however, because oxotremorine (a muscarinic agonist) was shown to increase the output of acetylcholine from nerve endings (Das *et al.* 1978), although this observation has been disputed (Gunderson and Jenden 1980; Abbs and Joseph 1981). More than one subtype of muscarinic receptor exists (Birdsall *et al.* 1974) and it is possible that herein may lie at least part of the explanation.

Prejunctional catecholamine receptors

Evidence for the existence of presynaptic alpha receptors is well established. The administration of noradrenalin or adrenalin increases acetylcholine output, an effect which can be antagonized by alpha-blocking agents (Bowman and Nott 1969; Kuba 1970). The function of these catecholamine receptors in unknown, but it has been postulated that their function is to modulate transmitter release in times of stress (Bowman and Nott 1969).

Prejunctional opioid receptors

Prejunctional opioid receptors have also been described although their function is unknown (Soteropoulos and Standaert 1973). It is possible that they respond to circulating enkephalins at times of stress, further modulating acetylcholine release.

CONCLUSION

The neuromuscular junction is the most extensively studied synapse and a great deal is known about its basic structure and function. Most of our knowledge so far comes from studies involving other species, in particular the electric eels. Our knowledge of the mammalian neuromuscular apparatus is, however, growing. The pieces of the jigsaw are slowly being assembled although there are still many gaps. More recent studies have given us yet further information and the story continues in Chapter 3 where the physiochemical aspects of the neuromuscular junction are examined.

REFERENCES

Abbs, E. T. and Joseph, D. N. (1981). The effects of atropine and oxotremorine on acetylcholine release in rat phrenic nerve–diaphragm preparations. *British Journal of Pharmacology*, **73**, 481–3.

Anderson, C. R. and Stevens, C. F. (1973). Voltage clamp analysis of acetylcholine produced end-plate current fluctuations at frog neuromuscular junction. *Journal of Physiology*, **235**, 655–91.

Anderson, D. C., King, S. C., and Parsons, S. M. (1983). Inhibition of [^{3}H]acetylcholine active transport by tetraphenyl-borate and other ions. *Molecular Pharmacology*, **24**, 55–9.

Ascher, P., Large, W. A., and Rang, H. P. (1979). Studies on the mechanism of action of acetylcholine antagonists on rat parasympathetic ganglion cells. *Journal of Physiology*, **295**, 139–70.

Barlow, R. B. and Ing, H. R. (1948). Curare-like action of polymethylene bis-quaternary ammonium salts. *Nature*, **161**, 718.

Beach, R. L., Vaca, K., and Pilar, G. (1980). Ionic and metabolic requirements for high-affinity choline uptake and acetylcholine synthesis in nerve terminals at a neuromuscular junction. *Journal of Neurochemistry*, **34**, 1387–98.

Bennett, A. E. (1968). The history of the introduction of curare into medicine. *Anesthesia and Analagesia*, **47**, 484–92.

Beranek, R. and Vyskocil, F. (1967). The action of tubocurarine and atropine on the normal and denervated rat diaphragm. *Journal of Physiology*, **188**, 53–66.

Bernard C. (1856). Analyse physiologique des proprietes des systèmes musculaire et nerveux au moyen du curare. *Compte Rendu de l'Academie de Science (Paris)*, **43**, 825–9.

Birdsall, N. J. M., Hulme, E. C., and Stockton, J. M. (1974). Muscarinic receptor heterogeneity. *Trends in Pharmacological Sciences*, Supplement, 4–8.

Birks, R. I. (1963). The role of sodium ions in the metabolism of acetylcholine. *Canadian Journal of Biochemistry and Physiology*, **41**, 2573–97.

Bittner, G. D. and Kennedy, D. (1970). Quantitative aspects of transmitter release. *Journal of Cell Biology*, **47**, 585–92.

Blaber, L. C. (1970). The effect of facilitatory concentrations of decamethonium on the storage and release of transmitter at the neuromuscular junction of the cat. *Journal of Pharmacology and Experimental Therapeutics*, **175**, 664–2.

Boheim, G., Hanke, W., Barrantes, F. J., Eibl, H., Sakman, B., Fels, G., *et al.* (1981). Agonist activated ionic channels in acetylcholine receptor reconstituted into planar lipid bilayers. *Proceedings of the National Acadamy of Sciences, USA* **78**, 3586–90.

Bowden, R. E. M. and Duchen, L. W. (1976). The anatomy and pathology of the neuromuscular junction. In *Neuromuscular junction*. (ed. E. Zaimis), *Handbook of experimental pharmacology*, Vol. 42, pp. 23–97. Springer-Verlag, Berlin.

Bowman, W. C. (1980). Prejunctional and postjunctional cholinoceptors at the neuromuscular junction. *Anesthesia and Analgesia*, **59**, 935–43.

Bowman, W. C. (1985). The neuromuscular junction: recent developments. *European Journal of Anaesthesia*, **2**, 59–93.

Bowman, W. C. and Nott, M. W. (1969). Actions of sympathomimetic amines and their antagonists on skeletal muscle. *Pharmacological Reviews*, **21**, 27–72.

Bowman, W. C. and Webb, S. N. (1976). Tetanic fade during partial transmission failure produced by non-depolarising neuromuscular blocking drugs in the cat. *Clinical and Experimental Pharmacology and Physiology*, **3**, 545–55.

Boyd, I. A. and Martin, A. R. (1956). The end-plate potential in mammalian muscle. *Journal of Physiology*, **132**, 74–91.

Brenner, H. R. and Sakmann, B. (1983). Neurotrophic control of channel properties at neuromuscular synapses of rat muscle. *Journal of Physiology*, **337**, 159–71.

Brooks, V. B. (1956). An intracellular study of the action of repetitive nerve volleys and of botulinum toxin on miniature end plate potentials. *Journal of Physiology*, **134**, 264–77.

Ceccarelli, B. and Hurlbut, W. P. (1980). Vesicle hypothesis of the release of quanta of acetylcholine. *Physiological Reviews*, **60**, 396–441.

Chang, C. C. and Lee, C. Y. (1963). Isolation of toxins from the venom of *Bungarus multicinctus* and their modes of neuromuscular blocking action. *Archives of International Pharmacodynamics*, **144**, 241–57.

Changeux, J. P., Benedetti, L., Bourgeois, J. P., Brisson, A., Cartaud, J., Devaux, P., *et al.* (1976). Some structural properties of the cholinergic receptor protein in its membrane environment relevant to its function as a pharmacological receptor. *Cold Spring Harbor Symposium on Quantitative Biology*, **40**, 211–30.

Ciani, S. and Edwards, C. (1963). The effect of acetylcholine on neuromuscular transmission in the frog. *Journal of Pharmacology and Experimental Therapeutics*, **142**, 21–3.

Clarke, A. J. (1913). The factors determining tolerance of glycosides of the digitalis series. *Journal of Pharmacology and Experimental Therapeutics*, **4**, 399–424.

Clarke, A. J. (1926). The reaction between acetyl choline and muscle cells. *Journal of Physiology*, **61**, 530–46.

Clarke, A. J. (1927). The reaction between acetyl choline and muscle cells. Part II. *Journal of Physiology*, **64**, 123–43.

Collier, B. and MacIntosh, F. C. (1969). The source of choline for acetylcholine synthesis in a sympathetic ganglion. *Canadian Journal of Physiology and Pharmacology*, **47**, 127–35.

Colquhoun, D., Dionne, V. E., Steinbach, J. H., and Stevens, C. F. (1975). Conductance of channels opened by acetylcholine-like drugs in muscle end-plate. *Nature*, **253**, 204–6.

Colquhoun, D., Dreyer, F., and Sheridan, R. E. (1979). The actions of tubocurarine at the frog neuromuscular junction. *Journal of Physiology*, **293**, 247–84.

Conti-Tronconi, B., Tzartos, S., and Lindstrom, J. (1981). Monoclonal antibodies as probes of acetylcholine receptor structure. 2. Binding to native receptor. *Biochemistry*, **20**, 2181–91.

Dale, H. H. (1914). The action of certain esters and ethers of choline and their relation to muscarine. *Journal of Pharmacology and Experimental Therapeutics*, **6**, 147–90.

Dale, H. H. (1934). Chemical transmission of the effects of nerve impulses. *British Medical Journal*, **1**, 835–41.

Dale, H. H. and Feldberg, W. (1933). The chemical transmitter of effects of the gastric vagus. *Journal of Physiology*, **80**, 16P–17P.

Dale, H. H., Feldberg, W., and Vogt. M. (1936). Release of acetylcholine at voluntary motor nerve endings. *Journal of Physiology*, **86**, 353–80.

Daniels, M. P. and Vogel, Z. (1975). Immunoperoxidase staining of alpha-bungarotoxin binding sites in muscle endplates shows distribution of acetylcholine receptors. *Nature*, **254**, 339–41.

Das, M., Ganguly, D. K., and Vedasiromoni, J. R. (1978). Enhancement by oxotremorine of acetylcholine release from the rat phrenic nerve. *British Journal of Pharmacology*, **62**, 195–8.

Davis, R. and Koelle, G. B. (1967). Electron microscopic localization of acetylcholinesterase and nonspecific cholinesterase at the neuromuscular junction by the gold-thiocholine and gold-thiolacetic acid methods. *Journal of Cell Biology*, **34**, 157–71.

Del Castillo, J. and Katz, B. (1954). Quantal components of the end-plate potential. *Journal of Physiology*, **124**, 560–73.

Del Castillo, J. and Katz, B. (1955). Local activity at a depolarized nerve-muscle junction. *Journal of Physiology*, **128**, 396–411.

Dixon, W. E. (1906). Vagus inhibition. *British Medical Journal*, **2**, 1807.

Dixon, W. E. (1909). On the mode of action of drugs. *Medical Magazine*, **16**, 454–7.

Dreyer, F. (1982). Acetylcholine receptor. *British Journal of Anaesthesia*, **54**, 115–30.

Dreyer, F., Peper, K., Akert, K., Sandri, C., and Moor, H. (1973). Ultrastructure of the factive zone, in the frog neuromuscular junction. *Brain Research*, **62**, 373–80.

Dreyer, F., Peper, K., and Sterz, R. (1978). Determination of dose response curves by quantitative ionophoresis at the frog neuromuscular junction. *Journal of Physiology*, **281**, 395–419.

Droz, B., Koenig, H. L., Di Giamberardino, L., Couraud, J. Y., Chretein, M., and Souyri, F. (1979). The importance of axonal transport and endoplasmic reticulum in the function of cholinergic synapse in normal and pathological conditions. *Progress in Brain Research*, **49**, 23–44.

Duncan, C. and Publicover, S. J. (1979). Inhibitory effects of cholinergic agents on the release of transmitter at the frog neuromuscular junction. *Journal of Physiology*, **294**, 91–103.

Dwyer, T. M., Adams, D. J., and Hille, B. (1980). The permeability of the endplate channel to organic cations in frog muscle. *Journal of General Physiology*, **75**, 469–103.

Edwards, C. (1979). The effects of innervation on the properties of acetylcholine receptors in muscle. *Neuroscience*, **4**, 565–84.

Ehrlich, P. (1900). On immunity with special reference to cell life. *Proceedings of the Royal Society of London, Series B*, **66**, 424–48.

Ekstrom, J. and Emmelin, N. (1971). Movement of choline acetyltransferase in axons disconnected from their cell bodies. *Journal of Physiology*, **216**, 247–56.

Eldefrawi, M. E., Eldefrawi, A. T., and Wilson, D. B. (1975). Tryptophan and cysteine residues of the acetylcholine receptors of Torpedo species. Relationship to binding of cholinergic ligands. *Biochemistry*, **14**, 4304–10.

Elliot, T. R. (1905). The action of adrenalin. *Journal of Physiology*, **32**, 401–67.

Ellisman, M. H., Rash, J. E., Staehelin, L. A., and Porter, K. R. (1976). Studies of exciteable membranes II. A comparison of specializations at neuromuscular junction and nonjunctional sarcolemmas of mammalian fast and BLOW twitch muscle fibres. *Journal of Cell Biology*, **68**, 752–74.

Elmqvist, D. and Quastel, D. M. J. (1965*a*). Presynaptic action of hemicholinium at the neuromuscular junction. *Journal of Physiology*, **177**, 463–82.

Elmqvist, D. and Quastel, D. M. J. (1965*b*). A quantitative study of end plate potentials in isolated human muscle. *Journal of Physiology*, **178**, 505–29.

Everett, A. J., Lowe, L. A. and Wilkinson, S. (1970). Revision of the structures of (+)-tubocurarine chloride and (+)-chondrocurine. *Journal of the Chemical Society,* D, 1020–1.

Fambrough, D. M. (1979). Control of acetylcholine receptors in skeletal muscle. *Physiological Reviews*, **59**, 165–227.

Fatt, P. and Katz, B. (1950). Some observations on biological noise. *Nature*, **166**, 597–8.

Fatt, P. and Katz, B. (1951). An analysis of the endplate potential recorded with an intracellular electrode. *Journal of Physiology*, **115**, 320–70.

Fatt, P. and Katz, B. (1952). Spontaneous subthreshold activity at motor nerve endings. *Journal of Physiology*, **117**, 109–28.

Feldberg, W. and Krayer, O. (1933). Das Auftreten eines azetylcholinartigen Stoffes in Herzvenenblut von Warmblutern bei Reizung der Nervi vagi. *Archiv für Experimentelle Pathologie und Pharmakologie* **172**, 170–93.

Feltz, A. and Trautmann, A. (1982). Desensitization of the frog neuromuscular junction: a biphasic process. *Journal of Physiology*, **322**, 257–72.

Fertuk, H. C. and Salpeter, M. M. (1974). Localization of acetylcholine receptor by 125 I-labelled alpha-bungarotoxin binding at mouse motor end plate. *Proceedings of the National Academy of Sciences of the USA*, **71**, 1376–80.

Fertuck, H. C. and Salpeter, M. M. (1976). Quantitation of junctional and extrajunctional acetylcholine receptors by electron-microscope autoradiography after 125 I-alpha-bungarotoxin binding at mouse neuromuscular junctions. *Journal of Cell Biology*, **69**, 144–58.

Fonnum, F. (1973). Recent developments in biochemical investigations of cholinergic transmission. *Brain Research*, **62**, 497–507.

Gage, P. W. and Hamill, O. P. (1980). Lifetime and conductance of acetylcholine-activated channels in normal and denervated toad sartorius muscle. *Journal of Physiology*, **298**, 525–38.

Gandiha, A. and Marshall, I. G. (1973). The effects of 2-(4-phenylpiperidino)-cyclohexanol (AH5183) on the acetylcholine content of, and output from, the chick biventer cervicis muscle preparation. *International Journal of Neuroscience*, **5**, 191–6.

Gibb, A. J. and Marshall, I. G. (1984). Pre- and post-junctional effects of tubocurarine and other nicotinic antagonists during repetitive stimulation in the rat. *Journal of Physiology*, **351**, 275–97.

Ginsborg, B. L., and Jenkinson, D. H. (1976). Transmission of impulses from nerve to muscle. In *Neuromuscular junction*. (ed. E. Zaimis). *Handbook of experimental pharmacology*, Vol. 42, pp. 229–364. Springer-Verlag, Berlin.

Glavinovic M. I. (1979). Presynaptic action of curare. *Journal of Physiology*, **290**, 499–506.

Grewaal, D. S. and Quastel, J. H. (1973). Control of synthesis and release of radioactive acetylcholine in brain slices from the rat. *Biochemical Journal*, **132**, 1–14.

Griffiths, H. R. and Johnson, G. E. (1942). The use of curare in general anesthesia. *Anesthesiology*, **3**, 418–20.

Grohavaz, F., Limbrick, A. R., and Miledi, R. (1982). Acetylcholine receptors at the rat neuromuscular junction as revealed by deep etching. *Proceedings of the Royal Society of London, Series B*, **215**, 147–54.

Gunderson, C. B. and Jenden, D. J. (1980). Oxotremorine does not enhance acetylcholine release from rat diaphragm preparations. *British Journal of Pharmacology*, **70**, 8–10.

Guy, H. R. (1984). A structural model of the acetylcholine receptor channel based on partition energy and helix packing calculations. *Biophysical Journal*, **45**, 249–61.

Guyton, A. C. (1976). Physiological classification of nerve fibres. In *Textbook of medical physiology* (5th edn), pp. 647–8. W. B. Saunders, Philadelphia.

Haga, T., and Noda, H. (1973). Choline uptake systems of rat brain synaptosomes. *Biochimica et Biophysica Acta*, **291**, 564–75.

Hebb, C. (1972). Biosynthesis of acetylcholine in nervous tissue. *Physiological Reviews*, **52**, 918–57.

Heidmann, T. and Changeux, J. P. (1978). Structural and functional properties of the acetylcholine receptor protein in its purified and membrane-bound states. *Annual Review of Biochemistry*, **47**, 317–57.

Heuser, J. E. and Reese, T. S. (1981). Structural changes after transmitter release at the frog neuromuscular junction. *Journal of Cell Biology*, **88**, 564–80.

Heuser, J. E. and Reese, T. S. (1973). Evidence for recycling of synaptic vesicle membrane during transmitter release at the frog neuromuscular junction. *Journal of Cell Biology*, **57**, 315–44.

Heuser, J. E. Reese, T. S., Dennis, M. J., Jan, Y., Jan, L., and Evans, L. (1979). Synaptic vesicle exocytosis captured by quick freezing and correlated with quantal transmitter release. *Journal of Cell Biology*, **81**, 275–300.

Heuser, J. E., and Salpeter, S. R. (1979). Organisation of acetylcholine receptors in quick-frozen deep-etched and rotary-replicated *Torpedo* postsynaptic membrane. *Journal of Cell Biology*, **82**, 150–73.

Hirokawa, N. and Heuser, J. E. (1983). Internal and external differentiations of the post-synaptic membrane at the neuromuscular junction. *Journal of Neurocytology*, **11**, 487–510.

Hobbiger, F. (1976). Pharmacology of anticholinesterase drugs. In *Neuromuscular junction*, (ed. E. Zaimis). *Handbook of experimental pharmacology*, Vol. 42, pp. 487–581. Springer Verlag, Berlin.

Hubbard, J. I. and Wilson, D. F. (1973). Neuromuscular transmission in a mammalian preparation in the absence of blocking drugs and the effect of *d*-tubocurarine. *Journal of Physiology*, **228**, 307–25.

Hubbard, J. I., Jones, S. F., and Landau, E. M. (1968). On the mechanism by which calcium and magnesium affect the release of transmitter by nerve impulses. *Journal of Physiology*, **196**, 75–86.

Hubbard, J. I., Schmidt, R. F., and Yokota, T. (1965). The effect of acetycholine upon mammalian motor nerve terminals. *Journal of Physiology*, **181**, 810–29.

Hurlbut, W. P. and Ceccarelli. B. (1979). Use of black widow spider venom to study the release of neurotransmitters. *Advances in Cytopharmacology*, **3**, 87–115.

Israel, M. and Dunant, Y. (1979). On the mechanism of acetylcholine release. *Progress in Brain Research*, **49**, 125–39.

Israel, M., Gautron, J., and Lesbats, B. (1968). Isolement des vesicules synaptiques de l'organe electrique de la Torpille et localisation de l'acétylcholine à leur niveau. *Comptes Rendus Hebdomadaires des Séances et Mémoirs de la Société de Biologie* (Series D), **266**, 273–5.

Israel, M., Dunant, Y., and Manaranche, R. (1979). The present status of the vesicular hypothesis. *Progress in Neurobiology*, **13**, 237–75.

Ito, Y., and Miledi, R. (1977). The effect of calcium-ionophores on acetylcholine release from Schwann cells. *Proceedings of the Royal Society of London, Series B*, **196**, 51–8.

James, R. W., Kato, A. C., Rey, M. -J., and Fulpius, B. W. (1980). Monoclonal antibodies directed against the neurotransmitter binding site of nicotinic acetylcholine receptor. *FEBS Letters*, **120**, 145–8.

Jones, S. F. and Kwanbunbumpen, S. (1970). The effects of nerve stimulation and hemi-cholinium on synaptic vesicles at the mammalian neuromuscular junction. *Journal of Physiology*, **207**, 31–50.

Jones, S. W. and Salpeter, M. M. (1983). Absence of I [125]-alpha-bungarotoxin binding to motor nerve terminals of frog, lizard and mouse muscle. *Journal of Neuroscience*, **3**, 326–31.

Karlin, A. (1969). Chemical modification of the active site of the acetylcholine receptor. *Journal of General Physiology*, **54**, 245S–64S.

Katz, B. (1966). *Nerve, muscle and synapse*. McGraw-Hill, New York.

Katz, B. and Miledi, R. (1977). Transmitter leakage from motor nerve endings. *Proceedings of the Royal Society of London, Series B*, **196**, 59–72.

Katz, B. and Miledi, R. (1979). Estimates of quantal content during, chemical potentiation, of transmitter release. *Proceedings of the Royal Society of London, Series B*, **205**, 369–78.

Katz, B. and Miledi, R. (1981). Does the motor nerve impulse evoke, non-quantal transmitter release? *Proceedings of the Royal Society of London, Series B*, **212**, 131–7.

King, H. (1935). Curare alkaloids, Part I. Tubocurarine. *Journal of the Chemical Society*, **2**, 1381–9.

Kloog, Y., Michaelson, D. M., and Sokolovsky M. (1980). Characterization of the presynaptic muscarinic receptor in synaposomes of Torpedo electric organ by means of kinetic and equilibrium binding studies. *Brain Research*, **194**, 97–115.

Koelle, G. B. (1962). A new general concept of the neurohumoral functions of acetylcholine and acetylcholinesterase. *Journal of Pharmacy and Pharmacology*, **14**, 65–90.

Koelle, G. B., Davis, R., and Gromadzki, C. G. (1967). Electron microscopic localization of cholinesterases by means of gold salts. *Annals of the New York Academy of Sciences*, **144**, 613–25.

Krnjevic, K. and Miledi, R. (1958). Some effects produced by adrenaline upon neuromuscular propagation in rats. *Journal of Physiology*, **141**, 291–304.

Kuba, K. (1970). Effects of catecholamines on the neuromuscular junction in the rat diaphragm. *Journal of Physiology*, **211**, 551–70.

Lambert, J. J., Durant, N. N., and Henderson E. G. (1983). Drug induced modification of ionic conductance at the neuromuscular junction. *Annual Review of Pharmacology and Toxicology*, **23**, 505–39.

Land, B. R., Salpeter, E. E., and Salpeter, M. M. (1980). Acetylcholine receptor site density affects the rising phase of miniature end plate currents. *Proceedings of the National Academy of Sciences of the USA*, **77**, 3736–40.

Langley, J. N. (1878). On the physiology of salivary secretion. Part II. On the mutual antagonism of atropin and pilocarpin, having especial reference to their relations in the submaxillary gland of the cat. *Journal of Physiology*, **1**, 339–69.

Langley, J. N. (1901). Observations on the physiological action of extracts of the supra-renal bodies. *Journal of Physiology*, **27**, 237–56.

Langley, J. N. (1906). Croonian Lecture 1906–On nerve endings and on special excitable substances in cells. *Proceedings of the Royal Society of London, Series B*, **78**, 170–94.

Langley, J. N. (1909). On the contraction of muscle chiefly in relation to the presence of 'receptive' substances. Part 4. The effect of curari and of some other substances on the nicotine response of the sartorius and gastrocnemius muscles of the frog. *Journal of Physiology*, **39**, 235–95.

Lawen, A. (1912). Ueber die Verbindung der Lokalanasthesie mit der Narkose, Über hohe Extraduralanastesie und epidurale Injektionen anästhesierender Lösungen bei tabischen Magenkrisen. *Beiträge Klinische Chirurgia*, **80**, 168–89.

Lawler, H. C. (1961). Turnover time of acetylcholinesterase. *Journal of Biology and Chemistry*, **236**, 2296–301.

Lee, C-M. (1975). Train of 4 quantitation of competitive neuromuscular block. *Anesthesia and Analgesia*, **54**, 649–53.

Lee, C. Y. (1972). Chemistry and pharmacology of polypeptide toxins in snake venoms. *Annual Review of Pharmacology*, **12**, 265–86.

Lehter, H. A. (1977). The response to acetylcholine. *Scientific American*, **236**, 106–18.

Lewandowsky, M. (1898). Ueber eine Wirkung des Nebennieren extractes auf das Auge. *Centralblatt für Physiologie*, **12**, 599–600.

Lilleheil, G. and Naess, K. (1961). A presynaptic effect of *d*-tubocurarine in the neuromuscular junction. *Acta Physiologica Scandinavica*, **52**, 120–36.

Lindstrom, J., Cooper, J., and Tzartos, S. (1980). Acetylcholine receptors from Torpedo and Electrophorus have similar subunit structures. *Biochemistry*, **19**, 1454–8.

Llinas, R. and Heuser, J. E. (1977). Depolarisation-release coupling systems in neurones. *Neurosciences Research Program Bulletin*, **15**, 577–687.

Loewi, O. (1921). Über humorale Übertragbarkeit der Herznervenwirkung. *Pflugers Archiv Gesamte Physiology*, **189**, 239–42.

Loewi, O. and Navratil, E. (1926). Über humorale Übertragbarkeit der Herznervenwirkung. X. Mitteilung. Über das Schicksal des Vagusstoffs. *Pflugers Archiv Gesamte Physiology*, **214**, 678–88.

Magleby, K. L., Pallotta, B. S., and Terrar D. A. (1981). The effect of tubocurarine on neuromuscular transmission during repetitive stimulation in the rat, mouse and frog. *Journal of Physiology*, **312**, 97–113.

Magelby, K. L. and Stevens, C. F. (1972). The effect of voltage on the time course of endplate currents. *Journal of Physiology* **223**, 151–71.

Magelby, K. L. and Terrar, D. A. (1975). Factors affecting the time course of decay of endplate currents: a possible cooperative action of acetylcholine on receptors at the frog neuromuscular junction. *Journal of Physiology*, **244**, 467–95.

Marchbanks, R. M. (1979). Role of storage vesicles in synaptic transmission. *Symposia of the Society for Experimental Biology*, **33**, 251–76.

Marchbanks, R. M. and Israel, M. (1972). The heterogeneity of bound acetylcholine and synaptic vesicles. *Biochemical Journal*, **129**, 1049–61.

Marshall, I. G. (1970). Studies on the blocking action of 2-(4-phenyl piperidino) cyclohexanol (AH5183). *British Journal of Pharmacology*, **38**, 503–16.

Martin, A. R. (1966). Quantal nature of synaptic transmission. *Physiological Reviews*, **46**, 51–66.

McIntyre, A. R., King, R. E., and Dunn, A. L. (1945). Electrical activity of denervated mammalian skeletal muscle as influenced by *d*-tubocurarine. *Journal of Neurophysiology*, **8**, 297–307.

Michaelson, D. M., Avissar, S., Kloog, Y., and Sokolovsky, M. (1979). Mechanism of acetylcholine release: possible involvement of presynaptic muscarinic receptors in regulation of acetylcholine release and protein phosphorylation. *Proceedings of the National Academy of Sciences of the USA*, **76**, 6336–40.

Michaelson, D. M., Avissar, S., Ophir, I., Pinchasi, I., Angel, I., Kloog, Y., *et al.* (1980). On the regulation of acetylcholine release: a study using Torpedo synaptosomes and synaptic vesicles. *Journal of Physiology (Paris)*, **76**, 505–14.

Miledi, R., Molenaar, P. C., and Polak, R. L. (1980). The effect of lanthanum ions on acetylcholine in frog muscle. *Journal of Physiology*, **309**, 199–214.

Mitchell, J. F. and Silver, A. (1963). The spontaneous release of acetylcholine from the denervated hemidiaphragm of the rat. *Journal of Physiology*, **165**, 117–29.

Nachmansohn, D. (1975). *Chemical and molecular basis of nerve activity*. Academic Press, New York.

Meubig, R. R., Boyd, N. D., and Cohen, J. B. (1982). Conformations of Torpedo acetylcholine receptor associated with ion transport and desensitisation. *Biochemistry*, **21**, 3460–7.

Palade, G. E. (1954). Electron microscope observations of interneuronal and neuromuscular synapses. *Anatomical Record*, **118**, 335–6.

Palay, S. L. (1954), Electron microscope study of the cytoplasm of neurons. *Anatomical Record*, **118**, 336.

Panella, A. (1907). Action du principe actif surrenal sur la fatigue musculaire. *Archivio Italiano di Biologia* **48**, 430–63.

Paton, W. D. M. and Waud, D. R. (1967). The margin of safety of neuromuscular transmission. *Journal of Physiology*, **191**, 59–90.

Paton, W. D. M. and Zaimis, E. J. (1948). Curare-like action of polymethylene bisquaternary ammonium salts. *Nature*, **161**, 718–9.

Paton, W. D. M. and Zaimis, E. J. (1952). The methonium compounds. *Pharmacological Reviews*, **4**, 219–53.

Pecot-Dechavassine, M. (1982). Synaptic vesicle openings captured by cooling and related to transmitter release at the frog neuromuscular junction. *Biological Cell*, **46**, 43–50.

Peper, K., Dreyer, F., Sandri, C., Akert K., and Moor, H. (1974). Structure and ultrastructure of the frog motor endplate. A freeze-etching study. *Cell Tissue Research*, **149**, 437–55.

Peper, K., Bradley, R. J., and Dreyer, F. (182). The acetylcholine receptor at the neuromuscular junction. *Physiological Reviews*, **62**, 1271–340.

Potter, L. T. (1970). Synthesis, storage and release of [^{14}C]acetylcholine in isolated rat diaphragm muscles. *Journal of Physiology*, **206**, 145–66.

Pumplin, D. W., and Fambrough, D. M. (1982). Turnover of acetylcholine receptors in skeletal muscle. *Annual Review of Physiology*, **44**, 319–35.

Raftery, M. A., Vandlen, R. L., Reed, K. L., and Lee, T. (1975). Characteristics of Torpedo acetylcholine receptor: its subunit composition and ligand-binding properties. *Cold Spring Harbor Symposia on Quantitative Biology*, **40**, 193–202.

Raftery, M. A., Hunkapiller, M. W., Strader, C. D., and Hood, L. E. (1980). Acetylcholine receptor: complex of homologous subunits. *Science*, **208**, 1454–7.

Raftery, M. A., Dunn, S. M. J., Conti-Tronconi, B. M., Middlemas, D. M., and Crawford R. D. (1983). The nicotinic acetylcholine receptor: subunit structure, functional binding sites and ion transport properties. *Cold Spring Harbor Symposia on Quantitative Biology*, **48**, 21–33.

Rama Sastry, B. V. and Sadavongvivad, C. (1979). Cholinergic systems in non-nervous tissues. *Pharmacological Reviews*, **30**, 65–132.

Rang, H. P. (1981). Drugs and ionic channels: mechanisms and implications. *Postgraduate Medical Journal*, **57**, Supplement 1, 89 91.

Reynolds, J. A. and Karlin, A. (1978). Molecular weight in detergent solution of acetylcholine receptor from Torpedo californica. *Biochemistry*, **17**, 2035–8.

Riker, W. F., Jr (1966). Actions of acetylcholine on mammalian motor nerve terminal. *Journal of Pharmacological Experimental Therapeutics*, **152**, 397–416.

Robertson, J. D. (1956). The ultrastructure of a reptilian myoneural junction. Journal of Biophysics, *Biochemistry and Cytology* **2**, 381–94.

Ross, M. J., Klymkowsky, M. W., Agard, D. A. and Stroud, R. M. (1977). Structural studies of a membrane-bound acetylcholine receptor from Torpedo californica. *Journal of Molecular Biology*, **116**, 635–59.

Sachs, F. and Lechar, H. (1977). Acetylcholine induced current fluctuations in tissue cultured muscle cells under voltage clamp. *Biophysical Journal*, **17**, 129–43.

Salpeter, M. M. (1967). Electron microscope radioautography as a quantitative tool in enzyme cytochemistry: I. The distribution of acetylcholinesterase at motor end plates of a vertebrate twitch muscle. *Journal of Cell Biology*, **32**, 379–89.

Sargent, P. B., Hedges, B. E., Tsaveler, L., Clemmons, L., Tzartos, S., and Lindstrom, J. M. (1984). Structure and transmembrane nature of the acetylcholine receptor in amphibian skeletal muscle as revealed by cross-reacting monoclonal antibodies. *Journal of Cell Biology*, **98**, 609–18.

Schmiedeberg, O. and Harnack, E. (1877). Über die Synthese des Muscarins und Über Muscarin-artig wirkende ammoniumbasen. *Archiv für Experimentele Pathologie und Pharmakologie*, **6**, 101–12.

Sobell, H. M., Sakore, T. D. Tavale, S. S. Canepa, F. G. Pauling, P. Patcher, T. J. (1972). Stereochemistry of a curare alkaloid: 0, 01, N-trimethyl-d-tubocurarine. *Proceedings of the National Academy of Sciences of the USA*, **69**, 2212–5.

Soteropoulos, G. C. and Standaert, F. G. (1973). Neuromuscular effects of morphine and naloxone. *Journal of Pharmacology and Experimental Therapeutics*, **184**, 136–42.

Standaert, F. G. (1964). The action of d-tubocurarine on the motor nerve terminal. *Journal of Pharmacology and Experimental Therapeutics*, **143**, 181–6.

Starke, K. (1981). Presynaptic receptors. *Annual Review of Pharmacology and Toxicology*, **21**, 7–30.

Steinbach, J. H. (1981). Neuromuscular junctions and alpha-bungarotoxin binding sites in denervated and contralateral cat skeletal muscle. *Journal of Physiology*, **313**, 513–28.

Strader, C. D. and Raftery, M. A. (1980). Topographic studies of Torpedo acetylcholine receptor subunits as a transmembrane complex. *Proceedings of the National Academy of Sciences of the USA*, **17**, 5807–11.

Strichartz, G. (1976). Molecular mechanisms of nerve block by local anesthetics. *Anesthesiology*, **45**, 421–41.

Stroud, R. M. (1983). Acetylcholine receptor structure. *Neuroscience Comment*, **1**, 124–8.

Sykes, W. S. (1982). Curare, or the Squire of Walton. In *Essays on the first 100 years of anaesthesia*, Vol. 1, pp. 86–98. Churchill Livingstone, Edinburgh.

Tauc, L. (1979). Are vesicles necessary for release of acetylcholine at cholinergic synapses? *Biochemistry and Pharmacology*, **28**, 3493–8.

Thesleff, S. and Molgo, J. (1983). A new type of transmitter release at the neuromuscular junction. *Neuroscience*, **9**, 1–8.

Trautmann, A. and Feltz, A. (1980). Open time of channels activated by binding of two distinct agonists. *Nature*, **286**, 291–3.

Tucek, S., and Cheng, S. C. (1974). Provenance of the acetyl group of acetylcholine and compartmentation of acetyl-CoA and Krebs cycle intermediates in the brain *in vivo*. *Journal of Neurochemistry*, **22**, 893–914.

Vaca, K. and Pilar, G. (1979). Mechanisms controlling choline transport and acetylcholine synthesis in motor nerve terminals during electrical stimulation. *Journal of General Physiology*, **73**, 605–28.

Van der Kloot, W. (1977). Quantal acetylcholine release: vesicles or gated channels? *General Pharmacology*, **8**, 21–5.

Vizi, E. S. and Viskocil, F. (1979). Changes in total and quantal release of acetylcholine in the mouse diaphragm during activation and inhibition of membrane ATPase. *Journal of Physiology*, **286**, 1–14.

Wallis, T. E. (1967). *Textbook of pharmacognosy*, (5th edn). Churchill, London.

Whittaker, V. P. and Luqmani, Y. A. (1980). False transmitters in the cholinergic system: implications for the vesicle theory of transmitter storage and release. *General Pharmacology*, **11**, 7–14.

Wray, D. (1980). Noise analysis and channels at the postsynaptic membrane of skeletal muscle. *Progress in Drug Research*, **24**, 9–54.

Yamamura, H. I. and Snyder, S. H. (1973). High affinity transport of choline into synaptosomes of rat brain. *Journal of Neurochemistry*, **21**, 1355–74.

3

Physio-chemical aspects of neuromuscular blockade

I. G. Marshall and R. D. Waigh

NEUROMUSCULAR TRANSMISSION

The basic physiology of the process of neuromuscular transmission — i.e. the process of transmission between somatic nerves and skeletal muscle — centres on acetylcholine, the chemical transmitter. The pharmacology of clinically useful muscle relaxants involves primarily, but possibly not entirely, interference with the postjunctional action of acetylcholine on nicotinic receptors. Neuromuscular transmission and its associated pharmacology have been comprehensively reviewed recently by Bowman (1990).

Acetylcholine is synthesized in the cytoplasm of the motor nerve terminal from the substrates choline and acetate, under the catalytic influence of the enzyme choline acetyltransferase. Choline is provided from extraterminal sources: plasma choline, and choline produced as the breakdown product of enzymatic hydrolysis of acetylcholine. The uptake of the charged quaternary choline is mediated by a high affinity sodium-dependent mechanism (Yamamura and Snyder 1972). Synthesized acetylcholine is then concentrated in its storage particles, the membrane-bound synaptic vesicles, by an ATP-dependent uptake process (see Marshall and Parsons 1987 for review). None of the clinically used muscle relaxants has significant effects on the choline uptake mechanism at normally achieved plasma concentrations, and the synaptic vesicle acetylcholine storage system, being intraterminal, is not normally accessible to non-lipid soluble quaternary ammonium compounds such as muscle relaxants.

Careful studies of transmitter release have indicated that not all stored acetylcholine has an equal chance of being released by nerve impulses. Thus, it appears that there are probably two readily or immediately releasable stores of acetylcholine, plus a depot or back-up store (Glavinović and Narahashi 1988). The translocation or movement of acetylcholine, or vesicles, towards the immediately releasable stores is the process known generally as transmitter mobilization. It is possible that phosphorylation of the synaptic vesicle-associated protein synapsin I in the presence of calcium is involved in the freeing of synaptic vesicles from the internal cytoskeleton of the nerve terminal, thus allowing movement towards the release sites (de Camilli and Greengard 1986).

The release process itself is exquisitely dependent upon calcium entry into the terminal subsequent to terminal depolarization. In some way, possible involving the fusion protein synaptotagnin, calcium induces the fusion of the synaptic vesicle membrane with the plasmalemma, leading to the release of quanta or packages of acetylcholine. At rest, individual quanta are released at random (Fatt and Katz 1951), but terminal depolarization results in the simultaneous release of many quanta (del Castillo and Katz 1954). At individual neuromuscular junctions the number of quanta released is related to the diameter, and hence the input resistance, of the muscle fibre innervated, small diameter fibres requiring only a small number of quanta for effective excitation.

Upon release, the acetylcholine diffuses across the junctional cleft and activates the postjunctional acetylcholine receptors. As will be discussed in greater detail later, the nicotinic receptor consists of five membrane spanning subunits, each of which crosses the membrane four or five times. The second membrane-spanning region (TM2) is the part of the subunit thought to be involved in ion permeation through the receptor–ion channel complex. Two of the five subunits are identical (alpha subunits); plus there are one beta, one delta, and one epsilon subunit in adult mammalian muscle. The recognition sites for acetylcholine are situated on the alpha subunits and activation of the receptor-channel complex is much more likely when both recognition sites are occupied (Colquhoun 1986). Occupation of the recognition sites induces a conformational change in the subunits comprising the receptor, leading to the opening of a pore, or channel, through the middle of the receptor. This channel conducts cations, mainly sodium and potassium, down their concentration and electrical gradients. The flow of ions reduces the normal membrane potential of the chemically excitable endplate region towards zero potential. The fall in membrane potential in the chemically excitable region leads to a disparity in potential with the adjacent electrically excitable area. As a result, local circuit current flow in the area between the chemically and electrically excitable regions. This has the effect of lowering the membrane potential, i.e. depolarizing the electrically excitable membrane. At a critical threshold potential, sodium channels open in the electrically excitable membrane and initiate an all-or-none action potential. This self-propagating muscle action potential results in muscle contraction. During the period occupied by the muscle action potential and the muscle contraction, transmitter acetylcholine is hydrolysed by the enzyme acetylcholinesterase; thus, one nerve action potential results in one muscle contraction. The process of chemical transmission involving acetylcholine acts as a mechanism for amplifying the signal in the tiny nerve terminal such that it is able to activate the very much larger muscle fibre.

NEUROMUSCULAR BLOCK

As indicated in the previous section, the prejunctional metabolism, synthesis, and storage of acetylcholine are not significantly affected by clinically used muscle relaxants. There is some evidence for a prejunctional action of relaxants on transmitter mobilization (see later), but the major established actions are on the postjunctional acetylcholine receptors. At the postjunctional site the muscle relaxant drugs can be divided into two major classes, agonists and antagonists. Agonists include transmitter acetylcholine itself, but also the depolarizing neuromuscular blocking agents, of which suxamethonium is the only example in widespread clinical use. Antagonists represent the non-depolarizing class of the relaxants such as tubocurarine, pancuronium, atracurium, and vecuronium. The action of both agonists and antagonists involves binding to the acetylcholine receptor recognition site. In the case of agonists this results in activation of the receptor; in the case of antagonists no activation is seen, but rather, by occupying the receptor, the antagonist prevents activation by an agonist. The antagonism of the activation of the receptor by transmitter acetylcholine results in failure of the level of postjunctional depolarization produced by released acetylcholine to reach the threshold level for firing of a muscle action potential; hence muscle contraction ceases. As the action potential that results in muscle contraction is an all-or-none response, the graded, concentration-dependent effect of the muscle relaxant on the graded endplate response eventually leads to an all-or-none response in the muscle fibre, i.e. the fibre either contracts or it does not contract. The time- and concentration-dependent gradations of neuromuscular block measured by tension-recording techniques (e.g. in clinical anaesthesia) are representations of the number of fibres in a muscle, or group of muscles, that contract in an all-or-none manner in response to nerve stimulation.

How does an agonist such as suxamethonium produce neuromuscular block? Initially, because of its acetylcholine-like agonist action, the compound produces receptor activation and muscle contraction; this is manifest as preblock fasciculation. However, unlike acetylcholine, suxamethonium is not hydrolysed by junctional acetylcholinesterase. Thus, relative to acetylcholine, suxamethonium produces persistent depolarization of the postjunctional endplate region. This is thought to lead to inactivation of the sodium channels in the electrically excitable membrane surrounding the endplate and hence to an insulation zone of electrical inexcitability through which impulses cannot pass. In this way muscle contraction fails. Like acetylcholine, suxamethonium is an ester and hence is susceptible to hydrolysis; in the case of suxamethonium this hydrolysis is catalysed, in humans at least, by plasma butyrylcholinesterase (pseudo-cholinesterase).

A second way in which nondepolarizing relaxants can produce block, in addition to the above-mentioned and well-documented competitive action on postjunctional receptors, is by a prejunctional action. As a result of this, transmitter release is diminished during the course of a high frequency burst of nerve activity (Bowman 1980; Bowman *et al.* 1976). Such high frequency activity underlies normal voluntary muscle movement, and hence such a mechanism has substantial potential clinical relevance. This action of nondepolarizing relaxants manifests itself as the well-known phenomenon of tetanic or train-of-four fade. It has been proposed that tetanic fade is produced by relaxants blocking a prejunctional autoreceptor which is normally activated by transmitter acetylcholine during high frequency activity to enhance transmitter mobilization — i.e. a positive feedback mechanism. Block of this mechanism results in a reduction of mobilization and hence a reduction in transmitter release, leading to a fading muscle response.

Another pharmacological mechanism that has been widely studied at the neuromuscular junction over the past 15 years is the phenomenon of ion channel block (see Colquhoun 1981, 1986; Lambert *et al.* 1983 for reviews). This occurs when drugs, generally carrying a positive charge and present in high concentrations in the extracelluar fluid, are driven into the endplate ion channel that has been opened as a result of the interaction of transmitter acetylcholine with the receptor recognition site. As a result of the molecules entering the lumen of the opened channel, the inward flow of sodium ions is prevented. The result is that the current flow is shut down and transmission is reduced; this is particularly evident in the time course of the current flow. At ion channel level, the manifestation of the phenomenon is crucially dependent upon the rate of dissociation of the channel blocking drug from the channel.

The kinetics of action of drugs that block the open ion channel can be described by the following sequential model (Adams 1975):

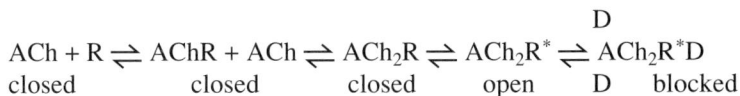

$$ACh + R \rightleftharpoons AChR + ACh \rightleftharpoons ACh_2R \rightleftharpoons ACh_2R^* \overset{D}{\underset{D}{\rightleftharpoons}} ACh_2R^*D$$

closed   closed   closed   open   blocked

If the dissociation of the drug (D) from the blocked receptor–channel complex is fast, then the channels will rapidly re-open, allowing the drug to block again, and so on (Neher and Steinbach 1978). This results in a longer, lesser, current flow than normal. If the dissociation rate is slow then the re-opening of the channels is so spread out in time that the secondary current flow is often indiscernible.

By its nature, channel block is non-competitive, i.e. increasing the concentration of acetylcholine will allow more channels to open, giving the drug more opportunity to block. Despite the fact that there are many published examples of non-characterized anticholinesterase-irreversible block in animals and humans being attributed to channel block, there is no definitive evidence that this phenomenon, although demonstrable *in vitro*, is relevant *in vivo*.

Structure–activity relationships in channel block

Open endplate ion channel block was first demonstrated with barbiturate (Adams 1976) and quaternary local anaesthetic drugs (Steinbach 1976). Subsequently, a wide range of chemically dissimilar compounds has been shown to include this property. Such compounds include volatile general anaesthetics, alcohols, atropine-like compounds, phencyclidine analogues, antidysrhythmic drugs, lincosamide, aminoglycoside, polymyxin and chloramphenicol-type antibiotics, and quaternary neuromuscular blocking agents, including tubocurarine, gallamine, and pancuronium analogues (see Colquhoun 1981, 1986; Lambert *et al.* 1983 for reviews).

Few structure–activity relationship studies have been performed, but the compounds that have been examined fall into two distinct groups that can be related to structure (Colquhoun 1981). The first group are the so-called voltage-dependent drugs; the kinetics of these compounds, and hence their affinity, are highly dependent upon the membrane potential of the endplate. These compounds carry a strong positive charge; most of them are quaternary salts. Thus, at hyperpolarized membrane potentials there is a strong electrical force driving the positively charged moiety towards the negatively charged inner side of the membrane, once the channel is opened. In contrast, the non-voltage-dependent drugs carry less positive charge.

Both voltage-dependent and non-voltage-dependent channel blocking drugs can vary in their rates of dissociation from the receptor–channel complex. Thus, both types can produce the secondary current tail described earlier, as a result of rapid dissociation and channel re-opening. However, in general, the quaternary, voltage-dependent channel blockers possess a blocking association rate of around an order of magnitude greater than the non-voltage dependent drugs. Given that both groups have variable dissociation rates, the affinity of the voltage-dependent group is, in general, greater.

One factor that seems to play a part in determining the dissociation rate is lipid solubility. Thus, in a study of lincosamide analogues, clindamycin, which is highly lipid soluble, possessed a much slower dissociation rate than that of lincomycin, which is less lipid soluble, and hence possesses a greater affinity for the channel binding site (Prior *et al.* 1990).

Channel block differs from receptor block in one very obvious characteristic, namely that whilst receptor block, and receptor interactions generally, are highly stereospecific, studies on several different chemical examples of channel blocking drugs, including perhydrohistrionicotoxin, disopyramide, lincosamide, and chloramphenicol-type antibiotics have illustrated that channel block is almost entirely non-stereospecific.

Other effects of neuromuscular blocking drugs

Neuromuscular blocking drugs have traditionally been synthesized to block post-junctional nicotinic-type acetylcholine receptors at the skeletal muscle neuromuscular junction. However, acetylcholine receptors are present at other synapses in the body and actions at these other synapses are responsible for the major side-effects of the muscle relaxant drugs (for reviews see Paton 1959; Marshall 1980; Bowman 1982). For example, nicotinic receptors are present at autonomic ganglia. As the cardiovascular system is normally under sympathetic tone, any blockade of the excitatory ganglionic nicotinic receptors will result in a fall in arterial blood pressure. Such an effect is seen with tubocurarine, in addition to its well-known histamine-releasing properties, which also result in hypotension. Another rather more curious action of quaternary muscle relaxants is at the muscarinic receptor of the sino-atrial node. Blockade of this muscarinic receptor results in a selective atropine-like action on the heart leading to tachycardia. Such an action is exemplified by gallamine which is now better known to many young researchers as an antagonist of a muscarinic receptor subtype than as a neuromuscular blocking drug.

Clearly, any programme aimed at the rational design of new muscle relaxants must take such side-effects into account and efforts made to understand the structure–activity relationships pertaining to the unwanted effects.

The binding of neuromuscular blocking agents to postjunctional acetylcholine receptors

The binding of an agonist to its receptor has some similarities with the binding of a substrate to an enzyme. Studies of enzymes at the molecular level have progressed rapidly in recent years, so that many aspects of small molecule/protein interactions are better understood than previously: it is becoming feasible with a number of well-studied enzymes to design inhibitors to fit their binding pockets from *a priori* considerations of shape and charge distribution, without substrate mimicry. The design of enzyme inhibitors in this fashion is technically very demanding, in that the conformation of the enzyme has to be fully characterized, either by X-ray crystallography or preferably in solution by nuclear magnetic resonance (NMR) spectroscopy. There is a practical limit on the size of enzyme receptor which can be fully characterized in this way — perhaps 20 kDa for NMR studies, and the enzyme has to be available in pure form in relatively large quantities. The nicotinic acetylcholine receptor satisfies none of these criteria. It is too large, by an order of magnitude, for NMR studies. It is not available in large quantities, it is difficult to purify, but above all it requires location in a lipid bilayer for its channel-like activity to function. The isolated 'receptor' therefore provides us with little functional information.

This observation is also true for membrane-dependent enzymes, whose function is catalysis of chemical reactions. Here enzyme function is a strictly passive process in which the substrate binds, not too strongly, then proceeds to a transition state which is strongly bound and after bond-making or bond-breaking releases the product(s) which are weakly bound. The nicotinic receptor binds acetylcholine, after which the channel opens. It is not sufficient therefore, to describe binding of acetylcholine to the nicotinic receptor as if it were an enzyme–substrate interaction, since after binding to the receptor, acetylcholine (the substrate) is released unchanged. When acetylcholine is bound the movement of cations is triggered, and the kinetics of channel opening and closing can be studied using single channel recording (patch clamp) techniques.

An extension of this approach to functional studies of the nicotinic receptor uses the techniques of genetic engineering (White 1985). Most of the information in the following section follows from the cloning and expression of nicotinic receptor proteins in cells, specifically *Xenopus* oocytes, which themselves do not produce such receptors (Mishina *et al.* 1986). It should be borne in mind that the *Xenopus* cells are being required to synthesize foreign proteins and process the products, particularly by glycosylation, into a form suitable for assembly into a functional complex. Without correct glycosylation the receptor will not form (Merlie *et al.* 1982). The receptor which apparently forms in *Xenopus* oocytes is therefore a composite of exogenous proteins and endogenous polysaccharides: the mechanism of assembly at the molecular level is a matter of surmise.

STRUCTURE OF THE NICOTINIC ACETYLCHOLINE RECEPTOR

Much of the work on nicotinic receptor constituents has been carried out for practical reasons on the receptors of the electric organ of the fish *Torpedo marmorata*, in which the electric organ is a bank of nicotinic cholinergic synapses. Recent work has shown that there is a high degree of homology between amino acid sequences in mammalian receptors and those of the electric fish (Takai *et al.* 1985; Mishina *et al.* 1986).

There is a consensus of opinion that the receptor consists of five glycosylated protein subunits, two of which (called alpha) are the same and have molecular weight of approximately 40 kDa. The other three units are designated beta (49 kDa), gamma (60 kDa), and delta (67 kDa) for the electric eel, and beta, delta, and epsilon for the mammalian (calf) receptor (Mishina *et al.* 1986). The epsilon subunit possibly has a similar function to the delta subunit of the electric eel receptor, but has only 53% amino acid homology, with more acidic and fewer basic amino acids. In *Torpedo* the receptors are linked in pairs via the delta subunit by

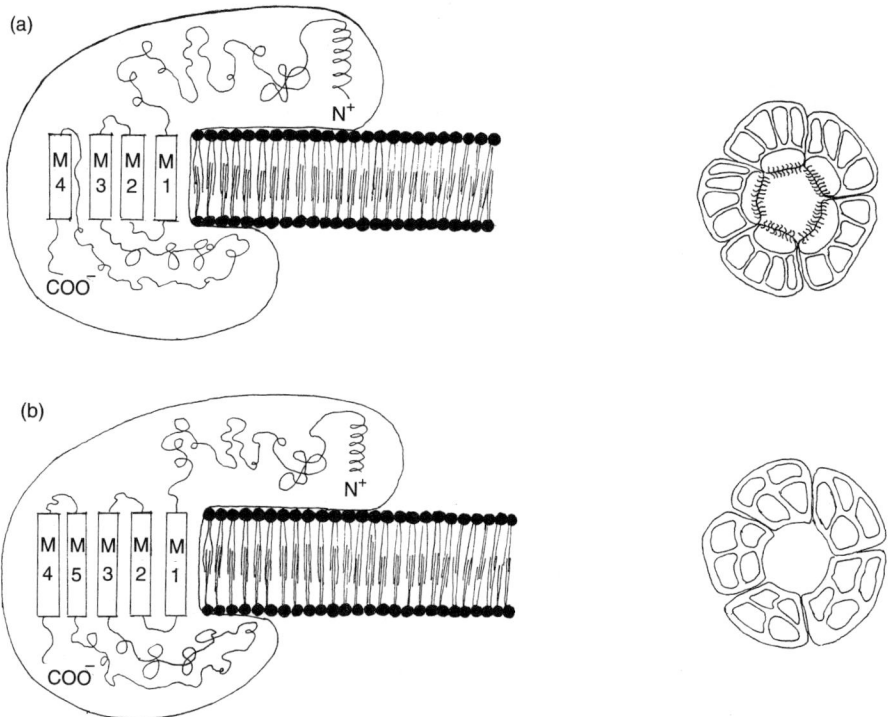

Fig. 3.1 Cross-sections through a nicotinic receptor as proposed by two different groups (see text), without (a) and with (b) the amphiphilic section of peptide embedded in the membrane. In each case the left side is a representation of one peptide, and the right side is a top view of the assembled receptor. In (b), the channel is lined by a hydrophilic surface.

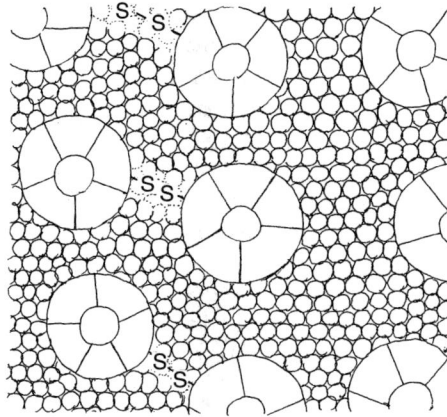

Fig. 3.2 Acetylcholine receptors embedded in the membrane of the mammalian postjunctional motor endplate, linked by disulphide bonds.

disulphide (-S-S-) bonds. It is not yet known whether this is also true for the calf receptors.

Each of the five subunits has alternating hydrophilic and hydrophobic regions. It is hypothesized that the latter are embedded in the cell membrane, in close contact with the lipid bilayer. There are four regions in each chain, designated M1–M4, with the typical amino acids of hydrophobic (alpha) helices. There is at present no clear consensus of opinion as to whether the hydrophobic regions themselves constitute the channel lining (Maelicke 1990) or whether a fifth segment, termed M5, performs an amphiphilic traverse of the membrane (Stevens 1985; Guy and Hucho 1987) (Fig. 3.1).

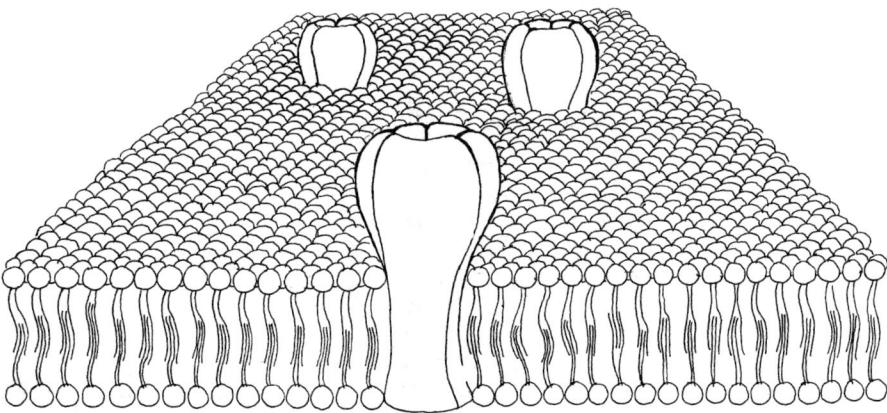

Fig. 3.3 Three-dimensional representation of the assembled nicotinic acetylcholine receptor. The external portion is both peptide and polysaccharide.

When all five subunits come together, the five M5 segments together may form a hydrophilic pore. For the *Torpedo* receptor this can be depicted as in Fig. 3.2, in which the pores are linked in pairs by disulphide bonds.

The hydrophilic parts of all five subunits are substantial, both between the 'M' regions and at the ends of the polypeptide chains, and include the glycosylated regions which contribute in no small measure to the bulk of the extracelluar part of the receptor. Based on an assessment of relative molecular dimensions it is possible to construct a supramolecular picture of the nicotinic receptor (Fig. 3.3).

When viewing such hypothetical diagrams it is easy to forget that we are describing structures at the molecular level and that molecules are subject to continuous thermal agitation. Even in crystallized proteins there are often surprisingly large translational motions (i.e. quite large sections change position fairly frequently), and there will be far more flexibility of movement of the molecules depicted in Fig. 3.3 than is conveyed by the diagram. We should not let artistic impressions lead us to an intuitive impression of the receptor as being a solid structure.

Protein conformation: binding of acetylcholine to the postjunctional receptor

An indirect way of deducing information about the structure of a receptor is to examine the effects of structural modification on agonist and antagonist activity. We can anticipate complementarity of structure, to some extent, so that for example a positive charge on the drug will be met by a negative charge on the receptor. Since all known agonists and antagonists at the neuromuscular junction are positively charged, it is highly likely that the specific area for binding bears at least one negative charge. This was originally guessed to be an array of phosphate groups (Cavallito 1967) but the information on protein structure described above does not encourage such a view. Although phosphate residues cannot be ruled out entirely, it seems more likely that the negative charge comes from an ionized acidic amino acid side chain, such as aspartate or glutamate.

It has been proposed that the binding site for acetylcholine is in a loop of the alpha subunit (Noda *et al.* 1982), with the requisite negative charge supplied by an aspartate residue (Fig. 3.4). The main problem with such a proposal is a lack of consequence. While acetylcholine may bind in such a pocket, there is no obvious reason why anything should happen as a result. It is possible that changes in conformation may occur as a result of changes in water structure; the solvent plays a vital role in maintaining protein tertiary and quaternary structure. A more obvious cause of conformational change in the receptor, leading eventually to membrane depolarization, would arise if acetylcholine disrupted a salt bridge between an acidic and a basic amino acid on different parts of the chain (Fig. 3.5), which might stimulate a major reversible change in conformation.

As our understanding of the forces governing protein conformation improves, it may be possible to make better predictions concerning the three-dimensional struc-

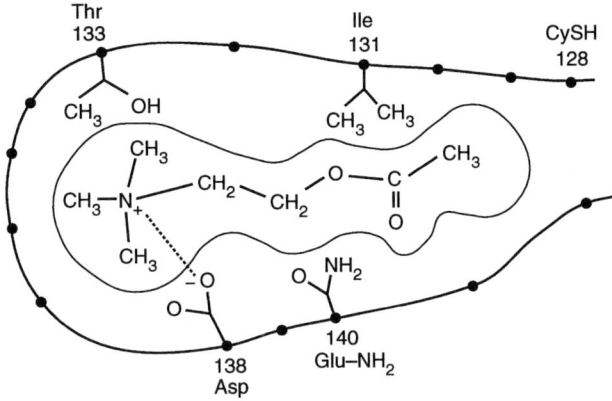

Fig. 3.4 Postulated binding pocket for acetylcholine in the alpha subunit of a postjunctional acetylcholine receptor.

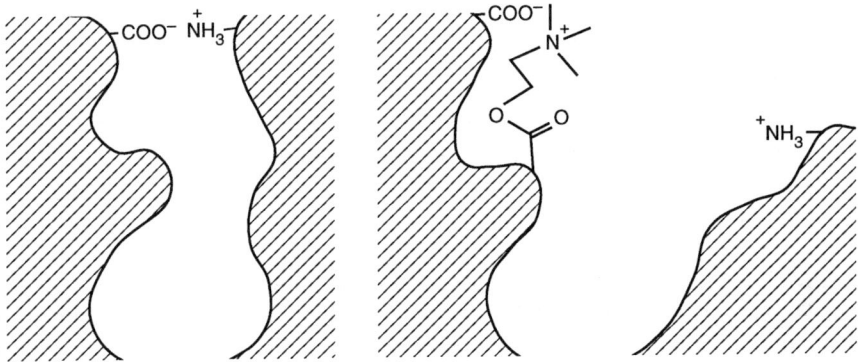

Fig. 3.5 Disruption of a hypothetical salt bridge leading to a major conformational change on binding of a molecule of acetylcholine to the postjunctional receptor.

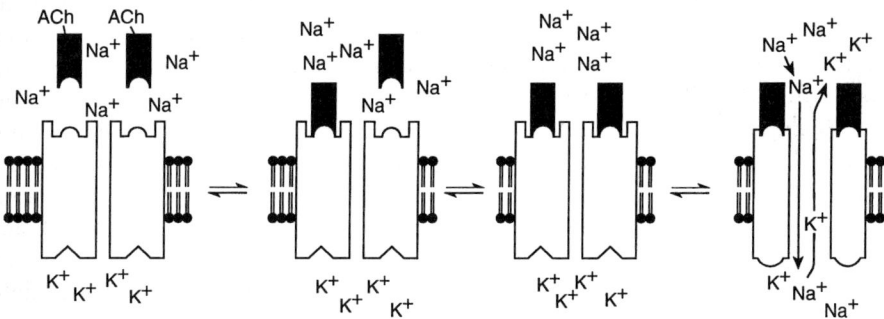

Fig. 3.6 Cooperative binding of two molecules of acetylcholine with endplate receptors leading to opening of the ion channel.

ture of the nicotinic receptor from a knowledge of amino acid sequence, not forgetting the effects of glycosylation and the proximity of the membrane. Until then we are restricted to a macroscopic picture of events which may be summarized as in Fig. 3.6.

BLOCKING AGENTS: SKELETAL MUSCLE RELAXANTS OF CLINICAL VALUE

Although there is no direct evidence, it seems highly likely that the binding site for acetylcholine bears a negative charge as a major feature. The two ways to block the action of acetylcholine at the neuromuscular junction are to occupy the binding site, either by an agent which does not effect depolarization but prevents the access of acetylcholine (an antagonist), or to cause prolonged depolarization which renders the receptor mechanism insensitive (an agonist). In either case, we would expect the blocking agent to possess a positive charge with affinity for the complementary negative charge on the acetylcholine receptor, and it is a fact that all clinically useful neuromuscular blocking agents bear positively charged nitrogens. It is less obvious why there should be a general requirement for two positive charges for a blocking agent to have high potency. We shall deal with the general structural requirements for potency first, in the context of the work on receptor structure described previously, and then the structural differences which confer depolarizing or nondepolarizing activity.

Bis-onium character and inter-onium distance

If we consider a generalized neuromuscular blocking agent, we can represent the structure as in Fig. 3.7.

It is broadly possible, comparing closely related structures only, to make the observation that if none of R^1–R^6 is H, one may achieve maximum potency in any given series. If one of R^1–R^6 is H, potency may be sufficiently high for the compound to be clinically useful; but if one of R^1–R^3 is H and one of R^4–R^6 is H, potency is likely to be very low. A probable explanation lies in the distribution of these compounds after intravenous injection.

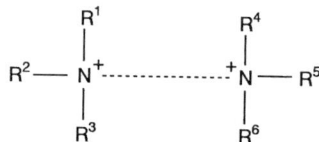

Fig. 3.7 Generalized structure of clinically useful neuromuscular blocking agents. For R^1–R^6, see specific structures.

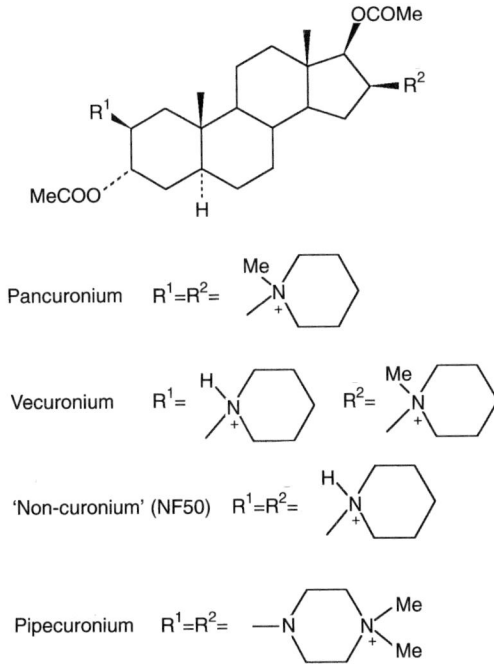

Fig. 3.8 Chemical structures of aminosteroid neuromuscular blocking drugs.

For argument's sake, let us take two clinically useful blocking agents, pancuronium and vecuronium, and one which is closely related (NF50) but has little activity, which we shall call non-curonium (Fig. 3.8).

At first sight there is little to choose between these three compounds. At physiological pH, all three will possess two positive charges, capable of bonding to a negatively charged receptor, and the remainder of the molecule is identical in each case, so the receptor must be able to accommodate all three structures with considerable affinity. However, the third compound, which is inactive (Savage 1980), has the ability to lose its charges completely when the situation demands.

It is normally difficult if not impossible for ionic compounds to pass through lipid barriers: non-curonium, however, can become detached from the two protons attached to nitrogen, becoming highly lipophilic in so doing. After diffusion through the barrier it can resume protonation (Fig. 3.9).

In this way, non-curonium is able to penetrate to any part of an intact animal, achieving a large volume of distribution. Pancuronium, in contrast, has two immutable positive charges and vecuronium has one, which will largely prevent access to most body tissues, retaining the material in blood and lymph. The only barrier which is required to be penetrated to achieve neuromuscular block is that presented by the walls of peripheral blood capillaries, which are leaky enough to allow rapid access to the neuromuscular junction.

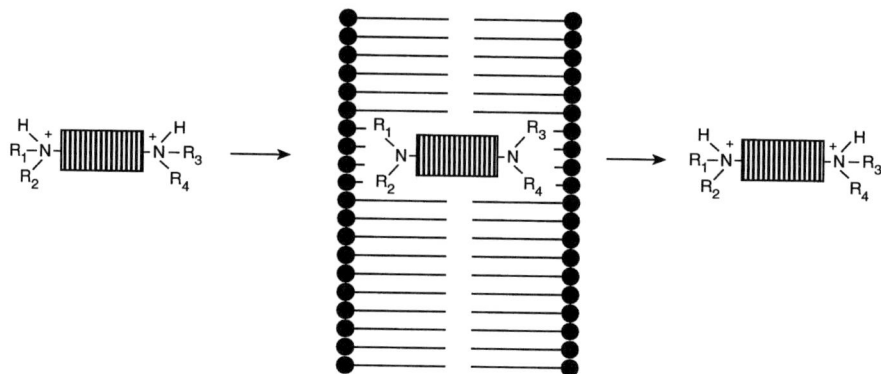

Fig. 3.9 Diffusion of a compound with two basic centres through a non-aqueous membrane. This process is governed by the relative free energies of protonated and non-protonated forms in the two environments and does not require selection of non-protonated material from the first (aqueous) compartment as implied by many authors.

In homologous series of compounds it appears that compounds with greater lipid solubility have a tendency to possess faster onset of action than do those of lower lipid solubility. This may be due to the ability of higher lipid soluble compounds to penetrate the Schwann cell enveloping the endplate region, and the basement membrane lying between the pre- and postjunctional elements, which pose a potential barrier.

So far we have explained why at least one quaternary nitrogen is necessary to achieve high potency, by confining the drug within a very restricted volume of distribution. It is less easy to explain why the possession of two positive charges should be significant. For many years it was assumed that the receptor possessed two negative charges (Stenlake 1963), a given distance apart: if this were the case then a drug which could fit both would gain enormously in binding affinity. The finding that there are two acetylcholine binding sites on each receptor acting cooperatively (see above) invites the conclusion that bis-onium compounds bind to both simultaneously. Unfortunately, the channel structure described above, with a pore sufficient to allow the passage of hydrated sodium ions after depolarization, suggests that the distance between the two acetylcholine receptors is too large to permit simultaneous binding by one neuromuscular blocking molecule. Even so, it should be remembered that the very large molecules which form the receptor are likely to be flexible and to a certain extent mobile; thus, we cannot rule out simultaneous binding altogether.

Such evidence as there is suggests that the role of the second 'onium' group may be on overall physicochemical properties rather than directly on receptor binding. Taking the series of compounds in Fig. 3.10, which differ only in the number of methylenes in the central chain, it is seen that potency varies in an apparently parabolic manner in cats as the chain is lengthened (Stenlake *et al.* 1981).

This is strongly reminiscent of many series of drugs which have been studied in detail by Hansch and co-workers (Hansch and Leo 1979), where physicochemical parameters, particularly hydrophobicity, play an important role. The data in Fig. 3.10 do not suggest that the receptor possesses two negative charges with a

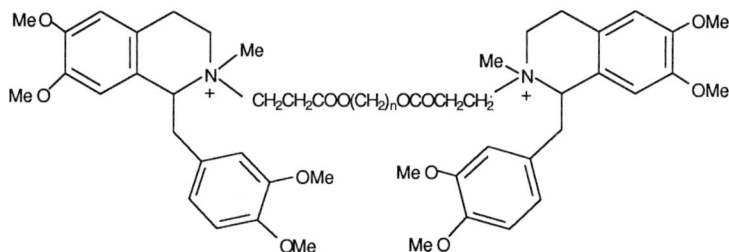

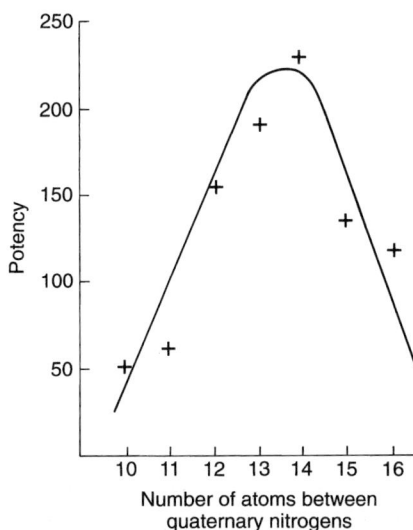

Fig. 3.10 Variation of neuromuscular blocking potency in cats (tubocurarine = 100) with number of atoms connecting the quaternary nitrogens in a series of homologues related to atracurium (in atracurium $n = 5$ and therefore 13 atoms connect the nitrogens).

preferred distance between them. Furthermore the inter-onium distance can be measured accurately from X-ray crystallographic data for the more rigid neuromuscular blocking agents and varies between 7.48 Å (Pointer *et al.* 1972) and 21 Å (Savarese and Kitz 1975). However, the clinically useful drugs represented in Fig. 3.8, 3.11, and 3.13 tend to have inter-onium distances of 9–11.5 Å, in those cases where there is sufficient rigidity for the distance to be accurately measured.

Examining these structures, it has to be said that these few preferred agents were arrived at in a largely empirical manner. Tubocurarine is the natural compound which stimulated much of the work on surgical muscle relaxants following its isolation and structural elucidation (King 1935), even though there was a small error in the structure assigned (Everett *et al.* 1970). Metocurine (Collier *et al.* 1948) is a simple methylated derivative of tubocurarine. The work on atracurium (Stenlake *et al.* 1981; Hughes 1985, 1986) adopted the benzylisoquinoline 'end-groups' from

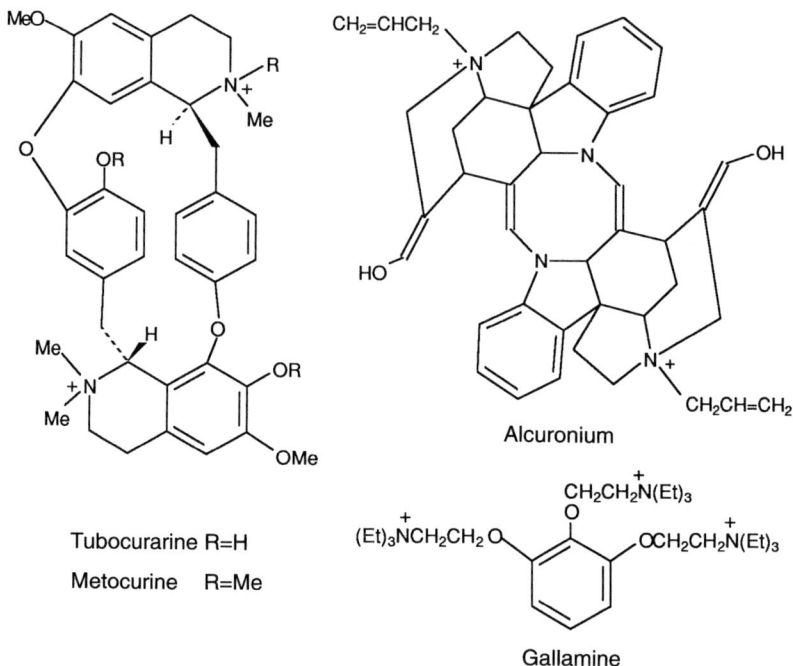

Fig. 3.11 Structures of some clinically useful neuromuscular blocking agents. Other structures are given in Figures 3.8, 3.12 and 3.13.

laudexium (Taylor and Collier 1951) which was itself based on tubocurarine. The design aspect of atracurium which was not empirical centred on its breakdown *in vivo*, rather than receptor fit. Alcuronium (Waser and Harbeck 1962) was the result of a minor modification to another natural compound, toxiferine 1. Gallamine triethiodide (Bovet *et al.* 1947) was synthesized following the empirical observation that ethyl, rather than methyl, *N*-substituents favoured the preferred nondepolarizing form of block (see below). Steroidal neuromuscular blocking agents such as pancuronium, pipecuronium, and vecuronium followed on from the original observation of the neuromuscular blocking action of malouétine (Quevauvillier and Lainé 1960), a naturally occurring steroid, and the suggestion that a rigid supporting moiety such as the steroid nucleus would allow accurate measurement of inter-onium distance, at a time when this was thought to be important. There was an attempt to mimic the structure of acetylcholine in the disposition of the acetate groups and quaternary centres around the nucleus in pancuronium (Buckett *et al.* 1973), but the subsequent development of vecuronium (Baird and Savage 1985) and pipecuronium (Biro *et al.* 1985) has progressed away from mimicry in an empirical manner.

Despite the empiricism inherent in the conception of drugs of this type they have evolved into very precise pharmacological agents: the better ones are very selective for the chosen receptor, with minimal side-effects and acceptable duration of action. However, there remains a need for an ultra short-acting nondepolarizing agent to replace succinylcholine (suxamethonium).

Structural requirements for depolarizing versus nondepolarizing blockade

Work in the 1940s showed that depolarization of the muscle endplate via acetylcholine receptors is very sensitive to the size of the nitrogen substituents, and also to the bulk of the inter-onium supporting structure. To achieve full potency as a depolarizing agent three methyl groups are usually best (Barlow and Ing 1948; Paton and Zaimis 1949), as with acetylcholine itself. The classic depolarizing drugs are decamethonium and suxamethonium, neither of which is broken down by the enzyme responsible for degradation of acetylcholine in the region of the muscle endplate, acetylcholinesterase. As the name implies, this enzyme is highly specific for the natural substrate. The depolarization produced by decamethonium or suxamethonium is thus prolonged and results in cessation of normal activity. Suxamethonium is readily hydrolysed in normal patients by plasma pseudocholinesterase (Fig. 3.12) and therefore has a much shorter duration of action than decamethonium. Problems arise where the patient is genetically deficient in the normal pseudocholinesterase, but despite this drawback suxamethonium is still widely used where rapid onset of relaxation is required, with short duration.

Any increase in size of the nitrogen substituents leads to a decrease in depolarizing activity and generally some decrease in potency, although this can be largely recovered by empirical modification of the 'end groups' as described in the previous section for atracurium, or by provision of a bulky hydrophobic central structure as in, for example, pancuronium. It is probable that these various agents act at the same part of the receptor, but that the nondepolarizing agents are unable to bring about the conformational change in the proteins which leads to opening of the ion channel. From a clinical point of view lack of depolarizing activity in a neuromuscular blocking agent is a positive advantage, since the muscle fasciculation which follows depolarization by suxamethonium may lead to post-operative muscle pain. In contrast to depolarization block, simple nondepolarizing competitive block is

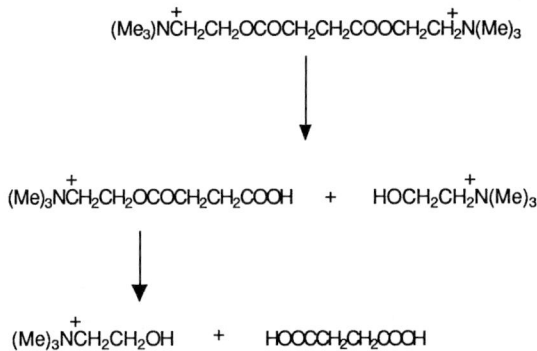

$$(Me_3)\overset{+}{N}CH_2CH_2OCOCH_2CH_2COOCH_2C\overset{+}{H}_2N(Me)_3$$

$$\downarrow$$

$$(Me)_3\overset{+}{N}CH_2CH_2OCOCH_2CH_2COOH \quad + \quad HOCH_2CH_2\overset{+}{N}(Me)_3$$

$$\downarrow$$

$$(Me)_3\overset{+}{N}CH_2CH_2OH \quad + \quad HOOCCH_2CH_2COOH$$

Fig. 3.12 Hydrolysis of suxamethonium by plasma pseudocholinesterase. The first hydrolytic step is sufficient to terminate the effect.

easily reversed, specifically by increasing the acetylcholine concentration with an esterase inhibitor. Such 'antidotes' must be use with care, since the half-life of the anticholinesterase may be shorter than that of the blocking agent, especially if one of the longer-acting drugs is used: paralysis may therefore return. The duration of block is thus of particular importance in the selection of the reversal agent.

METABOLISM OF NEUROMUSCULAR BLOCKING AGENTS IN CURRENT WIDESPREAD USE

These are listed in alphabetical order. All except suxamethonium are non-depolarizing. The approximate duration of action is given for 25% recovery from 98% block.

Alcuronium

Alcuronium is mostly excreted unchanged in urine (Raaflaub and Frey 1972) with a little in the bile which, alcuronium being a quaternary salt, is not then re-absorbed from the gastrointestinal tract. About 75% of a dose of alcuronium is bound to plasma albumin. The lack of metabolism means that alcuronium has a relatively long duration of action, at about 80 minutes.

Atracurium

Atracurium is designed to break down by a mechanism which depends only on pH, catalysed by OH^- ions (Stenlake *et al*. 1981) (Fig. 3.12). Atracurium is unique among neuromuscular blocking agents in requiring neither kidney nor liver function for its removal. Hydrolysis contributes to the decomposition, but the chemical reaction called Hofmann elimination accounts for most of the breakdown. Both elimination and hydrolysis lead to the formation of monoquaternary salts, which have very little pharmacological action. Laudanosine, an alkaloid present in opium, is formed as a product of elimination but also has very little biological activity. The other products are acrylates, which probably react quickly with glutathione, as the physiologically most abundant thiol, to give biologically inert metabolites. As a result of the reactions described in Fig. 3.13, a dose of atracurium lasts for about 20 minutes, and there is no cumulation with repeated doses even where kidney and liver function are compromised. About 80% is bound to plasma proteins.

Metocurine

Little of an injected dose of metocurine is metabolized, most appearing in the urine (Meijer *et al*. 1979), so that again the duration of action is not short, at about 80 minutes.

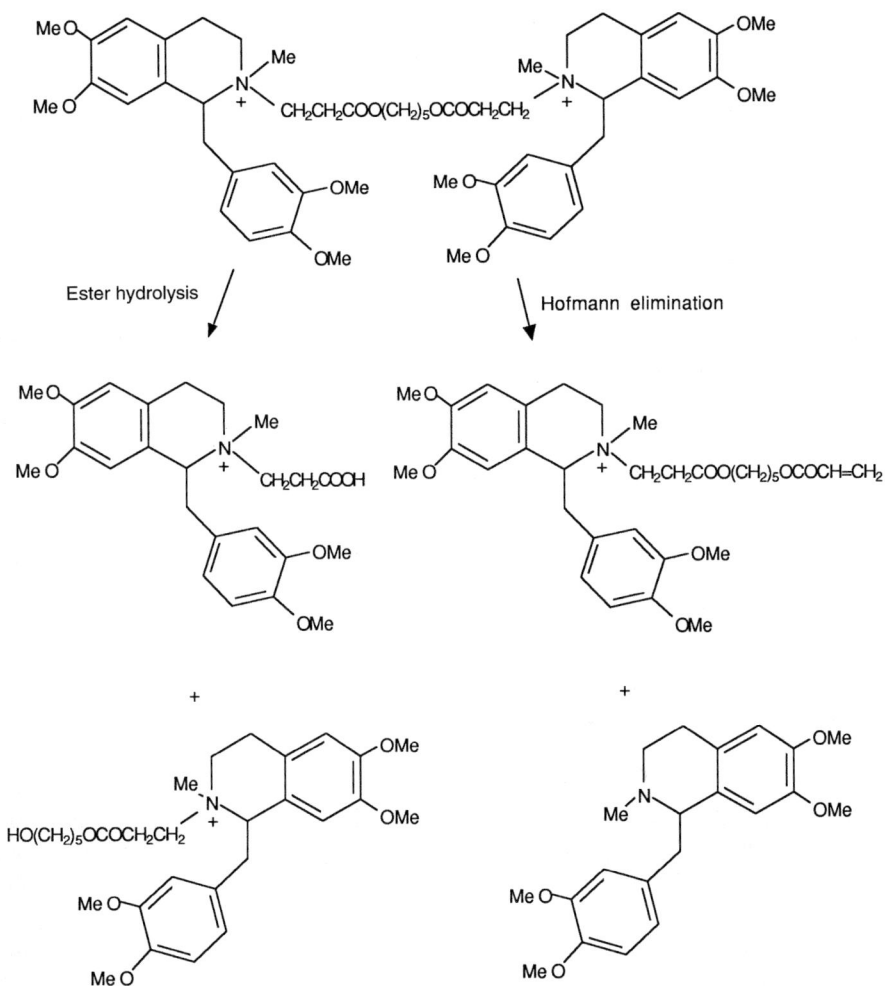

Fig. 3.13 *In vivo* degradation of atracurium by both Hofmann elimination, which is not enzyme-dependent, and esterases. Provided that pH is maintained at normal physiological values, Hofmann elimination will occur at a predictable rate. The drug is therefore unique in having no dependence in kidney, liver or enzyme function for its destruction after a normal paralysing dose.

Pancuronium

Although there may be some hydrolytic removal of the 3-acetyl group (Fig. 3.14), the product of this hydrolysis is still a bis-quaternary salt and a potent muscle relaxant, with about 50% of the activity of the parent compound (Miller *et al.* 1978; Marshall *et al.* 1983). Other than this hydrolysis there is little metabolic change and 60–80% is excreted unchanged in urine (Agoston *et al.* 1973). There is a rapid

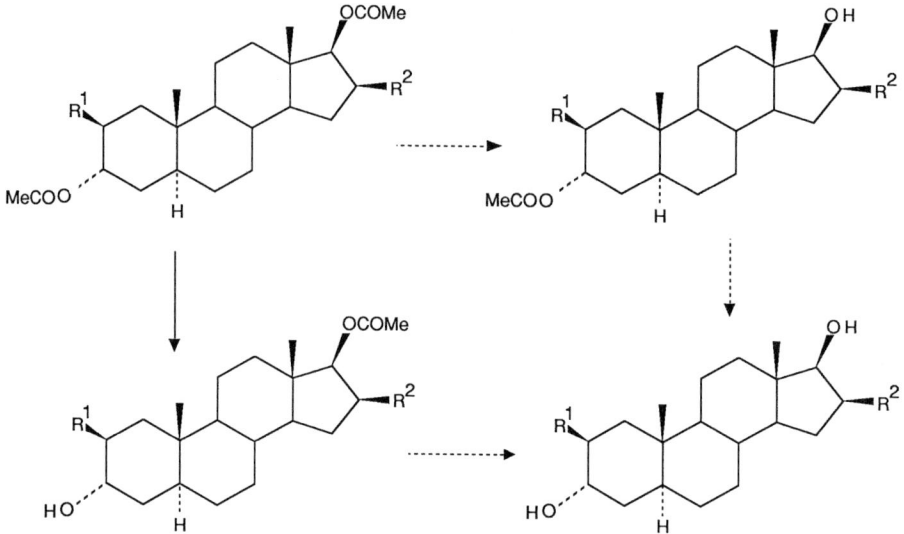

Fig. 3.14 Experimentally determined (→) and hypothetical (---->) degradation of aminosteroid neuromuscular blocking agents *in vivo*. Note that all of the hydrolysis products are bis-quaternary salts and therefore potentially muscle relaxants; it is not the hydrolysis *per se* which results in termination of action.

redistributive process in the first five minutes. As might be expected the duration of action is not short, at about 60 minutes.

Pipecuronium

Although pipecuronium may be hydrolysed, in a similar fashion to pancuronium (Fig. 3.14), the product is a bis-quaternary compound which is a potent muscle relaxant. Again, as expected, the result is a relatively long duration of action, at about two hours, with most eliminated via the kidneys.

Suxamethonium

As it is an excellent substrate for plasma pseudocholinesterase, most of a dose of suxamethonium is destroyed (Fig. 3.12) before it reaches the neuromuscular junction. Continued destruction ensures that the duration of action is only about 2–4 minutes in normal patients and that in these patients there is no cumulative effect. There are severe problems, of course, if the patient has abnormal or deficient pseudocholinesterase, since the dose which is given is then massively too large: in the worst case the block may last four hours or more. Various disease states may contribute to altered plasma enzyme levels, as well as genetically determined factors.

Tubocurarine

Again there are no obvious sites in the molecule for rapid metabolism, so the duration of action is about 80 minutes. Much of the dose is removed via the bile, with 30–40% excreted through the kidneys. Like gallamine and pancuronium the plasma concentration falls rapidly in the first few minutes by redistribution rather than destruction or excretion, so that there is the potential for cumulation with subsequent doses.

Vecuronium

Although there is no obvious reason for a shorter action than pancuronium, the reliable empirical observation is that the duration of action is about 20 minutes, i.e. comparable with that of atracurium. There is no obvious metabolic reason for loss of potency with time as the products of hydrolysis still have two positive charges (Fig. 3.14): the 3-OH derivative still has 60% of the potency of vecuronium. Elimination is mainly via the bile (Bencini *et al.* 1986) and repeated doses are only mildly cumulative. About 70% is bound to plasma proteins. Like tubocurarine, vecuronium is a monoquaternary compound, the other positively charged centre being a tertiary base which will be protonated at physiological pH.

NEW COMPOUNDS OF POTENTIAL CLINICAL INTEREST

Several new compounds are in advanced stage of clinical trial or have recently been marketed. Two of these compounds are of the bulky ester type. The bulky ester approach is an attempt to combine the suxamethonium-like lability of ester groupings with quaternary benzylisoquinolinium moieties. Mivacurium (Fig. 3.15) undergoes ester hydrolysis and is short-acting (recovery time mid-way between those of suxamethonium and atracurium), potent, and lacking in cardiovascular side effects (Ali *et al.* 1988). However, it is not as rapid in onset as is suxamethonium (Caldwell *et al.* 1989).

Doxacurium (Fig. 3.15) is a longer-acting compound, with duration of action in humans similar to that of tubocurarine (Murray *et al.* 1990). It appears not to be readily hydrolysed, despite the presence of two ester groups in the molecule.

Rocuronium (Org 9426) (Fig. 3.15) is a development from vecuronium, i.e. an aminosteroid with only the ring D nitrogen quaternized. Rocuronium was developed using the high potency and lack of side-effects of vecuronium as a template, introducing chemical changes to reduce neuromuscular blocking potency. The basis of this approach is that through reducing potency, i.e. increasing the dose, the rate of onset of the drug will be enhanced (Bowman *et al.* 1988). As long as this can be achieved without a marked increase in side-effects, it might produce an improved drug. Rocuronium has proven to be more rapid in onset than vecuronium in both experimental animals (Muir *et al.* 1989) and humans (Wierda *et al.* 1990).

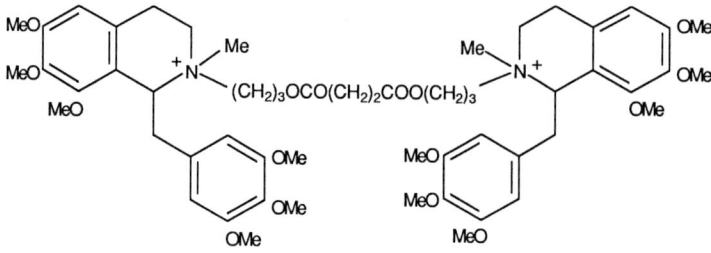

Doxacurium

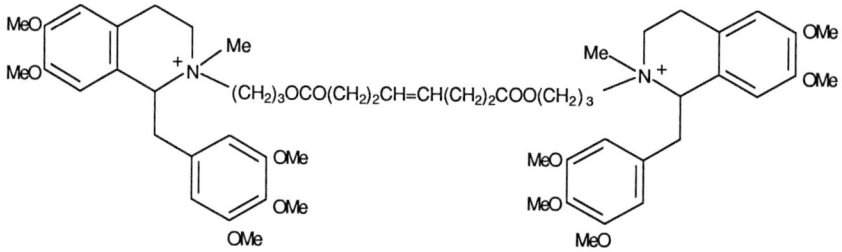

Mivacurium

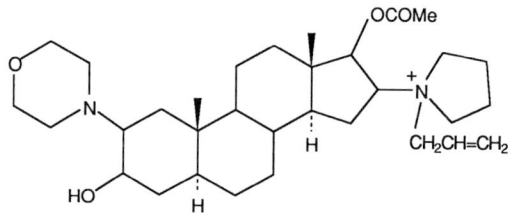

Org 9426 (rocuronium)

Fig. 3.15 Chemical structures of some newer neuromuscular blocking drugs.

FUTURE POSSIBILITIES

Ever since the first clinical use of tubocurarine by Griffith and Johnson (1942), fifty-two years ago, pharmacologists, medicinal chemists, and anaesthetists have been striving to achieve the 'gold standard' in muscle relaxants — a potent nondepolarizing agent with rapid onset and offset, and lacking cardiovascular side-effects. So far, efforts have been frustrated, despite the ease of prediction that a molecule carrying two nitrogens, with at least one a quaternary nitrogen, within a fairly wide range of inter-onium distances, will possess neuromuscular blocking activity. The fact that many thousands of compounds have been synthesized and tested in this quest stimulates the search for alternative approaches. One line is in the field of peptides, an area of great developmental activity in pharmacology at present. Ever since the discovery of the neuromuscular blocking activity of alpha-bungarotoxin (Chang and Lee 1963), a toxin derived from the venom of the elapid snake *Bungarus multicinctus*, it has been known that certain polypeptide toxins can block nicotinic receptors. Alpha-toxins from elapids are virtually irreversible in their antagonist action, and they have been widely used in the labelling and identification of receptors. However, because of their irre-versibility they have not been exploited as potential clinical muscle relaxants. It has, however, recently been shown that the alpha-neurotoxins from certain varieties of fish-eating snails of the *Conus* type possess reversible neuromuscular blocking activity (Hashimoto *et al.* 1985). *In vivo* these toxins have similar potency and time course to vecuronium and possess virtually no cardiovascular side-effects (Marshall and Harvey 1990). The alpha-conotoxins are very short chain polypeptides, containing 13–15 amino acid residues and are presumed to be substrates for circulating peptidases.

Amino acid variation in the molecules might increase susceptibility to the hydrolytic enzymes and represent a feasible approach to the development of new short-acting derivatives, perhaps with rapidity of onset comparable to that of suxamethonium.

ACKNOWLEDGEMENTS

The authors would like to acknowledge Professor W. C. Bowman, Dr E. Rowan and Dr J. Dempster for assistance with the literature searching and Dr T. Sleigh (Organon) for assistance with some of the chemical structures. The figures were skil-fully prepared by Mr A. J. Worsley. We thank Mrs E. Carruthers and Mrs J. Ronald for typing the manuscript.

REFERENCES

Adams, P. R. (1976). Drug blockade of open end-plate channels. *Journal of Physiology*, **260**, 532–52.

Adams, P. R. (1975). A model for the procaine endplate current. *Journal of Physiology*, **246**, 61–3P.

Agoston, S., Vermeer, G. A., Kersten, U. W., and Meijer, D. K. F. (1973). The fate of pan-curonium bromide in man. *Acta Anaesthesiologica Scandinavica*, **17**, 267–75.

Ali, H. H., Savarese, J. J. Embree, P. B., Basta, S. J., Stout, R. G., Bottros, L. H., and Weakly, J. N. (1988) Clinical pharmacology of mivacurium chloride (BW B1090U) infusion: com-parison with vecuronium and atracurium. *British Journal of Anaesthesia*, **61**, 541–6.

Baird, W. L. M. and Savage, D. S. (1985). Vecuronium — the first years. In *Clinics in anaes-thesiology*, Vol. 3, *Neuromuscular blockade* (ed. J. Norman), pp. 347–60. Saunders, London.

Barlow, R. B. and Ing, H. R. (1948). Curare-like action of polymethylene bis-quaternary ammonium salts. *British Journal of Pharmacology and Chemotherapy*, **3**, 298–304.

Bencini, A. F., Scaf, A. H. J., Sohn, Y. J., Kersten-Kleet, U. W., and Agoston, S. (1986). Hepatobiliary disposition of vecuronium bromide in man. *British Journal of Anaesthesia*, **58**, 988–95.

Biro, K., Karpati, E., and Szporny, L. (1986) Bisquaternary steroid derivatives. In *Neuromuscular blocking agents*, (ed. D. A. Kharkevich), *Handbook of experimental pharmacology*, Vol. 79, pp. 401–17. Springer-Verlag, Berlin.

Bovet, D., Depierre, F., and deLestrange, Y. (1947) Propriétés curarisantes des ethers phenoliques a fonctions ammonium quaternaires. *Comptes rendus hebdomadaires des seances de l'Academie des Sciences*, **225**, 74–76.

Bowman, W. C. (1980). Prejunctional and postjunctional cholinoreceptors at the neuromuscular junction. *Anesthesia and Analgesia*, **59**, 935–43.

Bowman, W. C. (1982). Non-relaxant properties of neuromuscular blocking drugs. *British Journal of Anaesthesia*, **54**, 147–60.

Bowman, W. C. (1990). *Pharmacology of neuromuscular function*. Wright, Bristol.

Bowman, W. C., Gibb, A. J., Harvey, A. L., and Marshall, I. G. (1976) Prejunctional actions of cholinoceptor agonists and antagonists, and of anticholinesterase drugs. In *New neuromuscular blocking agents* (ed. D. A. Kharkevich), pp. 141–70, *Handbook of experimental pharmacology*, Vol. 79. Springer-Verlag, Berlin.

Bowman, W. C., Rodger, I. W., Houston, J., Marshall, R. J., and McIndewar, L. I. (1988) Structure: action relationships among some desacetoxy analogues of pancuronium and vecuronium in the anaesthetized cat. *Anesthesiology*, **69**, 57–62.

Buckett, W. R., Hewett, C. L., and Savage, D. S. (1973) Pancuronium bromide and other steroidal neuromuscular blocking agents containing acetylcholine fragments. *Journal of Medicinal Chemistry*, **16**, 1116–24.

Caldwell, J. E., Heier, T., Kitts, J. B., Lynane, D. P., Fahey, M. R. and Miller, R. D. (1989) Comparison of the neuromuscular block induced by mivacurium, suxamethonium or atracurium during nitrous oxide-fentanyl anaesthesia. *British Journal of Anaesthesia*, **63**, 393–99.

Cavallito, C. J. (1967). Bonding characteristics of acetylcholine simulants and antagonists and cholinergic receptors. *Annals of the New York Academy of Sciences*, **144**, 900–12.

Chang, C. C. and Lee, C. Y. (1963) Isolation of neurotoxins from the venom of Bungarus multicinctus and their modes of neuromuscular blocking action. *Archives internationales de pharmacodynamie et de therapie*, **144**, 241–57.

Collier, H. O. J., Paris, S. K., and Woolf, L. T. (1948) Pharmacological activity in different rodent species of *d*-tubocurarine chloride and the dimethyl ether of *d*-tubocurarine iodide. *Nature*, **161**, 817–9.

Colquhoun, D. (1981). The kinetics of conductance changes at nicotinic receptors of the muscle end-plate and of ganglia. In *Drug receptors and their effectors* (ed. N. J. M. Birdsall), pp. 107–27. Macmillan, London.

Colquhoun, D. (1986) On the principles of postsynaptic action of neuromuscular blocking agents. In *New neuromuscular blocking agents* (ed. D. A. Kharkevich), *Handbook of experimental pharmacology*, Vol 79, pp. 59–113. Springer-Verlag, Berlin.

de Camilli, P. and Greengard, P. (1986) Synapsin 1: a synaptic vesicle-associated neuronal phosphoprotein. *Biochemical Pharmacology*, **35**, 4349–57.

del Castillo, J. and Katz, B. (1954) Quantal components of the endplate potential. *Journal of Physiology*, **124**, 560–573.

Everett, A. J., Lowe, L. A., and Wilkinson, S. (1970) Revision of the structures of tubocurarine chloride and (+)-chondrocurine. *Journal of the Chemical Society, Chemical Communications*, 1020–1.

Fatt, P. and Katz, B. (1951) An analysis of the endplate potential recorded with an intracellular electrode. *Journal of Physiology*, **115**, 320–70.

Glavinović, M. I. and Narahashi, T. (1988) Depression, recovery and facilitation of neuromuscular transmission during prolonged tetanic stimulation. *Neuroscience*, **25**, 271–81.

Griffith, H. R. and Johnson, G. E. (1942) The use of curare in general anaesthesia. *Anesthesiology*, **3**, 418–20.

Guy, H. R. and Hucho, F. (1987) The ion channel of the nicotinic acetylcholine receptor. *Trends in Neurosciences*, **10**, 318–21.

Hansch, C. and Leo, A. (1979) *Substituent constants for correlation analysis in chemistry and biology*. Wiley-Interscience, New York.

Hashimoto, K., Uchida, S., Yoshida, H., Nishiuchi, Y., Sakakibara, S., and Yukari, K. (1985) Structure–activity relations of conotoxins at the neuromuscular junction. *European Journal of Pharmacology*, **118**, 351–54.

Hughes, R. (1985) Atracurium — the first years. In *Neuromuscular blockade clinics in anaesthesiology*, Vol. 3 (ed. J. Norman), pp. 331–45. Saunders, London.

Hughes, R. (1986) Atracurium. In *New neuromuscular blocking agents* (ed. D. A. Kharkevich), *Handbook of experimental pharmacology*, Vol. 79, pp. 529–543. Springer-Verlag, Berlin.

King, H. (1935) Curare alkaloids, Part 1, Tubocurarine. *Journal of the Chemical Society*, **2**, 1381–9.

Lambert, J. J., Durant, N. N., and Henderson, E. G. (1983) Drug-induced modification of ionic conductance at the neuromuscular junction. *Annual Reviews of Pharmacology and Toxicology*, **23**, 505–39.

Maelicke, A. (1990) The nicotinic acetylcholine receptor. In *Monographs in anesthesiology – Muscle relaxants*, (ed. S. Agoston and W. C. Bowman), pp. 19–58. Elsevier, Amsterdam.

Marshall, I. G. and Parsons, S. M. (1987) The vesicular acetylcholine transport system. *Trends in Neurosciences*, **10**, 174–7.

Marshall, I. G. (1980) Actions of non-depolarizing blocking agents at cholinoceptors other than at the motor endplate. In *Curares and curarization* (ed. C. Conseiller *et al.*), pp. 257–74. Libraire Arnette, Paris.

Marshall, I. G., Gibb, A. J., and Durant, N. N. (1983). The neuromuscular and vagal blocking actions of pancuronium bromide, its metabolites, and vecuronium bromide and its potential metabolites in the anesthetized cat. *British Journal of Anaesthesia*, **55**, 703–14.

Marshall, I. G. and Harvey, A. L. (1990) Selective neuromuscular blocking properties of α-conotoxins *in vivo*. *Toxicon*, **28**, 231–4.

Meijer, D. K. F., Waitering, J. G., Vermeer, G. A., and Scaf, A. H. J. (1979). Comparative pharmacokinetics of *d*-tubocurarine and metocurine in man. *Anesthesiology*, **51**, 402–7.

Merlie, J. P., Sebanne, R., Tzartos, S., and Lindstrom, J. (1982). Inhibition of glycosylation with tunicamycin blocks assembly of newly synthesised acetylcholine receptor subunits in muscle cells. *Journal of Biological Chemistry*, **257**, 2694–701.

Miller, R. D., Agoston, S., Booij, L. D. H. J. Kersten, U. W., Crul, J. F., and Ham, J. (1978). Comparative potency and pharmacokinetics of pancuronium and its metabolites in anesthetized man. *Journal of Pharmacology and Experimental Therapeutics*, **207**, 539–43.

Mishina, M., Takai, T. and Imoto, K., Noda, M., Takahashi, T., Numa, S., *et al.* (1986) Molecular distinction between fetal and adult forms of muscle acetylcholine receptor. *Nature*, **321**, 406–11.

Muir, A. W., Houston, J., Green, K. L., Marshall, R. J., Bowman, W. C., and Marshall, I. G. (1989) Effects of a new neuromuscular blocking agent (Org 9426) in anaesthetized cats and pigs and in isolated nerve-muscle preparations. *British Journal of Anaesthesia*, **63**, 400–10.

Murray, D. J., Sokoll, M. D., Choi, W. W., Mehta, M. P., Forbes, R. B., Gergis, S. D. (1990) The neuromuscular blocking effect of doxacurium chloride during isoflurane anaesthesia. *European Journal of Anaesthesiology*, **7**, 395–402.

Neher, E. and Steinbach, J. H. (1978). Local anaesthetics transiently block currents through single acetylcholine-receptor channels. *Journal of Physiology*, **52**, 162–180.

Noda, M., Takahashi, H., Tanabe, T., Toyosato, M., Furatani, Y., Hirose, T. *et al.* (1982). Primary structure of α-subunit precursor of Torpedo californica acetylcholine receptor deduced from cDNA sequence. *Nature*, **299**, 793–7.

Paton, W. D. M. and Zaimis, E. J. (1949) The pharmacological actions of polymethylene bistrimethyl-ammonium salts. *British Journal of Pharmacology*, **4**, 381–400.

Paton, W. D. M. (1959). The effects of muscle relaxants other than muscular relaxation. *Anesthesiology*, **20**, 453–61.

Pointer, D. J., Wilford, J. B., and Bishop, D. C. (1972). Crystal structure of a novel curariform agent. *Nature*, **239**, 332–3.

Prior, C., Fiekers, J. F., Henderson, F., Dempster, J., Marshall, I. G. and Parsons, R. L. (1990). End-plate ion channel block produced by lincosamide antibiotics and their chemical analogs. *Journal of Pharmacology and Experimental Therapeutics*, **255**, 1170–6.

Quevauvillier, A. and Lainé, F. (1960). Sur la toxicité et le pouvoir curarisant du chlorure de malouétine. *Annals de Pharmacie Francaises*, **18**, 678–80.

Raaflaub, J. and Frey, P. (1972) Zur pharmacokinetic von Diallylnortoxiferin beim Menschen. *Arzneimittel-Forschung*, **22**, 73–78.

Savage, D. S. (1980). Mechanisms of action of muscle relaxants and relationships between structure and activity. In *Curares and curarization* (ed. C. Conseiller *et al.*), pp. 21–31. Libraire Arnette, Paris.

Savarese, J. J. and Kitz, R. J. (1975) Does clinical anesthesia need new neuromuscular blocking agents? *Anethesiology*, **42**, 236–9.

Steinbach, A. B. (1976). A kinetic model for the action of xylocaine on receptors for acetylcholine. *Journal of General Physiology*. **52**, 162–80.

Stenlake, J. B. (1963) Some chemical aspects of neuromuscular block. *Progress in Medicinal Chemistry*, **3**, 1–51.

Stenlake, J. B., Waigh, R. D., Dewar, G. H., Hughes, R., Chapple, D. J., and Coker, G. G. (1981) Biodegradable neuromuscular blocking agents. Part 4. Atracurium besylate and related polyalkylene diesters. *European Journal of Medicinal Chemistry*, **19**, 441–50.

Stevens, C. F. (1985) AChR structure: a new twist to the story. *Trends in Neurosciences*, **8**, 1–2.

Takai, T., Noda, M., Mishina, M., Shimizu, S., Furutani, Y., Kayano, T. *et al.* (1985) Cloning, sequencing and expression of cDNA for a novel subunit of acetylcholine receptor from calf muscle. *Nature*, **315**, 761–764.

Taylor, E. P. and Collier H. O. J. (1951) Synthetic curarizing agents structurally related to *d*-O, O-dimethyltubocurarine. *Nature*, **167**, 692.

Waser, P. G. and Harbeck, P. (1962) Pharmakologie und klinische anwendung des kurzdauernden Muskelrelaxans Diallyl-nor-Toxiferin. *Anaesthetist*, **11**, 33–7.

White, M. M. (1985) Designer channels: site directed mutagenesis as a probe for structural features of channels and receptors. *Trends in Neurosciences*, **8**, 364–9.

Wierda, J. M. K. H., de Wit, A. P. M., Knizenga, K., and Agoston, S. (1990) Clinical observations on the neuromuscular blocking action of Org 9426, a new steroidal nondepolarizing agent. *British Journal of Anaesthesia*, **64**, 521–3.

Yamamura, H. I. and Snyder, S. H. (1972) Choline: high affinity uptake by rat brain synaptosomes. *Science*, **178**, 626–8.

4

Onset of neuromuscular block

S. A. Feldman and N. Fauvel

Since the early studies in patients the difference between the rapid onset of depolarizing drugs and the slower onset of drugs like curare has been noticed (Feldman 1984; Zaimis and Head 1976). Whilst the nondepolarizing drugs presently available have a spectrum of onset times from about 4–6 minutes for doxacurium (Murray *et al.* 1988) to 90 seconds for ORG 9426 (Wierda *et al.* 1990), none has a speed of onset to match that of the depolarizing agents. The onset of suxamethonium varies between 40 and 60 seconds, and that for decamethonium between 60 and 80 seconds (Fig. 4.1) in a dose of twice the ED_{90} in anaesthetized patients.

Various theories have been advanced to explain these differences. One of the earliest was based upon the observation that all of the nondepolarizing neuromuscular blocking drugs were rigid bulky molecules (so-called pachycurares) whilst the depolarizing drugs were long flexible molecules, held stretched out, by the positively charged quaternary ammonium groups at each end (leptocurares). It was suggested that the thin molecules gained access to the synaptic cleft and receptor more easily than the bulky drugs. This led to the concept of limited access as an explanation of the difference in onset time.

It is noticeable that the smaller the dose of drug administered (Mirakhur *et al.* 1983; Jones *et al.* 1985; Rorvik *et al.* 1988), or the slower the rate of administration (Feldman *et al.* 1989), or the lower the blood flow (Goat *et al.* 1976), the longer the

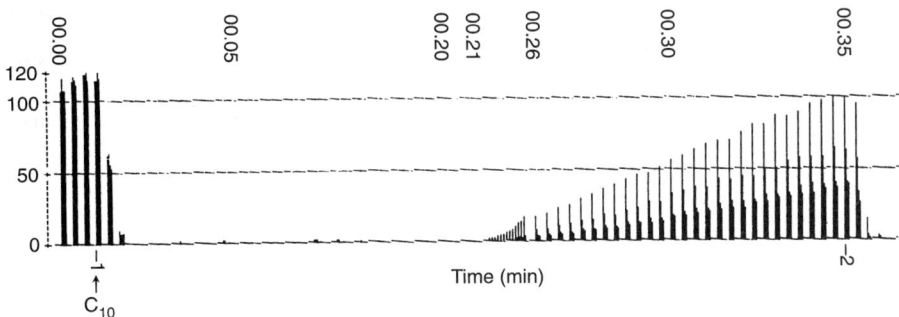

Fig. 4.1 Relaxograph recording showing the onset and recovery of blockade with decamethonium using a train-of-four stimulation pattern every 20 seconds. Note 90% block is reached within 40 seconds with minimal fade.

onset time. This led to a pharmacokinetic hypothesis to explain differences in onset time based upon the dose of drug administered. Further evidence in support of this theory came from the observation by Bowman *et al.* (1988) that there was an inverse correlation between potency of drugs in the aminosteroid series and the rapidity of onset of neuromuscular block. The more potent the drug and hence the smaller the dose given, the longer the onset time.

Another intriguing hypothesis was advanced by Donati (1988) who postulated that the rapid hydrolysis of suxamethonium by cholinesterase necessitated a high plasma to receptor concentration gradient to produce an effect and that this inevitably resulted in a rapid onset of block. This theory receives some support from the observation that low doses of suxamethonium administered to patients known to be deficient in plasma cholinesterase produced a slow onset of block (Cass *et al.* 1982).

The other hypothesis presented to explain the difference between the onset of nondepolarizing and depolarizing agents was advanced by Feldman *et al.* (1990). This was based upon a pharmacodynamic explanation which linked the slow onset of nondepolarizing drugs to the need for the drug to occupy many more binding sites than are required by suxamethonium or decamethonium in order to produce neuromuscular block. It was argued that with the same rate of delivery of molecules of drug the time to occupy the larger number of receptor sites resulted in a slower onset of block.

The various explanations can be categorized as:

(1) access limitation;
(2) plasma concentration effects;
(3) pharmacodynamic actions.

Before examining the evidence to support the various hypotheses it is useful to review the events leading to depolarization of the endplate and to nondepolarizing neuromuscular block.

Acetylcholine activates the receptor complex by simultaneously occupying the two acetylcholine receptor sites, one on each alpha subunit of the receptor pentamer. The activation of the receptor causes a shortening of the subunit in its longitudinal dimension and rotational distortion due the asymmetry of the structure. This results in dilatation of the central ionophore allowing the free inward passage of sodium ions from outside the cell, producing a chemical current. Activation of sufficient receptors produces an ion flux which in turn produces the endplate current which, if it exceeds threshold levels, will trigger off an action potential and muscle response. It follows that it is necessary to prevent transmitter access to only one of the two acetylcholine receptors in order to frustrate channel opening.

Assuming that depolarizing drugs produce their action by reacting directly with the acetylcholine recognition sites it is evident that in the absence of a large concentration of molecules that would swamp the site, the random chance of depolarizing drug reaching a pair of receptors would be less than that of a nondepolarizing drug occupying one or other receptor.

Paton and Waud (1967) calculated that tubocurarine would have to occupy approximately 80–90% of the potential receptors in the sartorius muscle of the cat in order to prevent the response to indirect sartorius nerve stimulation. These results can be interpreted as evidence that only 10–20% of receptors need to be activated in order to produce depolarization by suxamethonium. However, as the calculations are theoretical, being derived from dose ratio experiments using tubocurarine and other nondepolarizing drugs as the antagonist and suxamethonium as the agonist drug, they do not distinguish between prejunctional and postjunctional events or between acetylcholine receptor sites and other binding sites for tubocurarine. Paton and Waud (1967) interpreted their results as demonstrating the extent of the interference with the synaptic mechanism (dose of antagonist required relative to agonist) that can exist before transmission fails.

To generalize from a specialised muscle in a cat or dog to what happens in patients during anaesthesia is to some extent speculative. However, it is likely that a similar 'margin of safety' for nondepolarizing drugs occurs in humans although the exact dimensions may differ.

EXPLANATIONS FOR DIFFERENCES IN ONSET TIMES

Access limitation and pharmacokinetics

There is a good evidence to demonstrate that a slow circulation time (Fig. 4.2) (Harrison 1974; Goat *et al.* 1976) or the slow injection of drug into the blood (Feldman *et al.* 1989) results in a slow onset of block. This might be expected as peak plasma level would be achieved more slowly and the peak may not be as great

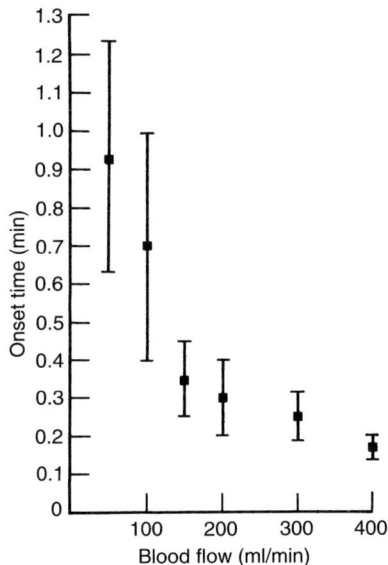

Fig. 4.2 The effect of blood flow on the onset of a gallamine block in the dog tibialis preparation. (From Goat *et al.* 1976.)

if redistribution begins during the injection. There would be a slower attainment of equilibrium between arterial blood and the neuromuscular junction. The slow onset of a neuromuscular block has been attributed to poor blood flow to muscle (Harrison and Junius 1972). However, although blood flow to various groups of muscles may differ (between 2.5 and 5.0 ml per minute per 100 g at rest) and indeed the flow may vary between the forearm and the wrist, the actual proportion of flow directed to the neuromuscular junction relative to the resting muscle is high. The neuromuscular junction enjoys luxury perfusion (Hennis and Stanski 1985) and blood flow should not limit access of drug. It has been demonstrated nevertheless that the peak plasma level of atracurium in venous blood leaving the forearm is achieved some 5–6 minutes before the neuromuscular block (Miller 1984), suggesting either that the drug's entry into the synapse is delayed or that its passage through the biophase to receptor introduces a temporal lag. This is in keeping with the observation made in the isolated arm that releasing the tourniquet which restricted the drug in the arm at 60 seconds does not prevent the establishment of full block in the following 3 minutes in spite of a rapidly failing plasma concentration of drug. This experiment is pharmacokinetically similar to those in which a small dose of drug has been injected intra-arterially. In those experiments, about 2–3 minutes elapse before complete neuromuscular block is produced.

It is the cause of this delay, found only with nondepolarizing drugs, that is intriguing. In an effort to compare the ability of a nondepolarizing drug to reach the receptor with that of depolarizing agents, a series of experiments was constructed in which vecuronium 0.1 mg per kilogram was administered at 10 seconds and 30

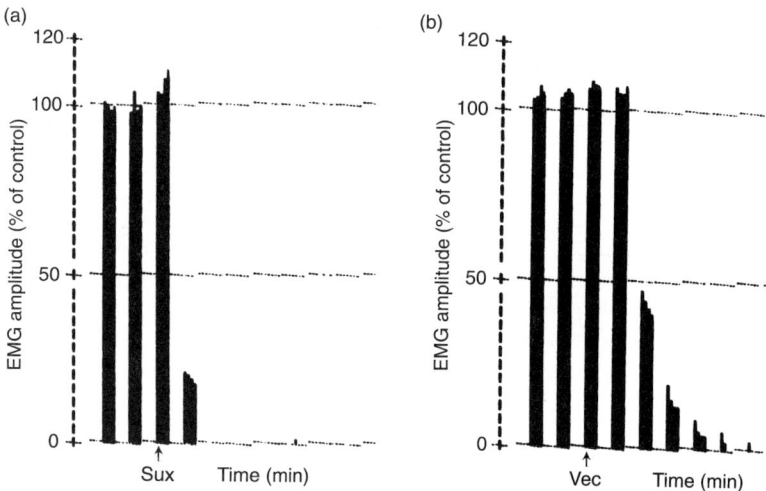

Fig. 4.3 The onset of block with (a) suxamethonium 1 mg/kg (relaxograph EMG) and (b) vecuronium 0.1 mg/kg followed after 10 seconds by suxamethonium 1 mg/kg. Note that the presence of vecuronium at the neuromuscular junction affected the onset of suxamethonium and produced train-of-four fade.

seconds before suxamethonium 1 mg per kilogram in patients who were receiving an isoflurane anaesthetic (Feldman *et al.* 1990). Figure 4.3 demonstrates that administering equipotent doses of suxamethonium approximately 10 seconds after vecuronium results in modification of the suxamethonium-induced block. This is even more clearly seen when the vecuronium is followed at 30 seconds by suxamethonium. The modification of the onset of the suxamethonium block can only be due to the simultaneous presence of vecuronium molecules in the region of the receptors. This experiment demonstrates that vecuronium is present at the receptor site within 10 seconds of suxamethonium. It also indicates that the presynaptic effect of vecuronium (indicated by train-of-four fade) occurs early. This simple experiment makes any explanation of the difference in onset time between nondepolarizing and depolarizing drugs in terms of access to receptors improbable and suggests that the variation in onset time is due to pharmacodynamic differences.

Effect of drug concentration

It is generally assumed that the passage of drug from the plasma to the synaptic cleft will follow first order kinetics within the extreme ranges of doses and will therefore be related to the logarithm of the concentration difference between plasma and receptor. Explaining a difference in onset time on the basis of the number of drug molecules circulating in the plasma requires that these be of very different dimensions. If one compares the ED_{95} doses of various drugs that have been reported (even allowing for the fact that they have been obtained using different background anaesthetics and different criteria for measurement) it is obvious that apart from suxamethonium (which undergoes metabolism or degradation in the plasma) all of the doses contain numbers of molecules of a similar order except for gallamine (Table 4.1). The explanation for the larger than anticipated number of

Table 4.1 Ratios of the number of molecules in one ED_{95} of neuromuscular blocking drugs

Drug	ED_{95} (mg/kg)	Ratio (number of vols) (vecuronium = 1)
Suxamethonium	0.2	8.8
Decamethonium	0.02	0.8
Tubocurarine	0.5	5.8
Gallamine	2.4	14.3
Pancuronium	0.05	1.1
Vecuronium	0.04	1.0
Atracurium	0.2	2.6
Alcuronium	0.15	2.6

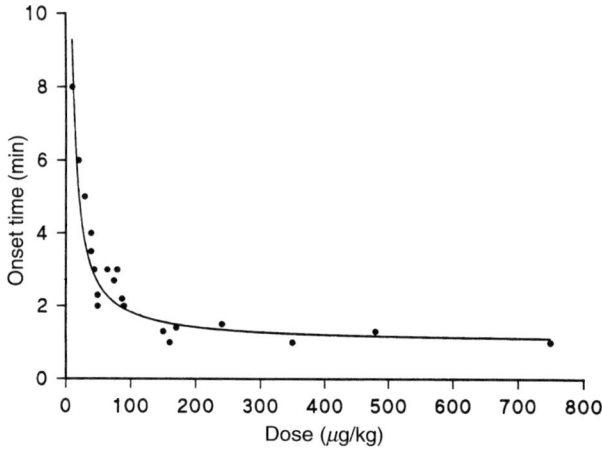

Fig. 4.4 Pooled data from various authors on the onset time of a vecuronium block using different initial dose regimes (note the asymptote at 90 seconds).

molecules of gallamine that are needed may lie in its uptake by red blood cells (Feldman *et al.* 1969). By calculating the number of molecules required and by taking into account the differences in distribution volume, it can be seen that, using vecuronium as a standard unit, fewer decamethonium molecules are required to produce an onset of 95% block than with vecuronium or pancuronium. The time to 95% block for decamethonium was, however, less than 60 seconds in our studies whereas using this dose of vecuronium or pancuronium gives 200–300 seconds onset time.

There is no doubt that increasing the dose of drug from one to two to three times the ED_{95} decreases the onset time, but even with doses of 10–15 times the ED_{95} the onset time to 95% block is longer than 90 seconds. Using pooled figures from reported studies it can be seen from Fig. 4.4 that there appears to be a barrier at 90 seconds onset time even using clinically unacceptably high doses.

A similar barrier to rapid onset is found when the number of molecules of aminosteroid neuromuscular blocking drug are increased as a result of reduced potency. Figure 4.5 illustrates that reducing potency in the aminosteroids is associated with more rapid onset but this is maximal at 90 seconds. Thus, when potency is reduced, there is a 90 second asymptotic level. Drug potency may relate to pharmacokinetic variables. However, it is likely that the main reason for the differences in potency is the rate of drug–receptor dissociation. Thus, the less potent the drug, the lower the dissociation constant. In effect, this makes more molecules available in the environment of the receptor and hence the dynamic effect is akin to the administration of a higher dose of a drug with the same potency. At the extreme of impotency there are drugs with a very low affinity with the receptor, which will only produce neuromuscular block for a few minutes unless they are infused at very high doses. However, even these have onset times longer than that of the depolarizing drugs.

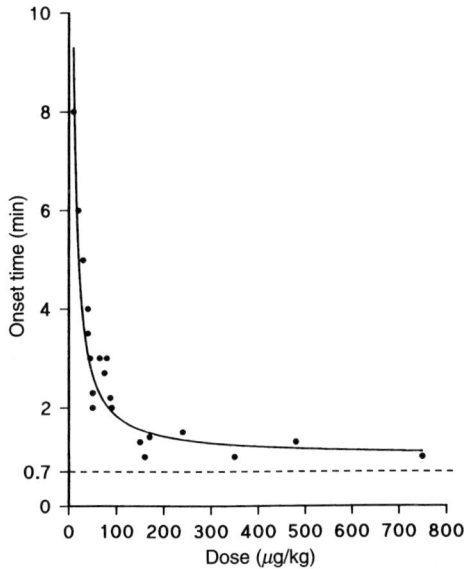

Fig. 4.5 The effect of potency in the aminosteroid neuromuscular blocking drugs on onset time (note the asymptote at 100 sec). (From Bowman *et al.* 1988.)

The general relationship between potency and rate of onset was demonstrated by Kopman (1989). Doses of drug that are subparalytic will result in a slow onset of block. Reduction in onset time results from increasing the dose of drug administered and reducing potency. The effect is, however, limited to a minimum onset time for a block of 90 seconds. Thus the concentration effect fails to explain why, if similar concentrations of drug molecules are administered, depolarizing drugs such as decamethonium and suxamethonium produce a more rapid onset than non-depolarizing agents.

The intriguing suggestion by Donati *et al.* (1991) that suxamethonium owes its rapid onset to rapid hydrolysis by cholinesterase is difficult to reconcile with the much slower onset of mivacurium which is metabolized at 80–90% of the rate of suxamethonium. Nor does it explain the rapid onset of decamethonium, which is not metabolized in patients.

Pharmacodynamic hypothesis

It would seem likely that a pharmacokinetic explanation of the difference in onset of neuromuscular block between nondepolarizing and depolarizing drugs is at best only part of the explanation. It is likely therefore that the reason for the delay between the arrival of nondepolarizing agents and the onset of block is pharmacodynamic. Feldman *et al.* (1990) attributed this difference to the need for drugs such as tubocurarine and vecuronium to achieve the interference in the synaptic mechanism that is

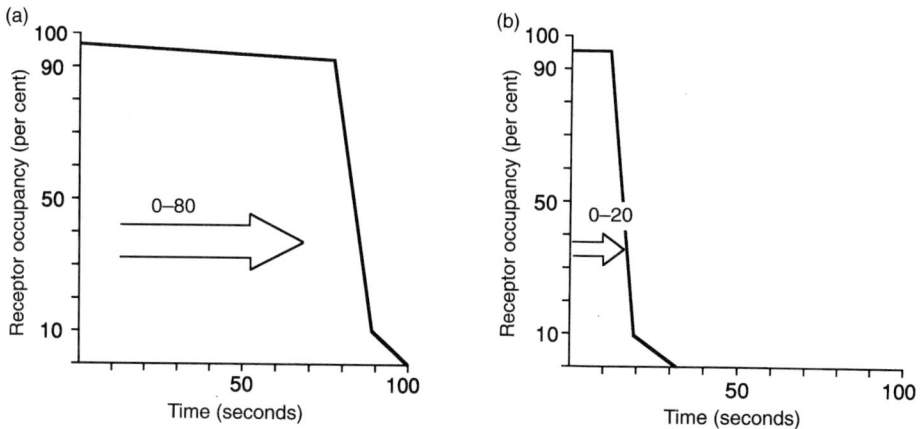

Fig. 4.6 Receptor dynamics as an explanation of the difference in onset time between depolarizing and nondepolarizing agents based on the requirement of nondepolarizing drugs to occupy > 80% of receptors (a) while depolarizing drugs only need to occupy < 20% of receptors (b).

calculated to be required to achieve transmission failure (Paton and Waud 1967). They referred to this apparent superfluity of binding sites for tubocurarine as the 'margin of safety of neuromuscular transmission'. Figures 4.6 illustrate that, using Paton and Waud's figures, over 80% of the binding sites have to be occupied by tubocurarine before it reduces the acetylcholine receptor population to a level that prevents activation by suxamethonium. The corollary of this is an agonist drug does not need to occupy these spare receptor sites in order to produce depolarization of the endplate. It follows from this observation that in order to achieve neuromuscular block with tubocurarine at least four times as many receptors require to be occupied as is necessary for an agonist drug such as suxamethonium. Therefore, even if the molecules of suxamethonium and vecuronium gained access to the receptor at the same rate it would take considerably longer for the necessary receptor occupancy to be achieved by the vecuronium. It is possible that the reason for the apparent excess of receptors for nondepolarizing drugs lies in the biophase binding sites (acceptor sites) suggested by Feldman (1992). It is envisaged that these binding sites, which may not be the acetylcholine receptors themselves, may be on the pentamer or nearby and have to be filled before the drug can produce block of transmission (see Chapter 6).

IMPROVING THE ONSET CHARACTERISTICS

The slow onset of action of the nondepolarizing neuromuscular blocking agents has always been a notable disadvantage. Strategies have therefore been developed in attempts to accelerate the onset of action with the goal of obtaining a speed of onset which was comparable to that of suxamethonium. The fact that such work continues testifies to the fact that a nondepolarizing agent with the rapidity of onset of suxamethonium is not yet available. Rocuronium is the only available nondepolarizing neuromuscular blocking agent which approaches that ideal at present. It does not, however, produce a block as intense as suxamethonium as rapidly as suxamethonium. Our desire to move away from suxamethonium relates to the multiplicity of undesirable side-effects seen with the depolarizing agents, most of which appear to be absent with the nondepolarizing agents.

The strategies which have been and are being employed principally fall into three groups: synthesis of new drugs, use of larger doses, and priming. None of the three strategies has yet been successful. It is possible to accelerate onset considerably in certain cases, although suxamethonium is still required, being unique in its rapidity of onset.

Synthesis of faster drugs

Chemists have been, and still are, attempting to synthesize and develop new agents which are intrinsically fast in onset. The rapidity of suxamethonium has not yet been reached, although some new drugs approach that goal. There are other exciting fields of development which may one day supply us with our rapid acting nondepolarizer (see Chapter 17). Much energy continues to be diverted into developing strategies to speed up the onset of the presently available drugs.

The effect of dose

The relevant molecules have to cross from the plasma into the neuromuscular junction and this movement will be at least partly dependent upon the concentration gradient from plasma to neuromuscular junction. A bolus dose will produce a peak concentration which then rapidly declines and the rate of transfer would be expected to depend upon this peak concentration.

It was shown by Healy *et al.* (1986) that as the dose of atracurium or vecuronium was increased from subparalytic levels to several times that needed to produce complete block, there were three distinct effects (Fig. 4.7). When in the subparalytic range the rate of onset did not change much with increases in the dose. Once the 'ED$_{100}$' had been exceeded, then increasing the dose led to a shortening of the onset time. There was, however, a limit beyond which any further increase in the intubating dose did not further shorten onset.

In the first case where a subparalytic dose of relaxant has been administered, the peak plasma concentration resulting from the bolus dose will be less than the concentration in the active biophase required to produce complete block. The rate of onset appears not to be completely dependent upon the concentration gradient. Once the peak plasma concentration is greater than that required to produce 100% block, the rate of transfer into the active biophase becomes dependent upon the concentration gradient. As the peak plasma concentration is increased further and further, the concentration gradient driving the relaxant into the active biophase shortens the time taken for the concentration to rise above that to produce 100% block; the rate of onset is dependent upon the peak plasma concentration. There is, however, a limit to this imposed by the finite time taken for the drug to get from the

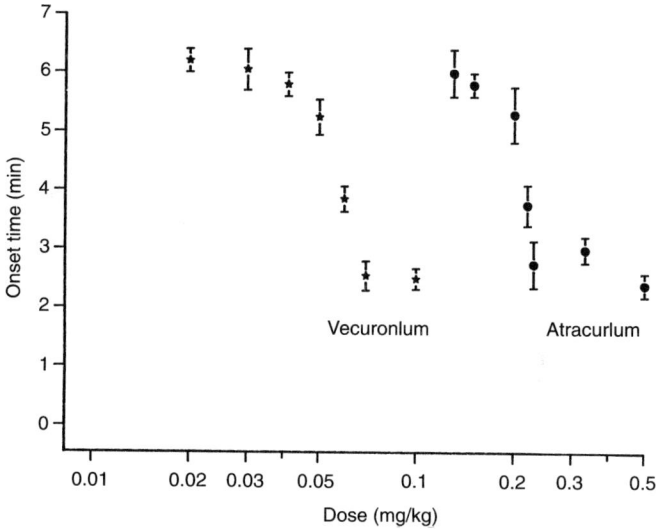

Fig. 4.7 The effect of increasing dose on the onset times of vecuronium and atracurium. (Healy *et al.* 1986).

site of injection to the muscles, coupled with the inbuilt biophase delay, and this places a minimum limit on the onset time.

This technique of accelerating the onset of a nondepolarizing neuromuscular blocking agent is only appropriate for those drugs which can be administered in doses several times the ED_{95} by virtue of their absence of cardiovascular side-events. It has been shown to be appropriate for atracurium (Healy *et al.* 1986), vecuronium (Casson and Jones, 1986; Healy *et al.* 1986; Rorvick *et al.* 1988), rocuronium (Quill *et al.* 1991) and mivacurium (Savarese *et al.* 1988).

Priming

It is likely that priming has its origins in a number of observations which date back to the 1960s. The observation was made that if a small dose of a muscle relaxant was administered, weakness was produced in many, but not all, muscle groups. Careful selection of the dose could reduce grip strength considerably while producing very little effect on respiration (Foldes *et al.* 1961). Part of the explanation for this observation came from work by Paton and Waud (1967). When an intubating dose of a neuromuscular blocking agent is administered there is a delay, typically between 1 and 3 minutes, before onset begins. Maximum block is reached after about 3 to 6 minutes. There is no observable effect on transmission until more than 75% of receptors have been blocked (Paton and Waud 1967) and so at least part of the delay at onset will be due to filling of this margin of safety. If a carefully calculated (priming) dose of neuromuscular blocking agent could be administered such that the margin of safety was just filled, there should theoretically be no observable effect on neuromuscular transmission. Administration of a second (intubating) dose would then only need to raise receptor occupancy from 75% to over about 95% for neuromuscular block to result, which should be more rapid (Fig. 4.8). However, it is difficult to reconcile the necessary delay between the administration of the priming dose and its effect on acceleration of block without proposing some mechanism to bind the drug in the active biophase while its plasma level is declining rapidly (Epstein and Bartkovoski 1993).

This theoretical concept has been borne out in clinical practice and the technique of priming has been examined in many studies and found to be effective. Most of the neuromuscular blocking agents in current clinical use have been examined, including tubocurarine (Donati *et al.* 1986; Pollard 1989), alcuronium (Black *et al.* 1986; Harrop-Griffiths *et al.* 1986; Pollard (1989), pancuronium (Bevan *et al.* 1985; Doherty *et al.* 1985; Mehta *et al.* 1985; Donati *et al.* 1986; Brady *et al.* 1987; Glass *et al.* 1989; Stanec *et al.* 1989), atracurium (Gergis *et al.* 1983; Nagashima *et al.*

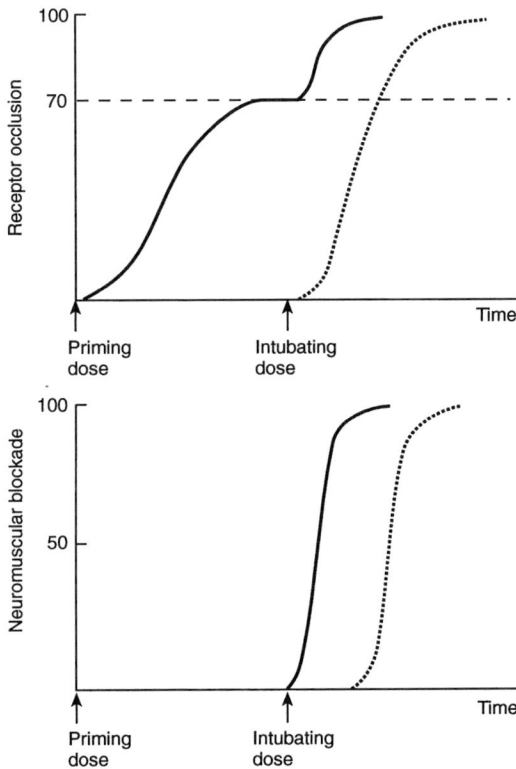

Fig. 4.8 Theoretical representation of priming. The upper trace shows the increased neuromuscular block, and the lower trace receptor occupancy. The administration of a priming dose occupies just less than 70% of receptors, but there is no effect on transmission. The intubating dose at I only has to increase receptor occupancy from 70–100% and so onset (upper trace) is rapid. When an intubating dose is given without priming (dotted lines), there is a delay until receptor occupancy has exceeded 70% before neuromuscular block begins.

1984; Mirakhur *et al.* 1986; Naguib 1986*a*, *b*; Brady *et al.* 1987; Davison and Holland 1989; Nielson *et al.* 1990; Karasic *et al.* 1992), vecuronium (Schwartz *et al.* 1985; Toboada *et al.* 1986; Fureya *et al.* 1991), mivacurium (Molbegott *et al.* 1992), and rocuronium (Foldes *et al.* 1991; Tryba *et al.* 1992). The great majority of these studies have demonstrated a shorter onset time for the main intubating dose following priming, although a small number of studies disagree and find very little difference. It is probable that these differences are related to methodological factors in the studies, including the size and timing of the dose of relaxant, other drugs administered at the same time, and the methods used to quantify relaxation. The efficacy of the priming technique is not now really called into question, with one possible exception, namely rocuronium (Foldes *et al.* 1991). It is possible that the rate of onset of rocuronium is sufficiently rapid for any further acceleration to be undetectable.

When two different nondepolarizing neuromuscular blocking agents are administered simultaneously, their combined effect may be greater than expected from simple addition of their separate actions (see Chapter 12). It would seem logical therefore to examine priming one agent with a different one to see if onset was even more rapid. This has been considered for tubocurarine and pancuronium (Mehta *et al.* 1985), tubocurarine and alcuronium (Pollard 1989), pancuronium and atracurium (Mehta *et al.* 1985), and tubocurarine and atracurium (Mehta *et al.* 1985). Although the use of synergistic pairs did have a small additional effect, the advantage was of a minor nature.

The priming dose

One of the problems with many of the studies on priming is that many different degrees of acceleration of onset have been described. The principal variables which have accounted for these differences include the size and timing of the priming doses. For example, when the priming dose might vary fourfold with intervals of between 2 and 16 minutes it is hardly surprising that differences in the effectiveness of the technique of priming have been reported.

The previous doses used and the time intervals separating priming and intubating doses are therefore of considerable importance. It is likely that the priming dose has to be greater than a certain minimum. What exactly is this minimum is not presently known and guidance only can be given. Furthermore, it is more logical to

Table 4.2 Suitable priming doses for the nondepolarizing neuromuscular blocking agents

Tubocurarine	50 μg/kg
Pancuronium	10 μg/kg
Alcuronium	30 μg/kg
Atracurium	50 μg/kg
Vecuronium	10 μg/kg

use a dose compensated for the patient's body weight rather than a fixed dose and Table 4.2 lists those doses which are generally suitable for use as priming doses. The optimum time interval between priming dose and intubating dose appears to be approximately four minutes.

The duration of action of the intubating dose does not appear to be affected by the presence of the priming dose (Brady *et al.* 1987; Martin *et al.* 1987).

Complications of priming

The aim with the priming dose is to just occupy those 76% of receptors which represent the margin of safety. Every patient is, however, different, and the same patient may not behave in an identical fashion on two separate occasions. It is therefore probably impossible to get the dose exactly correct every time. It is important to err on the side of a lower dose because of the clear potential problems of inducing a partial neuromuscular block from the priming dose alone. Indeed, side-effects and complications of varying severity have been observed following a priming dose of a nondepolarizing neuromuscular blocking agent. These include diplopia, ptosis, blurred vision, difficulty in swallowing, inability to raise the head, inability to protrude the tongue, and an overall feeling of weakness and heaviness (Baumgarten and Reynolds 1985; Engbaek *et al.* 1985; Taboada *et al.* 1986; Mirakhur *et al.* 1986; Sosis *et al.* 1987; Glass *et al.* 1989; Martin *et al*). These are clearly unpleasant for the patient and potentially hazardous. Aspiration of gastric contents has been reported following a priming dose (Musich and Walts 1986).

CONCLUSION

The difference in the time of onset between depolarizing and nondepolarizing neuromuscular blocking agents using equipotent doses cannot readily be explained on a pharmacokinetic basis. Indeed, evidence is presented that both drugs access the receptor complex with equal facility. It is likely that, in the doses at present used in clinical practice, the difference in onset time is primarily due to pharmacodynamic effects resulting from the greater receptor occupancy required to effect block by nondepolarizing drugs than block by suxamethonium or decamethonium.

Various strategies have been proposed to accelerate the onset of the presently available nondepolarizing neuromuscular blocking agents which include priming and the use of a larger intubating dose. None of these methods produces such a dense block as rapidly as suxamethonium.

There is a suggestion that the prejunctional blocking effects of the nondepolarizing drugs such as rocuronium appear earlier than the postjunctional effects. This is supported by the early appearance of fade in the train of four during the onset of nondepolarizing neuromuscular block and the late return of this indicator of presynaptic integrity. It would also explain the claimed early onset of neuromuscular block with rocuronium (Murray *et al.* 1988). It is interesting that the experimental nondepolarizing drug ANQ9040, which has a very rapid onset of action, demonstrates early marked TOF fade, indicating a prejunctional action (Munday and Jones 1993). If this is supported by further experiments it would seem reasonable to seek a nondepolarizing drug with specificity for the prejunctional nicotinic receptors if the ideal of a short onset drug is to be achieved.

REFERENCES

Baumgarten, R. K. and Reynolds, W. J. (1985). The priming principle and the open eye — full stomach. *Anesthesiology*, **63**, 561–2.

Bevan, J. C., Donati, F., and Bevan, D. R. (1985). Attempted acceleration of the onset of action of pancuronium. *British Journal of Anaesthesia*, **57**, 1204–8.

Black, A. M. S., Hutton, R., El-Hassan, K. M., Morgan, G., and Clutton-Brock, T. H. (1986). Priming and the onset of neuromuscular blockade with alcuronium. *British Journal of Anaesthesia*, **58**, 827–33.

Bowman, W. C., Marshall, I. G., Gibb, A. J., and Harborne, A. (1988). Feedback control of transmitter release at neuromuscular junction. *Trends in Pharmacological Sciences*, **9**, 16–20.

Brady, M. M., Mirakhur, R. K., and Gibson, F. M. (1987). Influence of priming on the potency of non-depolarizing neuromuscular blocking agents. *British Journal of Anaesthesia*, **59**, 1245–9.

Cass, N. M., Doolan, L. A., and Gutteridge, G. A. (1982). Repeated administration of suxamethonium in a patient with atypical cholinesterase. *Anaesthesia and Intensive Care*, **10**, 25–8.

Casson, W. R. and Jones, R. M. (1986). Vecuronium induced neuromuscular blockade. The effect of increasing dose on speed of onset. *Anaesthesia*, **41**, 354–7.

Davison, K. L. and Holland, M. S. (1989). A comparison study of vecuronium bromide and atracurium besylate for rapid sequence induction. *Journal of the American Association of Nurse Anaesthetists*, **57**, 37–40.

Doherty, W. G., Breen, P. J., Donati, F., and Bevan, D. R. (1985). Accelerated onset of pancuronium with divided doses. *Canadian Anaesthetists' Society Journal*, **32**, 1–4.

Donati, F. (1988). Onset of action of relaxants. *Canadian Journal of Anaesthesia*. **35**, S52–5.

Donati, F., Ducharme, J., Theoret, Y., and Bevan, D. (1991). Pharmacokinetics and pharmacodynamics of atracurium obtained with arterial and venous blood samples. *Clinical Pharmacology and Therapeutics*, **49**, 515–22.

Donati, F., Lahoud, J., Walsh, C. M., Lavelle, P. A., and Bevan, D. R. (1986). Onset of pancuronium and *d*-tubocurarine blockade with priming. *Canadian Anaesthetists' Society Journal*, 33, 571–7.

Engbaek, J., Howardy-Hansen, P., Ording, H., and Viby-Mogensen, J. (1985). Precurarization with vecuronium and pancuronium in awake, healthy volunteers: The influence on neuromuscular transmission and pulmonary function. *Acta Anaesthesiologica Scandinavica*, **29**, 117–20.

Epstein, R. H. and Bartkowski, R. R. (1993). Priming v. timing: predictions of a receptor binding model of the neuromuscular junction. *Anesthesia and Analgesia*, **76**, S97.

Feldman, S. A. (1984). Neuromuscular blocking drugs. In *A practice of anaesthesia* (5th edn), (ed. H. C. Churchill-Davidson), p. 680. Lloyd Luke, London.

Feldman, S. A. (1993). Neuromuscular blocking agents. In *Mechanisms of drugs in anaesthesia* (2nd edn), (ed. S. A. Feldman, W. Paton, and C. Scurr), p. 336–54. Edward Arnold, London.

Feldman, S. A., Cohen E. N., and Golling R. C. (1969). The excretion of gallamine in the dog. *Anesthesiology*, **30**, 593–8.

Feldman, S. A., Soni, N., and Kraayenbrink, M. A. (1989). Effect of rate of injection on the neuromuscular block produced by vecuronium. *Anesthesia and Analgesia*, **69**, 624–6.

Feldman, S. A., Fauvel, N., and Harrop-Griffiths, A. A. (1990). Onset of neuromuscular block. In *Neuromuscular blocking agents past, present and future*, (ed. W. C. Bowman, P. A. F. Denissen, and S. Feldman), pp. 44–51. Excerpta Medica, Amsterdam.

Foldes, F. F., Monte, A. P., Brunn, H. H., and Wolfson, B. (1961). Studies with muscle relaxants in unanesthetised subjects. *Anesthesiology*, **22**, 230–6.

Foldes, F. F., Nagishima, H., Nguyen, H., Schiller, W. S., Mason, M. M., and Ohta, Y. (1991). The neuromuscular effect of ORG9426 in patients receiving balanced anaesthesia. *Anesthesiology*, **75**, 191–6.

Furuya, T., Taniguchi, Y., Atarashi, K., Tachibana, C., Sato, K., and Ohe, Y. (1991). Clinical study on the priming principle of muscle relaxants: comparison of pancuronium with vecuronium. *Japanese Journal of Anesthesia*, **40**, 1659–65.

Gergis, S. D., Sokoll, M. D., Mehta, M., Kemmotsu, O., and Rudd, G. D. (1983). Intubation conditions after atracurium and suxamethonium. *British Journal of Anaesthesia*, **55**, 83S.

Glass, P. S. A., Wilson, W., Mace, J. A., and Wagoner, R. (1989). Is the priming principle both effective and safe? *Anesthesia and Analgesia*, **68**, 127–34.

Goat, V. A., Yeung, M. L., Blackeney, C., and Feldman, S. A. (1976). The effect of blood flow upon the activity of gallamine triethiodide. *British Journal of Anaesthesia*, **48**, 69–73.

Harrison, G. A. (1974). The relationship between the arm–arm circulation time and the neuromuscular action of pancuronium. *Anaesthesia and Intensive Care*, **2**, 91–4.

Harrison, G. A. and Junius, F. (1972). The effect of circulation time on the neuromuscular action of suxamethonium. *Anaesthesia and Intensive Care*, **1**, 33–40.

Harrop-Griffiths, A. W., Grounds, R. M., and Moore, M. (1986). Intubating conditions following pre-induction priming with alcuronium. *Anaesthesia*, **41**, 282–6.

Healy, T. E. J., Pugh, N. D., Kay, B., Sivalingam, T., and Petts, H. V. (1986). Atracurium and vecuronium: effect of dose on the time of onset. *British Journal of Anaesthesia*, **58**, 620–4.

Hennis, P. J. and Stanski, D. R. (1985). Pharmacokinetic and pharmacodynamic factors that govern the clinical use of muscle relaxants. In *Muscle relaxants* (ed. R. L. Katz), pp. 179–96. Grune and Stratton, Orlando.

Jones, R. M., Casson, W. R., and Lethbridge, J. R. (1985). Influence of dose on onset times of vecuronium induced neuromuscular blockade. *British Journal of Anaesthesia*, **57**, 828–9.

Karasic, L., Handlin, D. S., Patel, N., and Baker, T. (1992). Applying the priming principle to reduce atracurium intubating dose. *Anesthesiology*, **77**, A937.

Kopman, A. F. (1989). Pancuronium, gallamine and *d*-tubocurarine compared; its speed of onset inversely related to drug potency? *Anesthesiology*, **70**, 915–20.

Martin, C., Bonneru, J. J., Brun, J. P., Albanese, J., and Gouin, F. (1987). Vecuronium or suxamethonium for rapid sequence intubation: which is better? *British Journal of Anaesthesia*, **59**, 1240–4.

Martin, C., Guillen, J. C., Dupin, B., Ragni, J., Ankin, P., and Goiun, F. (1990). Lower oesophageal reflex during priming with vecuronium. *British Journal of Anaesthesia*, **64**, 33–5.

Mehta, M. P., Choi, W. S., Gergis, S. D., Sokoll, M. D., and Adelphson, A. (1985). Facilitation of rapid endotracheal intubation with divided doses of nondepolarizing neuromuscular blocking drugs. *Anesthesiology*, **62**, 392–5.

Miller, R. D. (1984). Pharmacokinetics of muscle relaxants. In *Pharmacokinetics of anaesthesia* (ed. C. Prys Roberts and C. C. Hug), pp. 246–69. Blackwell Scientific Publications, Oxford.

Mirakhur, R. K., Ferres, C. J., Clarke R. S. J., Bali I. M. and Dundee J. W. (1983). Clinical evaluation of ORG NC45. *British Journal of Anaesthesia*, **55**, 119–24.

Mirakhur, R. K., Lavery, C. G., Gibson, F. M., and Clarke, R. S. J. (1986). Intubating conditions after vecuronium and atracurium given in divided doses (the priming technique). *Acta Anaesthesiologica Scandinavica*, **30**, 347–50.

Molbegott, L., Flashburg, M., Patel, N., Handlin, D. S., and Baker, T. (1992). Speed and ease of endotracheal intubation: priming with mivacurium compared with succinylcholine. *Anesthesiology*, **77**, A967.

Munday, I. T. and Jones, R. M. (1993). ANQ9040: effect of twice the ED_{95} dose. *British Journal of Anaesthesia* **70**, 480P.

Murray, D. J., Mehta, M. P., Choi, W. W., Forbes, R. B., Sokoll, M. D., Gergis S. D. *et al.* (1988). The neuromuscular blocking and cardiovascular effects of doxacurium chloride in patients receiving nitrous oxide narcotic anesthesia. *Anesthesiology*, **69**, 472–7.

Musich, J. and Walts, L. F. (1986). Pulmonary aspiration after a priming dose of vecuronium. *Anesthesiology*, **64**, 517–9.

Nagashima, H., Nguyen, H. D., Lee, S., Kaplan, R., Duncalf, D., and Foldes, F. F. (1984). Facilitation of rapid endotracheal intubation with atracurium. *Anesthesiology*, **61**, A289.

Naguib, M., Abdullatif, M., and Absood, G. H. (1986a). The optimal priming dose for atracurium. *Canadian Anaesthetists' Society Journal*, **33**, 453–7.

Naguib, M., Gyasi, H. K., Abdulatif, M., and Absood, G. H. (1986b). Rapid tracheal intubation with atracurium — a comparison of priming intervals. *Canadian Anaesthetists' Society Journal*, **33**, 150–6.

Nielsen, H. K., May, O., and Back, V. (1990). Priming principle with atracurium. *Acta Anaesthesiologica Scandinavica*, **41**, 313–7.

Paton, W. D. M. and Waud, D. R. (1967). The margin of safety of neuromuscular transmission. *Journal of Physiology*, **191**, 59–90.

Pollard, B. J. (1989). Priming with alcuronium and tubocurarine accelerates the onset of neuromuscular block. *British Journal of Anaesthesia*, **63**, 7–11.

Quill, T. J., Begin, M., Glass, P. S. A., Ginsberg, B., and Gorback, M. S. (1991). Clinical response to ORG 9426 during isoflurane anesthesia. *Anesthesia and Analgesia*, **72**, 203–6.

Rorvik, K., Husby, P., Gramstad, L., Vamnes, J. S., Bitsch-Larsen, L. and Koller, M. E. (1988). Comparison of large dose of vecuronium with pancuronium for prolonged neuromuscular blockade. *British Journal of Anaesthesia*, **61**, 180–5.

Savarese, J. J., Ali, H. H., Basta, S. J., Embee, P. B., Scott, R. P. F., Sunder N., *et al.* (1988). The clinical neuromuscular pharmacology of mivacurium chloride (BW B1090U). *Anesthesiology*, **68**, 723–32.

Schwartz, S., Ilias, W., Lackner, F., Mayshofer, O., and Foldes, F. F. (1985). Rapid tracheal intubation with vecuronium: The priming principle. *Anesthesiology*, **62**, 388–91.

Sosis, M., Stiner, A., Larijani, G. E., and Marr, A. T. (1987). An evaluation of priming with vecuronium. *British Journal of Anaesthesia*, **59**, 1236–9.

Stanec, A., Nacino, I., and Baker, T. (1989). A five minute waiting period makes the priming dose effective. *Anesthesia and Analgesia*, **68**, S274.

Taboada, J. A., Rupp, S. M., and Miller, R. D. (1986). Refining the priming principle for vecuronium during rapid-sequence induction of anaesthesia. *Anesthesiology*, **64**, 243–7.

Tryba, M., Zorn, A., Thole, H., and Zenz, M. (1992). Crash-induction with ORG9426 vs succinylcholine — a randomized double blind study. *Anesthesiology*, **77**, A962.

Wierda, J. M. K. H., de Wit, A. P. M., Kuizenga, K., and Agoston S. (1990). Clinical observations on the neuromuscular blocking action of ORG 9426, a new steroidal non-depolarizing agent. *British Journal of Anaesthesia*, **64**, 521–3.

Zaimis, E. and Head, S. (1976). Depolarizing neuromuscular blocking drugs. In *Handbook of experimental pharmacology*, Vol. 42, (ed. E. Zaimis), Springer-Verlag, Berlin.

5

The maintenance of neuromuscular blockade

Hassan H. Ali and George D. Shorten

Before discussing the maintenance of neuromuscular block, we have to dwell on the important subject of the maintenance of anaesthesia in the clinical setting, since neuromuscular blocking drugs are an integral part of the term 'balanced anaesthesia'. Throughout this chapter, the maintenance of muscle relaxation will be considered as one component of a general anaesthetic technique, both influencing and influenced by the other components. In this way, the principles of muscle relaxant administration derived from a vast anaesthetic literature may be viewed in a way which is applicable in the operating room. While the usefulness of regional techniques in providing analgesia, immobilization, and muscle relaxation is acknowledged, this chapter will focus on the use of the peripherally acting neuromuscular blocking drugs.

HISTORICAL PERSPECTIVE

The concept of balanced anaesthesia began when George Washington Crile (1913) suggested that selection and combination of anaesthetic agents was preferable to the use of any one agent. He maintained that psychic stimuli might be obliterated by light general anaesthesia (nitrous oxide and/or diethyl ether) while the noxious impulses due to surgery might be blocked by local anaesthesia. This concept was called the theory of anoci-association or exclusion of noxious stimuli. Specifically, Crile recommended the combination of peripheral nerve block to provide analgesia, with inhalational anaesthesia to 'exclude the psychi stimulation of brain cells'. In 1926, John S. Lundy introduced the term 'balanced anaesthesia' for the combined effects of a moderate amount of preliminary hypnotic, a moderate amount of local anaesthesia, a moderate amount of nitrous oxide or ethylene, and a moderate amount of ether sufficient to obtain the desired result. He wrote that, 'It seems logical that a combination of the various agents might be used, each one in small enough amount so that it would produce no unsatisfactory effect; whereas collectively these agents produce a balanced anaesthesia'. When these are combined, they will usually produce satisfactory anaesthesia. Rees and Gray (1950) mentioned a balanced anaesthetic when a relaxant is used to complete a triad of narcosis, analgesia, and relaxation. Gray renamed the triad narcosis, reflex suppression, and relaxation. With selective drugs, it was possible to vary one component of the triad without affecting the others. The same author further suggested that a fourth component was necessary, namely controlled ventilation, and thus the 'triad' became a 'tetrad'.

If anaesthesia was regarded as the sum of individual and separate pharmacological effects, it was no longer necessary to administer excessive doses of any one agent. In this context, it was possible to avoid deep planes of anaesthesia with the concomitant undesirable respiratory, haemodynamic, central nervous system, and metabolic side-effects. Anaesthesia or analgesia is a process of modification of the normal physiological reflex response to surgical stimuli. The triad of anaesthesia may be considered to be:

(1) inhibition of the afferent limb of the reflex arc;

(2) depression of the central synaptic mechanism of coordination and awareness;

(3) inhibition of the efferent limb of the reflex arc.

Although curare was known for many years prior to its introduction to clinical anaesthesia, a real advance was made in 1851 when Benjamin Brody showed that animals poisoned with a curare preparation did not die if artificial ventilation was maintained (see Bryn Thomas 1951). Claude Bernard (1856) demonstrated that curare acted peripherally at the junction between the motor nerve and the muscle. West (1932) employed a highly purified fraction of curare in patients suffering from tetanus and other spastic disorders. Bennett (1940) was the first to use a standardized preparation of curare (Intocostrin) in patients to modify metrazol induced convulsive therapy, a precursor to electroconvulsive therapy. Griffith and Johnson (1942) introduced curare (Intocostrin) into anaesthetic practice to provide muscle relaxation. These authors opened their article with the sentence, 'Every anaesthetist has wished at times that he might be able to produce rapid and complete muscular relaxation in resistant patients under general anaesthesia'. Prior to this, intraoperative muscle relaxation could not be achieved independently, and very deep anaesthesia was necessary for major intraperitoneal procedures. This posed certain formidable problems. Knight (1944) considered that deep anaesthesia could be more dangerous and harmful than surgical shock. The advent of specifically acting muscle relaxant drugs overcame this problem. The introduction of curare made possible new surgical procedures (intrathoracic, intraperitoneal, and organ transplant surgery) and as Foldes (1990) has suggested, 'eliminated the concept of inoperability due to advanced pathology or extremes of age' (see Chapter 1). Cullen (1943) reported on 131 cases in which curare was used. Gray and Halton (1946*a*) published a paper entitled, 'A milestone in anaesthesia (*d*-tubocurarine chloride)'; this did much to establish the rational use of muscle relaxants in anaesthesia.

Following the introduction of curare into anaesthesia, medicinal chemists and pharmacologists began the search for synthetic substitutes. Gallamine triethiodide was first used clinically in 1948 in France. The same year, the semisynthetic curare (dimethyltubocurarine) was introduced into clinical anaesthesia. Decamethonium was described by Organe *et al.* (1949). Suxamethonium was next introduced by Thesleff (1951) and Foldes *et al.* (1952). Alcuronium was introduced by Hugin and Kissling (1961). Pancuronium was introduced in 1968, and in 1977 metocurine was revisited after being forgotten for a long period and became popular for cardiac anaesthesia (Savarese *et al.* 1977). The need for a neuromuscular blocking agent without side-effects prompted an extensive search to provide an ultra-short acting non-depolarizing agent to replace suxamethonium. The years 1980 and 1981 witnessed the successful clinical trails of two new intermediate-acting non-depolarizing relaxants, atracurium and vecuronium, which were later introduced to, and widely accepted by the anaesthesia community. In the late eighties, two long-acting non-depolarizing relaxants free from haemodynamic side-effects were introduced, pipecuronium (Arduan) and doxacurium (Nuromax). The most recent relaxant which has been released in the USA and the UK is mivacurium (Mivacron) which is a short-acting non-depolarizing relaxant, ideal for administration by continuous infusion. Rocuronium bromide (ORG 9426) is a new intermediate-acting nondepolarizing relaxant currently undergoing clinical trails. Its neuromuscular profile is similar to vecuronium with a faster onset.

OBJECTIVES OF MAINTENANCE OF MUSCLE RELAXATION

These may be summarized as follows:

1. To improve operating conditions under light planes of anaesthesia:
   (a) to allow adequate surgical exposure (e.g. laparotomy);
   (b) to secure patient immobilization (e.g. microsurgery);
   (c) to facilitate operative manipulation (e.g. shoulder surgery).

2. To facilitate controlled ventilation which permits:
   (a) prolonged procedures in patients with chronic obstructive or restrictive pulmonary disease;
   (b) hyperventilation of patients with increased intracranial pressure;
   (c) controlled ventilation in the intensive care unit, particularly when rapid wake-up and offset of the action of the relaxant is desirable for immediate evaluation of the neurological or pulmonary function.

3. To maintain a degree of neuromuscular block appropriate for the procedure, yet reliable reversibility when required.

4. To maintain balanced anaesthesia which is adequate, yet light enough to ensure quick recovery and early ambulation.

5. To reduce requirements for central depressant agents.

6. To employ available muscle relaxants in doses, and by modes of administration, which will minimize undesirable side effects, namely very profound

block (overdose), residual curarization, cardiovascular effects, histamine release, tachyphylaxis, and possibly to avoid the need for anticholinesterases by the proper choice of relaxant and the judicious choice of dose.

FACTORS INFLUENCING THE CHOICE AND RESPONSE TO MUSCLE RELAXANTS

We indicated at the outset that the maintenance of muscle relaxation should be regarded as one component of the overall anaesthetic technique. Evidence continues to accumulate of the interactions that occur between the commonly used anaesthetic agents and muscle relaxants.

It is inaccurate to regard the agents that are commonly administered by anaesthesiologists today as independent effectors. A synergism was observed to exist between inhalational agents, barbiturates, and curare as early as 1946. Gray and Halton (1946*b*) observed that 'administration of the combination of 15 mg of curare and a dose of barbiturate less than the minimal anaesthetic dose produces a completely anaesthetized and motionless patient'. Furthermore, 'if any inhalational anaesthetic is used to supplement this barbiturate–curare combination, only a minimal amount is required to produce deep anaesthesia'. Potent inhalational agents reduce muscle relaxant requirements in a concentration and duration of administration dependent fashion. In general, muscle relaxant doses may be reduced by 40% with halothane, and 50–60% with enflurane and isoflurane. The mechanisms of this effect include inhibition of presynaptic choline uptake (Johnson and Hartzell 1985), diminished acetylcholine mobilization and release at the motor nerve ending, postjunctional nicotinic acetylcholine receptor desensitization, decreased muscle contractility, and inhibitory effects on muscle spindles, spinal cord inter-neurons, and the cerebral cortex. Interestingly, the converse effect has also been demonstrated. Pancuronium has been shown to reduce the minimum alveolar concentration (MAC) of halothane by 25% (Forbes *et al.* 1979), although vecuronium has been shown to have no effect on the MACs of enflurane and isoflurane. Isoflurane-induced EEG burst suppression is potentiated by pancuronium (Schwartz *et al.* 1991). More interactions with relaxants are addressed in Chapter 12.

Thus, the well recognized interactions between analgesics, anaesthetics, and muscle relaxants dictate that intra-operative maintenance of muscle relaxation be regarded as an integral part of an anaesthetic technique rather than an independent function.

As the muscle relaxants available more closely approximate the ideal, the choice of a specific agent may appear less critical. In spite of this, many investigators have demonstrated that the incidence of residual post-operative neuromuscular block is unacceptably high, particularly when the long-acting muscle relaxants are used. Thirty (42%) of the 72 patients studied by Viby-Mogensen *et al.* (1979) were found to be inadequately recovered as evidenced by a train-of-four (TOF) ratio of less than 70%. These authors concluded that post-operative residual curarization was a significant problem, that anaesthetists tend to use high doses of muscle relaxants, and that neostigmine (2.5 mg) is an inadequate dose in some patients. They recommended that neuromuscular monitoring be used more extensively during anaesthesia. Lennmarken *et al.* (1984) and Beemer and Rozenthal (1986) in widely disparate settings have since demonstrated high incidences of post-operative residual neuromuscular block. The incidence of this potentially detrimental side-effect is highly dependent on the choice of muscle relaxant, being much less when atracurium or vecuronium is used than with pancuronium (Bevan *et al.* 1988; Andersen *et al.* 1988). This alone strongly emphasizes the need to plan the intra-operative maintenance of muscle relaxation carefully.

The following factors need to be considered:

The patient: any co-existing disease involving the neuromuscular, cardiovascular, pulmonary, and central nervous systems.

The procedure: the depth of block required, familiarity with the surgeon, duration of the procedure, surgical use of peripheral nerve stimulator to avoid neural injury, intra-operative 'wake-up' for neurological examination, monitoring of cranial nerve function (e.g. facial nerve during acoustic neuroma).

The anaesthetic technique chosen: whether a nitrous oxide/narcotic anaesthetic, a deep inhalational anaesthetic, or combined general anaesthesia and regional is used.

Others: experience of the anaesthetist, peri-operative monitoring of the neuromuscular function (see below), equipment available (infusion pumps, computerized feedback systems, electromyography (EMG), force transduction).

CLASSIFICATION OF RELAXANTS

The neuromuscular blocking agents may be classified in a number of ways. For the purpose of this chapter, they are all considered under three separate headings:

1. Mode of action:
   (a) depolarizing relaxants (suxamethonium);
   (b) nondepolarizing relaxants.

2. Duration of action:
   (a) ultra-short acting (suxamethonium);
   (b) short acting (mivacurium);
   (c) intermediate-acting (atracurium, vecuronium, rocuronium);
   (d) long-acting (tubocurarine, metocurine, gallamine, alcuronium, pancuronium, pipecuronium, and doxacurium).

3. Mode of administration:
   (a) infusion following a loading dose (suxamethonium, mivacurium);
   (b) intermittent bolus doses or infusion following a loading dose (atracurium, vecuronium);
   (c) intermittent bolus doses with or without a preceding loading dose (all the long-acting relaxants).

MONITORING NEUROMUSCULAR FUNCTION

The most clinically relevant pattern of stimulation is the train-of-four stimuli. It does not need the previous establishment of a control response and does not depend on sophisticated equipment for interpretation of the response.

The train-of-four count in response to supramaximal stimulation is commonly used in the following ways:

(1) The ulnar nerve is stimulated at the wrist with tactile evaluation of the response of the fully abducted thumb.

(2) The posterior tibial nerve is stimulated behind the medial malleolus of the tibia and assessment is made of the plantar flexion of the foot.

(3) The lateral popliteal or common peroneal nerve is stimulated at the neck of the fibula and dorsiflexion of the foot is assessed. A count of one or two responses will provide adequate surgical relaxation in most cases. Titrating the relaxant dose to maintain one or two responses will also provide surgical relaxation which is readily reversible when so desired.

Early detection of the development of phase II block following suxamethonium infusion is also possible using the train-of-four by identifying decrement in the ratio of the fourth to the first response.

Occasionally, a profound degree of neuromuscular block is required, usually for short periods. Under these circumstances, when no response is present following TOF stimulation, the number of responses detected following a brief tetanus may be used to quantify the degree of block. This post-tetanic count (PTC) is predictive of the time that must elapse before spontaneous recovery occurs to the extent that a response to single twitch stimulation can be detected. It was found that after repetitive tetanic stimuli at 50 Hz every six minutes, a PTC of one indicates that the mean time to first detectable response to TOF stimulation is about 30 minutes during a pancuronium-induced block and eight minutes after atracurium or vecuronium block (Viby-Mogensen *et al.* 1981). We believe that repeated tetanic stimulation every six minutes will lead to local recovery at the site of stimulation which does not reflect the systemic effect of the relaxant, although this view is not shared by all experts in the neuromuscular field. An occasional application of a five-second tetanus at 50 Hz may be used. The post-tetanic response will reveal the presence or absence of post-tetanic potentiation and thus indirectly determine the depth of block.

PRACTICAL APPLICATION

Gray and Halton (1946*b*) described three ways in which curare might be used to maintain muscle relaxation intra-operatively. For the short operation of endoscopy, it was suggested that a single dose of curare (15 mg) might be used. For longer procedures, increments of 2–4 mg were given 'from time to time' as well as intermittent injection of an intravenous barbiturate. A light level of general anaesthesia may be achieved with an inhalational agent and 'an intermittent fractional injection of a total dose of 15–30 mg of curare is utilized to produce relaxation for long procedures'.

Maintenance of muscle relaxation in current anaesthetic practice may be achieved in three ways.

An initial bolus or an intubating dose of an ultra-short or short acting relaxant followed by infusion

Following an intubating dose of suxamethonium, the suxamethonium infusion should be commenced at the first detection of a muscle response. In a dilution of 2 mg/ml, in 5% dextrose, an infusion rate of approximately 70–80 μg/kg/min is required initially and then titrated to maintain a barely detectable response. Tachyphylaxis develops early and heralds the development of phase II block (Lee and Katz 1975) after approximately 3–5 mg/kg under halothane anaesthesia. Phase II block develops at approximately 10–12 mg/kg under nitrous oxide-opioid anaesthesia with significant inter-individual variation (Ramsey *et al.* 1980). It is associated with an unpredictable duration of action. In 50% of patients who developed phase II block after discontinuation of the infusion, the recovery time to only 75% of control was over 30 minutes and this degree of residual block required reversal with anticholinesterases. As with a bolus dose, an unpredictably prolonged block will occur in patients with atypical plasma cholinesterase.

It has been argued that prolonged (greater than 1 hour) infusion of suxamethonium is a misuse of an ultra short-acting drug, when predictable, reversible non-depolarizing agents are available (Katz and Katz 1975). A high inter-patient variation in response is characteristic of a suxamethonium infusion. A range of 2–15 mg/kg/hr has been found necessary to maintain 90% neuromuscular block (Katz and Ryan 1969; Ramsey *et al.* 1980). Monitoring the TOF ratio is useful in the detection of phase II block. A T4/T1 ratio of less than 0.5 indicates an early development of phase II block and warns that prolonged spontaneous recovery may be imminent.

An initial bolus dose of a short-acting non-depolarizing relaxant (e.g. mivacurium chloride) followed by an infusion

Mivacurium chloride is a new short-acting nondepolarizing neuromuscular blocking agent. It is a synthetic bis-benzylisoquinolinium diester, which is hydrolysed rapidly by human plasma cholinesterase at 70–88% the rate of suxamethonium. The calculated ED$_{95}$ for inhibition of adductor pollicis twitch evoked at 0.15 Hz is 0.08 mg/kg (Savarese *et al.* 1988) in patients receiving nitrous oxide–opioid–barbiturate anaesthesia.

At 0.1 mg/kg, an onset of maximum block required 3.8 ± 0.5 (SE) min and recovery to 95% twitch height occurred 24.5 ± 1.6 (SE) min after injection. At 0.25 mg/kg, onset was 2.3 ± 0.3 min, and 95% recovery was reached within 30.4 ± 2.2 min. Comparative recovery indices from 5–95% or from 25–75% twitch heights did not differ significantly among all dosage groups from 0.1–0.3 mg/kg (range 12.9–14.7 and 6.6–7.2 min, respectively). Following recovery from doses of 0.1–0.3 mg/kg, an infusion of mivacurium was instituted when the evoked twitch recovered spontaneously to 5% of control (95% block). The infusion rate necessary to maintain 95 ± 4 (SE) % twitch suppression was 8.3 ± 0.7 μg/kg/min. The recovery time from termination of infusion to 25%, the 25–75% recovery time, and the 5–95% recovery time were 5.7 ± 5, 6.9 ± 0.3, and 14.5 ± 0.4 min, respectively and did not differ with duration of infusion (Ali *et al.* 1988).

Following an infusion of mivacurium chloride, the recovery times from 25–75%, 25–95%, and 5–95% did not differ significantly from those following single bolus doses ranging from 0.1–0.3 mg/kg. The recovery times of mivacurium are approximately half the times of atracurium and less than 50% those of vecuronium for a similar duration of infusion (Ali *et al.* 1988). In an earlier study with a suxamethonium infusion (Ramsey *et al.* 1980) it was found that in 50% of the patients who developed phase II block, the 25–95% and 5–95% recovery times were 12.7 ± 2.4 and 15.0 ± 3 min, respectively. These appear to be comparable to the corresponding times for mivacurium of 11.0 ± 0.5 and 14.5 ± 0.4 min for a similar duration of infusion. In the remaining 50% of the patients who developed phase II block, the time required to recover spontaneously from 5.0% to only 75% was 31.0 ± 5 min and this residual neuromuscular block necessitated antagonism with anticholinesterases. It appears that mivacurium chloride shows an excellent clinical profile for maintenance of neuromuscular block by continuous infusion because the block is non-cumulative with no haemodynamic changes. It is particularly useful during long procedures when rapid spontaneous recovery from neuromuscular block is desirable at the end of surgery or intra-operatively to assess neurological function.

Intermediate-acting relaxants: atracurium and vecuronium

Maintenance of neuromuscular block employing members of this class can be accomplished in two ways.

An initial intubating dose followed by small incremental bolus doses

The latter begins at the onset of spontaneous recovery or the appearance of two to three responses to TOF stimulation (i.e. approximately 20–25% recovery). For atracurium, the intubating dose is 0.4–0.5 mg/kg (2 × ED$_{95}$). A commonly practised technique is to administer an incremental bolus injection equivalent to one-fifth the intubating dose of 0.1 mg/kg approximately 30–40 minutes following intubation. The latter dose is generally repeated every 15–20 minutes to maintain a degree of surgical relaxation equivalent to 75–80% neuromuscular block under nitrous oxide

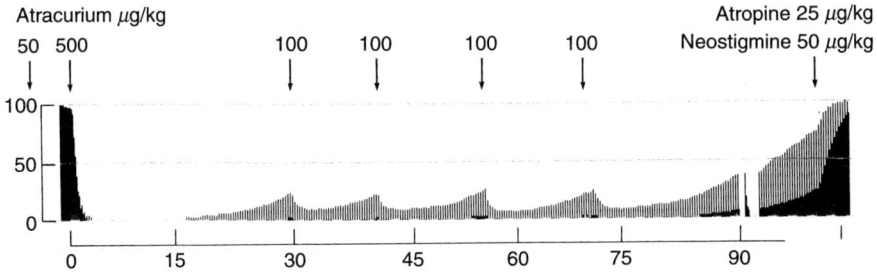

Fig. 5.1 Evoked integrated EMG of the adductor pollicis brevis muscle in response to supra-maximal ulnar nerve stimulation. Arrows indicate administration of drugs, from left to right, atracurium 50 and 500 μg/kg (priming and intubating doses, respectively), followed by four increments of 100 μg/kg, and reversal with atropine 25 μg/kg and neostigmine 50 μg/kg.

opioid anaesthesia (Fig. 5.1). Under inhalation anaesthesia with enflurane or isoflurane, these doses are decreased by 20–30%. For vecuronium, a similar proto-col can be employed with 0.1–0.12 mg/kg for intubation and supplemented with 20 μg/kg when spontaneous recovery reaches 20% of the control response (1–2 responses to TOF).

Generally, with repeated doses of vecuronium, a cumulative effect is more pro-nounced than with atracurium (Ali *et al.* 1983). Fisher and Rosen (1986) compared the duration of an initial dose of atracurium and vecuronium with the duration fol-lowing the fifth incremental dose. The initial bolus of atracurium varied from 150–400 μg/kg followed by five increments of 100 μg/kg each. For vecuronium, the initial dose was 30–80 μg/kg followed by 20 μg/kg increments repeated five times. The duration of action of atracurium boluses did not change, while the dura-tion of the fifth vecuronium increment was significantly greater than the first. These authors suggested that while the action of the initial vecuronium dose is terminated by distribution, recovery from subsequent doses occurs at a time when the initial dose has entered its elimination phase. This factor accounts for the decreased rate of decline of plasma concentration with repeated doses and hence decreased rate of recovery of neuromuscular function. In contrast, termination of effect of an initial atracurium bolus occurs when elimination is predominant. This is equally true of subsequent doses and recovery always occurs at a time when the plasma concentra-tion is falling at an equivalent rate and explains the lack of prolongation of effect with repeated doses of atracurium. There is evidence that the relatively constant and predictable recovery pattern of atracurium even after repeated doses, consti-tutes a real advantage over vecuronium in patients with liver disease (Ward and Neil 1983; Hunter *et al.* 1985; Lebrault *et al.* 1985, 1986; Arden *et al.* 1988), or renal failure (DeBros *et al.* 1986; Smith *et al.* 1987), and in elderly patients (d'Hollander *et al.* 1982, 1983; O'Hara *et al.* 1985; Bell *et al.* 1989; Kitts *et al.* 1990, Lien *et al.* 1991), and obese patients (Weinstein *et al.* 1988; Matteo *et al.* 1989).

The difference in the cumulative properties between atracurium and vecuronium results from their different modes of elimination. Neill *et al.* (1983) suggested that atracurium may be eliminated solely by Hofmann degradation and ester hydrolysis rather than by organ-based metabolism or excretion. Fisher and Rosen (1986), developed a model to describe the pharmacokinetic properties of atracurium. They argued that because elimination of atracurium occurs in both tissue and plasma, traditional pharmacokinetic models assuming elimination from a single central compartment are inaccurate for atracurium. The authors concluded that more than half of the clearance of atracurium occurs via pathways other than Hofmann elimination and ester hydrolysis. The fact that atracurium is eliminated through several pathways is an advantage in clinical use and explains why atracurium is an excellent muscle relaxant for patients with multi-organ failure or other clinical entities, such as extremes of age or obesity.

Vecuronium, on the other hand, having a tertiary amine attached to ring A of the steroid nucleus, is more lipophilic and thus more susceptible to uptake and metabolism by the liver microsomal enzymes. Bencini *et al.* (1988) found in the isolated perfused rat, that 70% of the administered dose was excreted in the bile within two hours and 22% remained in the liver. Of the vecuronium excreted into the bile, 57% was unchanged and 42% was present as 3-desacetylvecuronium. In cat and human studies, approximately 40% of the initial dose was excreted into the bile (Bencini *et al.* 1985, 1986). Pharmacokinetic and pharmacodynamic studies indicated that in patients with liver disease or cirrhosis, the duration of action of vecuronium was increased (Hunter *et al.* 1985). Duvaldestin *et al.* (1982) and Lebrault *et al.* (1985, 1986) found an increased elimination half-life due to decreased clearance and prolonged duration of action in patients with liver cirrhosis and in patients with cholestasis.

An initial intubating dose followed by continuous infusion

Vecuronium and especially atracurium are suitable for administration by infusion because they are minimally cumulative. A commonly practised technique is to achieve a clinically effective plasma concentration with an initial bolus dose and thereafter an infusion is titrated to effect, to maintain approximately 90% block or 1 to 2 responses to TOF stimulation. The initial infusion rates for atracurium or vecuronium are 10 μg/kg/min and 2 μg/kg/min, respectively, and these should be adjusted according to the neuromuscular response under nitrous oxide-opioid anaesthesia (Fig. 5.2). These rates are reduced by approximately 30% during inhalation anaesthesia.

Administration of these drugs by infusion can be accomplished by several methods. Among these are the gravity drip method using a dilution of atracurium of 500 μg/ml in 5% dextrose in water (100 μg/ml for vecuronium), or by using any of the commercially available infusion pumps. There are other infusion pumps which do not require dilution of the relaxant and can be set to give a bolus and/or continuous infusion by setting the patient's weight and the dose/kg and the infusion rate (μg/kg/min).

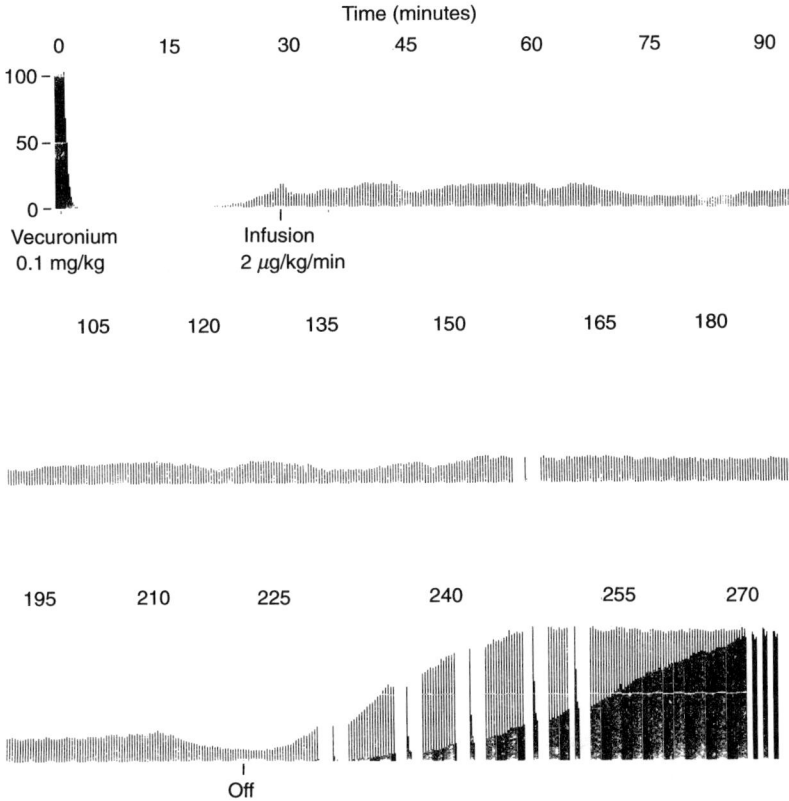

Fig. 5.2 Evoked integrated EMG of the adductor pollicis brevis muscle in response to an intubating dose of vecuronium 0.1 mg/kg. Infusion started after 30 min at 10% spontaneous recovery at a rate of 2 μg/kg/min. The infusion rate was adjusted to maintain approximately 90% neuromuscular block for 200 min followed by spontaneous recovery.

Feedback control systems for the delivery of muscle relaxants have been intro-duced to maintain a neuromuscular response at or close to a chosen set point. Each system consists of a controller which uses information obtained from a neuromus-cular function monitor (e.g. EMG response) to regulate the relaxant infusion rate. Methods for control included on–off (DeVries *et al.* 1986), proportional infusion (Asbury and Linkens 1986), state estimation (Bradlow *et al.* 1985), and propor-tional-integral-derivative (PID) (Ritchie *et al.* 1985; O'Hara *et al.* 1991). The PID system appears to minimize the overshoot and oscillation seen with other systems. It uses three components of the measured response to regulate the infusion rate. The error signal (proportional component) alters the drug infusion rate in proportion to the difference between the actual twitch height and the desired twitch height. The integral component integrates the area between the actual and desired values of the twitch height with time. The derivative component assesses how quickly the actual twitch height is approaching the desired value and makes an adjustment proportional to the rate of change. It must be emphasized that, since all control systems depend entirely on the measured twitch height for their information input, this measurement must be reliable to ensure success.

Both atracurium and vecuronium have minimal cardiovascular effects. Neuromuscular block induced by either drug can be easily reversed provided some evidence of spontaneous recovery is present. There is evidence that the recovery pattern of atracurium is more predictable than that of vecuronium in healthy patients. The 25–75% recovery time (recovery index) following atracurium is constant irrespective of the dose given or the duration of infusion (Gargarian *et al.* 1984; Basta *et al.* 1988). By contrast, Feldman (1987) found that the recovery index increased from 13.7 ± 5.7 min (mean ± SE) to 30 ± 11.8 min when the bolus dose of vecuronium was increased from 0.1 to 0.25 mg/kg. These findings were in agreement with Fahey *et al.* (1981); when the bolus dose of vecuronium was increased from 0.07 to 0.28 mg/kg, the recovery index changed from 8± 0.4 to 38.0 ± 0.5 min. With prolonged administration or following a high dose, vecuronium is more likely to demonstrate cumulative effects than atracurium. The TOF ratio at the point of recovery of the first twitch to 95% of the control height was significantly less after the final dose of vecuronium than after the first dose (Ali *et al.* 1983). It is apparent that the use of atracurium and vecuronium by infusion intra-operatively in normal healthy surgical patients is practical and may be beneficial (Eager *et al.* 1984; Gargarian *et al.* 1984). It has also, however, been demonstrated that the response to atracurium is more consistent and more predictable than vecuronium, particularly in patients with organ dysfunction (liver and kidney), the elderly, and obese patients.

The next issue to be addressed is the clinical use of atracurium and vecuronium for longer periods in critically ill patients in the intensive care unit (ICU) and the role of their metabolites in the contribution of undesirable side-effects.

For atracurium, clinical reports suggested that its administration by infusion is safe and useful in the management of the critically ill patients in the ICU (Griffiths *et al.* 1986; Wadon *et al.* 1986). Concern has, however, been expressed regarding possible cerebral excitatory activity induced by laudanosine, a metabolite of both Hofmann degradation and ester hydrolysis (Hennis *et al.* 1986). Yate *et al.* (1987) used an atracurium infusion in the ICU to facilitate mechanical ventilation. The duration of infusion was 38–219 hours and the average infusion rate was 0.76 mg/kg/hour. In six patients, maximum plasma concentration of laudanosine was 1.9–5 μg/ml which reached a plateau after two to three days. The latter concentration was far less than the 17 μg/ml, the threshold level for seizure activity in the dog and rat (Mercier and Mercier 1966; Scheepstra *et al.* 1986). The electroencephalogram in two patients at days 5 and 6 of the infusion showed no evidence of cerebral excitation. In 14 critically ill patients who received an initial bolus dose of atracurium of 0.6 mg/kg followed by infusion at a rate of 0.6 mg/kg/hour for a period of 11–47 hours, plasma laudanosine reached a plateau of about 1.2 μg/ml within 10 hours in seven patients with normal renal function. The other seven

Table 5.1 Ultrashort and short-acting relaxants

Drug	ED_{95} (mg/kg)	Intubating dose (mg/kg)	Recovery to 95% (min)
Suxamethonium	0.25	1.0	12–15
Mivacurium	0.09	0.15–0.25	24–30

patients were in renal failure and their plasma laudanosine was quite variable. The highest value measured was 4.3 μg/ml (Parker *et al*. 1988).

Vecuronium does not behave the same way when used in large doses or by infusion for long periods as it does when given by a bolus dose or very short infusion. Some reports have suggested that there is little difference between the pharmacokinetics of vecuronium in patients with and without renal failure (Fahey *et al*. 1981; Bencini *et al*. 1986). Other studies have reported that the duration of action of vecuronium is prolonged in the presence of renal failure (LePage *et al*. 1987; Slater *et al*. 1988). Recently, two cases have been reported where vecuronium was administered by continuous infusion (total dose 337 mg) or repeated bolus doses (total dose 83 mg). These two patients developed renal failure necessitating several haemodialysis courses but no liver failure. Prolonged neuromuscular block persisted for seven days following discontinuation of vecuronium infusion in the first patient and 40 hours after the last dose in the second patient (Segredo *et al*. 1990). These authors explained the prolonged neuromuscular block on persistent high level of a vecuronium metabolite 3-desacetylvecuronium which has approximately 50% of the potency of the parent compound vecuronium. It appears that contrary to earlier beliefs, this metabolite is eliminated via liver uptake and excretion. It was suggested that 3-desacetylvecuronium elimination is highly dependent on renal function. Segredo *et al*. (1991) went on to study the pharmacokinetics of 3-desacetylvecuronium in cats. They found that 70% of 3-desacetylvecuronium was recovered in the liver and bile and only 19% in the urine in cats, hence the liver is the primary organ of elimination of this vecuronium metabolite. This did not explain its accumulation in patients with kidney failure who have received vecuronium for a prolonged period. These findings may be due to species differences or to the fact that the cat data only represent the result after a single bolus of 3-desacetylvecuronium and not

Table 5.2 Intermediate-acting relaxants

Drug	ED_{95} (mg/kg)	$2 \times ED_{95}$[*] (mg/kg)	Clinical duration[**] (min)	Recovery to 95%[+] (min)
Atracurium	0.25	0.5	30–40	60–70
Vecuronium	0.05	0.1	30–40	60–80
ORG 9426	0.4	0.8	30–40	60–80

[*] A clinical intubating dose. [**] Duration from injection of intubating dose to 25% recovery. [+] At the intubating dose.

Table 5.3   Continuous infusion of relaxants under N_2O opioid–barbiturate anaesthesia

Drug	Infusion rate μg/kg/min mean (range)	Recovery index 25–75% (min)
Atracurium	7.9 (4.8–12)	11–12
Vecuronium	1.2 (0.9–4)	15–20
Mivacurium	8.3 (2–14)	6–7
Rocuronium	11.5 (8–15)	12–15

The infusion rate above is reduced by 20–30% under inhalation anesthesia (enflurane, isoflurane).

after chronic administration. The fact still remains that prolonged administration of vecuronium in ICU-type patients leads to persistent neuromuscular block which has not been experienced with prolonged infusions of atracurium.

Tables 5.1, 5.2, and 5.3 summarize the potency, intubating doses, recovery times and infusion rates of the ultrashort-, the short- and the intermediate-acting neuromuscular blocking drugs.

LONG-ACTING NEUROMUSCULAR BLOCKING DRUGS

These drugs range from the naturally occurring tubocurarine, through the semisynthetic relaxants, metocurine and alcuronium, to the synthetic nondepolarizing relaxants, gallamine, pancuronium, pipecuronium, and doxacurium. These drugs all share the common characteristics of being long acting, mostly cumulative, with a prolonged

Table 5.4   Long-acting relaxants

Drug	ED_{95}	Intubating dose	Clinical duration[*]
d-tubocurarine	0.51	0.5–0.6	80–100
Metocurine	0.28	0.3–0.4	80–100
Pancuronium	0.07	0.1	80–100
Alcuronium	0.2	0.2	80–100
Pipecuronium	0.05	0.1	60
Doxacurium	0.03	0.05–0.08	60–80

[*] Injection to 25% recovery at the ED_{95}.

At intubating dose, the onset is faster, usually at 3–5 minutes, and the clinical duration is longer (in the range of 80–120 minutes).

The supplemental dose is approximately a fifth of the intubating dose and more appropriately titrated to effect, to maintain one to two responses to train-of-four stimulation.

elimination half-life, a slow clearance, and a dependency on renal and hepatic elimination. Their potencies, onsets, and clinical durations are summarized in Table 5.4. The combination of direct histamine release and ganglion block following tubocurarine results in a significant reduction in peripheral resistance and a fall in arterial blood pressure at a dose close to the ED$_{95}$, especially if injected rapidly.

Metocurine is a trimethylated derivative of tubocurarine. It produces less ganglion block and histamine release than the parent compound and hence gained more acceptance in cardiovascular surgery (Savarese *et al.* 1977). Alcuronium is two to three times more potent than tubocurarine and has few undesirable side-effects. Gallamine has a strong vagolytic effect which occurs at every dose range (Bowman 1982), and indirect sympathomimetic effects (Brown and Crout 1970). Prolonged neuromuscular block may occur with repeated doses which are not readily reversible by anticholinesterases (Miller *et al.* 1972).

Pancuronium has certain similarities to gallamine, because it inhibits muscarinic acetylcholine receptors in the heart (Coleman *et al.* 1972). It also has an indirect cardiac sympathomimetic effect (Segerra-Domenech *et al.* 1976; Docherty and McGrath 1977). Its use is associated with a greater incidence of myocardial ischaemia during coronary artery bypass grafting (Thomson and Putnins 1985). Pancuronium also increases atrioventricular conduction and increases the incidence of premature ventricular beats (Geha *et al.* 1977). Pancuronium is partly metabolized (deacetylated) in the liver, but the kidney is responsible for eliminating the greater part of pancuronium administered.

Administration of a combination of pancuronium and metocurine or pancuronium and tubocurarine appears to produce a significantly greater effect than the sum of their individual effects. However, this potentiation has not been seen when metocurine is combined with tubocurarine (Lebowitz *et al.* 1980). Interestingly, the combination of the two relaxants yields a neuromuscular block of intermediate duration (Fig. 5.3) with minimal cardiovascular changes when compared with equipotent doses of each individual drug (Lebowitz *et al.* 1981).

Two new long-acting relaxants, pipecuronium bromide (a bisquaternary nondepolarizing steroid derivative) and doxacurium chloride (a bisquaternary benzylisoquinolinium diester), have recently become available. Their main advantage over the older long-acting relaxants is the absence of significant autonomic or histaminergic cardiovascular effects. Their potency, onset, and clinical durations are summarized in Table 5.4. The potency of pipecuronium appears to be increased during enflurane and isoflurane but not during halothane anaesthesia (Pittet *et al.* 1989; Foldes *et al.* 1990). During fentanyl–nitrous oxide–oxygen anaesthesia, a dose of 70 μg/kg provided intubating conditions in 3–4 min and a clinical duration of approximately one hour. No cardiovascular effects were seen in doses up to 3 × ED$_{95}$ (Tassonyi *et al.* 1988; Larijani *et al.* 1989), in patients undergoing coronary artery surgery or general surgery. Renal elimination is the primary route by which pipecuronium is cleared from plasma in humans and dogs (Caldwell *et al* 1989; Khuenl-Brady *et al.* 1989).

Doxacurium, like pipecuronium, undergoes little or no metabolism and the major route of elimination is the kidney (Dresner *et al.* 1990; Cook *et al.* 1991). At doses

Time (minutes)

| 0 | 15 | 30 | 45 | 60 | 75 | 90 |

dTC 12.0 mg   3.0   –   3.0   –
Panc 1.8 mg   0.5   0.5   –   0.5

| 105 | 120 | 135 | 150 | 165 | 170 | 175 | 180 | 183 |

          3.0   –   A 2.0 mg   A 0.5 mg
           –   1.0   N 4.0 mg   N 1.0 mg

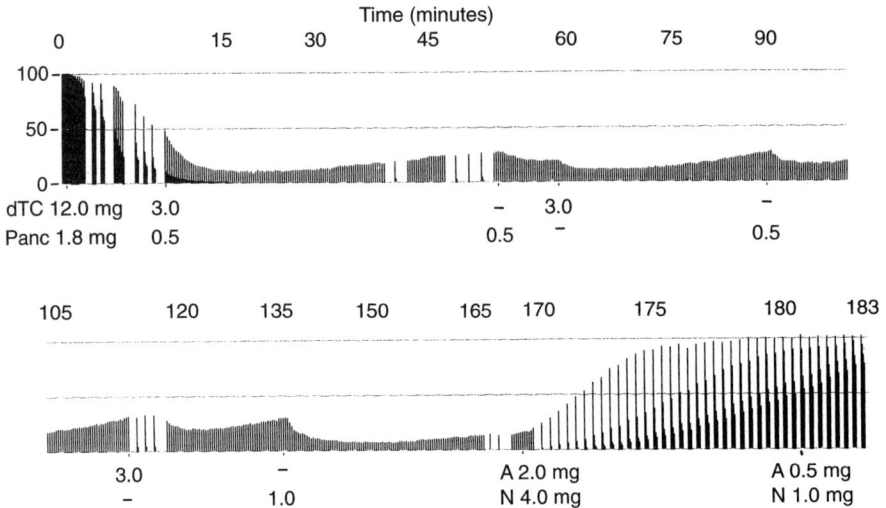

Fig. 5.3 Evoked integrated EMG of the adductor pollicis brevis muscle in response to a combination of *d*-tubocurarine (dTC) 0.15 mg/kg and pancuronium (Panc) 20 μg/kg, and increments of *d*-tubocurarine 3.0 mg alternating with pancuronium 0.5 mg. Reversal was induced with atropine (A) and neostigmine (N).

up to 2.7–3 $\times$ ED$_{95}$ (80 μg/kg), doxacurium produces no effect on heart rate or mean arterial pressure or any elevation in plasma histamine level (Basta *et al.* 1988; Murray *et al.* 1988). Doxacurium has been shown to be useful in patients undergoing coronary artery surgery or valve replacement, and for major vascular surgery in patients with cardiac disease (Stoops *et al.* 1988; Reich *et al.* 1989). Young adults and elderly patients have similar dose requirements, although in the elderly onset time and recovery times are slightly longer (Dresner *et al.* 1990). The likely role of doxacurium and pipecuronium is mostly in cardiac surgery, and long vascular and other procedures in which haemodynamic stability is particularly important.

The long-acting relaxants are generally administered as a bolus of 1–3 $\times$ ED$_{95}$ depending on the drug used and its haemodynamic profile. The maintenance of neuromuscular block is generally accomplished by using approximately a fifth of the original dose when a supplemental dose is indicated by monitoring data, generally at 20–25% twitch recovery or 2–3 responses to TOF stimulation.

IN SUMMARY

Neuromuscular block should be regarded as an integral component of a balanced anaesthetic technique to provide hypnosis, analgesia, and muscle relaxation, and complemented with controlled ventilation to maintain oxygenation and end-tidal carbon dioxide in the normal range. The maintenance of neuromuscular block can be accomplished in a way that ensures adequate surgical relaxation yet does not cover up for inadequate anaesthesia with the resultant recall or awareness during surgery. With adequate knowledge of the clinical pharmacology of the various classes of relaxants which include the ultrashort-, the short-, the intermediate- and the long-acting neuromuscular blocking drugs, we can choose the appropriate relaxant, and the mode of administration which is most suitable for the particular surgical procedure. Titrating the dose to effect, employing the currently available means of monitoring neuromuscular function, will avoid relaxant overdose, prolonged neuromuscular block, and inadequate reversal. This, in turn, will increase the efficiency of utilization of the operating rooms and post-anaesthesia recovery units, and consequently help to contain the staggering cost of medical care.

REFERENCES

Ali, H. H., Savarese . J. J., Embree, P. B., Basta, S. J., Stout, R. G., Bottros, L. H., *et al.* (1988). Clinical pharmacology of mivacurium chloride (BW B1090U) infusion: comparison with vecuronium and atracurium. *British Journal of Anaesthesia*, **61**, 541–6.

Ali, H. H., Savarese, J. J., Basta, S. J., Sunder, N., and Gionfriddo, M. (1983). Evaluation of cumulative properties of three new non-depolarizing neuromuscular blocking drugs BW A444U, atracurium and vecuronium. *British Journal of Anaesthesia*, **55**, 107–11S.

Andersen, B. N., Madsen, J. V., Schurizer, B. A., and Juhl, B. (1988). Residual curarization: a comparative study of atracurium and pancuronium. *Acta Anaesthesiologica Scandinavica*, **32**, 79–81.

Arden, J. R., Lynam, D. P., Castagnoli, B. A., Canfell, C., Cannon, J. C., and Miller, R. D. (1988). Vecuronium in alcoholic liver disease. A pharmacokinetic and pharmacodynamic analysis. *Anesthesiology*, **68**, 771–6.

Asbury, A. J. and Linkens, D. A. (1986). Clinical automatic control of neuromuscular blockade. *Anaesthesia*, **41**, 316–20.

Basta, S. J., Savarese, J. J., Ali, H. H., Embree, P. B., Schwartz, A. F., Rudd D., *et al.* (1988). Clinical pharmacology of doxacurium chloride. *Anesthesiology*, **69**, 478–86.

Beemer, G. H., and Rozenthal, P. (1986). Postoperative neuromuscular function. *Anaesthesia and Intensive Care*, **14**, 41–45.

Bell, P. F., Mirakhur, R. K., and Clarke, R. S. J. (1989). Dose response studies of atracurium, vecuronium and pancuronium in the elderly. *Anaesthesia*, **44**, 925–27.

Bencini, A. F., Houwertjes, M. C., and Agoston, S. (1985). Effects of hepatic uptake of vecuronium bromide and its putative metabolites on their neuromuscular blocking actions in the cat. *British Journal of Anaesthesia*, **57**, 789–95.

Bencini, A. F., Scaf, A. M. J., Sohn, Y. J., Meisterlman , C., Lienhart, A., Kersten, U. W., *et al.* (1986). Disposition and urinary excretion of vecuronium bromide in anaesthetized patients with normal renal function or renal failure. *Anesthesia and Analgesia*, **65**, 245–51.

Bencini, A. F., Mol, W. E. M., Scaf, A. H. J., Kersten, U. W., Wolters, K. T. P., Agoston, S., *et al.* (1988). Uptake and excretion of vecuronium bromide in the isolated perfused rat. *Anesthesiology*, **69**, 487–92.

Bennett A. E. (1940). Preventing traumatic complications in convulsive shock therapy by curare. *Journal of the American Medical Association*, **114**, 322–4.

Bernard, C. (1856). Analyse physiologique des properiétés des systemes musculaire et nerveux au majen due curare. *Compte Rendus de l'Acadademie de Science (Paris)*, **43**, 825–9.

Bevan, D. R., Smith, C. E., and Donati, F. (1988). Postoperative neuromuscular blockade: a comparison between atracurium, vecuronium and pancuronium. *Anesthesiology*, **69**, 272–6.

Bowman, W. C. (1982). Non-relaxant properties of neuromuscular blocking drugs. *British Journal of Anaesthesia*, **54**, 147–60.

Bradlow, H. S., Isys, P. C., and Rametti, L. B. (1985). On-line control of atracurium induced muscle relaxation. *Journal of Biomedical Engineering*, **8**, 72- 5.

Brown, B. R. and Crout, J. R. (1970). The sympathomimetic effects of gallamine on the heart. *Journal of Pharmacology and Experimental Therapeutics*, **172**, 266–73.

Bryn Thomas, K. (1951). *Curare: Its history and usage*, p. 34. Pitman Medical, London.

Caldwell, J. E., Canfell, P. C., Castagnoli, P. C., Lynam, D. M., Fahey, M. R., Fisher, D. M., *et al.* (1989). The influence of renal failure on the pharmacokinetics and duration of action of pipecuronium bromide in patients anesthetized with halothane and nitrous oxide. *Anesthesiology*, **70**, 7–12.

Coleman, A. J., Downing, J. W., Leary, W. P., and Style, M. (1972). The immediate cardiovascular effects of pancuronium, alcuronium and tubocurarine in man. *Anaesthesia*, **27**, 415–22.

Cook, D. R., Freeman, J. A., Lai, A. A., Robertson, K. A., Kang, Y., Stiller, R. L., *et al.* (1991). Pharmacokinetics and pharmaco dynamics of doxacurium in normal patients and in those with hepatic or renal failure. *Anesthesia and Analgesia*, **72**, 145–50.

Crile, G. W. (1913). The kinetic theory of shock and its prevention through anoci-association (shockless operation). *Lancet*, **2**, 7–16.

Cullen, S. C. (1943). The use of curare for improvement of abdominal relaxation during halothane anesthesia: report of 131 cases. *Surgery*, **14**, 261–6.

DeBros, F. M., Lai, A. A., Scott, R., DeBros, J., Batson, A. G., Goudsouzian, N., *et al.* (1986). Pharmacokinetics and pharmaco dynamics of atracurium during isoflurane anesthesia in normal and anephric patients. *Anesthesia and Analgesia*, **65**, 743–6.

DeVries, J. W., Ros, H. H., and Booij, L. H. D. (1986). Infusion of vecuronium controlled by a closed loop system. *British Journal of Anaesthesia*, **58**, 1100–3.

Docherty, J. R. and McGrath, J. C. (1977). Sympathomimetic effect of pancuronium bromide on the cardiovascular system of the pithed rat: a comparison with the effects of drugs blocking neuronal uptake of noradrenaline. *British Journal of Pharmacology*, **64**, 589–99.

Dresner, D. L., Basta, S. J., Ali, H. H., Schwartz, A. F., Embree, P. B., Wargin, W. A., *et al.* (1990). Pharmacokinetics and pharmacodynamics of doxacurium in young and elderly patients during isoflurane anesthesia. *Anesthesia and Analgesia*, **71**, 498–502.

Duvaldestin, P., Berger, J. L., Videcoq, M., and Desmonts, J. M. (1982). Pharmacokinetics and pharmacodynamics of ORG NC45 inpatients with cirrhosis. *Anesthesiology*, **57**, A238.

Eagar, B. M., Flynn, J., and Hughes, R. (1984). Infusion of atracurium for long surgical procedures. *British Journal of Anaesthesia*, **56**, 447–52.

Fahey, M. R., Morris, R. B., Miller, R.D., Nguyen, T. L., and Upton, R. A. (1981). Pharmacokinetics and ORG NC45 (Norcuron) in patients with and without renal failure. *British Journal of Anaesthesia*, **53**, 1049–53.

Feldman, S. A. (1987). Vecuronium — a variable dose technique. *Anaesthesia*, **42**, 199–201.

Fisher, D. M. and Rosen, J. L. (1986). A pharmacokinetic explanation for increasing recovery time following larger or repeated doses of non-depolarizing muscle relaxants. *Anesthesiology*, **65**, 286–91.

Foldes, F. F., McNall, P. G., and Borrego-Hinejosa, J. H. (1952). Succinylcholine: a new approach to muscular relaxation in anesthesiology. *New England Journal of Medicine*, **247**, 596–600.

Foldes, F. F. (1990). The impact of neuromuscular blocking agents on the development of anesthesia and surgery. In *Monographs in anesthesiology: Muscle relaxants.* (ed. S. Agoston and W. C. Bowman) p. 9. Elsevier, Amsterdam.

Foldes, F. F., Nagashina, H., Nguyen, H. D., Duncal, D., and Goldiner, P. L. (1990). Neuromuscular and cardiovascular effects of pipecuronium. *Canadian Journal of Anaesthesia*, **37**, 549–55.

Forbes, A. R., Cohen, N. H., and Egerm, E. I., II. (1979). Pancuronium reduces halothane requirements in man. *Anesthesia and Analgesia*, **58**, 497–9.

Gargarian, M. A., Basta, S. J., Savarese, J. J., Ali, H. H., Sunder, N., Scott, R., *et al.* (1984). The efficacy of atracurium by continuous infusion. *Anesthesiology*, **61**, A291.

Geha, D. G., Cozelle, B. C., Raessler, K. L., Groves, B. M., Wightman, M. A., and Blitt, C. D. (1977). Pancuronium bromide enhances atrioventricular conduction in halothane anesthetized dogs. *Anesthesiology*, **46**, 342–5.

Gray, T. C. and Halton, J. (1946a). A milestone in anesthesia (*d*-tubocurarine chloride). *Proceedings of the Royal Society of Medicine*, **34**, 400–10.

Gray, T. C. and Halton, J. (1946b). Technique for the use of *d*-tubocurarine chloride with balanced anaesthesia. *British Medical Journal*, **2**, 293–6.

Griffith, H. R. and Johnson, G. E. (1942). The use of curare in general anesthesia. *Anesthesiology*, **3**, 418–20.

Griffith, R. B, Hunter, J. M., and Jone, R. S (1986). Atracurium infusions in patient with renal failure in an ITU. *Anaethesia*, **41**, 375–81.

Hennis, P., Fahey, M. R., Canfel, P. C., Shi, W. Z., and Miller R. D. (1986). Pharmacology of laudanosine in dogs. *Anesthesiology*, **65**, 56–60.

d'Hollander, A. A., Massaux, F., Nevelsteen, M., and Agoston, S. (1982). Age dependent dose-response relationship of ORG NC45 in anaesthetized patients. *British Journal of Anaesthesia*, **54**, 653–7.

d'Hollander, A. A., Luyck, C., Barvais, L., and De Villa, A. (1983). Clinical evaluation of atracurium besylate requirement for a stable muscle relaxation during surgery: lack of age related effects. *Anesthesiology*, **59**, 237–40.

Hugin, V. W. and Kissling, P. (1961). A new relaxant drug Ro 4-3816 (Toxiferine). *Schweizerische MedizinischeWochenschrift*, **81**, 455.

Hunter, J. M., Parker, C. J. R., Bell, C. F., Jones, R. S., and Utting, J. E. (1985). The use of different doses of vecuronium in patients with liver dysfunction. *British Journal of Anaesthesia*, **57**, 758–64.

Johnson, G. V. and Hartzell, C. R. (1985) Choline uptake, acetylcholine synthesis, and release and halothane effects in synaptosomes. *Anesthesia and Analgesia*, **64**, 395–9.

Katz, R. L. and Katz, G. J. (1975). Clinical considerations in the use of muscle relaxants: In *Muscle relaxants* (ed. R. L. Katz), p. 313. Excerpta Medica, Amsterdam.

Katz, R. L. and Ryan, J. F. (1969). Neuromuscular effect of succinylcholine in man. *British Journal of Anaesthesia*, **41**, 381–90.

Khuenl-Brady, K. S., Sharma, M., Chung, K., Miller, R. D., Agoston, S., and Caldwell, J. E. (1989). Pharmacokinetics and disposition of pipecuronium bromide in dogs with and without ligated renal pedicles. *Anesthesiology*, **71**, 919–22.

Kitts, J. B., Fisher, D. M., Claver Canfell, P. C., Spellman, M. J., Caldwell, J. E., Heier, T., *et al.* (1990). Pharmacokinetics and pharmacodynamics of atracurium in the elderly. *Anesthesiology*, **72**, 272–5.

Knight, R. T. (1944). Use of curare in anesthesia. *Minneapolis Medicine*, **27**, 667–70.

Larijani, G. E., Bartkowski, R. R., Seltzer, J. L., Weinberger, M. J., Beach, C. A., and Goldberg, M. E. (1989). Clinical pharmacology of pipecuronium bromide. *Anesthesia and Analgesia*, **68**, 734–9.

LePage, J. Y., Malinge, M., Cozian, A., Pinaud, M., Blanloeil, Y. and Souron, R. (1987). Vecuronium and atracuronium in patients with end stage renal failure. *British Journal of Anaesthesia*, **59**, 1004–10.

Lebowitz, P. W., Ramsey, F. M., Savarese, J. J., and Ali, H. H. (1980). Potentiation of neuromuscular blockade in man produced by combinations of pancuronium and metocurine or pancuronium and *d*-tubocurarine. *Anesthesia and Analgesia*, **59**, 604–9.

Lebowitz, P. W., Ramsey, F. M., Savarese, J. J., Ali, H. H., and DeBros, F. M. (1981). Combination of pancuronium and metocurine: neuromuscular and cardiovascular advantages over pancuronium alone. *Anesthesia and Analgesia*, **60**, 12–7.

Lebrault, C., Berger, J. L., d'Hollander, A. A., Gomeni, R., Henzel, D., and Duvaldestin, P. (1985). Pharmacokinetics and pharmacodynamics of vecuronium (ORG NC45) in patients with cirrhosis. *Anesthesiology*, **62**, 601–5.

Lebrault, C., Duvaldestin, P., Henzel Chauvin, M., and Guesnon, P. (1986). Pharmacokinetics and pharmacodynamics of vecuronium in patients with cholestasis. *British Journal of Anaesthesia*, **58**, 983–7.

Lee, C. and Katz, R. L. (1975). Dose relationship of phase II, tachyphylaxis and train of four fade in suxamethonium induced dual neuromuscular block in man. *British Journal of Anaesthesia*, **47**, 481–5.

Lennmarken, C. and Lofstrom, J. B. (1984). Partial curarization in the postoperative period. *Acta Anaesthesiologica Scandinavica* **28**, 260–2.

Lien, C. A., Matteo, R. S., Ornstein, E., Schwartz, A. E., and Diaz, J. (1991). Distribution, elimination and action of vecuronium in the elderly. *Anesthesia and Analgesia*, **73**, 39–42.

Lundy, J. S. (1926). Balanced anesthesia. *Minnesota Medicine*, **9**, 99. Reprinted in Classical File. (1981) *Survey of Anesthesiology*, **25**, 272–8.

Matteo, R. S., Schwartz, A. E., Ornestein, E., Halevy, J., and Diaz, J. (1989). Pharmacokinetics and pharmacodynamics of vecuronium in the obese surgical patient. *Anesthesia and Analgesia*, **68**, S191.

Mercier, J. and Mercier, E. (1966). Action de quelques alcaloides secondaires de l'opium sur l'electrocorticogramme due chien. *Comptes Rendus des Sciences de la Société de Biologie*, **149**, 760–2.

Miller, R. D., Larson, C. P., and Way, W. C. (1972). Comparative antagonism of *d*-tubocurarine, gallamine and pancuronium induced neuromuscular blockade by neostigmine. *Anesthesiology*, **37**, 503–9.

Murray, D. J., Mehta, M. P., Choi, W. W., Forbes, R. B., Sokoll, M. D., Gergis, S. D., *et al.* (1988). The neuromuscular blocking and cardiovascular effects of doxacurium chloride in patients receiving nitrous oxide–narcotic anesthesia. *Anesthesiology*, **69**, 472–7.

Neill, E. A. M., Chappel, D. J., and Thompson, C. W. (1983). Metabolism and kinetics of atracurium: an overview. *British Journal of Anaesthesia*, **55**, 23–5S.

O'Hara, D. A., Fragen, R. J., and Shanks, C.A. (1985). The effects of age on the dose–response curves for vecuronium in adults. *Anesthesiology*, **63**, 542–4.

O'Hara, D. A., Derbyshire, G. J., Overdyk, F. J., Bogen, D. K., and Marshall B. E. (1991) Closed loop infusion of atracurium with four different anesthetic techniques. *Anesthesiology*, **74**, 258–63.

Organe, G. S. W., Paton, W. D., and Zaimes, E. I. (1949). Preliminary trials of bistrimethylammonium decane and pentane diodide (C10 and C5) in man. *Lancet*, **i**, 21–5.

Parker, C. J. R., Jones, J. E., and Hunter, J. M. (1988). Disposition of infusions of atracurium and its metabolite laudanosine, in patients in renal and respiratory failure in the ITU. *British Journal of Anaesthesia*, **61**, 531–40.

Pittet, J. F., Tassonyi, E., Morel, D. R., Gemperle, G., Richter, M., and Rouge, J. C. (1989). Pipecuronium-induced neuromuscular blockade during nitrous oxide–fentanyl, isoflurane and halothane anaesthesia in adults and children. *Anesthesiology*, **1**, 210–3.

Ramsey, F. M., Lebowitz, P. W., Savarese, J. J., and Ali, H. H. (1980). Clinical characteristics of long term succinylcholine infusion under balanced anesthesia. *Anesthesia and Analgesia*, **59**, 110–6.

Rees, G. J. and Gray, T. C. (1950). Methyl-*n*-propyl ether. *British Journal of Anesthesia*, **22**, 83–91.

Reich, D. L., Konstadt, S. N., Thys, D. M., Hillel, Z., Raymond, R., and Kaplan, J. A. (1989). The effects of doxacurium chloride on biventricular function in patients with cardiac disease. *British Journal of Anaesthesia*, **63**, 675–81.

Ritchie, G., Ebert, J. P., Jannett, T. C., Kissin, I., and Sheppard, L. C. (1985). A microcomputer based controller for neuromuscular blockade during surgery. *Annals of Biomedical Engineering*, **13**, 3–15.

Savarese, J. J., Ali, H. H., and Antonio, R. P. (1977). The clinical pharmacology of metocurine: dimethyl tubocurarine revisited. *Anesthesiology*, **47**, 277–84.

Savarese, J. J., Ali, H. H., Basta, S. J., Embree, P. B., Scott, R. P. F., Sunder, N., *et al.* (1988). The clinical neuromuscular pharmacology of mivacurium chloride (BW B1090U). *Anesthesiology*, **68**, 723–32.

Scheepstra, G. L., Vree, T. B., Crul, J. F., Van der Pol, F., Reekers-Ketting, J. (1986). Convulsive effects and pharmacokinetics of laudanosine in the rat. *European Journal of Anaesthesiology*, **3**, 371–83.

Schwartz, A. E., Navedo, A. T., and Berman, A. F. (1991). Pancuronium potentiates the EEG effect of isoflurane in dogs. *Anesthesiology*, **75**, A792.

Segarra-Domenech, J., Garcia, C. R., Sasiain, R. J. M., Loyola, Q., and Orez, J. S. (1976). Pancuronium bromide: an indirect sympathomimetic agent. *British Journal of Anaesthesia*, **48**, 1143–8.

Segredo, V., Matthay, M. A., Sharma, M. L., Gruenke, L. D., Caldwell, J. E., and Miller, R. D. (1990). Prolonged neuromuscular blockade after long-term administration of vecuronium in two critically ill patients. *Anesthesiology*, **72**, 566–70.

Segredo, V., Shin, Y. S., Sharma, M. L., Gruenke, L. D., Caldwell, J. E., Khuenl-Brady, K. S., *et al.* (1991). Pharmacokinetics, neuromuscular effects and biodisposition of 3-desacetylvecuronium (Org 7268) in cats. *Anesthesiology*, **74**, 1052–9.

Slater, R. M., Pollard, B.J., and Doran, B. R. H. (1988). Prolonged neuromuscular blockade with vecuronium in renal failure. *Anaesthesia*, **43**, 250–1.

Smith, C. L., Hunter, J. M., and Jones, R. S. (1987). Vecuronium infusion in patients with renal failure in an ITU. *Anaesthesia*, **42**, 387–93.

Stoops, C. M., Curtis, C. A., Kovach, D. A., McCammon, R. L., Stoelting, R. K., Warren, T. M., *et al.* (1988). Hemodynamic effects of doxacurium chloride in patients receiving oxygen-sufentanil anesthesia for coronary artery bypass or valve replacement. *Anesthesiology*, **69**, 365–70.

Tassonyi, E., Pittet, J. F., Morel, D. R., Gemperie, G., and Ronge, J. C. (1988). Cardiovascular effects of pipecuronium and pancuronium in patients undergoing coronary artery bypass grafting. *Anesthesiology*, **69**, 795–6.

Thesleff, S. (1951). Pharmacologic and clinical experiments with succinylcholine iodide. *Nordisk Medicinsk Tidskrift*, **46**, 1045–9.

Thomson, I. R. and Putnins, C. L. (1985). Adverse effects of pancuronium during high dose fentanyl anesthesia for coronary artery bypass grafting. *Anesthesiology*, **62**, 708–13.

Viby-Mogensen, J., Jorgensen, B. C., and Ording, H. (1979). Residual curarization in the recovery room. *Anesthesiology*, **50**, 539–41.

Viby-Mogensen, J., Howardy-Hansen, P., Chraemer-Jorgensen, B., Ording, H., Engbaek, J., and Nielsen, A. (1981). Post-tetanic count (PTC): a new method of evaluating an intense nondepolarizing neuromuscular blockade. *Anesthesiology*, **55**, 458–61.

Wadon, A. J., Dogra, S., and Anand, S. (1986). Atracurium infusions in the intensive care unit. *British Journal of Anaesthesia*, **58**, 64–7S.

Ward, S. and Neill, E. A. M. (1983). Pharmacokinetics of atracurium in acute hepatic failure (with acute renal failure). *British Journal of Anaesthesia*, **55**, 1169–72

Weinstein, J. A., Matteo, R. S., Ornstein, E., Schwartz, A. E., Goldstoff, M. and Thal, G. (1988). Pharmacodynamics of vecuronium and atracurium in the obese surgical patient. *Anesthesia and Analgesia*, **67**, 1149–53.

West, R. (1932). Curare in man. *Proceedings of the Royal Society of Medicine*, **25**, 1107–16.

Yate, P. M., Flynn, P. J., Arnold, R. W., Weatherly, B. C., Simmonds, R. J., and Dopson, T. (1987). Clinical experience and plasma laudanosine concentrations during the infusion of atracurium in the intensive therapy unit. *British Journal of Anaesthesia*, **59**, 211–17.

6

Recovery from a neuromuscular block

S. A. Feldman and N. Fauvel

In this chapter, the spontaneous recovery of a neuromuscular block will be considered. In the clinical practice of anaesthesia, it is common to accelerate recovery from a neuromuscular block by the use of an anticholinesterase drug, and this is considered in Chapter 7. If no reversal agent were given, there would eventually be a full recovery and it is this process which forms the subject of this chapter.

It has been suggested that the recovery from a nondepolarizing neuromuscular block results from the fall in plasma level of drug which is caused by redistribution, excretion, and metabolism. This results in a slow washout of drug from the junctional cleft along its concentration gradient. Thus the current view is that it is principally a pharmacokinetic effect which determines recovery from a neuromuscular block (Matteo *et al.* 1974; Ham *et al.* 1979; Shanks *et al.* 1979; Hull *et al.* 1980). This is, of course, directly analogous to the processes occurring during the onset of block (Chapter 4). Onset of block is relatively rapid as the drug enters the junctional cleft under the influence of a high concentration gradient between the plasma and the junction. Block is reversed by the slower washout of drug along a smaller concentration gradient as the level of drug in the plasma falls. This assumption was the basis of early pharmacokinetic studies in which an effort was made to associate the degree of neuromuscular block with a particular plasma level of drug (Matteo *et al.* 1974; Shanks *et al.* 1979).

Whilst this assumption is reasonable at an equilibrium state it is probable that it poorly reflects what is observed in clinical practice when a bolus dose of drug is given and its effects are allowed to wear off before further top-up doses are given. Under these circumstances, the recovery fails to explain the commonly observed lag between the rapid fall in plasma concentration of drug and the slower recovery of neuromuscular function (Hull *et al.* 1980; Hull 1982). The observation that the same degree of block can be achieved at very different plasma concentrations of drug is also very difficult to reconcile with this theory (Feldman 1973). It also fails to explain the differences observed in recovery rates from neuromuscular block produced by different drugs of similar physical properties and similar plasma half-lives. As a result of these deficiencies, it has been necessary to include a third 'buffer', 'effector' or 'biophase' compartment in the mathematical models of observed pharmacokinetic and pharmacodynamic events.

THE PHARMACOKINETICS OF NEUROMUSCULAR BLOCKING AGENTS

All of the neuromuscular blocking drugs in clinical use are water soluble, positively charged molecules, which do not readily cross physiological membranes, e.g. the blood–brain barrier. They can all be recovered from the urine although the proportion excreted unchanged may vary from less than 10% to greater than 80%. Following a bolus injection of neuromuscular blocking drug, there is a rapid decline in plasma concentration. This is largely due to rapid redistribution of the drug to the vessel-rich tissues, in particular the kidneys, liver, spleen, and neuromuscular junction. Muscle itself is relatively poorly perfused in the resting state and functions only as a late redistribution site for these drugs (Cohen *et al.* 1965). Autoradiographs of rats who had received radioactive (tritiated) tubocurarine (Fig. 6.1) demonstrate the rapid distribution of the drug to the liver and kidneys where it appears in high concentration. Certain other drugs — including gallamine, pancuronium, and vecuronium — are also rapidly distributed to cartilage, demonstrating that factors other than blood flow may influence tissue uptake. This effect only occurs following injection of a bolus dose of the drug when the plasma concentration is high; it is unlikely that mucopolysaccharide acts as a late sequestration or redistribution volume for these drugs.

The rate of hydrolysis of suxamethonium by plasma cholinesterase depends upon the logarithm of the substrate concentration. It will be most rapid at the time of high plasma concentration immediately following injection (Kalow and Gunn 1957). It is probable that over 50% of the injected bolus dose is hydrolysed before it reaches muscle and that possibly less than 20% of an injected dose actually reaches the neuromuscular junction. Mivacurium, which is reported to be hydrolysed by plas-

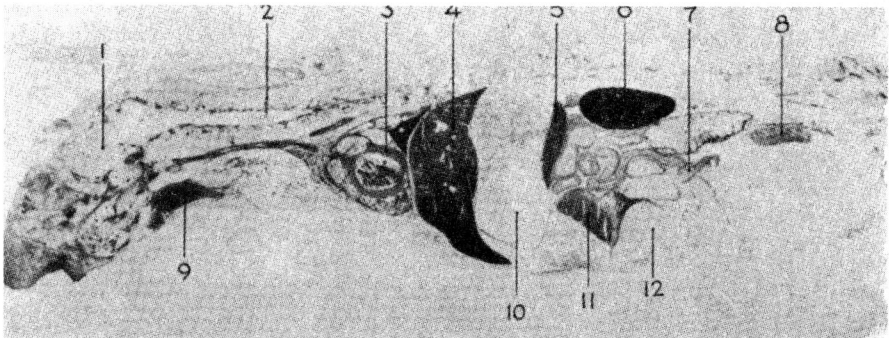

Fig. 6.1 Autoradiograph of rat 3 min after administration of ^{3}H tubocurarine. 1, brain; 2, spinal cord; 3, heart; 4, liver; 5, spleen; 6, kidney; 7, gut; 8, bladder; 9, salivary gland; 10. stomach; 11, placenta; 12, fetus.

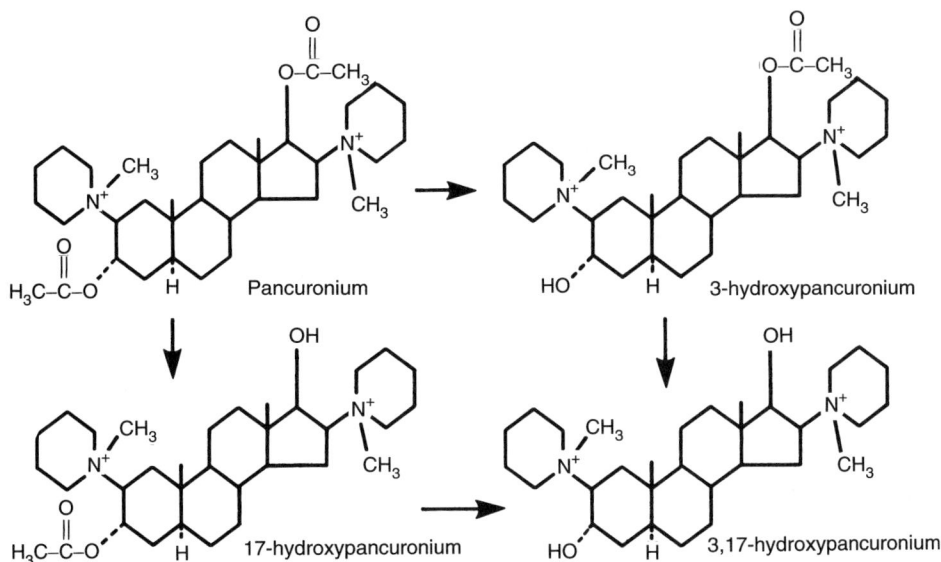

Fig. 6.2 Potential metabolic pathways for pancuronium.

macholinesterase at 80% of the rate of suxamethonium (Savarese *et al.* 1988), would be presumed to be affected in a similar manner. Following redistribution or metabolism, the plasma level of most neuromuscular blocking drugs is further reduced by renal excretion. Hepatic metabolism and biliary excretion play a part in the plasma clearance of some neuromuscular blocking agents, especially the aminosteroids. Gallamine (Feldman *et al.* 1969) and decamethonium are exclusively excreted unchanged in the urine. No biliary excretion or metabolites of either of these drugs has been identified. Pancuronium, alcuronium, and metocurine are largely excreted in the urine (more than 70%). Pancuronium is, however, excreted in the bile in a variable amount which may be up to 30% either as the parent drug or as metabolites. The metabolism of pancuronium and vecuronium occurs in the liver and the products are the 3-hydroxy, 17-hydroxy, or 3,17-dihydroxy derivatives (Fig. 6.2). Some of the urinary steroid excretion also consists of metabolites. In general the higher the lipid solubility, the greater the hepatic uptake and metabolism. Vecuronium is more readily distributed to the liver than pancuronium and this is reflected in a larger biliary excretion of the drug. The metabolites of vecuronium (also the 3-hydroxy, 17-hydroxy, and 3,17-dihydroxy derivatives) are largely excreted in the urine. Tubocurarine has not been demonstrated to undergo metabolism and is normally excreted unchanged in the urine. If the renal pedicles of animals are ligated, however, up to 35% of an injected dose can be recovered from the bile which provides an alternative excretory pathway (Cohen *et al.* 1967).

There are two pathways for the elimination of atracurium, namely ester hydrolysis in the liver and Hofmann degradation at physiological pH (Fig. 6.3). The

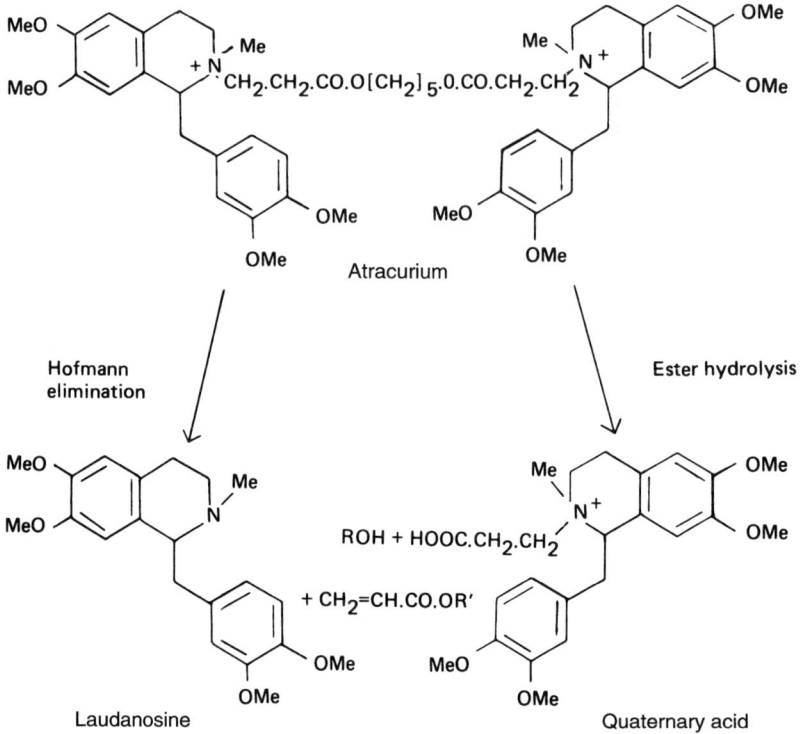

Fig. 6.3 Metabolism of atracurium by ester hydrolysis and Hofmann degradation.

products of breakdown include laudanosine, a tertiary base with a long half-life. There has been disagreement concerning the relative importance of the Hofmann pathway and ester hydrolysis. Hofmann degradation is a physical process with zero-order kinetics. The rate of degradation therefore parallels the plasma concentration of drug. The ester hydrolysis pathway is a first-order process and therefore its rate rapidly decreases as the plasma drug level falls. Laudanosine is largely conjugated in the liver and excreted in the urine. As a result of redistribution and metabolism, the plasma concentration of most drugs administered in a bolus dose of $1-2 \times ED_{95}$ is reduced to a level below that necessary to produce neuromuscular block in approximately 5–7 min. At this plasma concentration reversal of residual block at the end of the operation can be readily achieved with an anticholinesterase drug. The greater the total dose of drug administered, whether by intermittent bolus doses or by continuous infusion, the more likely are the non-active sequestration sites in the liver, kidneys, spleen, and other tissues to be saturated. When this has occured any further reduction of the plasma concentration of drug to subparalytic levels will rely upon the slower and less predictable excretory and metabolic pathways. In these circumstances reversal of neuromuscular block by an anticholinesterase is more difficult and may be incomplete.

INABILITY TO REVERSE A BLOCK

The ability of an agonist to reverse a block resulting from the presence of an antagonist is fundamental to the competition theory. The Schild equation describes the increasing dose of agonist needed, in the presence of an increased concentration of antagonist, to produce the same degree of interference with neuromuscular transmission. On this basis, increasing the dose of antagonist should cause a parallel shift to the right of the log dose–response curve of the agonist in the presence of an increasing concentration of antagonist. This is found to be true for low concentrations of antagonist but the parallelism is lost when larger doses are used. This suggests that some other, or additional, process is modifying the competition or that the action is noncompetitive. To explain these observations various hypotheses have been proposed.

It has been suggested that at higher levels of antagonist a state of quasi-equilibrium exists (Paton and Waud 1967). The inability of neostigmine to produce complete reversal of such a block has been reported with tubocurarine (Burchill 1957), gallamine (Montgomery and Bennett-Jones 1956), and pancuronium. In all these reports the circumstances suggest that the cause was a residual subparalytic but significant level of drug in the plasma. In one case report, lowering the plasma level by haemodialysis allowed complete reversal by neostigmine to be immediately effective (Feldman and Levi 1963). It is because of this phenomenon that the recommendation has been made that reversal of block with neostigmine should not be attempted before the return of 10% twitch response or two responses of the train-of-four. It is possible that this generally good advice is not necessary, or can be modified, with atracurium and mivacurium.

The inability to reverse a nondepolarizing block in the presence of a significant but subparalytic plasma level of drug, like the distortion of the Schild plot with higher concentrations of antagonist, is difficult to reconcile directly with the law of mass action and hence with the competition theory.

REVERSAL BY ANTICHOLINESTERASES

In most instances the residual action of nondepolarizing agents is reversed by an anticholinesterase. The basis of this action is the protection of the acetylcholine (ACh) in the junction from hydrolysis by cholinesterase, so increasing its effective concentration at the receptor site. It has been clearly demonstrated from patch-clamp experiments that ACh reverses nondepolarizing block in a competitive manner at the level of the individual receptor complex and in the absence of antagonist drug. This effect is an all-or-none phenomenon and is accomplished in milliseconds. Such a competitive interaction implies that lowering the antagonist drug concentration or increasing the ACh (agonist) concentration in the synapse will lessen the degree of neuromuscular block. This is undoubtedly true in general terms. In patch-clamp experiments this

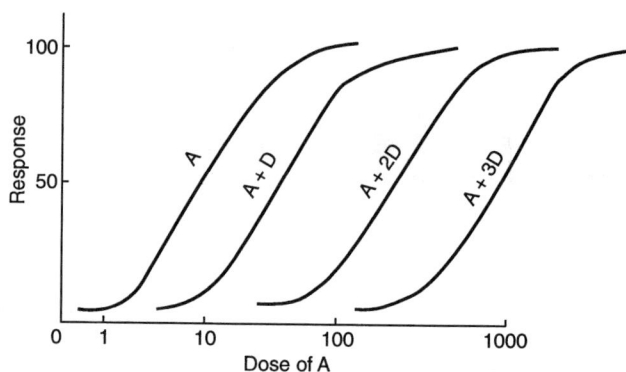

Fig. 6.4 Competitive antagonism — a parallel shift to the right of the log dose–response curve to agonist (A) in the presence of increasing doses of antagonist (D).

reversal of action is represented by an increase in the frequency of the generation of membrane currents implying the opening of sodium channels. When *in vitro* studies are considered, there is a parallel shift to the right of the log dose–response curve in the presence of increasing concentrations of antagonist (Fig. 6.4). There are, however, certain readily observed phenomena that are difficult to explain on the basis of simple competition and the law of mass action. This indicates the need to develop the concept if we are to understand the very much slower process of recovery from neuromuscular block in clinical practice. There are two observations to consider. Firstly, it is not always possible to reverse a neuromuscular block with neostigmine if the plasma concentration is high (Montgomery and Bennett-Jones 1956; Burchill 1957; Churchill-Davidson *et al.* 1967). Secondly, using the isolated arm or forearm to study recovery from neuromuscular block, it can be demonstrated that rapidly lowering the plasma drug concentration does not produce a rapid reversal of neuromuscular block (Feldman and Tyrrell 1970; Feldman 1976).

THE ISOLATED ARM

In 1970, Feldman and Tyrrell proposed a new theory of the termination of action of the muscle relaxants in which they suggested that antagonist agents such as tubocurarine had a high affinity for the receptor substance (the nature of the receptor was unknown at that time) whereas agonist drugs, such as decamethonium, did not. They interpreted their results in terms of Paton's rate theory which envisages antagonists as drugs which dissociate slowly from the receptors, thereby occupying the receptor for a relatively long period and consequently denying access to the biological transmitter. Agonist drugs are envisaged as freely associating and dissociating, enabling them rapidly to produce a continuing biological action at the receptor, which is related to the plasma concentration of drug. The theory was based on the isolated arm experiments in which a small dose of drug (3 mg of tubocurarine,

Vecuronium 0.3 mg

Pancuronium 0.3 mg

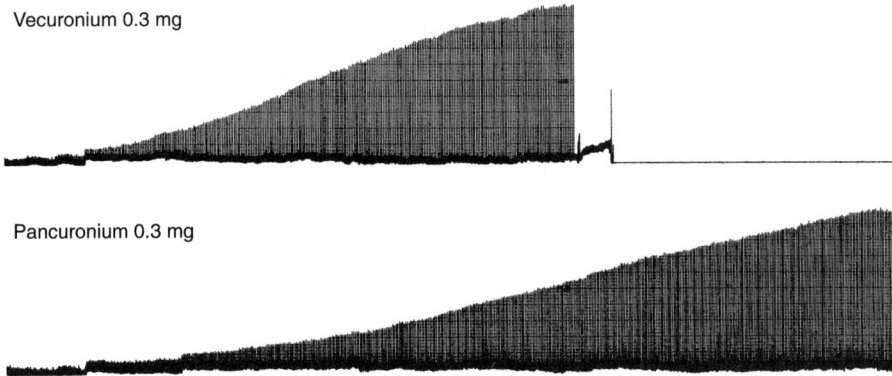

Fig. 6.5 Isolated arm recovery index (time from 25% to 75% recovery) for vecuronium (upper trace) and pancuronium (lower trace).

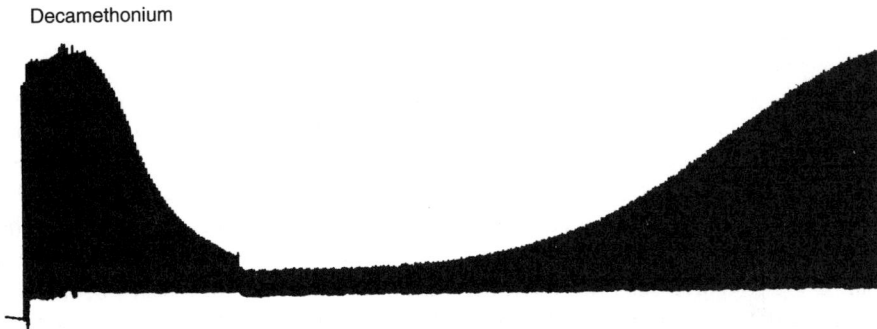

Decamethonium

Fig. 6.6 Isolated arm recovery index following decamethonium 1.0 mg.

8 mg of gallamine or 1 mg of decamethonium) was diluted in 40 ml of saline and injected into a vein on the back of the hand in an arm which was temporarily isolated from the circulation by means of an arterial tourniquet.

Three minutes after injection the tourniquet was released and the small amount of relaxant was diluted in the general circulation. By this means they produced a rapid onset of block followed, after the release of the tourniquet, by a sudden fall in plasma drug level. They argued that the isolated arm technique allowed the dynamic drug receptor process to be studied without any influence from changes in plasma drug concentration. They demonstrated that the block produced by antagonist drugs which included tubocurarine and pancuronium recovered only slowly (Fig. 6.5). This they attributed to drug binding at the receptor. Agonist drugs, for example decamethonium, produced blocks which recovered rapidly (Fig. 6.6) as the drug was washed out from the synapse along its concentration gradient. In subsequent experiments it was shown that the recovery index, which is defined as the time from

Table 6.1 The recovery index of five nondepolarizing neuromuscular blocking agents

Vecuronium	9.2 min /+ 1.8
Pancuronium	14.5 min /+ 2.4
Pipecuronium	13.6 min /+ 2.8
Atracurium	8.8 min /+ 2.1
Rocuronium	9.3 min /+ 1.3

25 to 75% recovery of the twitch response, was different for each drug. It was higher for longer acting drugs, for example pancuronium and tubocurarine and less for shorter acting drugs, for example vecuronium and atracurium. (Table 6.1).

These observations are difficult to reconcile with the competition theory of receptor interactions and the simple pharmacokinetic explanations which have been suggested. In order to explain these results, it has been suggested that the prolonged recovery index is the result of a low blood flow to muscle in the resting state (Waud 1975), residual circulating drug (Hull 1982) or portioning of drug between receptor and other tissues (Stanski and Sheiner 1979). It is difficult, however, to sustain any of these suggested explanations.

Effect of blood flow

In an early series of experiments, Churchill-Davidson and Richardson (1959) showed that there was a more rapid recovery from decamethonium neuromuscular block in the isolated arms of volunteers when there was an increased blood flow. This observation is in keeping with Feldman and Tyrell's theory which suggests that agonist drugs have a low affinity for receptors. It has also been clearly demonstrated that considerable alterations in blood flow (up to eight-fold) do not affect the recovery index from nondepolarizing drugs even when the perfusing blood is free of drug (Goat *et al.* 1976; Heneghan *et al.* 1978; White and Reitan 1984). These results strongly support the contention that nondepolarizing drugs are bound to the receptor whereas depolarizing agents such as decamethonium are not. The idea suggested by Waud (1975) that the long recovery index for tubocurarine in the isolated arm could be explained by blood flow rests on a somewhat tenuous proposition that a total fluid exchange between the plasma and extracellular space is required to effect drug clearance. This would seem to be difficult to reconcile with clinical experience. In addition, if it is assumed that the reverse process would be taking place during onset, this would make the onset of action of tubocurarine impossible in under 9 min.

The effect of residual drug in plasma

The suggestion has been made, on the basis of computer models for fazadinum, that the 0.6 mg of pancuronium released into the circulation when the tourniquet is

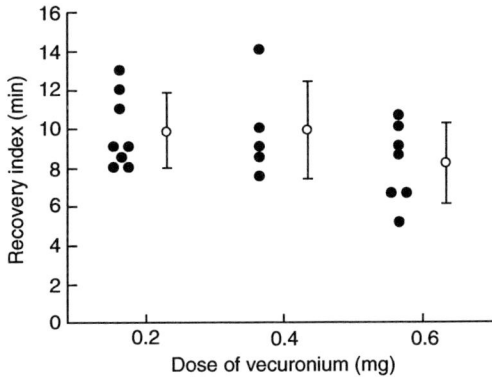

Fig. 6.7 The effect of reducing the dose of vecuronium under the tourniquet from 0.6 mg to 0.2 mg on the recovery index.

removed from an isolated arm produces a brief increase in plasma level of the drug which may account for the slow recovery from nondepolarizing drugs in isolated arm experiments (Hull 1982). The recovery index of vecuronium in the isolated arm has, however, been demonstrated to remain constant when the dose of drug used in the experiment is reduced from 0.6 mg to 0.2 mg and the tourniquet moved to the forearm (Fig. 6.7). It also fails to explain the different recovery indices of vecuronium and pancuronium when these drugs are administered at the same time, one in each isolated forearm of a volunteer, because any residual drug released into the circulation on simultaneous release of the tourniquet will affect both arms equally. Conclusive evidence that the small amount of drug released into the circulation at the time of the release of the tourniquet does not affect recovery of the twitch response comes from the observation that a systemic injection of a similar dose to that administered under the tourniquet at 50% recovery (when the sensitivity to alterations in drug concentration should be greatest) has no effect in the isolated forearm on the recovery index.

Partitioning

Stanski and Sheiner (1979) attributed the slow recovery of the neuromuscular block in the isolated arm to a 'partitioning' of drug between nonspecific tissue and receptor. If such a distribution volume were present then the drug concentration within the compartment would be expected to rise with increased plasma concentration. It has, however, been demonstrated that increasing the dose of vecuronium administered in the isolated arm from 0.2 mg to 2.0 mg does not prolong the time from release of the tourniquet to either 25% or 75% recovery. Had nonspecific partitioning been involved it would have been anticipated that the amount of drug 'partitioned in tissue' would have been greater as a result of a 10-fold greater concentration gradient and hence the recovery would have been delayed.

A further suggestion made by Stanski and Sheiner was that the drug might be partitioned between blood and muscle. The only neuromuscular blocking agent shown to enter muscle, however, is decamethonium and this drug exhibits the quickest recovery. This is not compatible with the theory: it would predict that decamethonium would have the lowest partitioning.

It would be expected that, if partitioning was the cause of the prolonged recovery, nondepolarizing drugs of similar physical characteristics would have a similar recovery index. Furthermore, vecuronium, which is relatively more lipophilic than pancuronium, should have a longer recover index because more drug would be partitioned. This is not the case. The recovery index of vecuronium is shorter than that of pancuronium.

One final consideration is blood flow. Increasing the blood flow would be expected to increase the rate of washout and therefore of recovery if physical partitioning were involved. The finding that an eight-fold increase in blood flow does not affect recovery from nondepolarizing block makes partitioning unlikely.

It is evident that blood flow, recirculation of drug, and partitioning fail to explain the observations in the isolated arm. It is necessary therefore to advance a further hypothesis to account for these observations. The evidence will next be considered with respect to the binding of nondepolarizing drugs in the effector compartment or biophase. This refers to the region at or near to the receptor pentamer where it can readily affect the acetylcholine recognition sites (receptors). Recent studies in our laboratory have suggested that, during recovery from a neuromuscular block, drug remains in the active biophase and that each drug has its own biophase dissociation constant. These studies have involved cross-over experiments using both arms of volunteers (Feldman *et al.* 1992). In these experiments, vecuronium was administered to one isolated forearm and pancuronium to the other at the same time. Both tourniquets were released simultaneously. At 50% recovery of the block in each arm, the tourniquet was reinflated and the drug originally given to the contralateral arm was injected. Three minutes later the tourniquet was released again. It was found that following vecuronium the recovery index of pancuronium was reduced, whilst the recovery index for vecuronium was increased when it was given after pancuronium (Fig. 6.8). This effect was not seen once full recovery from the initial

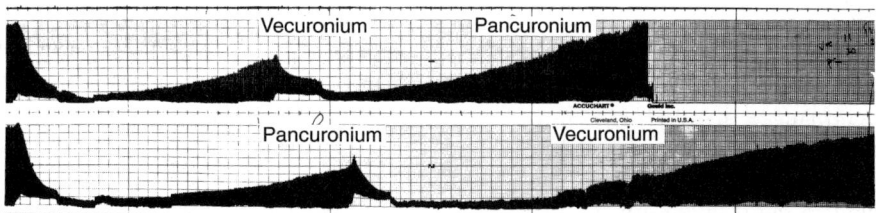

Fig. 6.8 The administration of 0.3 mg vecuronium in one isolated forearm (upper trace) and 0.3 mg pancuronium in the other (lower trace), followed by cross-over of drugs at 50% recovery. The second recovery index of vecuronium (lower trace) is prolonged and that of pancuronium shortened (upper trace).

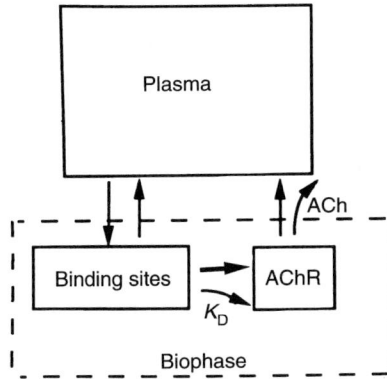

Fig. 6.9 A schematic representation of the relationship of the biophase compartment to plasma. AChR, acetylcholine receptor; K_D, affinity constant.

'conditioning' drug had occurred, suggesting that at the point of 100% recovery little drug remains bound in the biophase.

The ability of one drug to influence the recovery time of a subsequent agent, irrespective of the plasma concentration of either drug, suggests that at 50% recovery some of the initial drug remains bound in the biophase, thereby influencing the recovery of neuromuscular transmission following administration of a second, different agent. In order to explain these events it is necessary to postulate that drug is bound to some structure in the biophase and that either it is released at a rate dependent upon its physicochemical properties into the proximity of the acetylcholine receptor system, where it enters into competitive antagonism with acetylcholine, or it binds to ligand sites and affects the receptor by al allosteric mechanism. (Fig. 6.9). It is evident that the dynamic behaviour of each nondepolarizing drug in the biophase is the principal determinant of the recovery from neuromuscular block and not the blood concentration.

Only if the plasma concentration of drug is low will drug dissociating from the acetylcholine receptor be removed from the junction along its concentration gradient. This process will be accelerated by a high concentration of acetylcholine, such as might follow the use of neostigmine, provided that an adequate concentration gradient exists between the junction and the plasma. This will enhance the rundown of drug bound in the biophase. As reversal of the antagonist action will not occur until the biophase reservoir of drug is exhausted, the presence of a high plasma concentration of drug will frustrate reversal by acetylcholine because the biophase will be replenished from the plasma. It is probable that it is as a result of this mechanism that the linear relationship of the Schild plot is distorted. This also offers an explanation of the failure of reversal of block by neostigmine in patients with a significant plasma concentration of drug, as in these circumstances the concentration of drug in the biophase will be maintained and will continue to influence the acetylcholine receptor.

The ability of the biophase to fix drug regardless of elimination of drug from the plasma would offer a possible explanation for the duration of action of mivacurium.

Mivacurium is hydrolysed in the plasma by plasma cholinesterese at almost the same rate as suxamethonium. However, its duration of action at $2 \times ED_{95}$ is about 25 min, considerably longer than that of suxamethonium.

In addition to these possible mechanisms at the postjunctional receptor, it is necessary to bear in mind possible additional presynaptic effects which would not be readily observed with studies at slow rates of stimulation and which may influence recovery from a nondepolarizing block. Present evidence suggests that these presynaptic effects might last longer than those at the acetylcholine recognition sites.

The biophase

Although the anatomical site of the biophase is unknown, autoradiographs have demonstrated that non-competitive drugs do remain within the synapse after the preparation has been washed to remove unbound drug (Fig. 6.10). Experimental evidence suggests that the biophase may have certain individual characteristics:

1. It can be saturated by large doses of drug. It is therefore reasonable to assume it has a finite small volume.

2. The biophase is likely to be responsible for the slow onset of nondepolarizing block relative to decamethonium. This would suggest that the biophase is 5–10

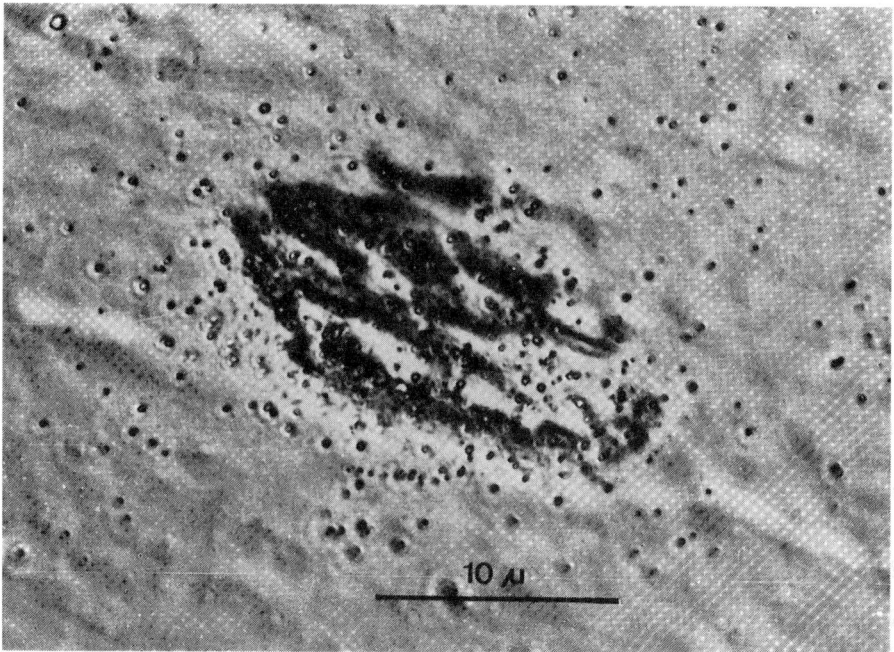

Fig. 6.10 Autoradiograph demonstrating the binding of radio labelled toxiferine in a synapse of mouse muscle.

times the size of the acetylcholine receptor pool. This slow onset is reduced by pretreatment with sufficient alpha-bungarotoxin to produce 50% block, suggesting that a reduction in the size of the biophase pool is associated with a more rapid onset of block.

3. The biophase dissociation constants, K_D, of various nondepolarizing drugs are characteristic for each individual agent. In general, more lipophilic drugs dissociate more rapidly, suggesting a predominantly liphobic binding site within the biophase.

4. Reduction in the size of the biophase or pretreatment with α-cobra venom causes an increased rate of recovery (Armstrong and Lester 1979). This suggests that the reduction in the size of the biophase produced by α-cobra venom results in a smaller pool of bound neuromuscular blocking drug and hence more rapid recovery.

5. The biophase is essentially empty when complete recovery of neuromuscular transmission occurs (no fade at 50 Hz and 100 Hz).

It is tempting to suggest that the reservoir of drug in the biophase is the cause of the apparent excess of receptors for tubocurarine that have to be occupied to prevent neuromuscular conduction. This has been described as the margin of safety of neuromuscular transmission (Paton and Waud 1967). If so it would also explain why the onset of a nondepolarizing block is relatively slow because time would be required to occupy these sites. This hypothesis would, however, necessitate postulating the removal of drug from this reservoir at 100% recovery from block. This is at variance with beliefs, on the basis of the margin of safety hypothesis, that up to 80% of receptors remain occupied at the time of recovery, the so-called 'iceberg effect'. Preliminary studies suggest that all the drug is indeed removed from the biophase (Campkin *et al.* 1993). In the isolated arm no tetanic fade (100 Hz) can be demonstrated following 100% recovery of twitch response, nor is there any change in sensitivity to subsequent doses of neuromuscular blocking agent following 100% recovery of twitch response. There is also no effect demonstrable upon the duration of a different drug administered after 100% recovery from the first. This suggests a low level of residual receptor occupancy once spontaneous recovery of neuromuscular conduction has been established in the presence of a low plasma drug concentration. Although minimal fade at 100 Hz stimulation is found following recovery from a systemic bolus of an ED_{90} dose of vecuronium, no fade at 50 Hz is seen. This may be due to additional factors including the background anaesthetic.

The significance of biophase binding

To accommodate the observations on the isolated arm, which are measured in minutes, with those in isolated tissues which also take place on a millisecond time-scale, similar to the competition between acetyl choline and antagonist drugs at the receptor level, the following hypothesis is proposed.

Following a bolus ED_{95} dose of a nondepolarizing drug it is suggested that molecules of drug enter the junctional cleft along a concentration gradient. Within the junction they bind rapidly to acceptor sites in the biophase and slowly to acetylcholine recognition sites. In order to reach a critical level of receptor occupation it is necessary to fill the large reservoir of acceptor sites in the biophase. As the plasma level falls, molecules acting at the receptor will diffuse out of the synaptic cleft to be replaced by those dissociating from the reservoir in the biophase. An alternative possibility is that the molecules bound to the acceptor sites in the biophase may directly affect the acetylcholine receptor by an allosteric mechanism. In both of these sets of circumstances, the duration of block will depend upon the dissociation rate of the drug from the biophase. This will be influenced by the rate of acetylcholine release from the nerve ending and also the concentration gradient of antagonist between the synapse and the plasma. The effect of the gradient of concentration between synapse and plasma was demonstrated by Agoston *et al.* (1979). They showed that the recovery from pancuronium neuromuscular block was twice as long when the concentration gradient was doubled. It is suggested that at 100% recovery of neuromuscular transmission the biophase concentration is too low to influence the acetylcholine receptor.

It follows that any delay in lowering the plasma level to produce a favourable gradient between the acetylcholine receptor and the plasma will delay recovery by impeding the removal of drug from the synapse and maintaining the biophase concentration by refilling the acceptor sites. Indeed, as long as a significant plasma concentration of drug remains, there will be an equilibrium between the plasma and the biophase which will prevent complete permanent reversal of neuromuscular block by neostigmine.

This fact, that it is not possible to safely reverse neuromuscular block in the presence of a sustained plasma concentration of neuromuscular blocking drug, exists as common ground between those who favour a pharmacokinetic explanation of the recovery of neuromuscular transmission and those who follow the concept of drug binding in a biophase compartment. It is evident therefore that these agents should be used in such a way that the plasma level is as low as possible at the end of the operation. This objective has been greatly helped by new drugs with rapid plasma clearance. It is the advent of these new drugs, for example vecuronium and atracurium, which has reduced the incidence of residual neuromuscular weakness in the recovery room (see Chapter 8).

REFERENCES

Armstrong, D. L. and Lester, H. A. (1979). The kinetics of tubocurarine action and restricted diffusion within the synaptic cleft. *Journal of Physiology*, **294**, 365–86.
Agoston, S., Feldman, S. A., and Miller, R. D. (1979). Plasma pancuronium and twitch response using the isolated arm; bolus injection and continuous infusion. *Anesthesiology*. **51**, 119–22.
Burchill, G. B. (1957). Irreversible curarisation. *British Journal of Anaesthesia*, **29**, 127–32.
Campkin, N. T. A. Hood, J. R., Fauvel, N. J. and Feldman S. A. (1993). The effect of residual receptor occupancy on sensitivity to repeated vecuronium. *Anaesthesia*, **48**, 572–4.

Churchill-Davidson, H. C. and Richardson, A. T. (1959). Decamethonium iodide (C10): some observations on its action using electromyography. *Proceedings of the Royal Society of Medicine*, **45**, 179–86.

Churchill-Davidson, H. C., Way, W. T. and DeJong, R. H. (1967). The muscle relaxants and renal excretion. *Anesthesiology*, **28**, 540–6.

Cohen, E. N., Corbascio, A. and Fleishli, G. (1965). The distribution and fate of *d*-tubocurarine. *Journal of Pharmacology and Experimental Therapeutics*, **147**, 120–8.

Cohen, E. N., Brewer, W. H., and Smith, D. (1967). The metabolism and elimination of *d*-tubocurarine H^3. *Anesthesiology*, **28**, 309–17.

Feldman, S. A. (1973). Termination of action of relaxants. In *Muscle relaxants*, (ed. S. A. Feldman), p. 68. Saunders, London.

Feldman, S. A. (1976). Affinity concept and the action of the muscle relaxants. *Acta Anesthesiologica Belgica*, **35**, 804–8.

Feldman, S. A. and Levi, J. A. (1963). Prolonged paresis following gallamine. *British Journal of Anaesthesia*, **35**, 804–6.

Feldman, S. A. and Tyrrell, M. F. (1970). A new theory of the termination of action of muscle relaxants. *Proceedings of the Royal Society of Medicine*, **63**, 692–5.

Feldman, S. A., Cohen, E. N., and Golling R. (1969). The excretion of gallamine in the dog. *Anesthesiology*, **30**, 593–8.

Feldman, S. A., Fauvel, N. J., and Hood, J. R. (1992). Recovery from pancuronium and vecuronium administered simultaneously in the isolated arm and the effect on recovery following administration after crossover of drugs. *Anesthesia and Analgesia*, **76**, 92–5.

Goat, V. A., Yeung, M. L., Blakeney, C., and Feldman, S. A. (1976). The effect of blood flow upon the activity of gallamine triethiodide. *British Journal of Anaesthesia*, **48**, 69–73.

Ham, J., Miller, R. D., Sheiner, L. B., and Matteo, R. S. (1979). Dosage schedule independence of *d*-tubocurarine pharmacokinetics and pharmacodynamics and recovery of neuromuscular function. *Anesthesiology*, **50**, 528–33.

Heneghan, C. P. A., Findley, I. L., Gilbe, C. E., and Feldman, S. A. (1978). Muscle blood flow and rate of recovery from pancuronium neuromuscular block in dogs. *British Journal of Anaesthesia*, **50**, 1105–8.

Hull, C. J. (1982). Pharmacodynamics of non-depolarizing neuromuscular blocking agents. *British Journal of Anaesthesia*, **54**, 169–82.

Hull, C. J., English, M. J., and Sibbald, A. (1980). Fazadinium and pancuronium: a pharmacodynamics study. *British Journal of Anaesthesia*, **58**, 1209–18.

Kalow, W. and Gunn, O. R. (1957). The relation between dose of succinylcholine and duration of apnoea in man. *Journal of Pharmacology and Experimental Therapeutics*, **120**, 203–14.

Matteo, R. S., Spector, S., and Horowitz, P. E. (1974). Relation of serum *d*-tubocuarine concentration to neuromuscular blockade in man. *Anesthesiology*, **41**, 440–3.

Montgomery, J. B. and Bennett-Jones, W. (1956). Gallamine triethiodide and renal disease. *Lancet*, **ii**, 1243.

Paton, W. D. M. and Waud, D. R. (1967). The margin of safety of neuromuscular transmission. *Journal of Physiology*, **191**, 59–90.

Savarese, J. J., Ali, H. H., Basta, S. J., Embree, P. B., Scott, R. P. F., Sunder, N., et. al. (1988). The clinical neuromuscular pharmacology of mivacurium chloride (BW B1090U). *Anesthesiology*, **68**, 723–32.

Shanks, C. A., Somogyi, A. A., and Triggs, E. K. (1979). Dose-response and plasma concentration–response relationships of pancuronium in man. *Anesthesiology*, **51**, 111–8.

Stanski, D. R. and Sheiner, L. B. (1979). Pharmacokinetics and dynamics of muscle relaxants. *Anesthesiology*, **51**, 103–5.

Waud, B. (1975). Serum *d*-tubocurarine concentration and twitch height. *Anesthesiology*, **43**, 381–2.

White, D. A. and Reitan, J. A. (1984). Effect of blood flow in the pharmacodynamics of non-depolarizing muscle relaxants using isolated limb model. *Anesthesiology*, **61**, A268.

7

Evoked reversal of neuromuscular block

Jan Bonde and Jorgen Viby-Mogensen

During anaesthesia neuromuscular block can be achieved by two different groups of drugs: the depolarizing (e.g. suxamethonium) and the nondepolarizing neuromuscular blocking agents (e.g. pancuronium, vecuronium, atracurium, and mivacurium). In this chapter reversal of neuromuscular block induced by these two groups of drugs will be discussed separately. Apart from a pharmacological and pharmacokinetic description of compounds used to reverse neuromuscular block, we shall focus on the appropriate time and the desired end-points of reversal and seek possible preferences for particular anticholinesterase agents when using different neuromuscular blocking agents. We shall also consider factors affecting reversal of neuromuscular block in general and in special groups of patients.

HISTORY

Anticholinesterase agents have an interesting history. The first report on these agents originates from a description by William Freeman Daniell. He observed the use of the calabar bean in a native judicial procedure in Africa about 1840. Prisoners suspected of capital offences and found guilty were forced to swallow a deadly poison, made from the seeds of an aquatic leguminous plant which rapidly destroyed life. The poison was later found to be physostigmine.

The plant was subsequently cultivated in the royal botanical gardens of Edinburgh in the late 1840s by John Hutton Balfour. Its first use as an antagonist (to atropine) was described by Thomas Richard Frazer in 1877. J. Pall was the first to demonstrate the ability of physostigmine to reverse the neuromuscular blocking effect of curare (in 1900). Its ability to treat the disease myasthenia gravis was demonstrated by Mary Walker in 1934, and its important role in identifying the cholinesterase enzymes was established in the laboratories of David Nachmansohn in the 1930s. Its less flattering use as a model for the development of nerve gases and later, insecticides, was established in the late 1930s.

PHARMACOLOGY

Classification of anticholinesterase agents

Anticholinesterase agents can be classified into four groups according to their chemical structure (Fig. 7.1) and modes of action (which are described later in this chapter):

(1) simple alcohols bearing one quaternary ammonium group (edrophonium);

(2) carbamic acid esters of alcohols bearing quaternary (neostigmine and pyridostigmine) or tertiary (physostigmine) ammonium groups;

(3) aminopyridines;

(4) organic derivatives of phosphoric esters.

   This chapter will only deal with edrophonium (group 1) and neostigmine and pyridostigmine (group 2). Being lipophilic, physostigmine readily penetrates biological membranes including the blood–brain barrier, thereby exerting CNS effects. The drug is consequently not used as a reversal agent in conjunction with anaesthesia. The mechanism of action of the aminopyridines is probably mediated through an increased release of acetylcholine from the motor nerve terminal. The drug decreases the efflux of potassium from the nerve terminal, thereby prolonging the depolarization phase. This in turn leads to an increase in the flux of calcium into the nerve ending and accordingly, an increase in the release of acetylcholine. The use of these drugs, however, is limited by their slow onset of action and potential for inducing CNS side-effects. The newer, more polar derivative, 2,4-aminopyridine is apparently devoid of CNS effects, but seems inferior to neostigmine in reversing a neuromuscular block (Beaufort *et al.* 1990). Because the aminopyridines act presynaptically, they have the potential for antagonizing drugs that act on the nerve ending, i.e. certain antibiotics. The clinical significance of these compounds is yet to be established. Compounds from group 4 are omitted because their use is restricted to agricultural and military purposes and they have no use in medicine.

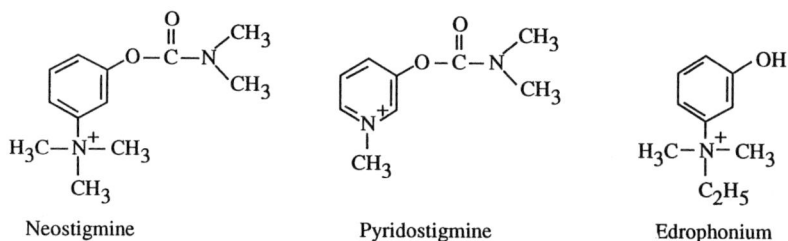

Fig. 7.1 Formulae for neostigmine, pyridostigmine, and edrophonium.

Mechanism of action

The main effects of anticholinesterase agents are exerted at three sites, the neuro-muscular junction, the autonomic cholinergic synapses, and the CNS.

Effects at the neuromuscular junction

The action of the neurotransmitter acetylcholine is terminated by enzymatic hydrolysis by acetylcholinesterase (true cholinesterase, acetylcholine-acetylhydrolase, EC 3.1.1.7.) to choline and acetic acid. Another enzyme, pseudocholinesterase or plasma cholinesterase (acetylcholine-acylhydrolase, EC 3.1.1.8.), is present in tissue and plasma and is also capable of hydrolysing acetylcholine. Pseudocholinesterase probably only plays a minor role in terminating the effect of acetylcholine.

The mode of action of edrophonium differs from that of neostigmine and pyridostigmine at the molecular level (Fig. 7.2). Edrophonium binds to the anionic site of the acetylcholinesterase by electrostatic attachment and to the esteratic site by hydrogen bonding. No chemical bonds are formed, and the bonds are easily broken, making the inhibition short lived. In contrast neostigmine and pyridostigmine are chemically bound to the acetylcholinesterase molecule as a carbamate group is transformed from the former to the esteratic site of the acetylcholinesterase. This binding causes a long-lasting inhibition of the enzyme (half-life approximately 30 min). The carbamate–enzyme complex is finally hydrolysed rendering the enzyme active again.

Acetylcholinesterase inhibitors have other effects at the neuromuscular junction. Prejunctionally they may influence the transport of calcium across the cell membrane, thereby increasing the release of acetylcholine from the nerve ending. The anticholinesterases may also cause repetitive firing in the motor nerve terminal in response to single action potentials. Postsynaptically, the drugs might have a direct cholinergic action on the nicotinic acetylcholine receptors (receptors located in autonomic ganglia and at skeletal neuromuscular junctions), which might add to the effectiveness of these compounds in reversing neuromuscular block. The main differences between the individual cholinesterases are, however, probably related more to chemical and pharmacokinetic properties than to pharmacodynamic properties and, irrespective of the mode of action, the net result of the inhibition of acetylcholinesterase is an accumulation of acetylcholine at the acetylcholine receptors.

Combinations of edrophonium and neostigmine have a simple additive effect on the reversal of neuromuscular block without signs of potentiation (Bevan *et al.* 1984; Breen *et al.* 1985), indicating that the mixture of the two does not offer any advantages over either drug alone.

The reversal of neuromuscular blocking agents by competitive antagonism is, by nature, limited in the sense that when maximal inhibition has been achieved, further administration of the drug does not add to its effectiveness (Fig. 7.3). Indeed, anticholinesterases have been reported to produce neuromuscular block (Payne *et al.* 1980; Sherby *et al.* 1985; Bartkowski 1987). Clinically significant neuromuscular block after anticholinesterases is, however, only seen after doses exceeding those used clinically. The point at which the cholinergic effect exceeds the anticholinergic

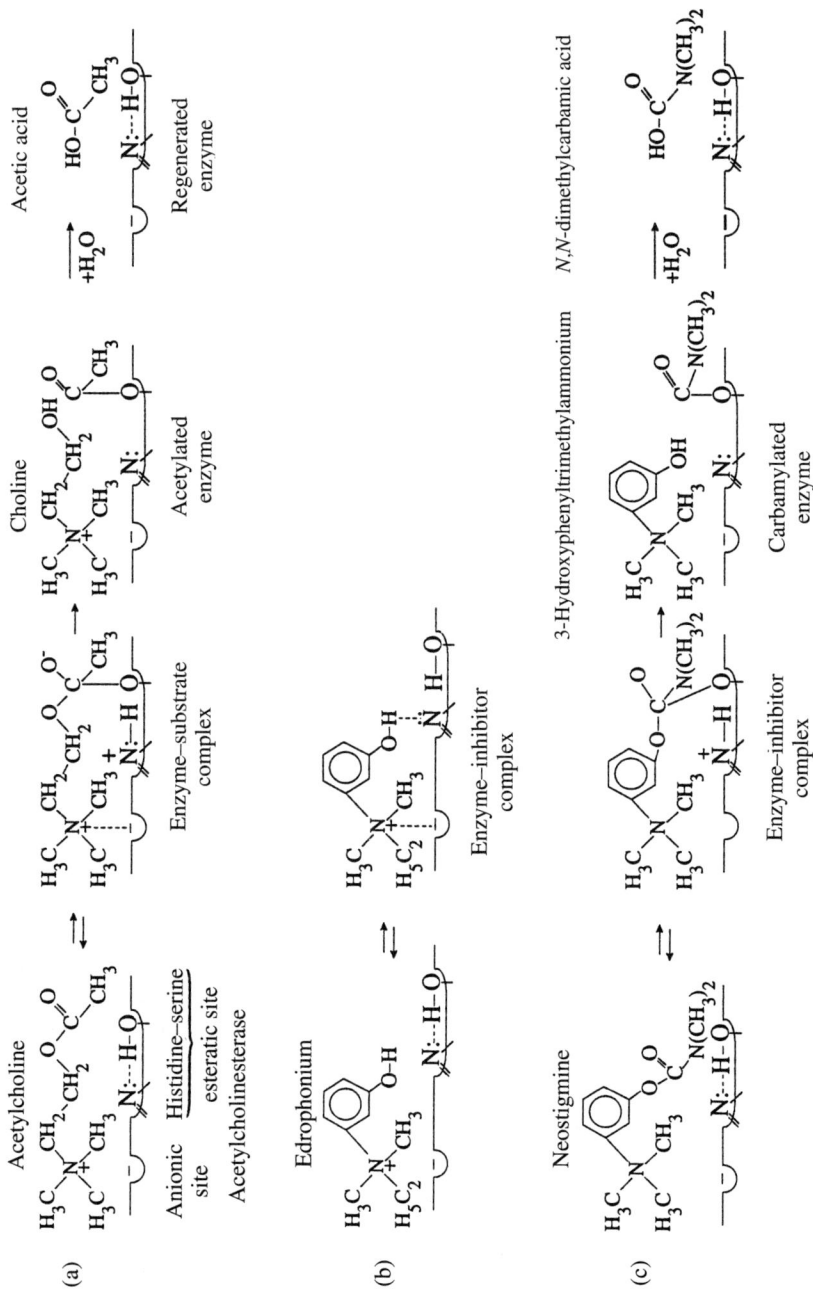

Fig. 7.2 (a) Reaction between acetylcholine and acetylcholinesterase, and regeneration of the enzyme. (b) Reaction of edrophonium with acetylcholinesterase. (c) Reaction of neostigmine with acetylcholinesterase.

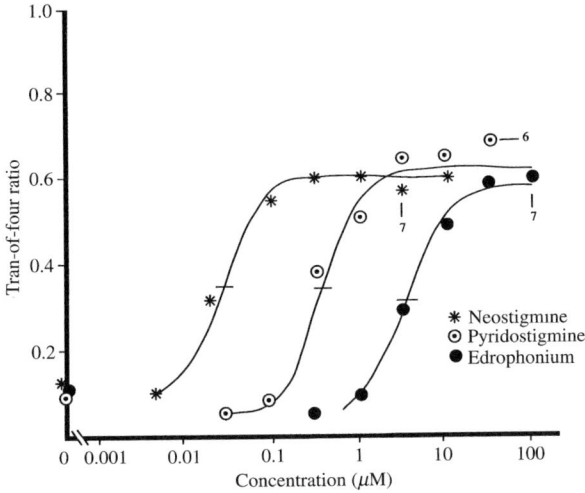

Fig. 7.3 Dose–response curves for neostigmine, pyridostigmine, and edrophonium showing the differences in potency of the three compounds and demonstrating the ceiling effect. The results are obtained in a rat phrenic nerve–diaphragm preparation. (From Bartkowski 1987, with permission.)

effect is yet to be established in humans. Normal neuromuscular transmission can take place when approximately 30% of the post-synaptic receptors are free (i.e. not occupied by a nondepolarizing agent) (Paton and Waud 1967). This implies an extensive 'margin of safety' in neuromuscular transmission.

Effects on autonomic cholinergic synapses

The autonomic effects mainly reflect an enhancement of acetylcholine activity at parasympathetic post-ganglionic synapses. The clinical impact is an increased secretion from exocrine glands, increased peristaltic activity, bronchoconstriction, bradycardia, hypotension, pupillary constriction, and difficulty in accommodation.

In equiantagonistic low doses it appears that edrophonium possesses fewer muscarinic side-effects (evaluated by the need for atropine to prevent the bradycardic effect of the anticholinesterase compounds) than neostigmine and pyridostigmine (Cronnelly *et al.* 1982). Using high doses of edrophonium (1.5 mg/kg), however, additional atropine may be required to avoid bradycardia (Engbæk *et al.* 1985).

Central effects

The tertiary compound physostigmine penetrates the blood–brain barrier and might therefore exert some CNS effects. The result is an initial excitation, which, following very high doses, might result in convulsions followed by CNS depression, unconsciousness, and respiratory failure.

Table 7.1   Pharmacokinetic parameters of neostigmine, pyridostigmine, and edrophonium in patients with normal renal function (N) and anephric patients (RF)

	Volume of distribution (l/kg)		Clearance (l/h/kg)		Elimination half-life (h)	
	N	RF	N	RF	N	RF
Edrophonium	0.9	0.7	0.5	0.2	1.9	3.4
Pyridostigmine	1.1	1.0	0.5	0.1	1.9	6.3
Neostigmine	1.4	1.6	1.0	0.5	1.3	3.0

Data from Morris *et al.* (1981) and Cronelly *et al.* (1979, 1980)

Pharmacokinetics

Table 7.1 shows the pharmacokinetic parameters of edrophonium, pyridostigmine, and neostigmine. The pharmacokinetics of the anticholinesterases has been reviewed by Aquilonius and Hartvig (1986).

Few pharmacokinetic data are available for edrophonium. The volume of distribution is approximately 0.9 l/kg and elimination clearance in the range of 0.5 l/kg/h. Approximately 67% of the plasma clearance is dependent on renal excretion and the remainder on nonrenal mechanisms. The half-life of edrophonium in patients with normal renal function is 1.9 hours (Morris *et al.* 1981). The volume of distribution of pyridostigmine is approximately 1.1 l/kg. Twenty per cent is metabolized in the plasma and 80% is excreted via the kidneys. Total elimination clearance is 0.5 l/kg/h. Pyridostigmine is extensively metabolized in plasma by plasma cholinesterase. The main metabolite is 3-hydroxy-*N*-methyl-pyridinum, which is rapidly glucuronidated. Excretion in the kidneys is accounted for by both tubular secretion and glomerular filtration.

The volume of distribution of neostigmine is approximately 1.4 l/kg. It is partly metabolized (50%) and partly eliminated by renal excretion (50%). The total elimination clearance is of the order of 1 l/kg/h. The renal clearance of the drug occurs by both glomerular filtration and tubular secretion. Nonrenal mechanisms of elimination are unclear, but possible modes of elimination include hepatic metabolism and hydrolysis by plasma cholinesterase.

DESIRED END-POINTS OF EVOKED REVERSAL OF NEURO-MUSCULAR BLOCK

The degree of neuromuscular block can be evaluated by bedside clinical tests and/or by the response to peripheral nerve stimulation (see Chapter 16). A train-of-four (TOF) ratio of 0.7–0.8 is normally considered to reflect adequate recovery of neuromuscular function (Brand *et al.* 1977; Engbæk *et al.* 1989*b*). When the ratio is only 0.6 the patient is able to lift the head for three seconds whereas vital capacity and inspiratory force may still be reduced. At a ratio of 0.70–0.75 the patient can open both eyes wide and stick out the tongue and the majority of patients can sustain a head-lift for at least five seconds. When the TOF ratio is 0.8, vital capacity and inspiratory force are normal and all patients can sustain a head-lift for five seconds (Engbæk *et al.* 1989*b*). Pavlin *et al.* (1989) showed that adequate ventilation in human volunteers recovering from a tubocurarine-induced neuromuscular block did not maintain a functionally intact airway. Only if the volunteers were able to sustain a head lift for five seconds could they perform what were considered to be satisfactory airway-protective manoeuvres (ability to swallow, to perform a valsalva manoeuvre, to prevent obstruction of the airway, and to approximate the teeth). One should also, however, recognize the fact that tactile and visual assessment of TOF (and tetanic) fade have limitations in sensitivity and accuracy (Viby-Mogensen *et al.* 1985; Dupuis *et al.* 1990), and that the above TOF-values refer to mean figures. The new stimulation pattern double burst stimulation (DBS) has improved the sensitivity of the tactile assessment of fade (Engbæk *et al.* 1989*a*), and tactile evaluation of the response to DBS is superior to tactile evaluation of the response to TOF stimulation. Absence of tactile fade in the response to DBS means that severe residual neuromuscular block can be excluded (Drenck *et al.* 1989).

The desired endpoints of the evoked reversal of neuromuscular block can be expressed as follows:

1. Clinical criteria:
    the patient should be able to
        – open the eyes widely;
        – sustain a hand grip;
        – sustain protrusion of the tongue;
        – sustain a head lift for five seconds;
        – cough effectively.
    The patient should have
        – an adequate tidal volume
        – a vital capacity $\geq$ 15–20 ml/kg
        – an inspiratory force $\geq$ 40–45 cm H_2O

2. Tactile evaluation of the response to peripheral nerve stimulation:
        no fade in response to train-of-four stimulation; and
        no fade in response to double burst stimulation.

3. Neuromuscular monitoring criteria:
        train-of-four ratio $\geq$ 0.7–0.8;
        double burst stimulation ratio $\geq$ 0.7–0.8.

REVERSAL OF NEUROMUSCULAR BLOCK INDUCED BY DEPOLARIZING DRUGS

The injection of a dose of suxamethonium sufficient for endotracheal intubation (1–1.5 mg/kg) normally causes a short depolarizing neuromuscular block because suxamethonium is rapidly hydrolysed by plasma cholinesterase. In patients with

Table 7.2   Treatment of prolonged neuromuscular block following
succinylcholine 1–1.5 mg/kg

Time from injection to first response	Most probable genotype	Possible treatment
< 20–25 min	1. Normal genotype but low enzyme activity	Edrophonium
		or
	2. Heterozygous	
≥ 30 min	Homozygote for two abnormal genes	neostigmine Mechanical ventilation + sedation

very low plasma cholinesterase activity, either because of depressed enzyme activity in a genotypically normal patient or because the patient has an inherited abnormal plasma cholinesterase genotype, the effect of suxamethonium is prolonged, sometimes for hours. In these patients the initial depolarizing block may change its characteristics to a so called phase II (or 'dual') block. This block is, though not nondepolarizing, characterized by fade in the TOF and the tetanic response. The treatment of a phase II block depends on whether the patient has a normal or an abnormal plasma cholinesterase genotype (Table 7.2). In genotypically normal patients the block may be reversed with an anticholinesterase drug. In patients with homozygous occurrence of the atypical or the silent plasma cholinesterase genes, the injection of an anticholinesterase drug may prolong the block significantly, unless purified human cholinesterase is injected prior to the anticholinesterase drug to hydrolyse any free suxamethonium in the plasma (Viby-Mogensen 1981). The genotype of the patient is not normally known, however, when an anaesthesiologist is suddenly faced with a case of prolonged apnoea following suxamethonium. It is therefore normally advised that no treatment is attempted and that the patient is kept ventilated and sedated until he or she has spontaneously regained sufficient muscle power to secure the airway (Viby-Mogensen 1983).

REVERSAL OF NEUROMUSCULAR BLOCK INDUCED BY NON-DEPOLARIZING DRUGS

The effect of a given dose of an anticholinesterase agent varies with the degree of block and with the type and dose of the neuromuscular blocking agent used. In the following, the effects of the anticholinesterases are considered separately for the long-acting, the intermediate-acting, and the short-acting neuromuscular blocking agents. Where possible, an attempt is made to establish a dose–response relationship for the different anticholinesterase drugs in the three groups of non-depolarizing neuromuscular blocking agents. Most emphasis is put on studies mimicking clinical settings, i.e. infusion studies or studies using repetitive bolus injections. When the pharmacodynamics of the anticholinesterase drugs are evaluated in these settings, it is important to realize that the observed apparent reversal effect of a drug is the net result of the pharmaceutical effect and the simultaneously occurring spontaneous recovery of the neuromuscular block, resulting from the spontaneous clearance of the drug from the plasma and hence the neuromuscular junction.

WHEN TO INITIATE REVERSAL

As Fig. 7.4 shows, intense neuromuscular block (the 'period of no response') is followed by a period of moderate or surgical block, defined by the presence of one, two, or three responses to TOF stimulation. Deep or profound surgical block is the period immediately following the period of intense block. During this period only one response to TOF stimulation is present, corresponding to a twitch height of ≤ 10% (T1/T0).

The effect of a given dose of an anticholinesterase agent varies with the degree of block at the time of attempted reversal (Katz 1971; Fig. 7.5). In clinical practice, reversal should not be attempted unless signs of spontaneous recovery have appeared, i.e. either spontaneous muscle movements or responses to peripheral nerve stimulation. Especially when using a long-acting neuromuscular blocking agent, two, three, or even better four responses to the TOF stimulation should be present before reversal is initiated. Antagonism should not be attempted when the block is intense, i.e. during the period of no response to TOF and single twitch stimulation (Fig. 7.4). Engbæk *et al.* (1990) and Gwinnutt *et al.* (1991) have shown that the total recovery time, which is defined as the sum of the spontaneous recovery time and the reversal time, cannot be shortened by injection of an anticholinesterase drug during this period.

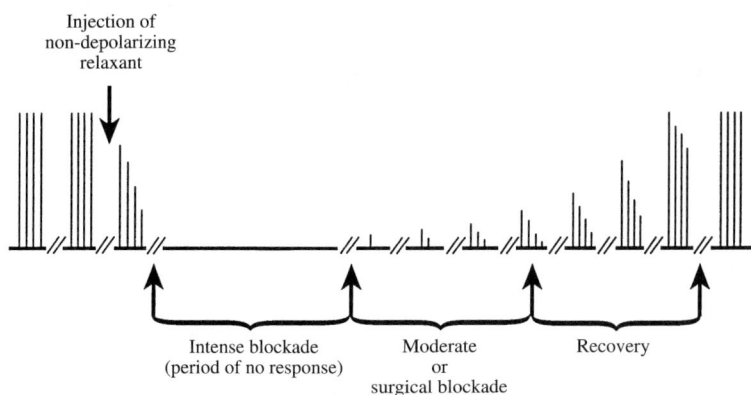

Fig. 7.4 Schematic illustration of the different degrees of neuromuscular blockade following injection of a non-depolarizing drug, as evaluated using train-of-four nerve stimulation (from Viby-Mogensen 1985, with permission.)

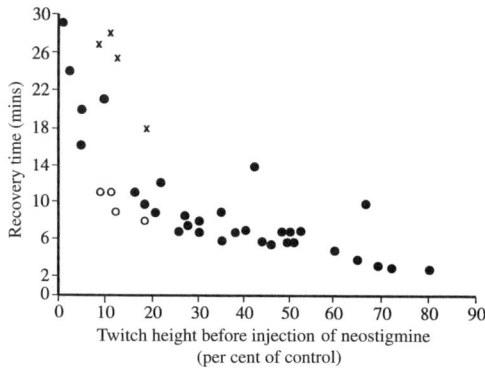

Fig. 7.5 Relationship between degree of neuromuscular blockade and recovery time. (From Katz 1971, with permission.)

Goldhill *et al.* (1986) evaluated the reversal effect of neostigmine during deep surgical block (T1/T0 < 5%). They gave three doses of neostigmine (0.03, 0.06, and 0.08 mg/kg) during a deep surgical pancuronium-induced block. The high doses of neostigmine produced a significantly faster reversal than the lower doses (to 95% recovery of T1). No significant differences were, however, found in the time to reach a TOF ratio of 0.75. In the majority of patients, recovery as evaluated by the TOF ratios was not satisfactory 30 min after neostigmine, irrespective of the dose of neostigmine administered. In another study of reversal from deep surgical block (T1/T0 = 1%) induced by pancuronium, Donati *et al.* (1987*a*) gave either neostigmine (0.04 or 0.08 mg/kg), pyridostigmine (0.2 or 0.38 mg/kg), or edrophonium (0.5 or 1.15 mg/kg) in a randomized order. The degree of reversal was evaluated at various time-points after the administration of the acetylcholinesterase inhibitor but not later than 10 min afterwards. In this study a dose-dependent effect seemed to exist. Comparing the efficacy of the high doses of the different compounds, neostigmine proved significantly better than the other two compounds (evaluated by T1/T0 values 10 min after reversal). These two studies thus indicate that neostigmine is superior to pyridostigmine and edrophonium for reversal of deep surgical block.

Priming technique

It has been suggested that reversal time may be shortened by injecting the anticholinesterase agent in divided doses, the so-called 'priming technique' (Abdulatif and Naguib 1986; Naguib and Abdulatif 1988). The efficacy of the priming technique has, however, been questioned. Donati *et al.* (1989) did not find an accelerated recovery when reversal was attempted at 90% block, and Magorian *et al.* (1990) could not demonstrate a shortened reversal time when using the priming technique in patients with deep neuromuscular block (T1/T0 < 1%) following vecuronium. These findings are in contrast to those of Abdulatif and Naguib (1986), and Naguib and Abdulatif (1988), who found a significant faster reversal from a 90% block.

As any time saving would be — at best — in the range of minutes, the technique is considered to be of limited clinical significance, irrespective of the degree of block at the time of reversal.

THE SIGNIFICANCE OF THE NEUROMUSCULAR BLOCKING AGENT ON THE ANTICHOLINESTERASE AGENT

The anticholinesterase agents have markedly different pharmacokinetic and pharmacodynamic characteristics and so have the neuromuscular blocking agents. It is therefore logical to consider the anticholinesterase agents with respect to the duration of action of the neuromuscular blocking agent in use.

Long-acting neuromuscular blocking agents

Ferguson *et al.* (1980) using different doses of neostigmine (2.5 and 5.0 mg/70 kg), edrophonium (50 and 100 mg/70 kg), and pyridostigmine (10 and 20 mg/70 kg) to reverse a low-dose pancuronium (3 mg/70 kg) block achieved a high and sustained degree of reversal ($T1/T0$ and $T4/T1$ of 0.9 and 0.75, respectively) using any one of the six reversal protocols initiated at 10% twitch height recovery. This result, however, cannot be extrapolated to situations where higher doses of long-acting neuromuscular blocking agents have been used. Bevan (1979) found, in accordance with Ferguson *et al.* (1980), satisfactory reversal (TOF > 0.7) following pancuronium 0.036 mg/kg using edrophonium 0.7 mg/kg. If the dose of pancuronium was increased to 0.086 mg/kg, however, the TOF ratio 30 min after injection of the same dose of edrophonium was only 0.41. Kopmann (1986) did not achieve satisfactory reversal of a pancuronium block (obtained by a steady-state infusion) using edrophonium 0.75 or 1.0 mg/kg (TOF ratio at 20 min 0.44 and 0.48, respectively) either. Neostigmine 0.05 mg/kg on the other hand produced a significantly higher TOF ratio (0.68). The differences observed in these three studies can be explained by the differences in doses of pancuronium given and the models employed. As the latter studies mimic the clinical situation the most, the results indicate that neostigmine possesses an advantage over edrophonium in reversing a neuromuscular block induced by clinical doses of pancuronium.

Donati *et al.* (1987*b*) performed a dose–response study in 120 patients each given a single dose of either pancuronium or tubocurarine. Four different doses of neostigmine, pyridostigmine or edrophonium were administered at a twitch height of 10%, and neuromuscular function was monitored using a train-of-four pattern of stimulation. The dose–response curve for edrophonium was found to be significantly flatter than that for neostigmine and also that for pyridostigmine. Similar results were found by Cronnelly *et al.* (1982) (Fig. 7.6). These investigations emphasize that the apparent potency of an anticholinesterase agent depends not only on the type, the dose, and the mode of administration of the neuromuscular blocking agent, but also the pharmacodynamic parameter used (single twitch or TOF

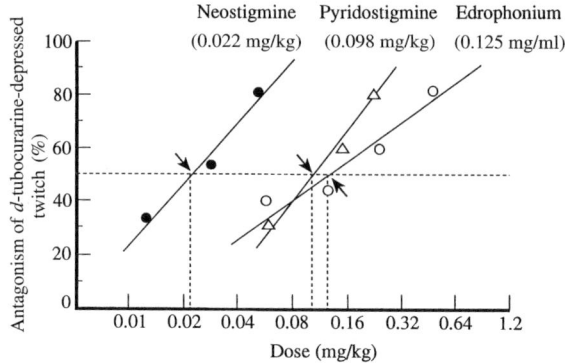

Fig. 7.6 Dose–response curves for neostigmine, pyridostigmine, and edrophonium. Values plotted are means and the lines determined linear regression by analysis. Figures in parentheses are ED_{50} values. (Reprinted with permission from the International Anesthesia Research Society (*Anesthesiology*, **57**, 261–6.)

stimulation). In addition, the potency ratio may vary with the dose range studied. This makes it difficult to produce any comparisons of the potency values of the individual anticholinesterases obtained in different studies. From the existing evidence it can, however, be concluded that edrophonium, neostigmine, and pyridostigmine cannot be used interchangeably when reversing neuromuscular block induced by long-acting nondepolarizing neuromuscular blocking drugs. In the everyday clinical practice, neostigmine appears to be superior to edrophonium, particularly if the block is still deep at the time of attempted reversal. Neostigmine also seems to be superior to edrophonium in reversing a block produced by one of the long-acting neuromuscular blocking drugs.

Intermediate acting neuromuscular blocking agents

When evaluating the efficacy of the anticholinesterase compounds in reversing a neuromuscular block induced by the intermediate-acting drugs one is confronted with the same methodological problems as mentioned in the section on long-acting neuromuscular blocking agents.

Caldwell *et al.* (1987) compared the effect of neostigmine 0.07 mg/kg and edrophonium 0.8 mg/kg following bolus injections of atracurium (150–200 μg/kg) and vecuronium (40–60 μg/kg). Reversal was attempted at deep surgical block (T1/T0 ≤ 5%) and the end-point for sufficient reversal was a TOF ratio of 0.7. Although the time to 25% twitch height was shorter following edrophonium, with atracurium and vecuronium the time to a TOF ratio of 0.7 was similar in the two groups. In addition, edrophonium was more unpredictable than neostigmine in reversing the vecuronium block.

In a more clinically relevant study, Kopman (1986) examined the reversal of a neuromuscular block which had been induced by an infusion of atracurium or vecuronium. Twenty minutes after the administration of neostigmine (0.05 mg/kg) there was a more complete reversal than after edrophonium (0.75 mg/kg). These results are in agreement with the observations of Engbæk *et al.* (1985), who found a significantly shorter onset and reversal time following neostigmine 0.04 mg/kg when compared with edrophonium 0.75 mg/kg following a vecuronium-induced block obtained by continuous infusion. If the dose of edrophonium was increased to 1.5 mg/kg, no significant difference was found between the effect of edrophonium and neostigmine 0.04 mg/kg. Using 1.5 mg/kg of edrophonium, however, supplementary atropine was necessary.

These studies have, as many other studies, demonstrated that edrophonium and neostigmine cannot be used interchangeably. Neostigmine seems to offer some advantages over edrophonium in reversing a vecuronium-induced block and also a deep surgical block following a continuous infusion of atracurium.

Short-acting neuromuscular blocking agents

Mivacurium is a new nondepolarizing neuromuscular blocking agent with short duration of action and short recovery time. It is eliminated mainly by hydrolysis in the plasma by plasma cholinesterase (Savarese *et al.* 1988; Ostergaard *et al.* 1992). Because this enzyme is inhibited by anticholinesterases, administration of an anticholinesterase agent, for example neostigmine, might theoretically inhibit the metabolism of mivacurium and prolong the neuromuscular block. In a study by Savarese *et al.* (1988), however, comprising a relatively small number of patients, administration of neostigmine in a dose of 0.06 mg/kg at a level of block of 67–93% actually shortened the time to 95% twitch height recovery to 6.3 min compared to 10.3 min in the control group. Goldhill *et al.* (1991) found that neostigmine and edrophonium produced a similar reduction in evoked recovery time following an infusion of mivacurium. Contrary to this Diefenbach *et al.* (1992) could not hasten recovery from a mivacurium induced block with neostigmine.

EDROPHONIUM VERSUS NEOSTIGMINE VERSUS PYRIDOSTIGMINE

As would appear from the above, neostigmine is superior to edrophonium for reversal of profound neuromuscular block irrespective of the neuromuscular blocking agent used. The alleged shorter duration of action of edrophonium — although not substantiated in clinical trials — may indicate caution when using the drug after high doses of long-acting neuromuscular blocking agents. Edrophonium has a faster onset time and, if given in low doses, has fewer muscarinic side-effects than neostigmine. In higher doses (≥ 1.0 mg/kg) the reduced atropine requirements of edrophonium are lost.

Pyridostigmine has a slower onset of action than neostigmine (Miller *et al.* 1974) and its longer duration of action makes it a less suitable compound for reversing one of the intermediate- or short-acting neuromuscular blocking agents. In the authors' opinion neostigmine is still the drug of choice.

FACTORS AFFECTING EVOKED REVERSAL OF NEUROMUSCULAR BLOCK

Acid–base and electrolyte status

Respiratory acidosis, but apparently not metabolic acidosis, impedes the capacity of neostigmine to reverse a pancuronium-induced block (Feldman 1963; Miller and Roderick, 1978). A metabolic alkalosis has been shown to prevent neostigmine antagonism of both tubocurarine- and pancuronium-induced blocks. Data on any pH-dependent sensitivity to reversal agents should, however, be interpreted with caution. Changes in pH are often associated with changes in electrolytes, and this may confound the picture. Electrolyte imbalance only seems to have a minor effect on the efficacy of neostigmine, however.

Interactions

No major, clinically significant interactions (pharmacokinetic or pharmacodynamic) exist between the anticholinesterase agents and other drugs (Ostergaard *et al.* 1989). The neuromuscular blocking agents are, however, potentiated by a variety of drugs including the potent volatile anaesthetics. As the reversal agents will only antagonize the neuromuscular block caused by the nondepolarizing agent itself, the reversal time may be prolonged in patients receiving potent inhalational agents. In a study by Delisle and Bevan (1982), it was demonstrated that antagonism of a pancuronium block with neostigmine was impaired during enflurane, but not during halothane anaesthesia. The apparent interaction between enflurane and the anticholinesterase agents was confirmed in a subsequent study with vecuronium and atracurium (Gill *et al.* 1990). Isoflurane also seems to impede the antagonistic potency of neostigmine (Dernovoi *et al.* 1987; Baurain *et al.* 1991).

REVERSAL OF NEUROMUSCULAR BLOCK IN SPECIAL GROUPS OF PATIENTS

Age

Age has an influence on the action of anticholinesterase compounds. In infants and children the dose of neostigmine required to reverse a tubocurarine-induced neuromuscular block is only half of that recommended for adults (Fisher *et al.* 1983), despite an unchanged volume of distribution and an increased clearance. This observation is suggestive of an altered pharmacodynamic response to neostigmine in children. In contrast, no significant differences could be demonstrated in antagonistic potency of edrophonium between children and adults in spite of a doubled elimination clearance and an unchanged volume of distribution (Fisher *et al.* 1984).

Increasing age has no effect on the edrophonium dose–response curve (Cronnelly and Miller 1984). The dose–response curve for neostigmine is, however, shifted significantly to the left in the elderly, indicating an increased sensitivity with increasing age (Miller 1990).

These two studies indicate that, in contrast to edrophonium, the pharmacodynamics of neostigmine are age dependent, suggesting a different mode of action of the two compounds.

The duration of action of pyridostigmine is prolonged in the elderly (Young *et al.* 1988).

Overall, a study of the literature suggests that the doses of neostigmine and pyridostigmine, but not that of edrophonium, can be reduced in the elderly.

Renal and hepatic disease

In anephric patients the elimination clearances of neostigmine, pyridostigmine, and edrophonium are reduced (Table 7.1) (Cronnelly *et al.* 1979, 1980; Morris *et al.* 1981). The dose of an anticholinesterase compound should therefore be adjusted according to renal function, bearing in mind the elimination characteristics of the neuromuscular blocking agent.

No pharmacokinetic data are available of the anticholinesterases in patients with hepatic disease.

Miscellaneous

Due to the cholinergic properties of the anticholinesterase agents, it has been suggested that they should be avoided in patients with bronchial asthma. As they are administered in conjunction with an anticholinergic drug, the risk of precipitating an acute asthmatic attack is probably minimal. The precise effect on the bronchi of the two compounds used in combination is, however, unclear.

Due to the muscarinic effects of neostigmine, ruptures of anastomoses following bowel surgery may occur (Bell and Lewis 1968). Neither atropine nor glycopyrrolate are able to alleviate these gastrointestinal effects (Wilkins *et al.* 1970; Child 1984). There is at present, however, no hard evidence to support the avoidance of neostigmine following surgery on the gastrointestinal tract.

ATROPINE AND GLYCOPYRROLATE AS ADJUNCTS TO REVERSAL BY ANTICHOLINESTERASES

Due to the cholinergic properties of the anticholinesterase compounds, an anticholinergic drug (atropine or glycopyrrolate) is usually coadministered. Traditionally, atropine is the anticholinergic drug employed in anaesthetic practice. Due to differences in physicochemical properties (atropine is a tertiary amine, glycopyrrolate is a quaternary ammonium compound), the pharmacodynamic profiles of the two drugs are different. Glycopyrrolate is alleged to influence cardiac rhythm less, to possess a better antisialagogue effect and not to penetrate the blood–brain barrier. Several comparative studies have been performed (Mirakhur *et al.* 1981; Kongsrud and Sponheim 1982; Mostafa and Vucevic 1984). Mirakhur *et al.* (1981) found a significant rise in heart rate following the combined administration of neostigmine 50 μg/kg and atropine 20 or 30 μg/kg. If neostigmine was given together with glycopyrrolate 5, 10, or 15 μg/kg, or atropine 10 μg/kg, no significant changes were seen in heart rate. When glycopyrrolate 5 μg/kg and atropine 10 μg/kg were given either before or in conjunction with neostigmine, additional anticholinergic drug had to be given due to an unacceptable decrease in heart rate. Glycopyrrolate 10 μg/kg was found to be associated with the most stable heart rates.

Mostafa and Vucevic (1984) found in a study of 100 patients with pre-existing heart disease that atropine (20 and 30 μg/kg) when used in conjunction with neostigmine was associated with a significantly higher incidence of ST-segment depressions, dysrhythmias and rise in rate–pressure product (used as an index of myocardial oxygen requirement) than glycopyrrolate (10 and 15 μg/kg). These results are in accordance with the observations of Kongsrud and Sponheim (1982). Haemodynamic changes may be tolerated in otherwise healthy patients but might represent a potential hazard in elderly patients or in patients with coexisting heart disease.

The required dose of the anticholinergic agent when used in conjunction with pyridostigmine (0.2 mg/kg) is approximately the same as for neostigmine (Fogdall and Miller 1973).

Atropine probably has a more rapid onset of action than glycopyrrolate and might consequently be preferred when used with edrophonium. There seems to be no advantage in interposing a time interval between the administration of glycopyrrolate/atropine and the anticholinesterase drug.

Glycopyrrolate and atropine produce a dose-related inhibition of salivary secretion, with the antisialogue potency of glycopyrrolate being five times that of atropine (Mirakhur and Dundee 1980). In a recent study by Wetterslev *et al.* (1991), however, no clinically significant differences were found in the salivary flow using relevant doses of atropine and glycopyrrolate.

Being a quaternary ammonium compound, glycopyrrolate is less lipophilic than atropine and thus devoid of central nervous system effects. One case has, however, been reported of a likely central anticholinergic syndrome following glycopyrrolate (Grum and Osborne 1991).

CONCLUSION

The mechanisms of action of the anticholinesterase agents neostigmine and pyridostigmine on the one hand, and edrophonium on the other hand, are different. The major difference in their pharmacological profile, however, is probably more related to differences in pharmacokinetic behavior. Irrespective of their mode of action, the net result of all three anticholinesterase agents is an accumulation of acetylcholine at the neuromuscular junction.

Edrophonium has a faster onset of action than neostigmine which is again faster than pyridostigmine. Pyridostigmine has the longest duration of action. Evoked reversal of neuromuscular block should not be attempted unless signs of neuromuscular recovery are present. Neostigmine is superior to edrophonium for reversal of deep surgical block, irrespective of the type of nondepolarizing agents used. If one has to choose only one anticholinesterase agent, neostigmine is still the drug of choice.

REFERENCES

Abdulatif, M. and Naguib, M. (1986). Accelerated reversal of atracurium blockage with divided doses of neostigmine. *Canadian Anaesthetists Society Journal*, **33**, 723–8.

Aquilonius, S. M. and Hartvig, P. (1986). Clinical pharmacokinetics of cholinesterase inhibitors. *Clinical Pharmacokinetics*, **11**, 236–9.

Bartkowski, R. R. (1987). Incomplete reversal of pancuronium neuromuscular blockage by neostigmine, pyridostigmine and edrophonium. *Anesthesia and Analgesia*, **66**, 594–8.

Baurain, M. J., d'Hollander, A. A., Melot, C., Dernovoi, B. S., and Barvais, L. (1991). Effects of residual concentrations of isoflurane on the reversal of vecuronium-induced neuromuscular blockade. *Anesthesiology*, **74**, 474–8.

Beaufort, T. M., Wierda, J. M. K. H., Kruyswijk, J. E., and Agoston, S. (1990). 2,4-diaminopyridine: clinical evaluation of a recently synthesized 4-aminopyridine derivative for reversal of competitive neuromuscular blockade. *European Journal of Anaesthesia*, **7**, 453–7.

Bell, C. M. A. and Lewis, C. B. (1968). Effect of neostigmine on integrity of ileorectal anastomoses. *British Medical Journal*, **iii**, 587–8.

Bevan, D. R. (1979). Reversal of pancuronium with edrophonium. *Anaesthesia*, **34**, 614–9.

Bevan, D. R., Doherty, W. G., Breen, P. J., and Donati, F. (1984). Mixtures of neostigmine and edrophonium are not synergistic. *Anesthesiology*, **61**, A298.

Brand, J. B., Cullen, D. J., Wilson, N. E., and Ali, H. H. (1977). Spontaneous recovery from nondepolarizing neuromuscular blockade: Correlation between clinical and evoked responses. *Anesthesia and Analgesia*, **56**, 55–8.

Breen, P. J., Doherty, W. G., Donati, F., and Bevan, D. R. (1985). The potencies of edrophonium and neostigmine as antagonists of pancuronium. *Anaesthesia*, **40**, 844–7.

Caldwell, J. E., Robertson, E. N., and Baird, W. L. M. (1987). Antagonism of vecuronium and atracurium: comparison of neostigmine and edrophonium administered at 5% twitch height recovery. *British Journal of Anaesthesia*, **59**, 478–81.

Child, C. S. (1984). Prevention of neostigmine-induced colonic activity. A comparison of atropine and glycopyrronium. *Anaesthesia*, **39**, 1083–5.

Cronelly, R. and Miller, R. D. (1984). Edrophonium: dose–response, onset and duration of antagonism in elderly patients. *Anesthesiology*, **61**, A303.

Cronnelly, R., Stanski, D. R., Miller, R. D., Sheiner, L. B., and Sohn, Y. J. (1979). Renal function and pharmacokinetics of neostigmine of neostigmine in anesthetized man. *Anesthesiology*, **51**, 222–6.

Cronnelly, R., Stanski, D. R., Miller, R. D., and Sheiner, L. B. (1980). Pyridostigmine kinetics with and without renal function. *Clinical Pharmacology and Therapeutics*, **28**, 78–81.

Cronnelly, R., Morris, R. B., and Miller, R. D. (1982). Edrophonium: Duration of action and atropine requirements in humans during halothane anaesthesia. *Anesthesiology*, **57**, 261–6.

Delisle, S. and Bevan, D. R. (1982). Impaired neostigmine antagonism of pancuronium during enflurane anaesthesia in man. *British Journal of Anaesthesia*, **54**, 441–4.

Dernovoi, B., Agoston, S., Barvais, L., Baurain, M., Lefevre, R., and d'Hollander, A. (1987). Neostigmine antagonism of vecuronium paralysis during fentanyl, halothane, isoflurane, and enflurane anesthesia. *Anesthesiology*, **66**, 698–701.

Diefenbach, C., Mellinghoff, H., Lynch, J., and Buzello, W. (1992). Mivacurium: dose–response relationship and administration by repeated injection or infusion. *Anesthesia and Analgesia*, **74**, 420–3.

Donati, F., Lahoud, J., McCready, D., and Bevan, D. R. (1987a). Neostigmine, pyridostigmine and edrophonium as antagonists of deep pancuronium blockade. *Canadian Journal of Anaesthesia*, **34**, 589–93.

Donati, F., McCarroll, S. M., Antzaka, C., McCready, D., and Bevan, D. R. (1987b). Dose–response curves for edrophonium, neostigmine, and pyridostigmine after pancuronium and D-tubocurarine. *Anesthesiology*, **66**, 471–6.

Donati, F., Smith, C. E., Wiesel, A., and Bevan, D. R. (1989). 'Priming' with neostigmine: failure to accelerate reversal of single twitch and train-of-four responses. *Canadian Journal of Anaesthesia*, **36**, 30–4.

Drenck, N. E., Ueda, N., Olsen, N. V., Engbæk, J., Jensen, E., Skovgård, L. T., and Viby-Mogensen, J. (1989). Manual evaluation of residual curarization using double burst stimulation: A comparison with train-of-four. *Anesthesiology*, **70**, 578–81.

Dupuis, J. Y., Martin, R., Tessonnier, J. M., and Tetrault, J. P. (1990). Clinical assessment of the muscular response to tetanic nerve stimulation. *Canadian Journal of Anaesthesia*, **37**, 397–400.

Engbæk, J., Ording, H., Ostergård, D., and Viby-Mogensen, J. (1985). Edrophonium and neostigmine for reversal of the neuromuscular blocking effect of vecuronium. *Acta Anaesthesiologica Scandinavica*, **29**, 544–6.

Engbæk, J., Ostergård, D., and Viby-Mogensen, J. (1989a). Double Burst Stimulation (DBS): A new nerve stimulation to identify residual neuromuscular blockade. *British Journal of Anaesthesia*, **62**, 274–8.

Engbæk, J., Ostergård, D., Viby-Mogensen, J., and Skovgård, L. T. (1989b). Clinical recovery and train-of-four ratio measured mechanically and electromyographically following atracurium. *Anesthesiology*, **71**, 391–5.

Engbæk, J., Ostergård, D., Skovgård, L. T., and Viby-Mogensen, J. (1990). Reversal of intensic neuromuscular blockade following infusion of atracurium. *Anesthesiology*, **72**, 803–6.

Feldman, S. A. (1963). Effect of changes in electrolytes, hydration and pH upon the reactions to muscle relaxants. *British Journal of Anaesthesia*, **35**, 546–51.

Ferguson, A., Egerszegi, P., and Bevan, D. R. (1980). Neostigmine, Pyridostigmine and edrophonium as antagonists of pancuronium. *Anesthesiology*, **53**, 390–4.

Fisher, D. M., Cronnelly, R., Miller, R. D., and Sharma, M. (1983). The neuromuscular pharmacology of neostigmine in infants and children. *Anesthesiology*, **59**, 220–5.

Fisher, D. M., Cronnelly, R., Sharma, M., and Miller, R. D. (1984). Clinical pharmacology of edrophonium in infants and children. *Anesthesiology*, **61**, 428–33.

Fogdall, R. P. and Miller, R. D. (1973). Antagonism of *d*-tubocurarine- and pancuronium-induced neuromuscular blockades by pyridostigmine in man. *Anesthesiology*, **39**, 504–9.

Gill, S. S., Bevan D. R., and Donati, F. (1990). Edrophonium antagonism of atracurium during enflurane anaesthesia. *British Journal of Anaesthesia*, **64**, 300–5.

Goldhill, D. R., Embree, P. B., Ali, H. H., and Savarese, J. J. (1986). Complete reversal of deep pancuronium block requires at lease 20 minutes. *Anesthesia and Analgesia*, **65**, S170.

Goldhill, D. R., Whitehead, J. P., Emmott, R. S., Griffith, A. P., Bracey, B. J., and Flynn, P. J. (1991). Neuromuscular and clinical effects of mivacurium chloride in healthy adult patients during nitrous oxide–enflurane anaesthesia. *British Journal of Anaesthesia*, **67**, 289–95.

Grum, D. F., and Osborne, L. R. (1991). Central anticholinergic syndrome following gly-copyrrolate. *Anesthesiology*, **74**, 191–2.

Gwinnutt, C. L., Walker, R. W. M., and Meakin, G. (1991). Antagonism of intense atracurium-induced neuromuscular block in children. *British Journal of Anaesthesia*, **67**, 13–6.

Katz, R. L. (1971) Clinical neuromuscular pharmacology of pancuronium. *Anesthesiology*, **34**, 550–6.

Kongsrud, F. and Sponheim, S. (1982). A comparison of atropine and glycopyrrolate in anaesthetic practice. *Acta Anaesthesiologica Scandinavica*, **26**, 620–5.

Kopman, A. F. (1986). Recovery times following edrophonium and neostigmine reversal of pancuronium, atracurium, and vecuronium steady-state infusions. *Anesthesiology*, **65**, 572–8.

Magorian, T. T., Lynam, D. P., Caldwell, J. E., and Miller, R. D. (1990). Can early adminis-tration of neostigmine, in single or repeated doses, alter the course of neuromuscular recovery from a vecuronium-induced blockade? *Anesthesiology*, **73**, 410–4.

Miller, R. D. (1990). Pharmacokinetics of reversal agents and clinical considerations in their use. In *Muscle relaxants*, (ed. S. Agoston and W. C. Bowman), pp. 503–14. Elsevier, Amsterdam.

Miller, R. D. and Roderick, L. (1978). Acid–base balance and neostigmine antagonism of pancuronium neuromuscular blockade. *British Journal of Anaesthesia*, **50**, 317–23.

Miller, R. D., Van Nyhuis, L. S., Eger, E. I., Vitez, T. S., and Way, W. L. (1974). Comparative times to peak effect and durations of action of neostigmine and pyridostig-mine. *Anesthesiology*, **41**, 27–33.

Mirakhur, R. K. and Dundee, J. W. (1980). Comparison of the effect of atropine and gly-copyrrolate on various end-organs. *Journal of The Royal Society of Medicine*, **73**, 727–30.

Mirakhur, R. K., Dundee, J. W., Jones, C. J., Coppel, D. L., and Clarke, S. J. (1981). Reversal of neuromuscular blockade: Dose determination studies with atropine and gly-copyrrolate given before or in a mixture with neostigmine. *Anesthesia and Analgesia*, **60**, 557–62.

Morris, R. B., Cronnelly, R., Miller, R. D., Stanski, D. R., and Fahey, M. R. (1981). Pharmacokinetics of edrophonium in anephric and renal transplant patients. *British Journal of Anaesthesia*, **53**, 1311–4.

Mostafa, S. M. and Vucevic, M. (1984). Comparison of atropine and glycopyrronium in patients with pre-existing cardiac disease. *Anaesthesia*, **39**, 1207–13.

Naguib, M. and Abdulatif, M. (1988). Priming with anticholinesterases — the effect of dif-ferent combinations of anticholinesterases and different priming intervals. *Canadian Journal of Anaesthesia*, **35**, 47–52.

Ostergaard, D., Engbæk, J., and Viby-Mogensen, J. (1989). Adverse reactions and interac-tions of the neuromuscular blocking drugs. *Medical Toxicology and Adverse Drug Experiences*, **4**, 351–68.

Ostergaard, D., Jensen, F. S., Jensen, E., Skovgaard, L. T., and Viby-Mogensen, J. (1992). Influence of plasma cholinesterase activity on recovery from mivacurium-induced neuro-muscular blockade in phenotypically normal patients. *Acta Anaesthesiologica Scandinavica*, **36**, 702–6.

Paton, W. D. and Waud, D. R. (1967). The margin of safety of neuromuscular transmission. *Journal of Physiology*, **191**, 59–90.

Pavlin, E. G., Holle, R. H., and Schoene, R. B. (1989). Recovery of airway protection com-pared with ventilation in humans after paralysis with curare. *Anesthesiology*, **70**, 381–5.

Payne, J. P., Hughes, R., and Azawi, S. A. (1980). Neuromuscular blockade by neostigmine in anaesthetized man. *British Journal of Anaesthesia*, **52**, 69–76.

Savarese, J. J., Ali, H. H., Basta, S. J, Embree, P. B., Scott, R. P. F., Sunder, N., *et al.* (1988). The clinical neuromuscular pharmacology of mivacurium chloride (BW B1090U). *Anesthesiology*, **68**, 723–32.

Sherby, S. M., Eldefrawi, A. T., Albuquerque, E. X., and Eldefrawi, M. E. (1985). Comparison of the actions of carbamate anticholinesterases on the nicotinic acetylcholine receptor. *Molecular Pharmacology*, **27**, 343–8.

Viby-Mogensen, J. (1981). Succinylcholine neuromuscular blockade in subjects homozygous for a typical cholinesterase. *Anesthesiology*, **55**, 429–34.

Viby-Mogensen, J. (1983). Cholinesterase and succinylcholine. *Danish Medical Bulletin*, **30**, 129–49.

Viby-Mogensen, J. (1985). Clinical measurement of neuromuscular function: An update. *Clinics in Anaesthesiology*, **3**, 467–82.

Viby-Mogensen, J., Jensen, N. H., Engbæk, J., Ording, H., Skovgaard, L. T., and Chræmmer-Jorgensen, B. (1985) Tactile and visual evaluation of the response to train-of-four nerve stimulation. *Anesthesiology*, **63**, 440–3.

Wetterslev, J., Jarnvig, I., Jorgensen, L. N., and Olsen, N. V. (1991). Split-dose atropine versus glycopyrrolate with neostigmine for reversal of gallamine-induced neuromuscular blockade. *Acta Anaesthesiologica Scandinavica*, **35**, 398–401.

Wilkins, J. L., Hardcastle, J. D., Mann, C. V., and Kaufman, L. (1970). Effects of neostigmine and atropine on motor activity of ileum, colon and rectum of anaesthetized subjects. *British Medical Journal*, **i**, 793–4.

Young, W. L., Matteo, R. S., and Ornstein, E. (1988). Duration of action of neostigmine and pyridostigmine in the elderly. *Anesthesia and Analgesia*, **67**, 775–8.

8

Post-operative sequelae of neuromuscular blocking agents

David R. Bevan

Within ten years of the introduction of curare (Griffith and Johnson 1942), it was being blamed for an increase in anaesthesia morbidity and mortality (Beecher and Todd 1954). Although initially ignored, it is now clear that the uncontrolled use of neuromuscular blocking agents may be associated with perioperative complications. Most of these are related to the presence of unrecognized residual neuromuscular block in the postoperative period. In addition, some of the complications of the use of muscle relaxants may present or persist in the postoperative period. The purpose of this chapter is to describe the continuing effects of neuromuscular blocking drugs which are seen after surgery, to discuss their recognition and importance, and to suggest how they may be prevented.

RESIDUAL NEUROMUSCULAR BLOCK

History

The first large-scale attempt to study deaths associated with anaesthesia was performed by Beecher and Todd (1954). Their study is important in relationship to the morbidity and mortality associated with the use of muscle relaxant drugs because it was performed within a few years after their introduction. The study examined all deaths in surgical patients over five years in 10 American university hospitals. Superficial examination of the data suggested that the use of 'curare' was associated with a six-fold increase in the mortality rate (Table 8.1). It should be remembered, however, that the non-curare group included patients undergoing minor procedures under local anaesthesia, but it proved impossible for the authors to relate the use of 'curare' to higher risk patients. There were insufficient numbers to demonstrate different mortality rates among the relaxants used at that time (tubocurarine, gallamine, suxamethonium, and decamethonium). The average doses of tubocurarine used (15 mg) and of gallamine (45 mg) are, however, much lower than the average dose of suxamethonium (197 mg). Most of the deaths were due to respiratory or cardiac failure and it was often difficult to differentiate between them.

Table 8.1   Incidence of deaths associated with the use of 'curare' (Beecher & Todd, 1954)

Number of anaesthetics	599 500
Anaesthetics with 'curare'	44 100
Death frequency with 'curare'	1 : 2100
Death frequency without 'curare'	1 : 370

From Beecher and Todd (1954)

Surprisingly, this condemnation of 'curare' had little general effect on the growth of the use of muscle relaxants during anaesthesia. In part, this reflects the greatly improved surgical conditions that could be achieved, but also greater care in their use. Several anaesthetists would have been influenced by Dripps' (1959) criticism of the survey, growing reports of the successful use of relaxants and the realization that much greater doses of tubocurarine had been given safely in England if the relaxants were reversed with anticholinesterases (Gray and Halton 1946). Nevertheless, warnings of the dangers of neuromuscular blocking drugs had been given.

Epidemiology

Several recent studies have demonstrated that neuromuscular relaxants contribute to anaesthetic morbidity and mortality. In the second of two studies conducted by the Association of Anaesthetists of Great Britain and Ireland, Lunn *et al.* (1983) showed that post-operative respiratory failure was the commonest single cause of postoperative death due to anaesthesia. Of 1897 deaths reported, 32 were due totally to anaesthesia: 11 were from postoperative respiratory failure. Neuromuscular relaxants were implicated directly in six of these deaths. In France, Tiret *et al.* (1986) examined major complications associated with anaesthesia in nearly 200 000 patients. Major complications occurred in 268 patients of whom 67 died, and in 16 coma persisted for more than 24 hr. Half of the deaths and coma directly attributed to anaesthesia were due to post-anaesthetic respiratory depression. Surprisingly, in a study of 112 000 anaesthetics in a single hospital in Winnipeg, Canada, death was rare and respiratory complications were reported less frequently as a postoperative complication than was hypotension (Cohen *et al.* 1986). In contrast, Cooper *et al.* (1989) reported on 53 patients admitted to the intensive care unit in Guildford, UK. The largest single group of admissions (24 of 53) was as a result of ventilatory failure after attempted reversal of nondepolarizing relaxants.

Thus, it seems that the first 24 hr after surgery is a time of high complication (Gamil and Fanning, 1991). Failure to provide adequate recovery room or intensive care facilities is likely to be associated with greater morbidity and mortality, a major portion of which is due to postoperative respiratory failure as a result of residual neuromuscular block.

Relaxants and respiration

Several studies have demonstrated that pulmonary ventilation is preserved until there is considerable weakness of peripheral musculature. This 'respiratory sparing' has been demonstrated for depolarizing and nondepolarizing relaxants (Foldes *et al.* 1961). When respiratory function is measured using a sensitive index — maximum inspiratory force (MIF) (Bendixen and Bunker 1962) — Wymore and Eisele (1978) showed that the intensity and duration of reduction in MIF is less intense and of shorter duration than the depression of thumb twitch after sequential small doses of tubocurarine. Similarly, Williams and Bourke (1985) demonstrated that, using a suxamethonium infusion, when grip strength was decreased by 50%, MIF and vital capacity (VC) were reduced by less than 15%.

During recovery from atracurium, spontaneous return of ventilation in patients whose tracheas were intubated occurred when there was less than 25% recovery of the tetanic response of the adductor pollicis (Hackett *et al.* 1986). Using train-of-four stimulation, Ali *et al.* (1975) demonstrated, in conscious volunteers given small doses of tubocurarine (0.05 mg/kg; total 0.164 mg/kg), that there was no change in VC until TOF reached 0.6 and that there was a measurable decrease in MIF when TOF was 0.7 (Fig. 8.1) Stanec *et al.* (1990), however, demonstrated that, in patients studied in the recovery room after anaesthesia, when TOF had recovered to 0.9–1, the MIF and VC were still reduced by 28 and 23% respectively. Nevertheless, a TOF ratio of 0.7 has become the 'gold standard' to be aimed for to demonstrate adequate return of neuromuscular function at the end of anaesthesia.

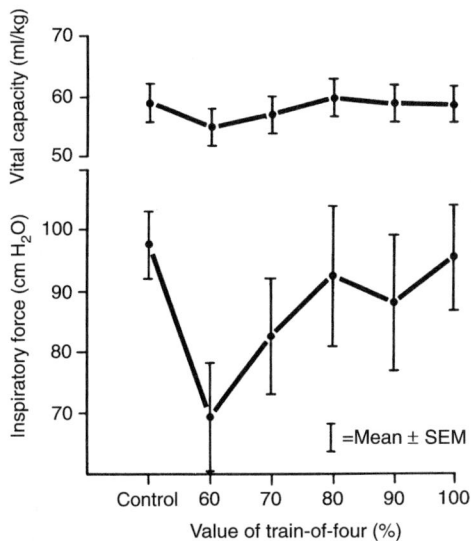

Fig. 8.1 Changes in vital capacity and inspiratory force in conscious volunteers during the administration of boluses of tubocurarine. (From Ali *et al.* 1975.)

Despite 'respiratory sparing', measurable decreases in ventilatory function have been observed after small, precurarizing, doses of alcuronium (Astley *et al.* 1987), atracurium (Howardy-Hansen *et al.* 1987), and pancuronium or vecuronium (Engbaek *et al.* 1985; Motsch *et al.* 1987). In addition, the respiratory effects of relaxants may be different in patients during anaesthesia and awake volunteers. For example, when repeated doses of tubocurarine were given until tidal volume was reduced in conscious subjects, this was usually associated with an increase in respiratory frequency (Gal and Smith 1976). When a similar experiment was performed during enflurane anaesthesia, not only was the neuromuscular blocking effect of pancuronium potentiated but the decrease in tidal volume was associated with a decrease in frequency (Nishindo *et al.* 1988). Thus it should not be assumed that ventilatory function has returned to normal when there is no clinical weakness of the peripheral musculature, particularly in the anaesthetized subject or in patients recovering from general anaesthesia.

In humans, under steady-state conditions, the ED_{50} of the diaphragm is approximately twice that of the adductor pollicis. This has been shown for suxamethonium (Smith *et al.* 1988), as well as for pancuronium (Donati *et al.* 1986), atracurium and vecuronium (Laycock *et al.* 1988*a*). Using intubating doses of suxamethonium (Pansard *et al.* 1987), vecuronium (Chauvin *et al.* 1987) or atracurium (Pansard *et al.* 1987; Derrington and Hindocha, 1988) onset and recovery at the diaphragm precedes that at the adductor pollicis. However, when subparalysing doses are administered the difference in potency may not be so apparent (Donati *et al.* 1990) probably because the preferential perfusion of the diaphragm, which is responsible for the earlier onset, also allows the delivery of a higher concentration of drug to the diaphragm after a bolus injection. Consequently, during onset of block the extent of paralysis of the adductor pollicis is a poor estimate of the effect at the diaphragm. Conversely, during recovery and particularly after the reversal of the block with anticholinesterase, recovery of the diaphragm precedes that of the adductor pollicis (Lebrault *et al.* 1988; 1989 *a*, *b*) (Fig. 8.2). In this situation, it can be assumed that when recovery of the adductor pollicis is complete, then

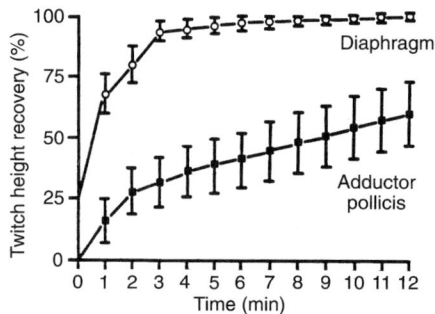

Fig. 8.2 Recovery of adductor pollicis and diaphragm after reversal of vecuronium neuromuscular block with edrophonium at 25% twitch recovery at the diaphragm. (From Lebrault *et al.* 1989*b*.)

recovery of the diaphragm is assured. Consequently, if ventilation is impaired at a time when the adductor pollicis is nearly fully recovered (TOF of 0.7), this is unlikely to be the result of diaphragmatic weakness.

The cause of the reduction of MIF and of respiratory impairment at mild levels of neuromuscular block as assessed at the adductor pollicis (TOF < 0.7) is uncertain. Circumstantial evidence suggests that it may be due to failure to maintain the patency of the upper airway. Firstly, before the use of muscle relaxants during anaesthesia, tubocurarine had been used to prevent bone fractures during convulsive therapy to psychiatric patients. Some deaths occurred and these were due to respiratory obstruction (Bennett 1968). Secondly, Pavlin *et al.* (1989) demonstrated that when tubocurarine was given in incremental doses to conscious volunteers greater muscle strength was required to protect the airway than to maintain maximum inspiratory pressure (MIP) greater than –25 cm H_2O (a value considered by Bendixen and Bunker (1962) to be adequate to support ventilation). Pavlin also demonstrated that even greater return of motor power was necessary to maintain a head lift for five seconds. Thirdly, Dodgson *et al* (1981) reported that when tubocurarine was given until hand grip strength was nearly abolished, MIP decreased only slightly, whereas upper airway resistance more than doubled. Finally, Isono *et al.* (1992) have demonstrated that the geniohyoid (a muscle which moves the hyoid bone forward and which may have a role in maintaining airway patency) was much more sensitive to vecuronium than the diaphragm, at least in dogs. Thus, the demonstration of sensitivity of at least one muscle in the upper airway to neuromuscular blocking drugs suggests that, until proved otherwise, the upper airway is the weak link in the respiratory chain.

The implication of these observations is that, if there is any doubt of the recovery of neuromuscular function, particular care should be directed towards maintenance of the airway. The appropriate precaution is to maintain tracheal intubation until adequate recovery can be demonstrated. If the patient can sustain a five second head lift, this implies that sufficient return of neuromuscular function has occurred to maintain airway patency and to support respiration.

RESIDUAL BLOCK AFTER ANAESTHESIA

Viby-Mogensen and his colleagues (1979) demonstrated a high incidence of residual neuromuscular block in patients in the recovery room. They examined 72 patients, who had received a variety of long-acting relaxants (tubocurarine, gallamine, and pancuronium), after the anaesthetist had left the patient to the care of the nursing staff. In 30 (42%), the TOF of the adductor pollicis was less than 0.7 even though 67 had received neostigmine to reverse the block. Of the 68 who were sufficiently awake and cooperative, 16 (24%) were unable to maintain a five-second head lift (Fig. 8.3). Other studies, performed in several countries, have reported a similar high incidence of residual paralysis (Lennmarken and Löfström 1984; Beemer and Rozental 1986; Andersen *et al.* 1988), although the incidence of weakness (TOF < 0.7) was reduced to less than 10% when the intermediate agents

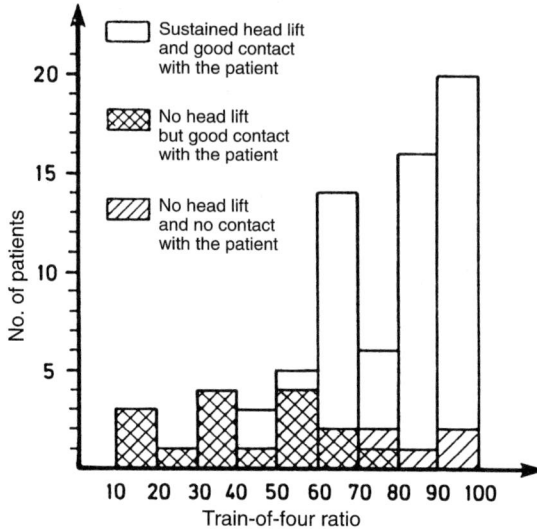

Fig. 8.3 Train-of-four ratio and ability to maintain five-second head lift in 72 patients after anaesthesia. (Adapted from Viby-Mogensen *et al.* 1979.)

atracurium and vecuronium were used (Bevan *et al.* 1988*b*; Brull *et al.* 1988; Howardy-Hansen *et al.* 1989; Jensen *et al.* 1990) (Table 8.2). Other objective measures of muscle strength — hand grip and expiratory and inspiratory forces — also recover more rapidly after using the intermediate agents during anaesthesia (Hutton *et al.* 1988; Kong and Cooper 1988) although some authors have been unable to confirm this (O'Connor and Russell 1988).

In those studies where clinical assessment of recovery was also made, most muscle groups had recovered when adductor pollicis TOF reached 0.7. However, to ensure that no weakness of head lift, hand grip, or tongue protrusion remains, the TOF should exceed 0.9 (Bevan *et al.* 1988*b*). Thus, to provide adequate recovery of neuromuscular function to maintain respiration, complete return of adductor pollicis function should be demonstrated.

Only in children less than 10 years old, studied 15–20 min after reversal of neuromuscular block was it not possible to demonstrate residual weakness (TOF < 0.7) (Baxter *et al.* 1991). The most likely reasons for the improved outcome after the use of relaxants in children are decreased potency of relaxants (Laycock *et al.* 1988*b*; Meakin *et al.* 1988; Meretoja *et al.* 1988), more rapid spontaneous recovery (Goudsouzian *et al.* 1983; Brandom *et al.* 1984), and quicker reversal (Fisher *et al.* 1983; Meakin *et al.* 1983). However, when atracurium and alcuronium were compared in children, Meretoja and Gebert (1990) did show a more rapid recovery after atracurium but, with both relaxants, recovery seemed to proceed more rapidly than in adults so that by the time the patients arrived in the recovery room no weakness

Table 8.2   Incidence of residual neuromuscular blockade after anesthesia
NMB, neuromuscular blocking drug; dTC, *d*-tubocurarine; P, pancuronium;
G, gallamine; Al, alcuronium; A, atracurium; V, vecuronium

Origin	NMB	TOF < 0.7	
		n	%
Copenhagen, Denmark	dTC/P/G	30/72	42
(Viby-Mogensen *et al.* 1979)			
Linköping, Sweden	P	12/48	25
(Lennmarken and Löfström 1984)			
Melbourne, Australia	dTC/P/G/Al	21/100	21
(Beemer and Rozental 1986)			
Aarhus, Denmark	P	6/30	20
(Andersen *et al.* 1988)	A	0/30	0
Montréal, Canada	P	17/47	36
(Bevan *et al.* 1988)	A	2/46	4
	V	5/57	9
New Haven, USA	P	14/29	48
(Brull *et al.* 1988)	V	2/24	8
Copenhagen, Denmark	G	5/10	50
(Howardy-Hansen *et al.* 1989)	A	0/9	0
Aarhus, Denmark	P	62/159	39
(Jensen *et al.* 1990)	A	3/171	2
	V	6/158	4
Montréal, Canada	P/A/V	0/91	0
(Children) (Baxter *et al.* 1991)			

NMB, ≠ neuromuscular blocking drug; dtc ≠ *d*-tubocurarine; P, ≠ pancuronium; G, ≠ gallamine; A1, ≠ alcuronium; A, ≠ atracurium; V, ≠ vecuronium

could be demonstrated. Residual neuromuscular block is unlikely after anaesthesia in children, particularly after the use of intermediate relaxants. These observations support the use of neuromuscular blocking drugs in the day-care setting, in which the majority of paediatric surgery is performed.

RECURARIZATION

There are many reports of patients who appeared to be awake and breathing adequately at the end of anaesthesia who, after settling in the recovery room, become drowsy and apnoeic (Feldman 1959; Jenkins 1961). Several occurred in patients with renal failure in whom it was assumed that the early recovery indicated adequate reversal of the block, but that this wore off and reparalysis occurred because of the kidney's failure to excrete the nondepolarizing relaxants (Miller and Cullen 1976). More careful monitoring of the block and its recovery has been unable to demonstrate 'recurarization' (Bevan *et al.* 1982). A more likely cause, particularly as the reports were characterized by the absense of neuromuscular monitoring, is that the stimulation of extubation and moving from the operating room table to a trolley is sufficient to rouse a partially anaesthetized, narcotized, and paralysed patient, but that in the peaceful environment of the recovery room, and after further narcotic analgesia is administered, this results in hypnosis and inadequate ventilation. In certain circumstances, 'recurarization' can be induced. Experimentally, the administration of reversal agents during the course of a continuous infusion of relaxant does result in an initial recovery of the block followed by reparalysis. In some clinical situations, for example after prolonged administration of pancuronium, tubocurarine, or gallamine to a patient with renal dysfunction, this may occur but it must be rare.

RESIDUAL PARALYSIS IN THE INTENSIVE CARE UNIT

Several reports of continued weakness after the prolonged use of nondepolarizing relaxants in intensive care patients have occurred recently. In two patients, this appears to have resulted from the accumulation of an active metabolite of vecuronium, 3-desacetyl-vecuronium, which was not eliminated because the patients had developed renal failure (Segredo *et al.* 1990). However, it is difficult to understand why the administration of relaxant was not reduced as the metabolite accumulated. Other reports have described a 'myopathy' producing continued weakness for several weeks (Gooch *et al.* 1991; Subramony *et al.* 1991). The aetiology is unclear and the reports lack characteristic features. It is easy to be cynical and to suggest that the incidence of such observations, as with those of 'recurarization', will decrease when monitoring becomes an integral part of the use of neuromuscular blocking drugs in the intensive care unit.

PREDISPOSING CAUSES

There are several causes of impaired antagonism of neuromuscular block (Bevan *et al.* 1992) (see Chapter 7). The most important include the intensity of neuromuscular block, choice of relaxant, and dose of reversal agent. The more intense the block, the longer will it take to achieve acceptable standards of reversal (Katz 1967; 1972) and the larger the dose of reversal agent that should be given. Intense neuromuscular block is reversed more easily with neostigmine than with edrophonium (Rupp *et al.* 1986; Donati *et al.* 1987). As restoration of neuromuscular function depends upon the combination of spontaneous recovery and reversal with anticholinesterases, reversal appears to be accomplished more easily with the intermediate-acting than the longer-acting agents (Gencarelli and Miller 1982). It is probably for this reason that residual curarization is seen infrequently in the recovery room after using atracurium or vecuronium (Jensen *et al.* 1990).

Recovery might be expected to be delayed in the elderly due to impaired renal excretion of the relaxants (Bevan *et al.* 1988*a*), but evidence for this is difficult to

Table 8.3 Principles of management of neuromuscular block

Anticipate abnormal reactions to relaxants and reversal agents

Monitor neuromuscular block

Titrate dose of relaxants to effect and maintain some muscular response to nerve stimulation

Avoid long-acting relaxants

Always reverse neuromuscular block

find (Marsh *et al.* 1980), in contrast to the more rapid recovery of neuromuscular block after reversal in children (Fisher *et al.* 1983; Meakin *et al.* 1983). Similarly, although several drug interactions have been described which prolong the duration of action of relaxants there are few convincing reports that such interactions hinder reversal. The reversal of pancuronium with neostigmine in the presence of enflurane (Delisle and Bevan 1982), or of vecuronium with enflurane or isoflurane (Dernovoi *et al.* 1987) is impaired. However, in clinical practice, the inhalational agent is stopped at the same time as or before reversal, and this reduces any effect on reversal (Gill *et al.* 1990). Failure to reverse neuromuscular block in the severely ill, cachectic patient probably results from several causes including acid–base disturbance (Brooks and Feldman 1962), hypothermia (Heir *et al.* 1991), fluid and electrolyte imbalance (Feldman 1968), and inadequate monitoring.

PREVENTION AND MANAGEMENT

The principles of management of residual neuromuscular block include its recognition by clinical and neuromuscular monitoring, reversal of detectable block, and maintenance of the airway and respiration until adequate return of neuromuscular function has been demonstrated (Table 8.3).

Clinical evaluation

In the conscious patient, the ability to head lift is the most sensitive sign of return of function. When head lift is sustained for five seconds, this is associated with near complete recovery of vital capacity and maximal voluntary ventilation (Walts *et al.* 1970). Engbaek *et al.* (1989) found that head lift could not be sustained at a TOF ratio of 0.5 and by only 50% of patients at a TOF ratio of 0.6. Other tests, including hand grip, leg lift, and the ability to open the eyes or protrude the tongue are less sensitive. The measurement of inspiratory force was developed as 'a vital capacity measurement in the unconscious'. Normal values, in conscious individuals are approximately –90 cm H_2O. At a maximum inspiratory pressure (MIP) of –25 cm H_2O or less, swallowing and the ability to maintain a patent airway were lost, head

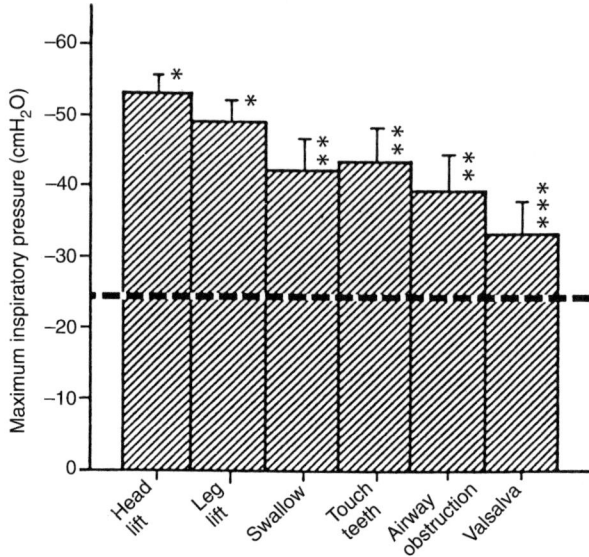

Fig. 8.4 Relationship between maximum inspiratory pressure and the ability to perform various clinical manoevres. Head lift is the most sensitive indicator of neuromuscular blockade. (From Pavlin *et al.* 1979.)

lift was affected at approximately –50 cm H_2O, and all subjects who could sustain a head lift could perform airway-protective manoeuvres (Pavlin *et al.* 1989) (Fig. 8.4).

Neuromuscular monitoring

Train-of-four stimulation of the ulnar nerve and measurement or observation of the force of contraction or electromyographic response of the adductor pollicis has become the standard for clinical practice. The aim is to achieve return of TOF ratio to greater than 0.7 at the end of anaesthesia. To ensure full return of respiratory function complete TOF recovery should be attempted (Stanec *et al.* 1990). Small degrees of TOF fade are difficult to recognize either by visual observation or by touch. Most anaesthetists are unable to recognize fade if the TOF ratio is 0.5 or greater (Viby-Mogensen *et al.* 1985). Double burst stimulation is more sensitive (Saddler *et al* 1990). In practice, however, full return of visual response to TOF stimulation appears to be an adequate guide particularly if intermediate-duration relaxants have been used and reversed with edrophonium or neostigmine.

Reversal of neuromuscular block

After using neuromuscular blocking drugs, reversal with anticholinesterases should be attempted unless complete recovery of neuromuscular block can be demonstrated. As it is not possible to assess small, but important, degrees of block by

Table 8.4 Recommended doses of neostigmine or edrophonium according to response to TOF stimulation

TOF visible twitches	Fade	Agent	Dose (mg/kg)
None	Postpone reversal until some evoked response		
≤ 2	++++	Neostigmine	0.07
3–4	+++	Neostigmine	0.04
4	++	Edrophonium	0.5

From Bevan *et al*. 1992

visual or tactile means, this is a recommendation always to reverse muscle relaxants. Several regimens have been proposed. In general, recovery is achieved more rapidly after edrophonium than after neostigmine. However, neostigmine is more effective in reversing an intense block. Thus, the choice and dose of reversal agents should be based upon the intensity of neuromuscular block (Table 8.4).

Failure of reversal

If it is not possible to achieve full recovery of neuromuscular block, ventilatory support and maintenance of a patent airway will be required until recovery can be demonstrated. In those situations, where some TOF fade is still obvious, the anaesthetist should consider retaining the endotracheal tube in position: it is not a sign of failure to return to the recovery room with a patient whose trachea is still intubated.

OTHER POST-OPERATIVE COMPLICATIONS

Some of the several complications associated with neuromuscular blocking drugs may persist or present in the post-operative period.

Suxamethonium

The most frequent and irritating complication of suxamethonium is the appearance of muscle pains on arousal from anaesthesia (Table 8.5). They occur particularly in the young and muscular who ambulate soon after surgery. They can be prevented or diminished by the prophylactic administration of a small dose of nondepolarizing relaxant, of which tubocurarine 3 mg appears to be the most effective if given three minutes before the suxamethonium (Erkola *et al*. 1983). The cause of the pains, and of the fasciculations with which they are usually associated, is not known nor is their relationship to the release of myoglobin clearly established.

Table 8.5   Complications associated with suxamethonium which present or
persist into the post-operative period

Muscle pains

Myoglobinaemia

Myoglobinuria

Hyperkalaemia

Phase II block

Reduced plasma cholinesterase activity

Malignant hyperthermia

Anaphylaxis

Small, transient increases in serum potassium concentration occur after administration of suxamethonium to normal individuals. The hyperkalaemia which occurs
in the burned (Tolmie *et al.* 1967), septic (Khan and Khan, 1983), or traumatized
(Birch *et al.* 1969) patient is probably the result of extrajunctional receptor duplica-
tion (Gronert and Theye 1975) which leads to prolonged depolarization and potassium leakage (and resistance to nondepolarizing relaxants).

Delayed recovery from suxamethonium may be due to the development of phase
II block after large doses (> 2.5 mg/kg), has the characteristic fade in response to
TOF stimulation, and can be reversed with small doses of edrophonium or neostigmine (Bevan *et al.* 1988*a*). Alternatively, reduced plasma cholinesterase activity
results in a very prolonged block and, although it may present with some fade in
response to TOF stimulation, it is not reversible with anticholinesterases (Bevan
and Donati 1983).

The most serious complication of suxamethonium, malignant hyperthermia, is
fortunately rare. Its early recognition and treatment with dantrolene ensure that
almost all patients now survive the syndrome.

Anaphylaxis to muscle relaxants is uncommon but has been reported more
frequently after suxamethonium than after any other relaxant. Treatment of the
bronchospasm and hypotension may persist into the post-operative period.

Non-depolarizing relaxants

Apart from residual neuromuscular block, effects of the nondepolarizing relaxants
are seldom seen in the postoperative period. The cardiovascular complications are
infrequent, mild, and transient. When due to histamine release, the cutaneous evidence may persist but the systemic effect will have disappeared or been treated.
Anaphylaxis is less common than after suxamethonium and the least frequently
implicated nondepolarizing relaxant is pancuronium.

CONCLUSION

The most common cause of anaesthetic-related morbidity and mortality is persistent postoperative neuromuscular block which results in respiratory failure and, rarely, in death. The individual response to neuromuscular blocking drugs is so variable that the only means of determining the appropriate dose is to titrate them with the help of neuromuscular monitoring. This will also allow residual paralysis to be detected and treated with the appropriate choice and dose of edrophonium or neostigmine. Safe practice dictates that muscle-relaxant drugs should always be reversed with anticholinesterases.

REFERENCES

Ali, H. H., Wilson, R. S., Savarese, J. J., and Kitz, R. J. (1975). The effects of tubocurarine on indirectly elicited train-of-four muscle response and respiratory measurements in humans. *British Journal of Anaesthesia*, **47**, 570–4.

Andersen, B. N., Madsen, J. V., Schurizek, B. A., and Juhl, B. (1988). Residual curarisation: a comparative study of atracurium and pancuronium. *Acta Anaesthesiologica Scandinavica*, **32**, 79–81.

Astley, B. A., Hughes, R., and Payne, J. P. (1987). Recovery of respiration after neuromuscular blockade with alcuronium. *British Journal of Anaesthesia*, **59**, 206–10.

Baxter, M. R. N., Bevan, J. C., Samuel, J., Donati, F., and Bevan, D. R. (1991). Postoperative neuromuscular function in pediatric day-care patients. *Anesthesia and Analgesia*, **72**, 504–8.

Beecher, H. K. and Todd, D. P. (1954). Study of deaths associated with anesthesia and surgery based on a study of 599,548 anesthesias in 10 institutions 1948–1952 inclusive. *Annals of Surgery*, **140**, 2–35.

Beemer, G. H. and Rozental, P. (1986). Postoperative neuromuscular function. *Anaesthesia and Intensive Care*, **14**, 41–5.

Bendixen, H. H. and Bunker, J. P. (1962). Measurement of inspiratory force in anesthetized dogs. *Anesthesiology*, **23**, 315–23.

Bennett, A. E. (1968). The history of the introduction of curare into medicine. *Anesthesia and Analgesia*, **47**, 484–92.

Bevan, D. R. and Donati, F. (1983). Succinylcholine apnoea: attempted reversal with anticholinesterases. *Canadian Anaesthetists' Society Journal*, **30**, 536–9.

Bevan, D. R., Archer, D. P., Donati, F., Ferguson, A., and Higgs, B. D. (1982). Antagonism of pancuronium in renal failure: no recurarization. *British Journal of Anaesthesia*, **54**, 63–8.

Bevan, D. R., Bevan, J. C., and Donati, F. (1988*a*) *Muscle relaxants in clinical anesthesia*, pp. 317–44. Year Book Medical Publishers, Chicago.

Bevan, D. R., Smith, C. E., and Donati, F. (1988*b*). Postoperative neuromuscular blockade: a comparison between atracurium, vecuronium, and pancuronium. *Anesthesiology*, **69**, 272–6.

Bevan, D. R., Donati, F., and Kopman, A. F. (1992). Reversal of neuromuscular blockade. *Anesthesiology*, **77**, 785–80.

Birch, A. A., Mitchell, G. D., Playford, G. A. and Lang, C. A. (1969). Changes in serum potassium response to succinylcholine following trauma. *Journal of the American Medical Association*, **210**, 490–3.

Brandom, B. W., Woelfel, S. K., Cook, D. R., Fehr, B. L., and Rudd, G. D. (1984). Clinical pharmacology of atracurium in infants. *Anesthesia and Analgesia*, **63**, 309–12.

Brooks, D. K. and Feldman, S. A. (1962). Metabolic acidosis: a new approach to 'neostigmine resistant curarization'. *Anaesthesia*, **17**, 161–9.

Brull, S. J., Silverman, D. G., and Ehrenwerth, J. (1988). Problems of recovery and residual neuromuscular blockade: pancuronium vs. vecuronium. *Anesthesiology*, **69**, A473.

Chauvin, M., Lebrault, C., and Duvaldestin, P. (1987). The neuromuscular blocking effect of vecuronium on the human diaphragm. *Anesthesia and Analgesia*, **66**, 117–22.

Cohen, M. M, Duncan, P. G, Pope, W. D. B, and Wolkenstein, C. (1986). A survey of 112,000 anaesthetics at one teaching hospital (1975–83). *Canadian Anaesthetists' Society Journal*, **33**, 22–31.

Cooper, A. L, Leigh, J. M., and Tring, I. C. (1989). Admissions to the intensive care unit after complication of anaesthetic techniques over 10 years. *Anaesthesia*, **44**, 953–8.

Delisle, S. and Bevan, D. R. (1982). Impaired neostigmine antagonism of pancuronium during enflurane anaesthesia in man. *British Journal of Anaesthesia*, **54**, 441–5.

Dernovoi, B., Agoston, S., Barvais, L., Baurain, M., Ufebvre, R. and d'Hollander, A. (1987). Neostigmine antagonism of vecuronium paralysis during fentanyl, halothane, isoflurane and enflurane anesthesia. *Anesthesiology*, **66**, 698–701.

Derrington, M. C. and Hindocha, N. (1988). Measurement of evoked diaphragm twitch strength during anaesthesia. *British Journal of Anaesthesia*, **61**, 270–8.

Dodgson, B. G., Knill, R. L., and Clement, J. L. (1981). Curare increases upper airway resistance while reducing ventilatory muscle strength. *Canadian Anaesthetists' Society Journal*, **28**, 505–6.

Donati, F., Antzaka, C., and Bevan, D. R. (1986). Potency of pancuronium at the diaphragm and the adductor pollicis muscle in humans. *Anesthesiology*, **65**, 1–5.

Donati, F., Lahoud, J., McCready, D., and Bevan, D. R. (1987). Neostigmine, pyridostigmine, and edrophonium as antagonists of deep pancuronium blockade. *Canadian Journal of Anaesthesia*, **34**, 589–93.

Donati, F., Meistelman, C., and Plaud, B. (1990). Vecuronium neuromuscular blockade at the diaphragm, the orbicularis oculi, and adductor pollicis muscles. *Anesthesiology*, **73**, 870–5.

Dripps, R. D. (1959). The role of muscle relaxants in anesthesia deaths. *Anesthesiology*, **20**, 542–5.

Engbaek, J., Howardy-Hansen, P., Ording, H., and Viby-Mogensen, J. (1985). Precurarization with vecuronium and pancuronium in awake, healthy volunteers: the influence on neuromuscular transmission and pulmonary function. *Acta Anaesthesiologica Scandinavica*, **29**, 117–20.

Engbaek, J., Ostergaard, D., Viby-Mogensen, J., and Skovgaard, L. T. (1989). Clinical recovery and train-of-four ratio measured mechanically and electromyographically following atracurium. *Anesthesiology*, **71**, 391–5.

Erkola, O., Salmenpera, A., and Kuoppamaki, R. (1983). Five nondepolarizing muscle relaxants in precurarization. *Acta Anaesthesiologica Scandinavica*, **27**, 427–32.

Feldman, S. A. (1959). An interesting case of recurarization. *British Journal of Anaesthesia*, **31**, 461–3.

Feldman, S. A. (1968). Effect of changes in electrolyte, hydration and pH upon the reactions to muscle relaxants. *British Journal of Anaesthesia*, **35**, 546–51.

Fisher, D. M., Cronnelly, R., Miller, R. D., and Sharma, M. (1983). The neuromuscular pharmacology of neostigmine in infants and children. *Anesthesiology*, **59**, 220–5.

Foldes, F. F., Monte, A. P., Brun, H. M., and Wolfson B. (1961). Studies with muscle relaxants in unanesthetised subjects. *Anesthesiology*, **22**, 230–6.

Gal, T. J. and Smith, T. C. (1976). Partial paralysis with *d*-tubocurarine and the ventilatory response to CO_2. *Anesthesiology*, **45**, 22–8.

Gamil, M. and Fanning, A. (1991). The first 24 hours after surgery. *Anaesthesia*, **46**, 712–5.

Gencarelli, P. J. and Miller, R. D. (1982). Antagonism of ORG NC45 (vecuronium) and pancuronium neuromuscular blockade by neostigmine. *British Journal of Anaesthesia*, **54**, 53–6.

Gill, S. S., Bevan, D. R. and Donati, F. (1990). Edrophonium antagonism of atracurium during enflurane anaesthesia. *British Journal of Anaesthesia*, **64**, 300–5.

Gooch, J. L., Suchyta, M. R., Balbierz, J. M., Petajan, J. H., and Clemmer, T. P. (1991). Prolonged paralysis after treatment with neuromusucular blocking agents. *Critical Care Medicine*, **19**, 1125–31.

Goudsouzian, N. G., Martyn, J. J. A., Liu, L. M., and Gionfriddo, M. (1983). Safety and efficacy of vecuronium in adolescents and children. *Anesthesia and Analgesia*, **62**, 1083–8.

Gray, T. C. and Halton, J. (1946). A milestone in anaesthesia? (*d*-tubocurarine chloride). *Proceedings of The Royal Society of Medicine*, **39**, 400–10.

Griffith, H. R. and Johnson, G. E. (1942). The use of curare in general anesthesia. *Anesthesiology*, **3**, 418–20.

Gronert, G. A. and Theye, R. A. (1975). Pathophysiology of hyperkalemia induced by succinylcholine. *Anesthesiology*, **43**, 89–99.

Hackett, G. H., Hughes, R., and Payne, J. P. (1986). Recovery of spontaneous breathing following neuromuscular blockade with atracurium. *British Journal of Anaesthesia*, **58**, 494–7.

Heir, T., Caldwell, J. E., Sessler, D. I., and Miller, R. D. (1991). Mild intraoperative hypothermia increases duration of action and spontanteous recovery of vecuronium blockade during nitrous oxide–isoflurane anesthesia in humans. *Anesthesiology*, **74**, 815–9.

Howardy-Hansen, P., Moller, J., and Hansen, B. (1987). Pretreatment with atracurium: the influence on neuromuscular transmission and pulmonary function. *Acta Anaesthesiologica Scandinavica*, **31**, 642–4.

Howardy-Hansen, P., Rasmussen, J. A., and Jensen, B. N. (1989). Residual curarization in the recovery room: atracurium versus gallamine. *Acta Anaesthesiologica Scandinavica*, **33**, 167–9.

Hutton, P., Bruchett, K. R., and Madden, A. P. (1988). Comparison of recovery after neuromuscular blockade by atracurium or pancuronium. *British Journal of Anaesthesia*, **60**, 36–42.

Isono, S., Kochi, T., Ide, T., Sugimori, K., Mizuguchi, T., and Nishino, T. (1992). Differential effects of vecuronium on diaphragm and geniohyoid muscle in anaesthetized dogs. *British Journal of Anaesthesia*, **68**, 239–43.

Jenkins, I. R. (1961). Three cases of apparent recurarization. *British Journal of Anaesthesia*, **33**, 314–7.

Jensen, E., Engbaek, J., Andersen, B. N. (1990). The frequency of residual neuromuscular blockade following atracurium (A), vecuronium (V) and pancuronium (P). A multicenter randomized study. *Anesthesiology*, **73**, A914.

Katz, R. L. (1967). Neuromuscular effects of *d*-tubocurarine, edrophonium and neostigmine in man. *Anesthesiology*, **28**, 327–36.

Katz, R. L. (1972). Clinical neuromuscular pharmacology of pancuronium. *Anesthesiology*, **34**, 550–6.

Khan, T. Z. and Khan, R. M. (1983). Changes in serum potassium following succinylcholine in patients with severe infections. *Anesthesia and Analgesia*, **62**, 327–31.

Kong, K. L. and Cooper, G. M. (1988). Recovery of neuromuscular function and postoperative morbidity following blockade by atracurium, alcuronium and vecuronium. *Anaesthesia*, **43**, 450–3.

Laycock, J. R. D., Donati, F., Smith, C. E., and Bevan, D. R. (1988*a*). Potency of atracurium and vecuronium at the diaphragm and the adductor pollicis muscle. *British Journal of Anaesthesia*, **61**, 286–91.

Laycock, J. R. D., Baxter, M. R. N., Bevan, J. C., Sangwan, S., Donati, F., and Bevan, D. R. (1988b). The potency of pancuronium at the adductor pollicis and diaphragm in infants and children. *Anesthesiology*, **63**, 309–12.

Lebrault, C., Chauvin, M., Guirimand, F., and Duvaldestin, P. (1988). Antagonism of vecuronium-induced diaphragmatic blockade by neostigmine. *Anesthesiology*, **69**, A513.

Lebrault, C., Chauvin, M., Guirimand, F., and Duvaldestin, P. (1989a). Relative potency of vecuronium on the diaphragm and the adductor pollicis. *British Journal of Anaesthesia*, 63, 389–92.

Lebrault, C., Chauvin, M., Alfonsi, P., Brusset, A., and Duvaldestin, P. (1989b). Antagonism of diaphragmatic neuromuscular block by edrophonium. *Anesthesiology*, **71**, A797.

Lennmarken, C. and Löfström, J. B. (1984). Partial curarization in the postoperative period. *Acta Anaesthesiologica Scandinavica*, **28**, 260–2.

Lunn, J. N, Hunter, A. R., and Scott, D. B. (1983). Anaesthesia-related surgical mortality. *Anaesthesia*, **38**, 1090–6.

Marsh, R. H. K., Chmielewski, A. T., and Goat, V. A. (1980). Recovery from pancuronium. A comparison between old and young patients. *Anaesthesia*, **35**, 1193–6.

Meakin, G., Shaw, E. A., Baker, R. D., and Morris, P. (1988). Comparison of atracurium-induced neuromuscular blockade in neonates, infants and children. *British Journal of Anaesthesia*, **60**, 171–5.

Meakin, G., Sweet, P. T., Bevan, J. C., and Bevan, D. R. (1983). Neostigmine and edrophonium as antagonists of pancuronium in infants and children. *Anesthesiology*, **59**, 316–21.

Meretoja, O. A., Wirtavuori, K., and Neuvonen, P. J. (1988). Age-dependence of the dose–response curve of vecuronium in pediatric patients during balanced anesthesia. *Anesthesia and Analgesia*, **67**, 21–6.

Meretoja, O. A. and Gebert, R. (1990). Postoperative neuromuscular block following atracurium or alcuronium in children. *Canadian Journal of Anaesthesia*, **37**, 743–6.

Miller, R. D. and Cullen, D. J. (1976). Renal failure and postoperative respiratory failure: recurarization? *British Journal of Anaesthesia*, **48**, 253–6.

Motsch, J., Fuchs, W., Hoch, P., Kaas, V., and Hutschenreuter, K. (1987). Side effects and changes in pulmonary function after fixed dose precurarization with alcuronium, pancuronium or vecuronium. *British Journal of Anaesthesia*, **59**, 1528–32.

Nishindo, T., Yokokawa, N., Hiraga, K., Honda, Y., and Mizuguchi, T. (1988). Breathing pattern of anesthetized humans during pancuronium-induced partial paralysis. *Journal of Applied Physiology*, **64**, 78–83.

O'Connor, M. and Russell, W. J. (1988). Muscle strength following anaesthesia with atracurium and pancuronium. *Anaesthesia and Intensive Care*, **16**, 255–9.

Pansard, J-L., Chauvin, M., Lebrault, C., Gauneau, P., and Duvaldestin, P. (1987). Effect of an intubating dose of succinylcholine and atracurium on the diaphragm and the adductor pollicis muscle in humans. *Anesthesiology*, **67**, 326–30.

Pavlin, E. G., Holle, R. F., and Schoene, R. B. (1989). Recovery of airway protection compared with ventilation in humans after paralysis with curare. *Anesthesiology*, **70**, 381–5.

Rupp, S. M., McChristian, J. W., Miller, R. D., Tabaoda, J. A., and Cronnelly, R. (1986). Neostigmine and edrophonium antagonism of varying intensity neuromuscular blockade induced by atracurium, pancuronium, or vecuronium. *Anesthesiology*, **64**, 711–7.

Saddler, J. M., Bevan, J. C., Donati, F., Bevan, D. R. and Pinto, S. R. (1990). Comparison of double-burst and train-of-four stimulation to assess neuromuscular blockade in children. *Anesthesiology*, **73**, 401–3.

Segredo, V., Matthay, M. A., Sharma, M. L., Gruenke, L. D., Cladwell, J. E., and Miller, R. D. (1990). Prolonged neuromuscular blockade after long-term administration of vecuronium in two critically ill patients. *Anesthesiology*, **72**, 566–70.

Smith, C. E., Donati, F. and Bevan, D. R. (1988). Potency of succinylcholine at the diaphragm and at the adductor pollicis. *Anesthesia and Analgesia*, **67**, 625–30.

Stanec, A., Nuesa, W., Akturk, A., Pillon, M., and Capek, K. (1990). Recovery of respiratory muscle function in surgical outpatients. *Anesthesiology*, **73**, A878.

Subramony, S. H., Carpenter, D. E., Raju, S., Pride, M. and Evans, O. B. (1991). Myopathy and prolonged neuromuscular blockade after lung transplant. *Critical Care Medicine*, **19**, 1580–2.

Tiret, L., Desmonts, J. M., Hatton, F., and Vourc'h, G. (1986). Complications associated with anaesthesia — a prospective survey in France. *Canadian Anaesthetists' Society Journal*, **33**, 336–44.

Tolmie, J. D., Joyce, T. H., and Mitchell, G. D. (1967). Succinylcholine danger in the burned patient. *Anesthesiology*, **28**, 467–70.

Viby-Mogensen, J., Jorgensen, B. C., and Ording, H. (1979). Residual curarization in the recovery room. *Anesthesiology*, **50**, 539–41.

Viby-Mogensen, J., Jensen, N. H., Engbaek, J., Ording, H., Skovgaard, L. T., and Chraemmer-Jorgensen, B. (1985). Tactile and visual evaluation of the response of train-of-four stimulation. *Anesthesiology*, **63**, 440–3.

Walts, L. F., Levin, N., and Dillon, J. B. (1970). Assessment of recovery from curare. *Journal of the American Medical Association*, **213**, 1894–6.

Williams, J. P. and Bourke, D. L. (1985). Effects of succinylcholine on respiratory and non-respiratory muscle strength in humans. *Anesthesiology*, **63**, 299–303.

Wymore, M. L. and Eisele, J. H. (1978). Differential effects of *d*-tubocurarine on inspiratory muscle and two peripheral muscle groups in anesthetized man. *Anesthesiology*, **48**, 360–2.

9

Relaxants for day-case and short-stay surgery

J. R. Barrie and T. E. J. Healy

Hypnosis, analgesia, and muscle relaxation form the classical triad of general anaesthesia. Historically, these elements of a general anaesthetic were provided by a single drug such as ether or chloroform, but with the introduction of tubocurarine into anaesthetic practice in 1942 (Griffith and Johnson 1942) and the development of balanced anaesthesia by Gray and Halton (1946), came the principle that drugs with selective actions might be used in combination to produce the individual components of general anaesthesia. The discovery of drugs with a high specificity of action enabled this principle to be realized.

The increasing availability of day-stay surgery has allowed an increased range of operative procedures to be considered suitable for this type of treatment. As recently as 1981 Thornton and Levy wrote that the intubation of day patients is a subject likely to arouse controversy (Thornton and Levy 1981). They related this to the morbidity associated with myalgia which often follows the use of suxamethonium. However, it is now regarded as safe and appropriate to use muscle relaxants when these are required for day-stay patients.

INDICATIONS

Indications for the use of muscle relaxants are similar to those applicable in general in-patient surgery, namely to provide muscle relaxation when required by the surgeon during the operative procedure and to provide relaxation for rapid, atraumatic intubation. This may be necessary to provide accessibility for the surgeon when a face mask may obstruct access or to provide a safe and secure airway when this is otherwise impossible, for example in the prone patient or the patient at risk of aspiration. The role of the laryngeal mask airway (Brain *et al.* 1985) remains to be fully evaluated, but it may reduce the need for intubation for minor head and neck surgery or airway maintenance (as opposed to airway protection) thus reducing the requirements for muscle relaxation with its concomitant morbidity.

Prolonged operative time is a relative indication for muscle relaxation and intra-operative positive pressure ventilation, particularly when endotracheal intubation is also indicated. Certainly, the use of an endotracheal tube reduces the diameter of the airway, thereby increasing the work of breathing (Bolder *et al*. 1986). Jones (1990), has suggested that muscle relaxants should be considered for use when the duration of surgery is likely to exceed 30 minutes. This is the maximum operative duration recommended by the Royal College of Surgeons to be performed as a day case (Royal College of Surgeons of England 1985). More recent guidelines from the UK Audit Commission (1989) are procedure based rather than time based and operations of longer duration than 30 minutes are now frequently performed on an out-patient basis.

The selection of an appropriate muscle relaxant for use in day-stay surgery is largely determined by taking into account the duration of effective action and, once recovery has commenced, the duration of that recovery. Further considerations in assessing the appropriateness of an individual agent include the speed of effective onset of the drug, the ease of reversibility, and the frequency and nature of side-effects. Side-effects are of particular relevance in day-stay patients who expect to feel relatively well post-operatively and return rapidly to normal life. In addition there may be factors pertaining to the patient which influence the decision to use muscle relaxation in the out-patient setting. Age *per se* has little effect on the onset or potency of vecuronium (Bell *et al*. 1989). Increased age (> 60 years) is associated with prolongation of spontaneous recovery from vecuronium-induced neuromuscular block (d'Hollander *et al*. 1982; Lien *et al*. 1991) but has little effect on reversiblilty once recovery has commenced. Conversely the duration of and recovery from vecuronium is reduced in children (Fisher and Miller 1983), a group which benefit greatly from the advantages of day-case treatment.

The interaction between the relaxant and the patient to whom it is given may be influenced by concomitant medication. Prolongation of the duration of action of nondepolarizing muscle relaxants has been described in patients taking verapamil (van Poorten *et al*. 1984), quinidine (Miller *et al*. 1967), and diltiazem (Chang *et al*. 1988), but has been demonstrated not to occur with nifedipine (Chang *et al*. 1988). This effect is secondary to the inhibition of acetylcholine release by these drugs. The situation regarding benzodiazepines is unclear. *In vitro* studies suggest a varying, concentration-dependent interaction between diazepam and pancuronium, with potentiation at low benzodiazepine concentrations and antagonism at high concentrations (Driessen *et al*. 1984). Clinically, diazepam has been reported to increase the intensity and duration of action of gallamine (Feldman and Crawley 1970) but to have no effect on the other long-acting agents (Bradshaw and Maddison 1979) or on vecuronium or atracurium (Driessen *et al*. 1986). These examples illustrate the danger of extrapolating data from specific studies involving particular drugs to the general situation. Interactions between neuromuscular blocking agents and other drugs are considered in more detail in Chapter 12. Such interactions are particularly relevant in out-patient anaesthesia; however, the disease for which these drugs are required may itself preclude day-case treatment. No muscle relaxant is ideal in all aspects and the choice of relaxant to use — or whether relaxation is required at all — is made in the light of the circumstances of the particular patient.

AGENTS

Muscle relaxants are generally considered under two headings defined by their mode of action, i.e. depolarizing and nondepolarizing.

Depolarizing agents

Drugs such as decamethonium have been used in the past (Paton and Zaimis 1952), but suxamethonium is the only depolarizing muscle relaxant presently available for clinical use. The chief advantages of suxamethonium for day-stay surgery are the rapidity of its onset of action and the brevity of its effect. It should therefore be the most appropriate agent to use to provide profound relaxation for intubation. This brevity of action, normally three to four minutes, ought also to suggest that it would be a most appropriate drug for use in the day-stay patient.

The usually brief action of suxamethonium is brought about by rapid hydrolysis through the action of pseudocholinesterase. However, the duration of the block due to suxamethonium may be prolonged in the presence of an atypical cholinesterase (Whittaker 1980). The incidence of the homozygous atypical cholinesterase is approximately one in 3000 patients. Suxamethonium should therefore be avoided in such patients or, if the indication for the use of suxamethonium is strong, the patient should be treated as an in-patient. Similarly, unanticipated prolonged apnoea following suxamethonium may require the patient to be transferred from day-stay to in-patient status. The normally brief action of suxamethonium may also be prolonged by concomitant medication, for example quinidine (in cats) (Miller *et al.* 1967), metoclopramide (Kao and Turner 1989), and lithium (Hill *et al.* 1976). This may be relatively unimportant in itself but may increase the ease with which phase II block develops (Hill *et al.* 1976) or aggravate the consequences of heterozygote atypical cholinesterases. These effects, whilst not in themselves precluding day-stay surgery, are of particular relevance in this group of patients.

The relatively minor side-effects of suxamethonium are of increased significance in day-stay patients who ambulate quickly. In this light, a major disadvantage the myalgia which frequently follows its use (Brindle and Soliman 1975). Indeed, Brodsky *et al.* (1979) report that the incidence may be as high as 89%. This is compounded by myalgia occurring more frequently when patients are young (Foster 1960) or ambulate soon after anaesthesia (Churchill-Davidson 1954), with up to 50% of out-patients receiving suxamethonium requiring analgesia or bed rest (Trépanier and Brousseau 1988). It has been suggested that the incidence and severity of myalgia can be reduced by pretreatment with a small dose of nondepolarizing relaxant before administration of suxamethonium. The evidence on this practice is contradictory. Beneficial effects have been claimed for pretreatment with pancuronium (Jansen and Hanson 1979), gallamine (Jansen and Hanson 1979), *d*-tubocurarine (Sosis *et al.* 1987), and atracurium (Sosis *et al.* 1987; Oxorn *et al.* 1992), whilst lack of benefit has been reported for pancuronium (Brodsky *et al.*

1979) and gallamine (Burtles and Tunstall 1961). Thus, the practice of pretreatment is of inconsistent benefit. It may also not be without hazard to the patient. Various post-operative side-effects have been reported following this technique (Engbaek and Viby-Mogensen 1984). Some of these consequences are potentially dangerous — weakness, respiratory impairment, impaired swallowing — whilst others, for example impaired speech and anxiety, are distressing to the patient who may therefore not benefit from attempts to minimize myalgia. Whilst the problem of myalgia is most severe following the use of suxamethonium, it can occur in over 20% of outpatients who receive vecuronium (Zahl and Apfelbaum 1989), atracurium or no relaxant at all (Trépanier and Brousseau 1988). Thus the aim of eliminating myalgia completely, whilst laudable, is probably unattainable without further understanding of its aetiology. A further minor but unpleasant side-effect, sore throat, is also more common in patients who have received suxamethonium (Capan *et al*. 1983) and may be related to myalgia or to the use of antisialogogues.

Suxamethonium is still used widely to provide relaxation for intubation, or by repeated injection or infusion to maintain muscle relaxation during the operative procedure. It must be remembered that, when used by repeated injection or by infusion, a sinus bradycardia may occur which responds to anticholinergic drugs, such as atropine or glycopyrollate. Moreover, the incidence and severity of myalgia increases with increasing number of bolus doses, and is further increased if the suxamethonium is allowed to wear off fully between increments (Waters and Mapleson 1971). Thus, if extended suxamethonium block is indicated, infusion may be preferable to repeated increments in day-case surgery. This however requires careful monitoring to compensate for initial tachphylaxis whilst minimizing the risk of the development of phase II block (Futter *et al*. 1983). The continuing development of short-acting, easily titratable nondepolarizing relaxants has reduced the necessity for this technique.

The main indication for suxamethonium in out-patient practice is to facilitate rapid control of the airway in patients with oesophageal reflux or otherwise at risk of aspiration. Despite the problems associated with its use, the rapidity of onset of suxamethonium renders it the agent of choice in this situation. It also still has a role in providing relaxation for procedures of 10–20 minute duration, for which no nondepolarizing agent is currently ideal.

Nondepolarizing agents

The difficulties associated with the use of suxamethonium together with the increasing frequency and scope of day-case surgery have lead to the use of nondepolarizing agents in these patients. Tubocurarine, alcuronium, and pancuronium are traditionally regarded as long-acting muscle relaxants. The clinical profile of the newer agents doxacurium (Lennon *et al*. 1989) and pipercuronium (Wierda *et al*. 1989) are such that they too must be included in this group. In general these drugs are unsuitable for use for day-stay surgery, the major problem being that residual curarization may still be present during the immediate post-operative period (Viby-Mogensen *et al*. 1979).

A second group of relaxants are of intermediate duration and are therefore more suitable for day-case anaesthesia. Vecuronium and atracurium fall into this group and are comparable in their pharmacokinetics. Their onset times are similar at equipotent doses (Healy *et al.* 1986) but, even at large doses, do not approach the rapidity of onset of suxamethonium. At $3 \times ED_{95}$, atracurium has an onset time of 1.2 min (Payne and Hughes 1981), and $4 \times ED_{95}$ of vecuronium has an onset time of 1.3 min (Viby-Mogensen *et al.* 1980).

Both drugs show a biphasic plasma concentration–time curve. The redistribution $(T_{1/2\alpha})$ and elimination $(T_{1/2\beta})$ half-lives of vecuronium are over twice as long as the corresponding values for atracurium $(T_{1/2\alpha}$ 3.4 min and $T_{1/2\beta}$ 21 min) and vecuronium $(T_{1/2\alpha}$ 8.5 min and $T_{1/2\beta}$ 79 min) (Fahey *et al.* 1983, 1984). The duration of action of the two agents are similar, with a $3 \times ED_{95}$ dose of atracurium lasting 34–64 min (Payne and Hughes 1981; Savarese *et al.* 1982) and a comparable dose of vecuronium having a duration of action of 44–60 min (Agoston *et al.* 1980). Recovery from the two agents is also comparable, with the recovery rate from 75% to 25% twitch suppression being 8–11 min for vecuronium (Agoston *et al.* 1980; Fahey *et al.* 1981) and 12 min for atracurium (Basta *et al.* 1982).

These pharmacokinetic and clinical profiles render atracurium and vecuronium much more suitable for short surgical procedures than the agents which preceded them and they are widely used for such operations. Despite this, these drugs are unsuitable in certain circumstances. The first of these is as an alternative to suxamethonium when rapid airway protection is required. Pretreatment with a small dose of the nondepolarizing agent (priming) prior to the induction of anaesthesia does hasten the onset of effective neuromuscular block. However when a priming dose of 15% of the total dose of relaxant is given, the incidence of diplopia, impaired head lift and impaired swallowing are each over 20% (Glass *et al.* 1989). This may in itself put the patient at risk of aspiration and is unpleasant.

The recently developed nondepolarizing relaxant rocuronium (ORG 9426) is being investigated as an alternative to suxamethonium in these circumstances. Initial studies in animals indicated that rocuronium had an onset time considerably shorter than that of vecuronium and similar to that of suxamethonium (Muir *et al.* 1989). Clinical studies of dose–responsiveness suggest an ED_{90} of 0.25–0.4 mg kg^{-1} but with much inter-individual variation (Lambalk *et al.* 1991; Quill *et al.* 1991). Onset time to maximum block also shows marked inter-individual variation, with a range of 0.7–4.3 min being reported in one study (Booij and Knape 1991) but is, however, relatively unaffected by the anaesthetic technique used (Lambalk *et al.* 1991). Intubation is feasible at one minute after an ED_{90} dose of rocuronium (Wierda *et al.* 1990) although with some coughing. At higher doses $(2 \times ED_{95})$, intubating conditions following rocuronium have compared favourably with those following suxamethonium at one minute in outpatients, although the study samples were small (Cooper *et al.* 1992; Pühringer *et al.* 1992). If these studies are substantiated, rocuronium may be a useful alternative to suxamethonium to facilitate rapid intubation. A technique of rapid intubation without the administration of a muscle relaxant has also been described (Davidson and Gillespie 1993). Whilst this technique, based on propofol, alfentanil, and lignocaine, is not appropriate for all cases the avoidance of paralysis may also help minimize awareness.

The second circumstances in which vecuronium or atracurium are not ideal is in operations of 10–20 min duration. Rocuronium, with a duration of action of 20–30 min and recovery time from 25% to 75% block of 5–15 min (Booij and Knape 1991; Quill *et al.* 1991), may be more suitable for these circumstances. A second agent undergoing investigation, mivacurium (BW B1090U), which has been recently released in the UK and the USA, is also showing potential for short procedures. This drug produces nondepolarizing muscle relaxation with an onset time of 1.5–2.3 min after a dose of 0.25 mg kg^{-1} (Goldberg *et al.* 1989; Savarese *et al.* 1988), with onset being faster during nitrous oxide–fentanyl anaesthesia than during isoflurane anaesthesia (Weber *et al.* 1988). Its duration of action, 13–20 min, is thus intermediate between suxamethonium and atracurium/vecuronium (Caldwell *et al.* 1989; Goldberg *et al.* 1989). Mivacurium is readily reversible by both neostigmine and edrophonium after bolus dose and infusion (Goldberg *et al.* 1989; Wrigley *et al.* 1992).

Mivacurium is metabolized by plasma cholinesterase and thus its duration of action would be expected to be increased in patients with atypical cholinesterases. Both the potency of and recovery from mivacurium are related to cholinesterase activity, although the effect is inconsistent and an alternative metabolic pathway has been suggested (Ali *et al.* 1988; Weber *et al.* 1988). Mivacurium is thus, like suxamethonium, subject to the potential problem of an unexpectedly long duration of action with the disadvantages that implies for out-patient use. A further problem with mivacurium is that of histamine release which, following rapid injection, may increase histamine levels by 33% with a concomitant decrease in blood pressure (Ali *et al.* 1988). This degree of histamine release is, however, less than that seen following atracurium, when histamine levels may double (Basta *et al.* 1983).

TECHNIQUE

Muscle relaxants may be administered in three ways: by injection of a dose sufficient to maintain adequate neuromuscular block for the whole period during which relaxation is required; by incremental small bolus administration; or by continuous infusion. These techniques are discussed in more detail in Chapter 5 and 10. Most out-patient surgical procedures are of short duration and so the recovery characteristics and the ease with which relaxants may be reversed is of particular importance in these patients. Hillgenberg (1983) showed that, following either atracurium or vecuronium, a rapid reversal of neuromuscular block could be achieved using an anti-cholinesterase. Similarly rapid reversal has been demonstrated with the newer relaxants described above. Reversibility appears to require some degree of initial recovery however, as administration of neostigmine during profound block does not hasten ultimate recovery (Magorian *et al.* 1990). Both neostigmine and edrophonium may be less potent at profound than at moderate block (Donati *et al.* 1989; Rupp *et al.* 1986). The relative potencies of the two agents vary with the intensity of block to be antagonized (Donati *et al.* 1989) with neostigmine being more effective than edrophonium in antagonizing profound block (Beemer *et al.* 1991).

Once recovery has commenced edrophonium, in doses of 0.5–1.0 mg/kg, has a shorter reversal time than neostigmine (Beemer *et al.* 1991; Cronnelly and Morris 1982; Jones *et al.* 1984; Sanfilippo *et al.* 1988) and is more specific to the nicotinic receptor (Jones *et al.* 1984) but the effect of edrophonium on antagonism of a neuromuscular block is less predictable especially when antagonizing vecuronium (Lavery *et al.* 1985; Smith *et al.* 1989). Whilst the shorter onset time of edrophonium may make it attractive for use in out-patient surgery, benefits in terms of increased patient turnover or more rapid recovery to street fitness have not been demonstrated.

The quality of recovery from neuromuscular block is of particular importance in day-case patients. Monitoring and assessing the quality of this recovery is difficult however. Miller (1989), in an editorial, advocates a five second head lift as being equivalent to an inspiratory pressure of –50 cm H_2O which he regards as being necessary to ensure airway protection and adequate ventilation (Miller 1989). It has also been suggested that a train of four ratio of 0.5 can be regarded as safe recovery from atracurium (Jones *et al.* 1984). Whilst in one study 80% of patients could protrude their tongue satisfactorily, no patient could sustain a head lift at this degree of recovery (Engbaek *et al.* 1989) and extubation at this stage is unwise. The situation is further complicated by the differential effect of relaxants on different muscle groups, with the diaphragm being less sensitive to the effects of vecuronium than the adductor pollicis (Lebrault *et al.* 1989). The onset of and recovery from neuromuscular block occurrs in the diaphragm before the adductor pollicis (Bencini and Newton 1984; Derrington and Hindocha 1990). Similarly, restoration of sustained head lift is associated with reduced hand grip both in patients who have and in those who have not received relaxants (Russell and Serle 1987). The criteria of Jones (1990) for assessing the adequacy of return of muscle power are as follows:

(1) forceful cough;

(2) sustained head lift of 5 seconds;

(3) a sustained response to a 5 s 50 Hz tetanic stimulus;

(4) TOF ratio of 0.7, measured electromyographically (TOF ratio cannot be estimated satisfactorily by look or feel alone).

These are valuable, but the factors outlined above must be borne in mind when assessing the adequacy of recovery from neuromuscular block.

CONCLUSION

The use of muscle relaxants in day-case surgery is well attested and has allowed the range of procedures which may be performed as day-cases to be extended. The safe use of muscle relaxants in these patients requires that anaesthetists have a detailed knowledge of the pharmacology of the agents available and the clinical circumstances of patients. In addition, they must have the skill to select and use the most appropriate drug in the most appropriate manner with all care and attention to the patient.

REFERENCES

Agoston, S., Salt, P., Newton, D., Bencini, A., Boomsma, P., and Erdmann, W. (1980). The neuromuscular blocking action of ORG NC45, a new pancuronium derivative, in anaesthetized patients. A pilot study. *British Journal of Anaesthesia*, **52 (Suppl. 1)**, 53–9S.

Ali, H. H., Savarese, J. J., Embree, P. B., Basta, S. J., Stout, R. G., Bottros, L. H., *et al.* (1988). Clinical pharmacology of mivacurium chloride (BW B1090U) infusion: comparison with vecuronium and atracurium. *British Journal of Anaesthesia*, **61**, 541–6.

Audit Commission. (1989). *A short cut to better services: day surgery in England and Wales*, HMSO.

Basta, S. J., Ali, H. H., Savarese, J. J., Sunder, N. Gionfriddo, M., Cloutier, G., *et al.* (1982). Clinical pharmacology of atracurium besylate (BW 33A): A new non-depolarising muscle relaxant. *Anesthesia and Analgesia*, **61**, 723–9.

Basta, S. J., Savarese, J. J., Ali, H. H., Sunder, N., Moss, J., Giofriddo, M., *et al.* (1983). Vecuronium does not alter serum histamine within the clinical dose range. *Anesthesiology*, **59**, A273.

Beemer, G. H., Bjorksten, A. R., Dawson, P. J., Dawson, R. J., Heenan, P. J., and Robertson, B. A. (1991). Determinants of the reversal time of competitive neuromuscular block by anticholinesterases. *British Journal of Anaesthesia*, **66**, 469–75.

Bell, P. F., Mirakhur, R. J., and Clarke, R. S. J. (1989). Dose–response studies of atracurium, vecuronium and pancuronium in the elderly. *Anaesthesia*, **44**, 925–7.

Bencini, A. and Newton, D. E. F. (1984). Rate of onset of good intubating conditions, respiratory depression and hand muscle paralysis after vecuronium. *British Journal of Anaesthesia*, **56**, 959–65.

Bolder, P. M., Healy, T. E. J., Bolder, A. R., Beatty, P. C. W., and Kay, B. (1986). The extra work of breathing through adult endotracheal tubes. *Anesthesia and Analgesia*, **65**, 853–9.

Booij, L. H. D. J. and Knape, H. T. A. (1991). The neuromuscular blocking effect of ORG 9426. *Anaesthesia*, **46**, 341–3.

Bradshaw, E. G. and Maddison, S. (1979). Effect of diazepam at the neuromuscular junction. *British Journal of Anaesthesia*, **51**, 955–60.

Brain, A. I., McGhee, T. D., McAteer, E. J., Thomas, A., Abu Saad, M. A. and Bushman, J. A. (1985) The laryngeal mask airway. *Anaesthesia*, **40**, 356–61.

Brindle, G. and Soliman, M. G. (1975). Anaesthetic complications in surgical outpatients. *Canadian Anaesthetists' Society Journal*, **22**, 613–9.

Brodsky, J. B., Brock-Utne, J. G., and Samuels, S. I. (1979). Pancuronium pre-treatment and post-succinylcholine myalgias. *Anesthesiology*, **51**, 259–61.

Burtles, R. and Tunstall, M. E. (1961). Suxamethonium chloride and muscle pains. *British Journal of Anaesthesia*, **33**, 24–8.

Caldwell, J. E., Heier, T., Kitto, J. B., Lynam, D. P., Fahey, M. R., and Miller, R. D. (1989). Comparison of the neuromuscular block induced by mivacurium, suxamethonium or atracurium during nitrous oxide–fentanyl anaesthesia. *British Journal of Anaesthesia*, **63**, 393–9.

Capan, L. M., Bruce, D. L., Patel, K. P., and Turndorf, H. (1983). Succinyl-choline-induced postoperative sore throat. *Anesthesiology*, **59**, 202–6.

Chang, C. C., Lin, S. O., Hong, S. J., and Chiou, L. C. (1988). Neuromuscular block by ver-apamil and diltiazem and inhibition of acetylcholine release. *Brain Research*, **454**, 332–9.

Churchill-Davidson, H. C. (1954). Suxamethonium (succinylcholine) chloride and muscle pains. *British Medical Journal*, **ii**, 74–5.

Cooper, R., Mirakhur, R. K., Clarke, R. S. J., and Boules, Z. (1992). Comparison of intubating conditions after administration of ORG 9426 (Rocuronium) and suxamethonium. *British Journal of Anaesthesia*, **69**, 269–73.

Cronnelly, R. and Morris, R. B. (1982). Antagonism of neuromuscular blockade. *British Journal of Anaesthesia*, **54**, 183–94.

Davidson, J. A. H. and Gillespie, J. A. (1993). Tracheal intubation after induction of anaes-thesia with propofol, alfentanil and intravenous lignocaine. *British Journal of Anaesthesia*, **70**, 163–6.

Derrington, M. C. and Hindocha, N (1990). Comparison of neuromuscular block in the diaphragm and hand after administration of tubocurarine, pancuronium and alcuronium. *British Journal of Anaesthesia*, **64**, 294–9.

d'Hollander, A., Massaux, F., Neuelsteen, M., and Agoston, S. (1982). Age-dependent dose–response relationship of ORG NC45 in anaesthetized patients. *British Journal of Anaesthesia*, **54**, 653–7.

Donati, F., Smith, C. E., and Bevan D. R. (1989). Dose–response relationships of edropho-nium and neostigmine as antagonists of moderate and profound atracurium blockade. *Anesthesia and Analgesia*, **68**, 13–9.

Driessen, J. J., Vree, T. B., van Egmond, J., Booji, L. H. D., and Crul, J. F. (1984). *In vitro* interaction of diazepam and oxazepam with pancuronium and suxamethonium. *British Journal of Anaesthesia*, **56**, 1131–7.

Driessen, J. J., Crul, J. F., Vree, T. B., van Egmond, J., and Booji, L. H. D. (1986). Benzodiazepines and neuromuscular blocking drugs in patients. *Acta Anaesthesiologica Scandinavica*, **30**, 642–6.

Engbaek, J. and Viby-Mogensen, J. (1984). Precurarisation — a hazard to the patient? *Acta Anaesthesiologica Scandinavica*, **28**, 61–2.

Engbaek, J., Østergaard, D., Viby-Mogensen, J., and Skovgaard, L. T. (1989). Clinical recovery and train of four ration measured mechanically and electromyographically fol-lowing atracurium. *Anesthesiology*, **71**, 391–5.

Fahey, M. R., Morris, R. B., Miller, R. D., Sohn, Y. J., Cronnelly, R., and Gencarelli, P. (1981). Clinical pharmacology of ORG NC45, a new pancuronium derivative, in anaes-thetized patients. *Anesthesiology*, **55**, 6–11.

Fahey, M. R., Morris, R. B., Miller, R. D., Nguyen T-L., and Upton, R. A. (1983). Pharmacokinetics of ORG NC45 (Norcuron) in patients with and without renal failure. *British Journal of Anaesthesia*, **53**, 1049–53.

Fahey, M. R., Rupp, S. M., Fisher, D. M., Miller, R. D., Sharma, M., Castagnoli, K., *et al.*, (1984). The pharmacokinetics and pharmacodynamics of atracurium in patients with and without renal failure. *Anesthesiology*, **61**, 699–702.

Feldman, S. A. and Crawley, B. E. (1970). Interaction of diazepam with muscle-relaxant drugs. *British Medical Journal*, **ii**, 336–8.

Fisher, D. M. and Miller, R. D. (1983). Neuromuscular effects of vecuronium (ORG NC45) in infants and children during N_2O (sic), Halothane anaesthesia. *Anesthesiology*, **58**, 519–23.

Foster, C. A. (1960). Muscle pains that follow administration of suxamethonium. *British Medical Journal*, **ii**, 24–5.

Futter, M. E., Donati, F., and Bevan, D. R. (1983). Prolonged suxamethonium infusion during nitrous oxide anaesthesia supplemented with halothane or fentanyl. *British Journal of Anaesthesia*, **55**, 947–53.

Glass, P. S. A., Wilson, W., Mace, J. A., and Wogoner, R. (1989). Is the priming principle both effective and safe? *Anesthesia and Analgesia*, **68**, 127–34.

Goldberg, M. E., Larijani, B. D., Azad, S. S., Sosis, M., Seltzer, J. L., Ascher, J., *et al.* (1989). Comparison of tracheal intubating conditions and neuromuscular blocking profiles after intubating doses of mivacurium chloride or succinylcholine in surgical outpatients. *Anesthesia and Analgesia*, **69**, 93–9.

Gray, T. C. and Halton, J. (1946). A milestone in anaesthesia (d-tubocurarine). *Proceedings of the Royal Society of Medicine*, **39**, 400–8.

Griffith, H. R. and Johnson, G. E. (1942). The use of curare in general anaesthesia. *Anesthesiology*, **3**, 418–20.

Healy, T. E. J., Pugh, N. D., Kay, B., Sivalingham, T., and Petts, H. V. (1986). Atracurium and vecuronium: Effect of dose on the time of onset. *British Journal of Anaesthesia*, **58**, 620–4.

Hill, G. E., Wong, K. C., and Hodges, M. R. (1976). Potentiation of suxamethonium induced neuromuscular blockage by lithium carbonate. *Anesthesiology*, **44**, 439–42.

Hillgenberg, J. C. (1983). Comparison of the pharmacology of vecuronium and atracurium with that of other currently available muscle relaxants. *Anesthesia and Analgesia*, **62**, 524–31.

Jansen, E. C. and Hanson, P. H. (1979). Objective measurement of succinylcholine-induced fasciculations and the effect of pre-treatment with pancuronium or gallamine. *Anesthesiology*, **51**, 159–60.

Jones, R. M. (1990). Muscle relaxants for day-stay surgery. *Baillière's Clinical Anaesthesiology*, **4**, (3), 679–89.

Jones, R. M., Pearce, A. C., and Williams J. P. (1984). Recovery characteristics following antagonism of atracurium with neostigmine or edrophonium. *British Journal of Anaesthesia*, **56**, 453–7.

Kao, Y. K. and Turner, D. R. (1989). Prolongation of succinylcholine block by metoclopramide. *Anesthesiology*, **70**, 905–8.

Lambalk, L. M., de Wit, A. P. M., Wierda, J. M. K. H., Hennis, P. J., and Agoston, S. (1991). Dose–response relationship and time course of action of ORG 9426. *Anaesthesia*, **46**, 907–11.

Lavery, G. G., Mirakhur, R. K., and Gibson, F. M. (1985). A comparison of edrophonium and neostigmine for the antagonism of atracurium-induced neuromuscular blockade. *Anesthesia and Analgesia*, **64**, 867–70.

Lebrault, C., Chawin, M., Guirimand, F., and Duvaldestin, P. (1989). Relative potency of vecuronium on the diaphragm and the adductor pollicis. *British Journal of Anaesthesia*, **63**, 389–92.

Lennon, R. L., Hosking, M. P., Houck, P. C., Rose, S. H., Wedel, D. J., Gibson, B. E., *et al.* (1989). Doxacurium chloride for neuromuscular blockade before tracheal intubation and surgery during nitrous oxide–oxygen–narcotic–enflurane anaesthesia. *Anesthesia and Analgesia*, **68**, 255–60.

Lien, C. A., Matteo, R. S., Ornstein, E., Schwartz, A. E., and Diaz, J. (1991). Distribution, elimination and action of vecuronium in the elderly. *Anesthesia and Analgesia*, **73**, 39–42.

Magorian, T. T., Lynam, D. P., Caldwell, J. E., and Miller, R. D. (1990). Can early administration of neostigmine, in single or repeated doses alter the course of neuromuscular recovery from vecuronium-induced neuromuscular blockade? *Anesthesiology*, **73**, 410–4.

Miller, R. D. (1990). How should residual neuromuscular blockade be detected? *Anesthesiology*, **70**, 379–80.

Miller, R. D., Way, W. L. and Katzung, B. G. (1967). The potentiation of neuromuscular blocking agents by quinidine. *Anesthesiology*, **28**, 1036–41.

Muir, A. W., Houston, J., Green, K. L., Marshall, R. J., Bowman, W. C., and Marshall, I. G. (1989). Effects of a new neuromuscular blocking agent (ORG9426) in anaesthetized cats and pigs and in isolated nerve–muscle preparations. *British Journal of Anaesthesia*, **63**, 400–10.

Oxorn, D. C., Whatley, G. S., Knox, J. W. D., and Hooper, J. (1992). The importance of activity and pretreatment in the prevention of suxamethonium myalgias. *British Journal of Anaesthesia*, **69**, 200–1.

Paton, W. D. M. and Zaimis, E. J. (1952). The methonium compounds. *Pharmacology Review*, **4**, 219–53.

Payne, J. P. and Hughes, R. (1981). Evaluation of atracurium in anaesthetized man. *British Journal of Anaesthesia*, **53**, 45–54.

P#uhringer, F. K., Khuenl-Brady, K. S., Keller, J., and Mitterschuffthaler, G. (1992). Evaluation of the endotracheal intubating conditions of rocuronium (ORG 9426) and succinylcholine in outpatient surgery. *Anesthesia and Analgesia*, **75**, 37–40.

Quill, T. J., Begin, M., Glass, P. S. A., Ginsberg, B., and Gorback, M. S. (1991). Clinical responses to ORG 9426 during isoflurane anaesthesia. *Anesthesia and Analgesia*, **72**, 203–6.

Royal College of Surgeons of England. (1985). *Guidelines for day case surgery*. Report of the Commission on the Provision of Surgical Services. Royal College of Surgeons, London.

Rupp, S. M., McChristian, J. W., Miller, R. D., Taboada, J. A., and Connelly, R. (1986). Neostigmine and edrophonium antagonism of varying intensity neuromuscular blockade induced by atracurium, pancuronium or vecuronium. *Anesthesiology*, **64**, 711–7.

Russell, W. J. and Serle, D. G. (1987). Hand grip force as an assessment of recovery from neuromuscular block. *Journal of Clinical Monitoring*, **3**, 87–9.

Sanfilippo, M., Vilardi, V., Fierro, G., Rosa, G., Pelaia, P., and Gasparetto, A. (1988). Neostigmine and edrophonium as antagonists of atracurium and pancuronium. *Acta Anaesthesiologica Scandinavica*, **32**, 437–40.

Savarese, J. J., Basta, S. J., Ali, H. H., Sunder, N., and Moss, J. (1982). Neuromuscular and cardiovascular effects of BW 33A (atracurium) in patients under halothane anaesthesia. *Anesthesiology*, **57**, A262.

Savarese, J. J., Ali, H. H., Basta, S. J., Embree, P. E., Scott, R. P. F., Sunder, N., *et al.* (1988). The clinical neuromuscular pharmacology of mivacurium chloride (BW B1090U). *Anesthesiology*, **68**, 723–32.

Smith, C. E., Donati, F., and Bevan, D. R. (1989). Dose–response relationships for edrophonium and neostigmine as antagonists of atracurium and vecuronium neuromuscular blockade. *Anesthesiology*, **71**, 37–43.

Sosis, M., Broad, T., Larijani, G. E., and Marr, A. T. (1987). Comparison of atracurium and *d*-tubocurarine for prevention of succinylcholine myalgia. *Anesthesia and Analgesia*, **66**, 657–9.

Thornton, J. A. and Levy, C. J. (1981). *Techniques of anaesthesia*, (2nd edn). Chapman and Hall, London.

Trépanier, C. A. and Brousseau, C. (1988). Myalgia in outpatient surgery: a comparison of atracurium and succinylcholine. *Canadian Journal of Anaesthesia*, **35**, 255–9.

van Poorten, J. F., Dhasmara, K. M., Kuypero, R. S. M. and Erdmann, W. (1984). Verapamil and reversal of vecuronium neuromuscular blockade. *Anesthesia and Analgesia*, **63**, 155–7.

Viby-Mogensen, J., Chraemmer-Jorgensen, B., and Ording, H. (1979). Residual curarization in the recovery room. *Anesthesiology*, **50**, 539–41.

Viby-Mogensen, J., Jørgensen, B. C., Engbaek, J., and Sørensen, B. (1980). On ORG NC45 and halothane anaesthesia. Preliminary results. *British Journal of Anaesthesia*, **52** *(Suppl. 1)*, 67–9S.

Waters, D. J. and Mapleson, W. W. (1971). Suxamethonium pains: hypothesis and observation. *Anaesthesia*, **26**, 127–41.

Weber, S., Brandom, B. W., Powers, D. M., Sarner, J. B., Woelfel, S. K., Cook, D. R., *et al.* (1988). Mivacurium chloride (BW B1909U) induced neuromuscular blockade during nitrous oxide–isoflurane and nitrous oxide–narcotic anaesthesia in adult surgical patients. *Anesthesia and Analgesia*, **67**, 495–9.

Whittaker, M. (1980). Plasma cholinesterase variants and the anaesthetist. *Anaesthesia*, **35**, 174–97.

Wierda, J. M. K. H., Richardson, F. J., and Agoston, S. (1989). Dose response relation and time course of action of pipercuronium bromide in humans anaesthetized with nitrous oxide and isoflurane, halothane or droperidol and fentanyl. *Anesthesia and Analgesia*, **68**, 208–13.

Wierda, J. M. K. H., de Wit, A. P. M., Kuizenga, K., and Agoston, S. (1990). Clinical observations on the neuromuscular blocking action of ORG 9426, a new steroidal non-depolarising agent. *British Journal of Anaesthesia*, **64**, 521–3.

Wrigley, S. R., Jones, R. M., Harrop-Griffiths, A. W. and Platt, M. W. (1992). Mivacurium chloride: a study to evaluate its use during propofol–nitrous oxide anaesthesia. *Anaesthesia*, **47**, 653–7.

Zahl, K. and Apfelbaum, J. L. (1989). Muscle pain occurs after outpatient laparoscopy despite the substitution of vecuronium for succinylcholine. *Anesthesiology*, **70**, 408–11.

10

Muscle relaxation for long surgical procedures

G. J. McCarthy and R. K. Mirakhur

The use of neuromuscular blocking agents has become routine in clinical anaesthesia since their introduction by Griffith and Johnson in 1942. This was soon hailed as a milestone in anaesthesia (Gray and Halton 1946) and their use has no doubt facilitated the conduct of more and more complicated surgery. In more recent years this has enabled long surgical procedures to be carried out without the necessity for profound central nervous system depression for prolonged periods with consequent adverse effects for the patient.

FACTORS IN THE CHOICE OF MUSCLE RELAXANT

When dealing with muscle relaxation for long surgical procedures, the rational choice is not simply to administer a long-acting agent. It is likely that larger amounts of the drug will need to be administered for a long surgical procedure and thus it is important that the drug has certain desirable characteristics. These include cardiovascular stability, a favourable profile of metabolism and elimination thus avoiding cumulation, safety in the presence of impaired hepatic and renal function, absence of significant histamine release, and the ability to be antagonized promptly and reliably (Jones 1985). It is important that any metabolites have no harmful or unpredictable effects. A rapid onset of action is desirable although not critical unless it is necessary to perform a rapid tracheal intubation.

Savarese and Kitz (1975) suggested that muscle relaxants with three different profiles of action should be available, these being the short-, intermediate-, and long-duration drugs. It is clear that any of these agents could be used for provision of relaxation for long surgical procedures with each having advantages and disadvantages of its own. The use of each of these is discussed later. The effects of relaxants during long procedures may also be modified by other factors which might include the background anaesthetic technique, the age of the patient, any deviation from normal body temperature, blood loss, arterial hypotension, and the presence of concomitant disease. In general, the choice will be between using a long-acting agent, or a larger dose of an intermediate-acting agent, or an infusion of an intermediate- or short-acting agent.

LONG-ACTING AGENTS

The use of muscle relaxants in anaesthesia began with the use of the long-acting relaxant tubocurarine. This agent is still used today although the frequency of use has declined considerably (Mirakhur 1990). Although other agents including gallamine and alcuronium have been introduced since then, the most popular alternative to tubocurarine has been pancuronium. Tubocurarine is generally used in a dose of 0.5–0.6 mg/kg which is close to its ED_{95} value. The onset of action is relatively slow, taking between five and six minutes (Savarese *et al.* 1977; Blackburn and Morgan 1978). The duration of clinical relaxation (to 25% recovery of twitch height) of this dose is about 80 minutes. Further doses of the relaxant can usually be administered following recovery from the initial dose but this often results in a longer duration of block and cumulation (Walts and Dillon 1968). Although the long duration of action is convenient for long operations, cumulation after repeated administration is a clear disadvantage because the recovery, whether spontaneous or anticholinesterase-induced, will become progressively slower. Moreover, the drug frequently releases histamine and produces block of autonomic ganglia, which may result in arterial hypotension, a common occurrence with this agent. The effects of the drug are prolonged in patients with renal and hepatic disease and as a result the use of this agent is not considered suitable in these patients.

Pancuronium, one of the first aminosteroid muscle relaxants, became popular soon after its introduction owing to its lack of any histamine-releasing potential. The onset of action of equipotent doses of pancuronium is similar to that of tubocurarine (Norman *et al.* 1970). In practice, however, the onset of pancuronium is slightly faster because doses of one and a half times the ED_{95} (approximately 0.1 mg/kg) are generally used, in contrast to one ED_{95} dose of tubocurarine. As with tubocurarine, the duration of clinical relaxation is long and the total overall recovery slow (Norman *et al.* 1970). Pancuronium demonstrates true cumulation after repeated administration (Fahey *et al.* 1981) and problems may therefore arise during antagonism. In view of this, pancuronium should be used with care for very long surgical procedures particularly if it is planned to antagonize the block at the end of surgery. Like tubocurarine, pancuronium also possesses significant cardiovascular effects. These, however, present as tachycardia, hypertension, and increased cardiac output (Stoelting 1972). Pancuronium has been implicated in the production of myocardial ischaemia (Thomson and Putnins 1985). The cardiovascular effects are not a specific problem except when the initial bolus dose is administered, however, and the problems with pancuronium during prolonged use are related to its long duration of action.

An alternative to tubocurarine and pancuronium is one of the newer long-acting agents, pipecuronium or doxacurium (Mirakhur 1992). Because both are more potent than any other nondepolarizing agents, they are also relatively slow in onset since higher potency has been linked to a longer onset time (Minsaas and Stovner 1980; Bowman *et al.* 1988; Kopman 1989). Pipecuronium is a bisquaternary steroid which is almost devoid of any significant cardiovascular side-effects (Agoston and Richardson 1985; Stanley *et al.* 1991*a*). It differs little from pancuronium in its onset and duration of action; in other words it is slow in onset and has a long duration of action (Foldes *et al.* 1990; Stanley *et al.* 1991*b*). Higher doses may hasten the onset, but result in an even longer duration of action Caldwell *et al.* 1988; Stanley *et al.* 1991*b*; Sanfilippo *et al.* 1992). In normal patients when used as the relaxant for long procedures, not only is pipecuronium slower in onset than large doses of vecuronium for the same duration of relaxation, but it is also associated with marked cumulation (Harrop-Griffiths *et al.* 1992). The prolongation in duration of action is more profound in patients with renal disease even when the drug is given in similar doses (Caldwell *et al.* 1989). The prolongation of effect in a patient with renal failure was demonstrated recently when an inadvertent overdose of pipecuronium produced neuromuscular paralysis for three days, although without haemodynamic side-effects (Cabellero and Johnstone 1992). Antagonism of a neuromuscular block with pipecuronium is satisfactory only when considerable spontaneous recovery has taken place and may well be prolonged if repeated or if large doses have been administered over a long period.

Doxacurium, a new benzylisoquinolinium diester compound, is currently the most potent nondepolarizing relaxant available and also the slowest in onset and the longest acting (Lennon *et al.* 1989; Scott and Norman 1989). The duration of action is greater than 90 minutes after a single ED_{95} dose (Basta *et al.* 1988). In keeping with the high potency of the drug, a dose of 50 $\mu g/kg$ (approximately twice the ED_{95} required five minutes after administration for successful intubation, and 80 $\mu g/kg$ reduced this time by only one minute. The duration of action of these doses in terms of time to 25% spontaneous recovery ranged from 85 to 164 minutes. A characteristic feature of this drug is the extreme variability in the neuromuscular response making it unpredictable even after prolonged use (Maddineni *et al.* 1992). Although there is no direct evidence for cumulation (the drug is far too long acting to enable this to be studied), this is a feature which would be expected in a drug with the characteristics of doxacurium. Reversal even from a block where the first contraction of the train of four has risen to 25% of control was reported to be slow, taking more than 20 minutes to reach a train of four ratio of 0.7 in the presence of enflurane anaesthesia (Lennon *et al.* 1989). Thus, the longer the surgical procedure and the greater the amount of doxacurium given, the more difficult and prolonged the reversal may be. Since the drug is primarily eliminated via the kidneys, the effects are even more prolonged in patients with renal failure, although its administration is not associated with significant cardiovascular effects (Cashman *et al.* 1990). Like pipecuronium, the principal advantage of doxacurium is the extreme cardiovascular stability it provides (Stoops *et al.* 1988; Emmott *et al.* 1990).

It thus appears that in spite of excellent cardiovascular profiles neither pipecuronium nor doxacurium fits the desirable criteria of the ideal muscle relaxant as suggested by Savarese and Kitz (1975). These agents may be suitable for surgical procedures of moderately long duration (about two hours) where they could be given as a single bolus. Although they may be convenient, repeated administration is likely to result in cumulation and difficulties in antagonism. In addition it has been demonstrated that longer-acting agents in general are associated with a higher incidence of residual post-operative curarization (Bevan *et al.* 1988). Furthermore the use of long-acting neuromuscular blocking drugs, in general, is going out of fashion, the present trend in anaesthetic practice being to use shorter-acting agents for more control of drug effect.

The approach to the provision of muscle relaxation for long procedures could therefore be based more logically on using relaxants with an intermediate or short duration of action. These include atracurium, vecuronium, rocuronium, and mivacurium. These agents could be administered in a variety of ways.

THE 'BIG BANG' APPROACH

The simplest clinical approach to a long procedure would be to administer a single large bolus of such a size that the plasma concentration of the drug would maintain relaxation for the duration of the procedure, albeit waning during the procedure. This approach, however, requires that large doses of the relaxant do not release significant amounts of histamine, nor result in significant cardiovascular problems. Unfortunately most muscle relaxants — with the possible exception of vecuronium — have the potential for producing such undesirable side-effects. Although atracurium has a lower propensity for releasing histamine than tubocurarine, it can release significant amounts of histamine when given in larger doses (Basta *et al.* 1983; Lavery *et al.* 1985; Mirakhur *et al.* 1985; Scott *et al.* 1986). Mivacurium has the same limitation to the use of larger doses (beyond 0.15–0.2 mg/kg) which release significant amounts of histamine and may lead to decrease in arterial pressure (Savarese *et al.* 1989). Vecuronium has a dose-related onset and duration of action and even in high doses is relatively free from side-effects such as histamine release or ganglion block (Marshall *et al.* 1980; Mirakhur *et al.* 1983; Morris *et al.* 1983; Rorvik *et al.* 1988; Ginsberg *et al.* 1989).

Using larger doses of an agent such as vecuronium would also be helpful in accelerating the onset of block. In the study of Rorvik *et al.* (1988) a 0.3 mg/kg dose of vecuronium resulted in complete block in 81 seconds with a duration of clinical relaxation of 86 minutes which was similar to the duration of clinical relaxation of 0.1 mg/kg of pancuronium. Ginsberg *et al.* (1989) similarly reported the duration of clinical relaxation of vecuronium to increase from 37 to 138 minutes as the dose was increased from 0.1 to 0.4 mg/kg. These doses of vecuronium obviously result in a block of relatively long duration which is similar to that produced by a moderate dose of a longer-acting agent and with some loss of flexibility. However there are no significant cardiovascular side-effects from such a large dose and recovery is comparatively fast once it starts to take place.

It must also be noted that when using this technique of a large initial dose, the pharmacokinetics of the drug may be different and not based on the initial rapid redistribution. This may mean that the duration of action is not as easy to predict as after prolonged fixed rate infusions (Segredo *et al.* 1990). Furthermore because vecuronium shows a variation in duration of action with age (d'Hollander *et al.* 1982*b*), the consequences in different age groups of a single large bolus are not clear.

The newer agent rocuronium (Org 9426) has almost the same duration of action as vecuronium but is associated with a much faster onset of action (Cooper *et al.* 1993). This agent however may give rise to some tachycardia when administered in large doses and its cumulative potential is not yet clearly defined.

It has been suggested that the large bolus dose approach is preferable in pharmacokinetic terms because the duration of effect then becomes dependent upon the time necessary to reduce acetylcholine receptor occupancy to below the accepted 70–80% above which block begins (Paton and Waud 1967). At this point the plasma levels of the relaxant would be low and this might theoretically permit easier reversal (Feldman 1973). However, a clinical study indicated no such advantage for the bolus method (Ham *et al.* 1979).

A further disadvantage of this method is that the level of neuromuscular block is not constant and is not titrated to effect thus raising the possibility of an unexpectedly short or long duration of block. In addition this method suffers from the well known disadvantage of marked individual variation in response to muscle relaxants (Katz 1967; d'Hollander *et al.* 1982*a*). In conclusion therefore, this method of relaxant administration would appear to be principally suited to moderately long procedures only and has only marginal advantages over the longer acting relaxants except in terms of side-effects. It is therefore preferable to use other approaches for maintaining relaxation for longer procedures.

ADMINISTRATION OF REPEATED DOSES

The administration of single doses of muscle relaxants (even when large) is useful only for moderately long procedures. For procedures lasting several hours initial doses have to be followed up by further increments of relaxant. It is an advantage in this situation to use the intermediate-duration relaxants which might include vecuronium or atracurium — or perhaps rocuronium when enough experience has accumulated with it — since there is less cumulation which these agents (Buzello and Noldge 1982; Mirakhur *et al.* 1983, 1985). Mivacurium might find a place in these techniques although many would regard its duration of action as being too short for use by repeated increments.

The size of the incremental doses to maintain block is important. It is generally accepted that they should be about 20–33% of the initial bolus (Hughes and Chapple 1981; Hughes and Payne 1983). It was suggested that the incremental dose to re-establish a 95% block is about 20% of the ED_{95} when this is administered at 25% recovery from the previous dose (Brull and Silverman 1993). Another proposal was, however, made by Khuenl-Brady *et al.* (1991) whose scheme is to administer about half the ED_{95} dose as a maintenance increment of agents such as atracurium and vecuronium. This is claimed to give a further 15–20 minutes of adequate relaxation with a low risk of cumulation.

In general not only is it inconvenient to have to administer bolus doses of muscle relaxants frequently during a long surgical procedure but it also provides relaxation which is not constant unless the doses are repeated when the block is still very deep. In this situation there is always a risk of overdose or underdose (d'Hollander *et al.* 1982*a*). In addition, if long-acting agents such as pancuronium have been given intermittently, antagonism of block takes longer to achieve (Beattie *et al.* 1992). To avoid this fluctuating relaxation, it is better to administer the relaxants by a continuous infusion.

ADMINISTRATION BY INFUSION

Theoretically a good way of providing adequate and constant relaxation is to induce relaxation with a bolus dose of the drug and then maintain a steady plasma concentration and a constant state of relaxation by the use of continuous infusion. This approach, which has become popular in recent years with the introduction of the relatively shorter-acting relaxants, had been described even before the introduction of these new drugs (Ryan 1964; Somogyi *et al.* 1978; Ramzan *et al.* 1980). It is based on the observation of a highly significant linear correlation between the serum concentration and the twitch tension (Matteo *et al.* 1974).

The initial bolus dose should be sufficiently large to achieve the target concentration and fill the initial volume of distribution. If that situation is reached, the plasma concentration never falls below the target concentration as the infusion builds up. The rationale and method for calculating the initial bolus dose and the maintenance requirements were reviewed by Shanks (1986). The question of the size of the initial bolus dose is interesting, because it is determined by the volume of distribution of the drug and may be difficult to predict accurately. With muscle relaxants, however, it is possible to adjust the rate of the subsequent infusion to the degree of block by using some system of neuromuscular monitoring unlike, for example, the case for intravenous anaesthetic agents. This allows a smaller initial bolus to be used, followed by maintenance infusion tailored to the patient's requirements. It is also possible to use a closed-loop pharmacological control system. Pancuronium, vecuronium, and atracurium have all been administered in this way (Asbury and Linkens 1986; De Vries *et al.* 1986; Wait *et al.* 1987).

Automatic control systems of this general type depend on the error or difference between the output of the control system and a resultant feedback or input from some sensor. The system usually consists of some form of evoked compound electromyogram monitoring device (input) linked to a control system and then to an infusion device (output), although systems based on mechanomyography have also been described (Uys *et al.* 1988).

Several types of control systems have been used. A simple one is the 'flick-flack' device (Wait *et al.* 1987). This is an on-off control system which responds to the sign of the difference between the actual response and the target level. As such it is prone to oscillations, like physiological hunting, but nevertheless performs well. In order to improve on this system, more sophisticated systems have been developed such as the 'proportional plus derivative' (Webster and Cohen 1987) and the 'proportional plus integral' (MacLeod *et al*. 1989). In these cases the idea is to achieve adequate paralysis for surgery rapidly, without waiting for a long 'hunting' period. The 'integral' term is a common control system feature to remove steady-state error by reducing the output or infusion rate according to the time integral of the error signal.

A yet more subtle method of control is to adapt the closed-loop feedback of neuromuscular blocker by making it 'self-tuning'. In this the control system starts by using established mean pharmacokinetic and pharmacodynamic data but then modifies these kinetic parameters according to the discrepancy between its model-based theoretical expectation and the measured effect. When used for vecuronium this system was found to adapt successfully to wide variations in vecuronium requirements to produce stable neuromuscular block at a set level (Olkkola and Schwilden 1991).

An advantage of self-tuning control of neuromuscular block is that it allows some compensation to be made for alterations in the pharmacokinetics and pharmacodynamics of the relaxant which may occur during long surgical procedures. Clearly the disadvantage is that it demands greater attention to detail than simpler methods, and is more time consuming to establish. The quality of post-operative recovery facilities, and the availability of high dependency or intensive care must also have an influence on the final choice of technique.

Although closed-loop feedback systems provide good control of muscle relaxation, many investigators have been able to use intraoperative infusions of intermediate-action muscle relaxants without such equipment using simple manual control. It is, of course, essential to be able to monitor the neuromuscular block under these circumstances (Mirakhur and Ferres 1984; Hunter *et al*. 1987; Cannon *et al*. 1987; Ali *et al*. 1988). These workers have been able to maintain relaxation using infusions in this manner for up to six hours. The average rates of relaxant administration for maintenance of 90–95% block of the twitch height are approximately 0.5 mg/kg/h for atracurium and 0.1 mg/kg/h for vecuronium. Vecuronium requirements are reduced by almost two-thirds when using enflurane or isoflurane for maintenance of anaesthesia in comparison to a narcotic-based technique. The recovery following the use of infusions is usually rapid in healthy patients, of the order of 20–25 minutes to 20–25% of control levels, at which stage antagonism of the block using an anticholinesterase is achieved quickly.

Mivacurium, which has a short duration of action because of its metabolism by plasma cholinesterase, is ideally administered by a continuous infusion if it is used for maintenance of relaxation. The dosage of mivacurium required to maintain a constant level of block has been reported to be about 0.5 mg/kg/h during balanced anaesthesia (Ali *et al*. 1988). These workers also reported that recovery following mivacurium infusions was twice as rapid as that after infusions of atracurium or vecuronium. A recent study with rocuronium showed the maintenance requirements by infusion to be about 0.6 mg/kg/h during balanced anaesthesia and reduced by about 40% in the presence of enflurane or isoflurane (Shanks *et al*. 1993). In all of these manually controlled schemes using the intermediate- and short-acting drugs, the patients received an initial bolus of the relaxants equivalent to between one and a half and twice the ED_{95} dose. The infusions in most cases were commenced at 5–10% recovery of the twitch height. Once stable it has been relatively easy to maintain steady-state relaxation.

It is important to recognize that, while the use of neuromuscular blocking agents by infusion provided good steady-state relaxation at any desired level, the requirements of individual patients may vary widely (Mirakhur and Ferres 1984). For this reason it is of paramount importance that the relaxation is monitored carefully in order to optimize the dose for each patient. This may be done using only a nerve stimulator as long as the degree of relaxation is such that only first response in a train-of-four stimulation is felt.

Apart from steady-state relaxation, another advantage of using infusions of intermediate-acting relaxants is the feasibility of relatively easy reversal and recovery if for some reason the surgery is terminated abruptly. Not being able to do this is a serious disadvantage of the use of large bolus doses. Since the use of infusions entails only the use of moderately large doses at the beginning, there is a reduced likelihood of the occurrence of undesirable side-effects. The titration of effect also takes into account the individual variations in response to the relaxants.

When large doses of muscle relaxants are used it is important to consider any potential problems with their metabolites. Although muscle relaxants are eliminated unchanged for the most part, some do undergo considerable metabolism. The metabolites may have neuromuscular activity (as is possible with pancuronium and vecuronium), or they may have the potential to produce other effects. In recent years there has been much debate on laudanosine which is an end-product of the breakdown of atracurium. It is a tertiary compound capable of crossing into the central nervous system and might give rise to central stimulation, as has been suggested by increased anaesthetic requirements in experimental studies (Shi *et al.* 1985). Concentrations capable of inducing convulsions or even cardiovascular effects are unlikely to result after a few hours use in the operating room. Measurements of plasma laudanosine have shown that levels rise to approximately 5 μg/ml after infusing atracurium for about five days (Yate *et al.* 1987). Concentrations higher than these have also been reported without problems in animal species.

FACTORS MODIFYING RELAXATION DURING LONG PROCEDURES

As has been noted, the effects of muscle relaxants are modified by many factors and this is more likely to occur during long procedures where larger doses are likely to be used. One problem with the use of muscle relaxants was recognized by Gray (1948) soon after their introduction:

I have repeatedly seen experienced anaesthetists returning patients to the ward after operation still partially curarized. They often appear to be breathing fairly adequately

… but a little closer observation would show that their respirations are depressed and inadequate.

This spectre of residual curarization has not been banished by simple neuromuscular monitoring. The reason is that this does not prevent or always rule out residual neuromuscular block, which is reported to be common (Viby-Mogensen *et al.* 1979; Beemer and Rozental 1986; Bevan *et al.* 1988). Furthermore the problem may be underestimated as the standard train-of-four ratio of 0.7 may not be adequate to rule out clinically significant post-operative weakness of the airway musculature (Miller 1989).

Background anaesthesia

The choice of background anaesthetic technique will have an influence on the requirements for neuromuscular block. It is well established that the action of the nondepolarizing muscle relaxants is prolonged by the addition of volatile anaesthetic agents, in particular enflurane (Miller *et al.* 1972; Fogdall and Miller 1975). This does not appear to be on the basis of changes in nerve conduction velocity or acetylcholine release, but rather a change in endplate potential generated by acetylcholine (Kennedy and Galindo 1975).

When using enflurane for long surgical procedures there appears to be a time-dependent alteration in the sensitivity of the neuromuscular junction at least to tubocurarine. This is manifest as a liner increase in paralysis with enflurane of about 9% per hour over the first two hours of anaesthesia. The complete explanation for this is not clear, but may involve a change in the sensitivity of the neuromuscular junction and a simple pharmacokinetic effect based on a muscle equilibration half-time of 40 minutes for enflurane (Stanski *et al.* 1980). It is not known whether a total intravenous anaesthetic technique based on propofol would show such changes, but for short infusions there appears to be no significant potentiation of neuromuscular block (McCarthy *et al.* 1992*b*).

Age

There is well documented evidence that the effects of nondepolarizing neuromuscular blocking agents are prolonged in the elderly. This holds true for both the long- and the intermediate-acting agents with the possible exception of atracurium (Duvaldestin *et al.* 1982; Matteo *et al.* 1985; Lien *et al.* 1991; McCarthy *et al.* 1992*a*; Bevan *et al.* 1993). Since most of the differences in the elderly are based on kinetic differences rather than on any differences in sensitivity to the neuromuscular blocking agents, it is highly likely that the effects would last even longer after administration over prolonged periods. The requirements of infusions of vecuronium for steady-state relaxation have been shown to be reduced in the elderly even over relatively short periods (d'Hollander *et al.* 1982*b*). The duration of action of mivacurium is also prolonged in the elderly and its requirements during steady-state infusion reduced (Maddineni *et al.* personal communication).

Hypothermia

A potential feature of prolonged surgery is unintentional hypothermia. Some workers have shown that 60% of patients may have a reduced body temperature in the recovery ward following a range of surgical procedures (Vaughan *et al.* 1981). This may have both pharmacokinetic and pharmacodynamic consequences. In the cardiovascular system, hypothermia causes a fluid shift from the vascular space which may increase blood viscosity to the detriment of cardiac output. All metabolic processes are slowed. This is a situation in which the elimination of many drugs could be expected to be prolonged and indeed hypothermia is known to decrease the plasma clearance and elimination of muscle relaxants including tubocurarine (Ham *et al.* 1978).

A pharmacodynamic effect also exists. Thornton *et al.* (1976) have shown in animals that cooling results in a partial failure of acetylcholine release which will enhance the sensitivity of the neuromuscular junction. Miller and his colleagues (1975) have also shown that the infusion rate necessary to maintain 90% depression of twitch height is directly related to temperature. Hypothermia will also reduce the rate of breakdown of more modern agents such as atracurium (Merrett *et al.* 1983). This may result in a 50% reduction in the requirement of atracurium during cardiopulmonary bypass (Flynn *et al.* 1983, 1984). The net result of the effects of hypothermia may be a prolongation of neuromuscular block or even recurarization during rewarming, although this has not been found to be so in an animal model (McKlveen *et al.* 1973).

Temperature is also important when attempting to monitor neuromuscular block during prolonged surgery. If an exposed arm is being used to represent the rest of the musculature then it must not be allowed to cool or there will be an apparent prolongation in the duration of relaxation of a nondepolarizing muscle relaxant.

Haemorrhage and hypotension

A contributory factor in hypothermia is blood loss and its subsequent replacement with inadequately warmed cold blood. Massive blood transfusion can in theory be associated with citrate toxicity, especially in the presence of hypothermia, resulting in hypocalcaemia which might temporarily alter muscle contraction. In some craniofacial operations it is common for blood loss to be greater than the patients total blood volume, or even a multiple of this in paediatric cases.

Induced hypotension has been recognized as a way of minimizing blood loss during long surgical procedures (Schaberg *et al.* 1976). These periods of hypotension which reduce renal and hepatic blood flow could be expected to alter the duration of action of some relaxants. Possible mechanisms for the facilitation of neuromuscular block during deliberate hypotension may not only involve reductions in organ blood flow, but also include some direct drug interaction at the neuromuscular junction. Nitroglycerine has, for example, been shown in animals to potentiate pancuronium, while trimetaphan has been reported to have neuromuscular blocking properties in dogs even when noradrenalin had been used to maintain blood pressure (Deacock and Hargrove 1962; Glisson *et al.* 1980).

Attempts to maintain urinary output in the face of hypotension by administering diuretics such as frusemide can also result in significant interactions. At low doses (under 10 μg/kg) frusemide potentiates the action of nondepolarizing neuromuscular blocking drugs while at higher doses it may actually antagonize the block (Azar *et al.* 1980). Beta adrenergic blocking agents have also been used for hypotensive anaesthesia and their administration may also result in a prolongation in the duration of action of relaxants.

Disease

Altered responses to muscle relaxants may also be due to the underlying pathology. Patients suffering from muscular disorders, for example, are frequently sensitive to the actions of nondepolarizing neuromuscular blocking agents. Sensitivity is also classically seen in the Eaton–Lambert syndrome. This myasthenic-like condition is usually associated with oat cell carcinoma of the bronchus, and results in a prejunctional disorder of acetylcholine release.

Not all conditions will, of course, enhance the sensitivity of the neuromuscular junction to nondepolarizing muscle relaxants. In patients with burns there is a well established effective denervation of muscle resulting in nicotinic receptors becoming spread over the surface of muscle so that there is an increased dose requirement of nondepolarizing muscle relaxants (Martyn *et al.* 1980). It is therefore important to monitor neuromuscular block in such patients away from the site of pathology. Further details concerning the effect of various disease states on the action of the neuromuscular blocking agents are discussed in Chapter 18.

REFERENCES

Agoston, S. and Richardson, F. J. (1985). Pipecuronium bromide (Arduan) a new long-acting non-depolarizing neuromuscular blocking drug. *Clinics in Anesthesiology*, **3**, 351–69.

Ali, H. H., Savarese, J. J., Embree, P. B., Basta, S. J., Stout, R. G., Bottros, L. H., *et al.* (1988). Clinical pharmacology of mivacurium chloride (BW B1090U) infusion: Comparison with vecuronium and atracurium. *British Journal of Anaesthesia*, **61**, 541–6.

Asbury, A. J. and Linkens, D. A. (1986). Clinical automatic control of neuromuscular blockade. *Anaesthesia*, **41**, 316–21.

Azar, I., Cottrell, J., Gupta, B., and Turndorf, H. (1980). Furosemide facilitates recovery of evoked twitch response after pancuronium. *Anesthesia and Analgesia*, **59**, 55–7.

Basta, S. J., Savarese, J. J., Ali, H. H., Moss, J., and Gionfriddo, M. (1983). Histamine-releasing potencies of atracurium, dimethyltubocurarine and tubocurarine. *British Journal of Anaesthesia*, **55**, 105–6S.

Basta, S. J., Savarese, J. J., Ali, H. H., Embree, P. B., Schwartz, A. F., Rudd, G. D., *et al.* (1988). Clinical pharmacology of doxacurium chloride. A new long-acting nondepolarizing muscle relaxant. *Anesthesiology*, **69**, 478–86.

Beattie, W. S., Buckley, D. N., and Forrest, J. B. (1992). Continuous infusions of atracurium and vecuronium, compared with intermittent boluses of pancuronium: dose requirements and reversal. *Canadian Journal of Anaesthesia*, **39**, 925–31.

Beemer, G. H. and Rozental, P. (1986). Postoperative neuromuscular function. *Anaesthesia and Intensive Care*, **14**, 41–5.

Bevan, D. R., Smith, C. E., and Donati., F. (1988). Postoperative neuromuscular blockade: a comparison between atracurium, vecuronium, and pancuronium. *Anesthesiology*, **69**, 272–6.

Bevan, D. R., Fiset, P., Balendran, P., Law-Min, J. C., Ratcliffe, A., and Donati, F. (1993). Pharmacodynamic behaviour of rocuronium in the elderly. *Canadian Journal of Anaesthesia*, **40**, 127–32.

Blackburn, C. L. and Morgan, M. (1978). Comparison of speed of onset of fazadinium, pancuronium, tubocurarine and suxamethonium. *British Journal of Anaesthesia*, **50**, 361–4.

Bowman, W. C., Rodger, I. W., Houston, J., Marshall, R. J., and McIndewar, I. (1988). Structure: action relationships among some desacetoxy analogues of pancuronium and vecuronium in the anesthetized cat. *Anesthesiology*, **69**, 57–62.

Brull, S. J. and Silverman, D. G. (1993). Intraoperative use of muscle relaxants. *Anesthesiology Clinics of North America*, **11**, 325–44.

Buzello, W. and Noldge, G. (1982). Repetitive administration of pancuronium and vecuronium (Org NC45, Norcuron) in patients undergoing long-lasting operations. *British Journal of Anaesthesia*, **54**, 1151–7.

Caballero, P. A. and Johnstone, R. E. (1992). Long lasting neuromuscular blockade from pipecuronium. *Anesthesiology*, **76**, 154–5.

Caldwell, J. E., Castagnoli, A. P., Canfell, D. C., Fahey, M. R., Lynam, D. P., Fisher, D. M., *et al.* (1988). Pipecuronium and pancuronium: comparison of pharmacokinetics and duration of action. *British Journal of Anaesthesia*, **61**, 693–7.

Caldwell, J. E., Canfell, P. C., Castagnoli, K. P., Lynam, D. P., Fahey, M. R., Fisher, D. M., *et al.* (1989). The influence of renal failure on the pharmacokinetics and duration of action of pipecuronium bromide in patients anaesthetized with halothane and nitrous oxide. *Anesthesiology*, **70**, 7–12.

Cannon, J. E., Fahey, M. R., Castagnoli, Y. P., Furuta, T., Canfell, P. C., Sharma, M., *et al.* (1987). Continuous infusion of vecuronium: The effect of anesthetic agents. *Anesthesiology*, **67**, 503–6.

Cashman, J. N., Luke, J. J., and Jones, R. M. (1990). Neuromuscular block with doxacurium (BW A938U) in patients with normal or absent renal function. *British Journal of Anaesthesia*, **64**, 186–92.

Cooper, R. A., Mirakhur, R. K., and Maddineni, V. R. (1993). Neuromuscular effects of rocuronium bromide (Org 9426) during fentanyl and halothane anaesthesia. *Anaesthesia*, **48**, 103–5.

Deacock, A. R. and Hargrove, R. L. (1962). The influence of certain ganglion blocking agents on neuromuscular transmission. *British Journal of Anaesthesia*, **34**, 357–62.

d'Hollander, A. A., Czerucki, R., Deville, A., and Covelier, F. (1982*a*). Stable muscle relaxation during abdominal surgery using combined intravenous bolus and demand infusion: clinical appraisal with ORG NC45. *Canadian Anaesthetists' Society Journal*, **29**, 136–41.

d'Hollander, A., Massaux, F., Nevelsteen, M., and Agoston, S. (1982*b*). Age-dependent dose–response relationship of ORG NC45 in anaesthetized patients. *British Journal of Anaesthesia*, **54**, 653–7.

De Vries, J. W., Ros, H. H., and Booij, L. H. D. J (1986). Infusion of vecuronium controlled by a closed-loop system. *British Journal of Anaesthesia*, **58**, 1100–3.

Duvaldestin, P., Saada, J., Berger, J. L., d'Hollander, A., and Desmonts, J. M. (1982). Pharmacokinetics, pharmacodynamics and dose–response relationships of pancuronium in control and elderly subjects. *Anesthesiology*, **56**, 36–40.

Emmott, R. S., Bracey, B. J., Goldhill, D. R., Yate, P. M., and Flynn, P. J. (1990). Cardiovascular effects of doxacurium, pancuronium and vecuronium in anaesthetized patients presenting for coronary artery bypass surgery. *British Journal of Anaesthesia*, **65**, 480–6.

Fahey, M. R., Morris, R. B., Miller, R. D., Sohn, Y. J., Cronnelly, R., and Gencarelli, P. (1981). Clinical pharmacology of ORG NC45 (Norcuron): a new nondepolarizing muscle relaxant. *Anesthesiology*, **55**, 6–11.

Feldman, S. A. (1973). The rational use of muscle relaxants. In *Muscle relaxants*, (ed. S. A. Feldman), pp. 149–55. Saunders, London.

Flynn, P. J., Hughes, R., Walton, B., and Jothilingham, S. (1983). Use of atracurium for general surgical procedures including cardiac surgery with induced hypothermia. *British Journal of Anaesthesia*, **55**, 135–8S.

Flynn, P. J., Hughes, R., and Walton, B. (1984). Use of atracurium in cardiac surgery involving cardiopulmonary bypass with induced hypothermia. *British Journal of Anaesthesia*, **56**, 967–71.

Fogdall, R. P. and Miller, R. D. (1975). Neuromuscular effects of enflurane alone and combined with *d*-tubocurarine, pancuronium, and succinylcholine in man. *Anesthesiology*, **42**, 173–8.

Foldes, F. F., Nagashima, H., Nguyen, H. D., Duncalf, D., and Goldiner, B. L. (1990). Neuromuscular and cardiovascular effects of pipecuronium. *Canadian Anaesthetists' Society Journal*, **37**, 549–55.

Ginsberg, B., Glass, P. S., Quill, T., Shafron, D., and Ossey, K. D. (1989). Onset and duration of neuromuscular blockade following high-dose vecuronium administration. *Anesthesiology*, **71**, 201–5.

Glisson, S. N., Sanchez, M. M., El-Etr, A. A., and Lim, R. A. (1980). Nitroglycelin and the neuromuscular blockade produced by gallamine, succinylcholine, *d*-tubocurarine, and pancuronium. *Anesthesia and Analgesia*, **59**, 117–22.

Gray, T. C. (1948). *d*-Tubocurarine chloride. *Proceedings of the Royal Society of Medicine*, **41**, 559–68.

Gray, T. C. and Halton, J. (1946). A milestone in anaesthesia (*d*-tubocurarine chloride). *Proceedings of the Royal Society of Medicine*, **34**, 400–6.

Griffith, H. R. and Johnson, G. E. (1942). The use of curare in general anesthesia. *Anesthesiology*, **3**, 418–20.

Ham, J., Miller, R. D., Benet, L. Z., Matteo, R. S., and Roderick, L. L. (1978). Pharmacokinetics and pharmacodynamics of *d*-tubocurarine during hypothemia in the cat. *Anesthesiology*, **49**, 324–9.

Ham, J., Miller, R. D., Sheiner, L. B., and Matteo, R. S. (1979). Dosage schedule independence of *d*-tubocurarine pharmacokinetics and pharmacodynamics, and recovery of neuromuscular function. *Anesthesiology*, **50**, 528–33.

Harrop-Griffiths, W., Fauvel, N., Plumley, M., and Feldman, S. (1992). Pipecuronium versus high dose vecuronium I. A comparison of speed of onset and cumulation during isoflurane anaesthesia. *Anaesthesia*, **47**, 105–6.

Hughes, R. and Chapple, D. J. (1981). The pharmacology of atracurium: a new competitive neuromuscular blocking agent. *British Journal of Anaesthesia*, **53**, 31–44.

Hughes, R. and Payne, J. P. (1983). Clinical assessment of atracurium using the single twitch and tetanic responses of the adductor pollicis muscles. *British Journal of Anaesthesia*, **55**, 47S–52S.

Hunter, J. M., Kelly, J. M., and Jones, R. S. (1987). Atracurium infusions in major ophthalmic surgery. *European Journal of Anaesthesiology*, **4**, 9–15.

Jones, R. M. (1985). Neuromuscular transmission and its blockade: Pharmacology, monitoring and physiology updated. *Anaesthesia*, **40**, 964–76.

Katz, R. L. (1967). Neuromuscular effects of d-tubocurarine, edrophonium, and neostigmine in man. *Anesthesiology*, **28**, 327–36.

Kennedy, R. D. and Galindo, A. D. (1975). Comparative site of action of various anaesthetic agents at the mammalian myoneural junction. *British Journal of Anaesthesia*, **47**, 533–40.

Khuenl-Brady, K. S., Scharz, S., Richardson, F. J., and Mitterschiffthaler, G. (1991). Maintenance of surgical muscle relaxation by repeated doses of vecuronium and atracurium at three different dose levels. *European Journal of Anaesthesiology*, **8**, 1–6.

Kopman, A. F. (1989). Pancuronium, gallamine, and *d*-tubocurarine compared: Is speed of onset inversely related to drug potency? *Anesthesiology*, **70**, 915–20.

Lavery, G. G., Boyle, M. M., and Mirakhur, R. K. (1985). Probable histamine liberation with atracurium. *British Journal of Anaesthesia*, **57**, 811–3.

Lennon, R. L., Hosking, M. P., Houck, P. C., Rose, S. H., Wedel, D. J., Gibson, B. E., *et al.* (1989). Doxacurium chloride for neuromuscular blockade before tracheal intubation and surgery during nitrous oxide–oxygen–narcotic–enflurane anesthesia. *Anesthesia and Analgesia*, **68**, 255–60.

Lien, C., Matteo, R., Ornstein, E., Schwartz, A., and Diaz, J. (1991). Distribution, elimination, and action of vecuronium in the elderly. *Anesthesia and Analgesia*, **73**, 39–42.

McCarthy, G., Elliott, P., Mirakhur, R. K., Cooper, R., Sharpe, T. D. E, and Clarke, R. S. J. (1992*a*). Onset and duration of action of vecuronium in the elderly: comparison with adults. *Acta Anaesthesiologica Scandinavica*, **36**, 383–6.

McCarthy, G. J., Mirakhur, R. K., and Pandit, S. K. (1992*b*). Lack of interaction between propofol and vecuronium. *Anesthesia and Analgesia*, **75**, 536–8.

MacLeod, A. D., Asbury, A. J., Gray, W. M., and Linkens, D. A. (1989). Automatic control of neuromuscular block with atracurium. *British Journal of Anaesthesia*, **63**, 31–5.

McKlveen, J. R., Sokoll, M. D., Gergis, S. D., and Dretchen, K. L. (1973). Absence of recuratization upon rewarming. *Anesthesiology*, **38**, 153–6.

Maddineni, V. R., Cooper, R., Stanley, J. C., Mirakhur, R. K., and Clarke, R. S. J. (1992). Clinical evaluation of doxacurium chloride. *Anaesthesia*, **47**, 554–7.

Marshall, R. J., McGrath, J. C., Miller, R. D., Docherty, R. J., and Lamar, J-C. (1980). Comparison of the cardiovascular actions of ORG NC45 with those produced by other non-depolarizing neuromuscular blocking agents in experimental animals. *British Journal of Anaesthesia*, **52**, 21S–32S.

Martyn, J. A. J., Szyfelbein, S. K., Ali, H. H., Matteo, R. S., and Savarese, J. J. (1980). Increased *d*-tubocurarine requirement following major thermal injury. *Anesthesiology*, **52**, 352–5.

Matteo, R. S., Spector, S., and Horowitz, P. E. (1974). Relation of serum *d*-tubocurarine concentrations to neuromuscular block in man. *Anesthesiology*, **41**, 440–3.

Matteo, R. S., Backus, W. W., McDaniel, D. D., Brotherton, W. P., Abraham, R., and Diaz, J. (1985). Pharmacokinetics and pharmacodynamics of *d*-tubocurarine and metocurine in the elderly. *Anesthesia and Analgesia*, **64**, 23–9.

Merrett, R. A., Thompson, C. W., and Webb, F. W. (1983). *In vitro* degradation of atracurium in human plasma. *British Journal of Anaesthesia*, **55**, 61–6.

Miller, R. D. (1989). How should residual neuromuscular blockade be detected? *Anesthesiology*, **70**, 379–80.

Miller, R. D., Way, W. L., Dolan, W. M., Stevens, W. C., and Eger, E. I. (1972). The dependence of pancuronium- and *d*-tubocurarine-induced neuromuscular blockades on alveolar concentrations of halothane and forane. *Anesthesiology*, **37**, 573–81.

Miller, R. D., Van NyHuis, L. S., and Eger, E. I. (1975). The effect of temperature on a *d*-tubocurarine neuromuscular blockade and its antagonism by neostigmine. *Journal of Pharmacology and Experimental Therapeutics*, **195**, 237–41.

Minsaas, B. and Stovner, J. (1980). Artery-to-muscle onset time for neuromuscular blocking drugs. *British Journal of Anaesthesia*, **52**, 403–7.

Mirakhur, R. K. (1990). Drug usage by anaesthetists. *Anaesthesia*, **45**, 500–1.

Mirakhur, R. K. (1992). Newer neuromuscular blocking drugs. An overview of their clinical pharmacology and therapeutic use. *Drugs*, **44**, 182–99.

Mirakhur, R. K. and Ferres, C. J. (1984). Muscle relaxation with an infusion of vecuronium. *European Journal of Anaesthesiology*, **1**, 353–9.

Mirakhur, R. K., Ferres, C. J., Clarke, R. S. J., Bali, I. M., and Dundee, J. W. (1983). Clinical evaluation of Org NC45. *British Journal of Anaesthesia*, **55**, 119–24.

Mirakhur, R. K., Lavery, G. G., Clarke, R. S. J., Gibson, F. M., and McAteer, E. (1985). Atracurium in clinical anaesthesia: effect of dosage on onset, duration and conditions for tracheal intubation. *Anaesthesia*, **40**, 801–5.

Morris, R. B., Cahalan, M. K., Miller, R. D., Wilkinson, P. L., Quasha, A. L., and Robinson, S. L. (1983). The cardiovascular effects of vecuronium (ORG NC45) and pancuronium in patients undergoing coronary artery bypass grafting. *Anesthesiology*, **58**, 438–40.

Norman, J., Katz, R. L., and Seed, R. F. (1970). The neuromuscular blocking action of pancuronium in man during anaesthesia. *British Journal of Anaesthesia*, **42**, 702–9.

Olkkola, K. T. and Schwilden, H. (1991). Adaptive closed-loop feedback control of vecuronium-induced neuromuscular relaxation. *European Journal of Anaesthesiology*, **8**, 7–12.

Paton, W. D. M. and Waud, D. R. (1967). The margin on safety of neuromuscular transmission. *Journal of Physiology*, **191**, 59–90.

Ramzan, M. I., Shanks, C. A., and Triggs, E. J. (1980). Pharmacokinetics of tubocurarine administered by combined IV bolus and infusion. *British Journal of Anaesthesia*, **52**, 893–9.

Rorvik, R. P. F., Husby, P., Gramstad, L., Vamnes, J. S., Bitsch-Larsen, L., and Koller, M-E. (1988). Comparison of large dose of vecuronium and pancuronium for prolonged neuromuscular blockade. *British Journal of Anaesthesia*, **61**, 180–5.

Ryan, A. R. (1964). Tubocurarine administration based upon its disappearance and accumulation curves in anaesthetized man. *British Journal of Anaesthesia*, **36**, 287–94.

Sanfilippo, M., Fierro, G., Vilardi, V., Rosa, G., Licia De Gregorio, A., and Gasparetto, A. (1992). Clinical evaluation of different doses of pipecuronium bromide during nitrous-oxide–fentanyl anaesthesia in adult surgical patients. *European Journal of Anaesthesiology*, **9**, 49–53.

Savarese, J. J. and Kitz, P. J. (1975). Does clinical anesthesia need new neuromuscular blocking agents? *Anesthesiology*, **42**, 236–9.

Savarese, J. J., Ali, H. H., and Antonio, R. P. (1977). The clinical pharmacology of metocurine: Dimethyltubocurarine revisited. *Anesthesiology*, **47**, 277–85.

Savarese, J. J., Ali, H. H., Basta, S. J., Scott, R. P. F., Embree, P. B., Wastila, W. B., *et al.* (1989). The cardiovascular effects of mivacurium chloride (BW B1090U) in patients receiving nitrous oxide–opiate–barbiturate anesthesia. *Anesthesiology*, **70**, 386–94.

Schaberg, S. J., Kelly, J. F., Terry, B. C., Posner, M. A., and Anderson, E. F. (1976). Blood loss and hypotensive anaesthesia in oral-facial corrective surgery. *Journal of Oral Surgery*, **34**, 147–56.

Scott, R. P. F. and Norman, J. (1989). Doxacurium chloride, a preliminary clinical trial. *British Journal of Anaesthesia*, **62**, 373–7.

Scott, R. P. F., Savarese, J. J., Basta. S. J., Embree, P., Ali, H. H., Sunder, N., *et al.* (1986). Clinical pharmacology of atracurium given in high dose. *British Journal of Anaesthesia*, **58**, 834–8.

Segredo, V., Caldwell, J. E., Matthay, M. A., Sharma, M. L., Gruenke, L. D., and Miller, R. D. (1990). Pharmacokinetics of vecuronium after long-term administration. *Anesthesia and Analgesia*, **70**, S360.

Shanks, C. A. (1986). Pharmacokinetics of the nondepolarizing neuromuscular relaxants applied to calculation of bolus and infusion dosage regimens. *Anesthesiology*, **64**, 72–86.

Shanks, C. A., Fragen, R. J., and Ling, D. (1993). Continuous intravenous infusion of rocuronium (Org 9426) in patients receiving balanced, enflurane, or isoflurane anesthesia. *Anesthesiology*, **78**, 649–51.

Shi, W.-Z., Fahey, M. R., Fisher, D. M., Miller, R. D., Canfell, C., and Eger, E. I. (1985). Laudanosine (a metabolite of atracurium) increases the minimum alveolar concentration of halothane in rabbits. *Anesthesiology*, **63**, 584–8.

Somogyi, A. A., Shanks, C. A., Triggs, E. J. (1978). Combined i.v. bolus and infusion of pancuronium bromide. *British Journal of Anaesthesia*, **50**, 575–82.

Stanley, J. C., Carson, I. W., Gibson, F. M., McMurray, T. J., Elliot, P., Lyons, S. M., *et al.* (1991a). Comparison of the haemodynamic effects of pipecuronium and pancuronium during fentanyl anaesthesia. *Acta Anaesthesiologica Scandinavica*, **35**, 262–6.

Stanley, J. C., Mirakhur, R. K., Bell, P. F., Sharpe, T. D. E., and Clarke, R. S. J. (1991b). Neuromuscular effects of pipecuronium bromide. *European Journal of Anaesthesiology*, **8**, 151–6.

Stanski, D. R., Ham, J., Miller, R. D., and Sheiner, L. B. (1980). Time-dependent increase in sensitivity to *d*-tubocurarine during enflurane anesthesia in man. *Anesthesiology*, **52**, 483–7.

Stoelting, R. K. (1972). The haemodynamic effects of pancuronium and d-tubocurarine in anesthetized patients. *Anesthesiology*, **36**, 612–5.

Stoops, C. M., Curtis, C. A., Kovach, D. A., McCammon, R. L., Stoelting, R. K., Warren, T. M., *et al.* (1988). Hemodynamic effects of doxacurium chloride in patients receiving oxygen–sufentanil anesthesia for coronary artery bypass grafting or valve replacement. *Anesthesiology*, **69**, 365–70.

Thomson, I. R. and Putnins, C. L. (1985). Adverse effects of pancuronium during high-dose fentanyl anesthesia for coronary artery bypass grafting. *Anesthesiology*, **62**, 708–13.

Thornton, R. J., Blakeney, C., and Feldman, S. A. (1976). The effect of hypothermia on neuromuscular conduction. *British Journal of Anaesthesia*, **48**, 264.

Uys, P. C., Morrell, D. F., Bradlow, H. S., and Rametti, L. B. (1988). Self-tuning, micro-processor-based closed-loop control of atracurium-induced neuromuscular blockade. *British Journal of Anaesthesia*, **61**, 685–92.

Vaughan, M. S., Vaughan, R. W., and Cork, R. C. (1981). Postoperative hypothermia in adults: Relationship of age, anesthesia and shivering to rewarming. *Anesthesia and Analgesia*, **60**, 746–51.

Viby-Mogensen, J., Jorgensen, B. C., and Ording, H. (1979). Residual curarization in the recovery room. *Anesthesiolgy*, **50**, 539–41.

Wait, C. M., Goat, V. A., and Blogg, C. E. (1987). Feedback control of neuromuscular blockade: A simple system for infusion of atracurium. *Anaesthesia*, **42**, 1212–7.

Walts, L. F. and Dillon, J. B. (1968). *d*-Tubocurarine cumulation studies *Anesthesia and Analgesia*, **47**, 696–701.

Webster, N. R. and Cohen, A. T. (1987). Closed-loop administration of atracurium: Steady-state neuromuscular blockade during surgery using a computer controlled closed-up atracurium infusion. *Anaesthesia*, **42**, 1085–91.

Yate, P. M., Flynn, P. J., Arnold, R. W., Weatherly, B. C., Simmonds, R. J., and Dopson, T. (1987). Clinical experience and plasma laudanosine concentration during the infusion of atracurium in the intensive therapy unit. *British Journal of Anaesthesia*, **59**, 211–7

11

Neuromuscular blocking agents in intensive therapy

Jennifer M. Hunter

Although it may be thought that there are few indications for the use of neuromuscular blocking agents in intensive therapy, — indeed, some feel strongly that they are inappropriate (Willatts 1985) — most anaesthetists practising in this speciality acknowledge the small, but vital, part these drugs play in the management of the critically ill patient. Neuromuscular blocking agents are used in two different ways in the intensive therapy unit (ITU). The first is in bolus form, often in only one or two doses: no one would question the use of a muscle relaxant such as suxamethonium for facilitating tracheal intubation on first establishing artificial ventilation (IPPV). The more contentious issue is the repeated use of nondepolarizing neuromuscular blocking agents when continued management of IPPV becomes difficult (Table 11.1). The continued tolerance of IPPV is usually achieved with the use of sedatives and analgesics, but if it proves impossible to achieve adequate oxygenation using these techniques alone, nondepolarizing neuromuscular blocking agents are often introduced. Miller-Jones and Williams (1980) in a retrospective analysis of fifty admissions to a district general hospital ITU, were surprised to find that

Table 11.1 Indications for the use of neuromuscular blocking agents in intensive therapy

---

Endotracheal intubation

During technical procedures, e.g. bronchoscopy, gastroscopy

Transfer of patients, e.g. to the operating theatre, for investigations, between hospitals

To aid oxygenation in patients with a poor lung compliance and marked respiratory drive, e.g. Adult Respiratory Distress Syndrome (ARDS)

To prevent an increase in intracranial pressure from straining, especially after neurosurgery, head injuries, cardiac arrest

Difficulty in controlling muscle tone, e.g. tetanus, status epilepticus

Impossibility of achieving synchrony with IPPV from sedatives and analgesics, especially in large, healthy, adult males

---

96% of all the patients had at some stage received pancuronium. Although subsequent reports have suggested that the use of muscle relaxants in intensive therapy is decreasing and is possibly as low as 16% (Merriman 1981; Bion and Ledingham 1987), a more recent study by our department has revealed that, in 49% of admissions to the 14 general ITUs of Mersey Region and North Wales over a three week period, it was deemed necessary to use a nondepolarizing neuromuscular blocking agent for purposes other than tracheal intubation.

It would thus seem that the assumption that muscle relaxants are now rarely used in intensive care is incorrect, and in certain discrete areas, including neonatal and neurosurgical intensive care, they are in routine use.

Table 11.2 Pathophysiological changes which potentiate the action of neuromuscular blocking agents in intensive care

---

1. Acid–base disturbances
  Metabolic acidosis
  Respiratory acidosis
  ? Metabolic alkalosis
  Hypothermia

2. Electrolyte imbalance
  Hypokalaemia ⎫
  Hypernatraemia ⎬ hyperpolarize muscle membrane
  Hypocalcaemia ⎫ decrease presynaptic
  Hypermagnesaemia ⎰ acetylcholine release

3. Drug interactions
Suxamethonium
  Inhibitors of plasma cholinesterase, e.g. organophosphosphorus compounds, ecothiopate, tetrahydroaminoacridine, hexafluorenium, alkylating agents, ester local anaesthetic agents, trimetaphan
  Metoclopramide

Nondepolarizing neuromuscular blocking agents
  Calcium channel blockers, e.g. verapamil, diltiazem
  Antibiotics, e.g. aminoglycosides (neomycin, gentamycin, vancomycin, kanamycin), erythromycin, tetracycline, metronidazole
  Local anaesthetic agents, quinidine
  Immunosuppressant drugs, e.g. cyclosporin, azathioprine
  H_2 receptor antagonists
  Frusemide
  Trimetaphan
  Lithium carbonate

4. Pre-existing neuromuscular disease
  Myasthenia gravis
  Myasthenic syndrome
  Muscle disorders, e.g. muscular dystrophy, myotonia, familial periodic paralysis

---

From Hunter (1987)

The role of individual neuromuscular blocking agents in the ITU will be discussed in this chapter. It must be remembered that many pathophysiological changes which occur commonly in intensive care can potentiate any neuromuscular blocking agent. These changes include acid–base disturbances, electrolyte imbalance, drug interactions, and pre-existing neuromuscular disease (Table 11.2).

SUXAMETHONIUM

This is the only depolarizing neuromuscular blocking agent available in the UK. It must be stressed that suxamethonium has a faster rate of onset than any of the nondepolarizing neuromuscular blocking agents, a dose of 50 mg having been shown to ablate the train-of-four (TOF) twitch response in a group of healthy adults in a mean time of 59 sec; in contrast atracurium (0.5 mg kg^{-1}) has a mean time to maximum depression of 110 sec (Hunter *et al.* 1982). Even the use of a 'priming' dose of a nondepolarizing agent, prior to a bolus dose of the same drug, cannot be relied upon to achieve such a rapid onset of neuromuscular blockade.

A rapid sequence induction with pre-oxygenation, cricoid pressure, and the use of an intravenous barbiturate and suxamethonium is frequently indicated for emergency intubation in the ITU, even if a nasogastric tube is already in place and a drug which promotes gastric emptying, such as metoclopramide has been given. The benefits of using suxamethonium are especially pertinent to a new admission to an ITU for two reasons. It is frequently not known when the patient last ate; and it is recognized that severe stress, such as trauma, infection, and acute renal failure, delays gastric emptying, as does the use of opioids.

Suxamethonium has important side-effects. It is recognized that it will increase the serum potassium by approximately 0.5 mmol/l in healthy, anaesthetized patients (Paton 1959). The increase is similar in magnitude in patients in renal failure but as such cases may well have a raised serum potassium prior to the dose of suxamethonium, the increased plasma concentration may be sufficient to cause ventricular arrhythmias, even cardiac arrest. Just as important is the fact that this increase in serum potassium after suxamethonium may be exaggerated in several acute conditions which may be present on admission to the ITU and thus put the patient at an increased risk of cardiac arrest (Table 11.3). These include burns, where its use is contraindicated, since increases of serum potassium of over 7 mmol/l have been reported (Tolmie *et al.* 1967).

It is also now recognized that patients who have a prolonged period of artificial ventilation, of the order of more than two weeks, may develop profound muscle weakness, even when a neuromuscular blocking agent has not been used. This is thought to be due to axonal degeneration in the peripheral nerves and has been referred to as 'critical illness neuropathy' (Zochodne *et al.* 1987). It is associated with the development of multiple postsynaptic acetylcholine receptors over the surface of the diseased muscle and, as in other cases of denervation sensitivity, these diseased muscles will 'leak' potassium in response to a dose of suxamethonium, causing a

Table 11.3 Clinical conditions in which an exaggerated rise in serum potassium may occur after suxamethonium

Acute burns

Neuromuscular disorders
    Duchenne muscular dystrophy
    Myotonia dystrophica
    Malignant hyperthermia
    Hemiplegia, paraplegia

Critical illness neuropathy
Acute abdomen
Head injuries, encephalitis, ruptured cerebral aneurysm
Tetanus

marked rise in serum concentration, again sufficient to cause cardiac arrest. This phenomenon has also been reported in septicaemic patients undergoing artificial ventilation for between 17 and 31 days (Horton and Ferguson 1988; Coakley 1991). Further work is required in this area. In all these conditions it is unfortunately impossible to significantly reduce this rise by the prior use of a nondepolarizing agent. The lesson from all this is clear: it is absolutely essential to measure the serum potassium concentration immediately before using suxamethonium in the ITU.

Once tracheal intubation has been effected, the further use of suxamethonium in the ITU must therefore be questioned. There is little place for the use of a constant infusion of suxamethonium in these circumstances.

NONDEPOLARIZING NEUROMUSCULAR BLOCKING AGENTS

For many years the older generation of neuromuscular blocking agents, such as tubocurarine, pancuronium, and alcuronium, were given, together with opioid analgesics, in bolus doses to aid artificial ventilation. These techniques were cheap (Table 11.4) and in many instances produced satisfactory conditions, although neither adequate sedation nor muscle relaxation were consistently and constantly achieved. In addition, in the critically ill patient with multisystem organ failure such factors as reduced metabolism of the drug due to liver dysfunction, and delayed excretion of active breakdown products due to renal dysfunction, could lead to cumulation of active agent after repeated doses, even if the total dose given was only small. Persistent neuromuscular blockade then prolonged weaning from artificial ventilation.

One of the advances in the care of the critically ill has been the development of techniques for the constant infusion of short-acting drugs, such as inotropic agents. This has spread to the use of drugs with a longer elimination half-life, such as analgesics and sedatives, and to the constant infusion of muscle relaxants, with an

Table 11.4   The approximate cost per vial of the various neuromuscular blocking agents in July 1993 in the UK (including VAT)

Suxamethonium	(100 mg/2 ml)	£0.38
Tubocurarine	(15 mg/1.5 ml)	£0.83
Pancuronium	(4 mg/2 ml)	£0.79
Alcuronium	(10 mg/2 ml)	£0.68
Atracurium	(250 mg/25 ml)	£17.07
	(50 mg/5 ml)	£3.97
	(25 mg/2.5 ml)	£2.18
Vecuronium	(10 mg)	£4.64

increased incidence of cumulative effects. The effects of this cumulation have become more obvious because of the increased number of patients with multisystem organ failure who are treated in the ITU — and those are the very patients most likely to require a neuromuscular blocking agent (Table 11.1). The use of constant infusions of nondepolarizing neuromuscular blocking agents in the ITU has therefore become more frequent, despite the risks of cumulation, which will be an important part of the ensuing discussion.

It is perhaps also surprising that, despite the increased use of invasive monitoring in intensive therapy, very little thought seems to be given to the routine monitoring of neuromuscular function when a nondepolarizing neuromuscular blocking agent is infused, even if only by using a clinical nerve stimulator and visual assessment (Pollard 1990). More attention to this detail in the routine care of ITU patients would reduce the problems of residual curarization in the critically ill. The elimin-

Table 11.5   The elimination half-life ($T^{1}/_{2\beta}$), routes of excretion and active metabolites of some of the nondepolarizing neuromuscular blocking agents

	$t^{1}/_{2}\beta$ (min)	Excretion		Active metabolite
		Bile	Kidney	
Tubocurarine	119	12%	44%	–
Pancuronium	132.5	10%	46%	3-desacetyl pancuronium
Alcuronium	199	20%	80%	–
Atracurium	20	–	10%	*
Vecuronium	79.5	12%	30%	3-desacetyl vecuronium

* The metabolic degradation of atracurium yields laudanosine which has no action at the neuromuscular junction but is a central stimulant in certain laboratory animals.

From Stanski *et al.* 1979; Walker *et al.* 1980; Fahey *et al.* 1981; Duraldestin *et al.* 1985; Parker and Hunter 1989

ation half-lives of the commonly used nondepolarizing muscle relaxants and the routes of clearance are given in Table 11.5

Tubocurarine

Although tubocurarine was the first nondepolarizing neuromuscular blocking agent to be employed in intensive care, its current use in these circumstances is probably now confined to a few paediatric centres where it is given by repeated bolus dose. A prolonged length of action (Table 11.5), which is increased further in the presence of renal or hepatic dysfunction — together with largely unfounded concerns about histamine release causing profound hypotension in the critically ill — has led to a decreased use in these circumstances. It is also expensive (Table 11.4).

Pancuronium

This cheap (Table 11.4) steroidal muscle relaxant has long enjoyed popularity in intensive care, due in part to its cardiovascular effects. The vagolytic and direct sympathetic stimulant effects of pancuronium increase pulse rate and help to maintain blood pressure, even in the hypovolaemic, critically ill patient. Being almost devoid of histamine-releasing effects has also been thought to be beneficial, because of the low risk of bronchospasm.

Pancuronium is, however, metabolized in the liver and excreted in part through the kidney (Table 11.5). It has a metabolic breakdown product (3-desacetyl pancuronium) with about 40% of the neuromuscular blocking activity of the parent drug, which is also excreted through the kidney. In the critically ill patient with renal and liver dysfunction, clearance of this long-acting drug may be prolonged, producing persistent neuromuscular blockade, even if the drug is only given in bolus doses. It would seem, therefore, inappropriate to use pancuronium by constant infusion in intensive care, and this has been confirmed by the clinical findings of Vanderbrom and Wierda (1988). These workers reported the case of a patient who underwent emergency repair of an aortic aneurysm. He was given bolus doses of pancuronium pre-operatively and electively ventilated post-operatively, during which time pancuronium was given by constant infusion. The patient developed acute renal failure within 24 hours of surgery. He received pancuronium 105 mg over a 96-hour period. Both the parent drug and the 3-desacetyl metabolite could be detected in the plasma and haemofiltrate fluid for three days after stopping the infusion; indeed the metabolite was still detectable on the fourth day. It is not surprising that difficulty was experienced with 'weaning' from artificial ventilation. It is more appropriate to administer pancuronium in bolus doses to the critically ill.

Alcuronium

This synthetic derivative of tubocurarine was, for a considerable time, the main competitor to pancuronium in intensive care. ITUs used bolus doses of either one of these drugs consistently, without appraising their pharmacological properties.

Alcuronium has less effect on the cardiovascular system than tubocurarine but may cause some histamine release, with subsequent tachycardia and hypotension. In eight years of regular usage of this drug in the general ITU of the Royal Liverpool Hospital, two patients developed anaphylactic shock. Although this is a rare event, it is a major hazard in a patient who is already critically ill. This drug is also cheap, and, unlike pancuronium, does not require refrigeration.

Alcuronium depends on the kidney for excretion to a larger extent than pancuronium (Table 11.5). It is inevitable that, if alcuronium is given by constant infusion to the patient with renal dysfunction, problems of cumulation will occasionally be experienced. Smith *et al.* (1987*a*) have reported such a case. The patient had received an infusion of alcuronium 10 mg per hour for $4\frac{1}{2}$ days, in the presence of undetected renal dysfunction (serum creatinine 576 μmol/1). Despite three periods of haemodialysis, haemofiltration for 72 hours, and plasma exchange, neuromuscular function took nine days to recover fully, as assessed by a clinical nerve stimulator. The authors suggest that plasma exchange made the most significant contribution to neuromuscular recovery, indicating that little of the drug is removed across the membrane during haemodialysis or haemofiltration, although there is no direct evidence for this conclusion. As with pancuronium, it is more appropriate to administer alcuronium by bolus doses in the critically ill.

With the advent of nondepolarizing neuromuscular blocking agents of intermediate duration, such as atracurium and vecuronium, the use of muscle relaxants in the ITU by constant infusion has become more popular, despite the fact that the technique is more expensive than giving drugs in bolus doses. Initially it was thought that the shorter length of action of these two drugs would mean that it was impracticable to give them by bolus dose. With vecuronium, however, this has proved not to be the case. Because these newer agents offer some advantages over the older ones and because there is more recent work on them, the remainder of this review will be mainly devoted to more detailed discussion of atracurium and vecuronium.

Atracurium

This unique neuromuscular blocking agent was designed to break down in the plasma at body temperature and pH, independently of the liver or kidney, by Hofmann degradation and ester hydrolysis (Stenlake *et al.* 1983). This property suggested, at an early stage, that atracurium would be useful in the management of the critically ill patient. It is now appreciated that in health, about 60% of a dose of atracurium undergoes organ elimination, but that Hofmann degradation acts as a sort of 'safety net' when organ function is impaired (Fisher *et al.* 1986).

Griffiths *et al.* (1986) reported the use of a constant infusion of atracurium given for 11–37 hours to five ITU patients in renal and respiratory failure. Neuromuscular function was monitored during the infusion and until full recovery of the TOF after the infusion had been stopped. Even without the use of an anticholinesterase, recovery of neuromuscular function was rapid, the first twitch of the TOF taking a mean time of 60 minutes to return to control values (Fig. 11.1). This is similar to the

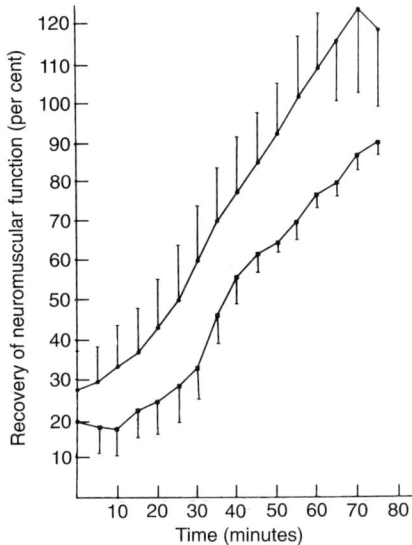

Fig. 11.1 The mean recovery rates of the first response of the train of four compared to control (A′/A) (●——●) and the train of four ratio (D′/A′) (■——■) in five multiorgan system failure patients after an atracurium infusion had been stopped at time zero. (From Griffiths *et al.* 1986; published with kind permission of the editor of *Anaesthesia*.)

recovery time after a bolus dose of atracurium without the use of neostigmine. No adverse cardiovascular effects were noted, despite the use of large doses of atracurium (0.6–1.0 mg/kg/h).

Breakdown products — the laudanosine controversy

Concern was expressed that the metabolite produced by Hofmann degradation, laudanosine, is known to be a cerebral irritant in animals and, as it is excreted in many species through the kidney, it might accumulate in the critically ill. Fahey *et al.* (1985) reported significantly higher levels of laudanosine after a bolus dose of atracurium (0.5 mg/kg) in renal failure compared with healthy patients, but the plasma levels of laudanosine were of the order of only 0.2 μg/ml. The level required to produce cerebral irritation in dogs is around 14 μg/ml (Chapple *et al.* 1987), although in cats it is lower — about 8 μg/ml (Ingram *et al.* 1985). Because of this evidence of wide species variation, it was realized that it would be necessary to perform pharmacokinetic studies on atracurium and laudanosine in intensive care patients.

Yate *et al.* (1987) reported the first estimations of plasma laudanosine levels in ITU patients receiving a constant infusion of atracurium. These patients were mainly neurosurgical, though some were in renal failure. The infusions of atracurium were given for up to six days. The highest recorded level of laudanosine (which was in a patient with normal renal function) was 5.1 μg/ml. This, as expected, was higher than that recorded during general anaesthesia, but not as high as the toxic level in dogs.

Parker *et al.* (1988) have reported similar values in a pharmacokinetic study of atracurium and laudanosine in two groups of ITU patients, one with normal renal function, the other in acute renal failure. These received a bolus dose of atracurium 0.6 mg/kg followed by a constant infusion of 0.6 mg/kg/h for up to 48 hours. There was no difference in the mean clearance of atracurium (7.5 ml/kg/min) between the two groups of patients, and the clearance value obtained was similar to that reported after bolus doses of atracurium. Although the clearance of laudanosine was not significantly different between the two groups, the elimination half-life of the metabolite in renal failure was prolonged, with an increased volume of distribution. It was postulated that renal elimination only contributes in part to the clearance of laudanosine in humans and that the liver may also be responsible in part for the breakdown of the metabolite.

At present, pharmacokinetic data on ITU patients in severe liver failure are not available. Those in Parker's study (1988) had some degree of hepatic dysfunction, compatible with a septicaemic state, but none was in complete liver failure. The highest recorded laudanosine level in an ITU patient receiving atracurium (1.0 mg/kg/hr) is 8.6 μg/ml, although this is an isolated, unsubstantiated recording (Gwinnutt *et al.* 1990). All other reports are below 5.1 μg/ml.

Shearer *et al.* (1991*a*) have studied the clearance of atracurium and laudanosine in the urine in ITU patients with relatively normal renal function receiving atracurium 0.6 mg/kg/hr. They found that about 10% of a dose of atracurium and about 10% of the metabolite, laudanosine are excreted in the urine.

In the same study clearance of both substances across the haemofiltrate membrane was recorded in a second group of more critically ill patients with renal and respiratory failure, receiving the same dosage regime. It was found that venovenous haemofiltration was less efficient than the kidney at clearing atracurium and laudanosine; only about 2% of a dose was excreted by this route. The plasma clearances of atracurium and laudanosine were similar to those found previously. The more critically ill were receiving high doses of inotropes such as dobutamine and noradrenalin. Thus they would have been expected to have decreased hepatic blood flow and therefore decreased clearances of any drug metabolized in the liver, which may be relevant to laudanosine, but this was not found to be the case (Table 11.6).

Table 11.6 The plasma, urinary, and notional continuous venovenous haemofiltration (CVVH) clearances of atracurium and laudanosine in artificially ventilated ITU patients

	Atracurium clearance (ml/kg/min)		Laudanosine clearance (ml/kg/min)	
	Plasma	Urine	Plasma	Urine
Normal renal function	7.2	0.55	3.8	0.33
	Plasma	CVVH	Plasma	CVVH
Acute renal failure	6.7	0.11	4.5	0.09

From Shearer *et al.* (1991*a*)

In none of these pharmacokinetic studies was any evidence of epileptiform activity reported. In the pharmacodynamic study (Griffiths *et al.* 1986), one patient was noted to have had a series of epileptiform movements during the infusion of atracurium. The plasma laudanosine at that time was less than 1.0 μg/ml, and as the patient was known to have herpes simplex encephalitis and to be hypoxic from intercurrent pneumonia, it was thought that there were more obvious reasons for the cerebral irritability.

It is impossible to know the toxic level of laudanosine in humans and, although there can now be no concern of any side-effects from this metabolite in general anaesthesia, it is possible to construct a hypothetical situation in an ITU where laudanosine accumulation might be a problem. If large doses of atracurium had been given for several days to a patient with multisystem organ failure — perhaps with a low epileptic threshold — epileptogenic activity due to laudanosine could be a possibility. There is however no clinical evidence for this at present, despite extensive use of this drug by constant infusion in intensive care in the UK.

Atracurium has the benefit of no cumulation even when given for several days to a critically ill patient. This makes it a very flexible drug to use, allowing rapid assessment of both cerebral and respiratory function after it has been discontinued, even when large doses have been used. There is no evidence of delayed recovery, unlike all other nondepolarizing muscle relaxants. Indeed, Yate *et al.* (1987) postulated that tolerance to the drug developed over many hours. Although this has been suspected by other ITU workers, it has not yet been proven. It is now the most commonly used muscle relaxant in intensive care in the UK.

Vecuronium

When this drug was introduced, at a similar time to atracurium, it was thought that it was short-acting and suitable for administration by constant infusion. However, vecuronium has a long elimination half-life of about 80 min (Table 11.5) and one of the main metabolites, 3-desacetyl vecuronium (produced after de-acetylation in the liver), has at least 50% of the neuromuscular blocking properties of the parent compound and is excreted in the urine (Bencini *et al.* 1985). Soon after the drug was introduced, reports appeared describing a cumulative effect when it was used in repeated doses or by constant infusion in multisystem organ failure patients (Cody and Dormon 1987; Sinclair *et al.* 1987). This does not seem to occur when the agent is used in the less severely ill with normal renal and hepatic function, as for example in those admitted to an ITU for routine monitoring post-operatively or those who have suffered head injuries (Darrah *et al.* 1987).

Smith *et al.* (1987*b*), in a pharmacodynamic study of seven multisystem organ failure patients given a bolus of vecuronium 0.1 mg/kg followed immediately by a constant infusion of 0.05 mg/kg/hr, found a prolonged and unpredictable recovery, which could not be related to the degree of liver dysfunction present. Monitoring by the TOF twitch technique showed a much longer recovery both of the first twitch of the TOF and of the TOF ratio, than was the case after atracurium. Indeed, recovery took several hours (Figs. 11.2 and 3). This prolonged effect of vecuronium when

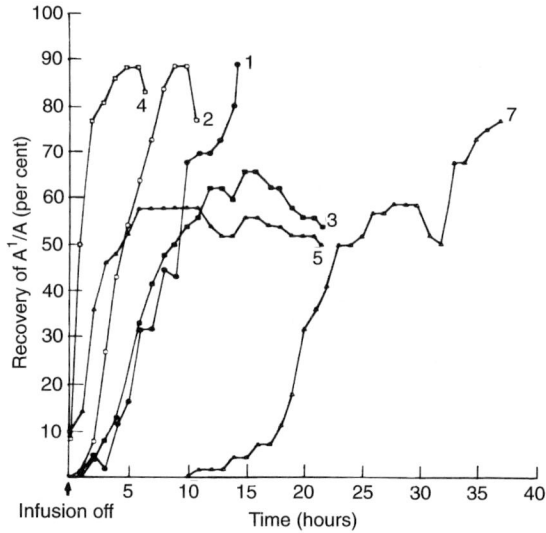

Fig. 11.2 The rate of recovery of A'/A in six patients after an infusion of vecuronium had been stopped at time zero. (From Smith *et al.* 1987*b*; published with kind permission of the editor of *Anaesthesia*.)

given by constant infusion in the critically ill, may be due, in large part, to the cumulation of the active metabolite. Segredo *et al.* (1990) have demonstrated the presence of 3-desacetylvecuronium in the plasma of multisystem organ failure patients for seven days after a constant infusion of vecuronium.

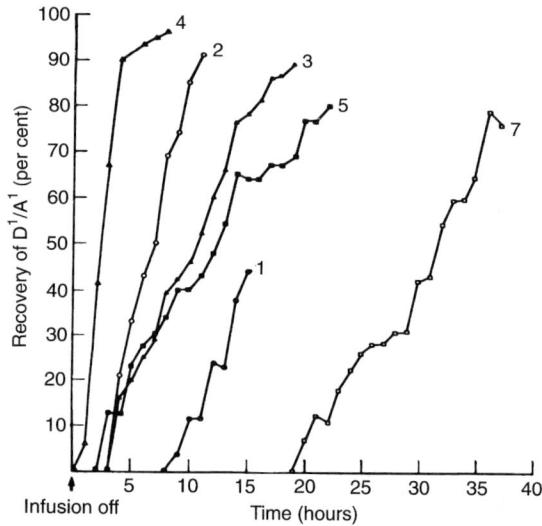

Fig. 11.3 The rate of recovery of D'/A' in six patients after an infusion of vecuronium had been stopped at time zero. (From Smith *et al.* 1987*b*; published with kind permission of the editor of *Anaesthesia*.)

This drug does have the advantages of having little or no effect on the cardiovascular system and not causing histamine release. It is, however, probably more appropriate to administer it in bolus doses in the critically ill.

Newer nondepolarizing neuromuscular blocking agents: mivacurium, doxacurium, and pipecuronium

There are, as yet, no studies reported of the use of these newer agents in the ITU. Although mivacurium has a short elimination half-life (17 min) (de Bros *et al.* 1987), it is thought to be metabolized in the plasma by pseudocholinesterase, an enzyme synthesized in the liver. Production of this enzyme may well be reduced in critically ill patients with liver dysfunction, prolonging the action of mivacurium. Drug interaction with pseudocholinesterase may also potentiate it (Table 11.2). It will be interesting to see if mivacurium finds a role in the case of the patient with multisystem organ failure.

Doxacurium and pipecuronium are longer-acting drugs, comparable to pancuronium, although devoid of cardiovascular effects. They are also excreted in part through the kidney (Cashman *et al.* 1990; Caldwell *et al.* 1987). It is difficult to imagine that they will be useful adjuncts to intensive care.

DISADVANTAGES OF NEUROMUSCULAR BLOCKING AGENTS IN INTENSIVE CARE

These have been highlighted by Willatts (1985). Disconnection from the ventilator is obviously a major hazard, although with the allocation of a nurse to every patient in modern day intensive care practice and alarms on all ventilators, the risk must have been reduced. Pulmonary emboli were thought to be more common in the paralysed ITU patient, but this has not been substantiated. Willatts (1985), also noted that immobility predisposes to infection, although with active physiotherapy and regular patient turning this should not represent an increased hazard. It must be stressed that adequate sedation and analgesia should always be established before neuromuscular blocking agents are introduced, as it is essential to reduce the risk of awareness in the partially paralyzed patient. Recent developments in cerebral function monitoring in the ITU are undoubtedly helping to alleviate this problem (Shearer *et al.* 1991*b*).

REFERENCES

Bencini, A. F., Houwertjes, M. C., and Agoston, S. (1985). Effects of hepatic uptake of vecuronium bromide and its putative metabolites on their neuromuscular blocking actions in the cat. *British Journal of Anaesthesia*, **57**, 789–95.
Bion, J. F. and Ledingham, I. McA. (1987). Sedation in intensive care — a postal survey. *Intensive Care Medicine*, **13**, 215–6.

Caldwell, J. E., Canfell, P. C., Castagnoli, B. A., Lynam, D. P., Fahey, M. R., Fisher, D. M., *et al*. (1987). The influence of renal failure on the pharmacokinetics and duration of action of pipecuronium bromide. *Anesthesiology*, **67**, A612.

Cashman, J. N., Luke, J. J., and Jones, R. M. (1990). Neuromuscular block with doxacurium (BW A938U) in patients with normal or absent renal function. *British Journal of Anaesthesia*, **64**, 186–92.

Chapple, D. J., Miller, A. J., Ward, J. B., and Wheatley, P. L. (1987). Cardiovascular and neurological effects of laudanosine studies in mice and rats and in conscious and anaesthetised dogs. *British Journal of Anaesthesia*, **59**, 218–25.

Coakley, J. (1991). Suxamethonium and intensive care. *Anaesthesia*, **46**, 330.

Cody, M. W. and Dormon, F. M. (1987). Recurarization after vecuronium in a patient with renal failure. *Anaesthesia*, **42**, 993.

Darrah, W. C., Johnston, J. R., and Mirakhur R. K. (1987). Vecuronium infusions for prolonged muscle relaxation in the intensive care unit. *Critical Care Medicine*, **17**, 1297–300.

de Bros, F., Baston, S. J., Ali, H. H., Wargin, W., and Welch, R. (1987). Pharmacokinetics and pharmacodynamics of BW1090U in healthy surgical patients receiving N20/02 isoflurane anesthesia. *Anesthesiology*, **67**, A609.

Duvaldestin, P., Lebrault, C., and Chauvin, M. (1985). Pharmacokinetics of muscle relaxants in patients with liver disease. In *Clinics in anaesthesiology*, Vol. 3, No. 2, (ed. J. Norman), pp. 293–306. Saunders, London.

Fahey, M. R., Morris, R. B., Miller, R. D. Nguyen, T., and Upton, R. A. (1981). Pharmacokinetics of Org NC45 (Norcuron) in patients with and without renal failure. *British Journal of Anaesthesia*, **53**, 1049–53.

Fahey, M. R., Rupp, S. M., Canfell, C., Fisher, D. M., Miller, R. D., Sharma, M., *et al*. (1985). Effect of renal failure on laudanosine excretion in man. *British Journal of Anaesthesia*, **57**, 1049–51.

Fisher, D. M., Canfell, P. C., Fahey, M. R., Rosen, J. I., Rupp, S. M., Sheiner, L. B., and Miller, R. D. (1986). Elimination of atracurium in humans. Contribution of Hofmann elimination and ester hydrolysis versus organ based elimination. *Anesthesiology*, **65**, 6–12.

Griffiths, R. B., Hunter, J. M., and Jones, R. S. (1986). Atracurium infusions in patients with renal failure on an ITU. *Anaesthesia*, **41**, 375–81.

Gwinnutt, C. L., Eddleston, J. M., Edwards, D., and Pollard, B. J. (1990). Concentrations of atracurium and laudanosine in cerebrospinal fluid and plasma in three intensive care patients. *British Journal of Anaesthesia*, **65**, 829–32.

Horton, W. A. and Ferguson, N. V. (1988). Hyperkalaemia and cardiac arrest after the use of suxamethonium in intensive care. *Anaesthesia*, **43**, 890–1.

Hunter, J. M. (1987) Adverse effects of neuromuscular blocking drugs. *British Journal of Anaesthesia*, **59**, 46–60.

Hunter, J. M., Jones, R. S., and Utting, J. E. (1982). Use of atracurium during general surgery monitored by the train-of-four stimuli. *British Journal of Anaesthesia*, **54**, 1243–50.

Ingram, M. D., Sclabassi, R. J., Stiller R. L., Cook, D. R., and Bennett, M. H. (1985). Cardiovascular and electroencephalographic effects of laudanosine in nephrectomised cats. *Anesthesia and Analgesia*, **64**, 232.

Merriman, M. H. (1981). The techniques used to sedate ventilated patients. *Intensive Care Medicine*, **7**, 217.

Miller-Jones, C. M. H. and Williams, J. H. (1980). Sedation for ventilation. A retrospective study of fifty patients. *Anaesthesia*, **35**, 1104–7.

Parker, C. J. R. and Hunter, J. M. (1989). Pharmacokinetics of atracurium and laudanosine in patients with hepatic cirrhosis. *British Journal of Anaesthesia*, **62**, 177–83.

Parker, C. J. R., Jones, J. E., and Hunter, J. M. (1988). Disposition of infusions of atracurium and its metabolite, laudanosine, in patients in renal and respiratory failure in an ITU. *British Journal of Anaesthesia*, **61**, 531–40.

Paton, W. D. M. (1959). The effects of muscle relaxants other than muscle relaxation. *Anesthesiology*, **20**, 453–63.

Pollard, B. J. (1990). Paralysis after long-term administration of vecuronium: I. *Anesthesiology*, **73**, 364.

Segredo, V., Matthay, M. A., Sharma, M. L., Gruenke, L. D., Caldwell, J. E., and Miller, R. D. (1990). Prolonged neuromuscular blockade after long-term administration of vecuronium in two critically ill patients. *Anesthesiology*, **72**, 566–70.

Shearer, E. S., O'Sullivan, E. P., and Hunter, J. M. (1991*a*). Clearance of atracurium and laudanosine in the urine and by continuous venovenous haemofiltration. *British Journal of Anaesthesia*, **67**, 569–73.

Shearer, E. S., O'Sullivan, E. P., and Hunter, J. M. (1991*b*). An assessment of the Cerebrotrac 2500 for continuous monitoring of cerebral function in the intensive care unit. *Anaesthesia*, **46**, 750–5.

Sinclair, J. F., Malcolm, G. A., Stephenson, B. P., and Hallworth, D. (1987). Prolonged neuromuscular blockade in an infant. *Anaesthesia*, **42**, 1020.

Smith, C. L., Hunter, J. M., and Jones, R. S. (1987*a*). Prolonged paralysis following an infusion of alcuronium in a patient with renal dysfunction. *Anaesthesia*, **42**, 522–5.

Smith, C. L., Hunter, J. M., and Jones, R. S. (1987*b*). Vecuronium infusions in patients with renal failure in an ITU. *Anaesthesia*, **42**, 387–93.

Stanski, D. R., Ham, J., Miller, R. D., and Sheiner, L. B. (1979). Pharmacokinetics and pharmacodynamics of *d*-tubocurarine during nitrous oxide–narcotic and halothane anesthesia in man. *Anesthesiology*, **51**, 235–41.

Stenlake, J. D., Waigh, R. D., Unwin, J., Dewar, G. H., and Coker, G. G. (1983). Atracurium: conception and inception. *British Journal of Anaesthesia*, **55**, 3S–10S.

Tolmie, J. D., Joyce, T. H., and Mitchell, G. D. (1967). Succinylcholine danger in the burned patient. *Anesthesiology*, **28**, 467–70.

Vanderbrom, R. H. G. and Wierda, J. M. H. K. (1988). Pancuronium bromide in the intensive care unit. A case of overdose. *Anesthesiology*, **69**, 996–7.

Walker, J., Shanks, C. A., and Triggs, E. T. (1980). Clinical pharmacokinetics of alcuronium chloride in man. *European Journal of Clinical Pharmacology*, **17**, 449–57.

Willatts, S. M. (1985). Paralysis for ventilated patients: yes or no? *Intensive Care Medicine*, **11**, 2–4.

Yate, P. M., Flynn, P. M., Arnold, R. W., Weatherley, B. C., Simmonds, R. J., and Dopson, T. (1987). Clinical experience and plasma laudanosine concentrations during atracurium infusion in the intensive therapy unit. *British Journal of Anaesthesia*, **59**, 211–7.

Zochodne, D. W., Bolton, C. F., Wells, G. A., Gilbert, J. J., Hahn, A. F., Brown, J. D., *et al.* (1987). Critical illness polyneuropathy. A complication of sepsis and multiple organ failure. *Brain*, **110**, 819–42.

12

Interactions involving relaxants

B. J. Pollard

When more than one drug is used at the same time in any patient, there is the potential for one drug to be affected by the other(s). Very few anaesthetics require the use of only one drug and if a relaxant is being used, then there must already be at least one drug in use — the anaesthetic agent. In reality, it is common to use several drugs simultaneously during an anaesthetic, e.g. systemic analgesics, local anaesthetics, and antibiotics. In addition, the patient is likely to be receiving therapy for one or more pre-existing medical disorders. Antihypertensive agents, diuretics, steroids, and anticonvulsants are all commonly used and with each of these there is the potential for interactions. Furthermore, as the number of drugs in use at the same time increases, so the potential for interactions increases. Polypharmacy is common.

There are a large number of drugs on the market and it is certain that the number will not fall. There are many textbooks available on drug interactions. This book is devoted to the muscle relaxant family and therefore only interactions concerning the muscle relaxants will be considered.

GENERAL CONSIDERATIONS

Drug interactions in general fall into three main categories and these can be summarized as follows:

1. Logical and expected
   These are interactions which should have been readily anticipated. It should therefore be possible to avoid them or to adapt a technique in anticipation of their appearance. It may also be possible to turn them to the anaesthetist's advantage.

2. Theoretically possible but does not occur
   In these cases, an interaction might be expected and all preparations are made for its management. It either does not occur, or is very much less serious than expected. It is possible that other mechanisms (or indeed other interactions) are at work which have prevented the interaction.

3. Unexpected

    These interactions are the most worrying. They are usually isolated incidents which are quite unpredictable. It may often be difficult or even impossible to determine the underlying mechanism. There is the potential for serious consequences to trap the unwary anaesthetist.

This chapter will not consider drug effects which are caused by allergies or anaphylactic mechanisms. Those are covered in Chapter 13. Where possible, the mechanism will be outlined if it is known or suspected. In many cases the mechanism is not known.

SITE OF DRUG INTERACTION

It is appropriate first to consider where possible interactions concerning the neuromuscular blocking agents might take place. The desired pharmacological action of the neuromuscular blocking agents lies within the neuromuscular junction and so this must clearly be considered as a primary location for interactions. Acetylcholine is released from the prejunctional nerve ending and crosses the synaptic cleft to interact with the receptors on the postjunctional membrane. An action to increase to decrease the release, mobilization, storage, or synthesis of acetylcholine will alter neuromuscular block. An action on the breakdown of acetylcholine by inhibiting or accelerating the action of cholinesterase is also a potential site for interactions.

Released acetylcholine crosses the synaptic cleft to combine with the receptors on the postjunctional membrane. The two alpha-subunits lie in different environments, surrounded by different protein molecules, and drugs may act differentially on one or other alpha-subunit. Binding to other parts of the receptor–ion channel complex may also occur, and these may result in closed channel block, open channel block, or simply a distortion of the receptor's milieu. Receptors are constantly being synthesized and replaced and it is conceivable that a drug could affect this process, although the onset of action would be slow (hours to days).

The release of acetylcholine is triggered by an impulse arriving down the nerve. Any agent which blocks or slows the impulse generation or passage along the nerve will therefore affect the neuromuscular block. When the receptors on the postjunctional membrane have been activated an impulse travels across the muscle and activates the contractile mechanism. There is scope here also for an effect on the passage of the impulse or on excitation contraction coupling to modify the action of a neuromuscular blocking agent.

There are many possible sites of interaction of drugs which do not lie within or near to the neuromuscular junction. These mainly involve pharmacokinetic factors and may be modified by a number of processes. Changes in protein binding or binding to other nonspecific acceptor sites, alterations in the volume of distribution, and changes in the rate of metabolism and/or elimination might be included here.

Having considered the possible sites where drugs can theoretically interact, it is now appropriate to examine known interactions which are of importance concerning the neuromuscular blocking agents. The most logical system is to divide the drugs into their principal families and subdivide from there. Interactions between the neuromuscular blocking agents and ions, including acid–base changes, are also considered in this chapter, although these are not drug interactions in the strict sense of the definition.

VOLATILE AGENTS

Every anaesthetist is taught from an early stage that there is an interaction between the volatile anaesthetic agents and the neuromuscular blocking agents. This interaction is useful clinically and it is likely that most anaesthetists make use of the potentiating action of the volatile agents on a neuromuscular block almost every day. The extent of the interaction depends upon the volatile agent and relaxant combination.

At high concentrations volatile agents alone will depress neuromuscular transmission (Lebowitz et al. 1970; Pollard and Miller 1973; Caldwell et al. 1991), although at lower concentrations certain of the volatile agents may augment twitch height (Pollard and Miller 1973). The existence of potentiation between the volatile agents and the neuromuscular blocking agents is therefore hardly surprising. Numerous studies have demonstrated this interaction in various ways from simple observation of responses to formal analysis of dose–response relationships (Watland et al. 1957; Sabawala and Dillon 1958; Katz and Gissen 1967; Padfield 1968; Lebowitz et al. 1970; Walts and Dillon 1970; Katz 1971a; Miller et al. 1971a, b, 1972; Vitez et al. 1974; Fogdall and Miller 1975; Hughes and Payne 1979; Chapple et al. 1983; Rupp et al. 1984a, b; Bennett and Hahn 1985; Caldwell et al. 1991). These include clinical studies and both in vivo and in vitro animal studies.

The extent of the potentiation depends upon the exact volatile agent–neuromuscular blocking agent combination. Isoflurane and enflurane potentiate a tubocurarine and pancuronium neuromuscular block more than does halothane (Fogdall and Miller 1975; Miller et al. 1972). Enflurane is however more potent than either halothane or isoflurane on a vecuronium neuromuscular block (Foldes et al. 1980; Rupp et al. 1984a; Swen et al. 1985). All of the three volatile agents enflurane, isoflurane, and halothane appear to potentiate an atracurium block to a similar degree (Rupp et al. 1983, 1984b, 1985). A suxamethonium neuromuscular block is also potentiated by volatile agents (Donati and Bevan 1982, 1983) and it has been suggested that the characteristics of the depolarizing block may change with time from a phase I to a phase II type in the presence of a volatile agent (Hilgenberg and Stoelting 1981). It is interesting to note that there may be changes in the extent of potentiation with time. That due to an enflurane block becomes greater with time, whereas the effects due to halothane appear to remain constant (Stanski et al. 1979, 1980).

The presence of enflurane has been reported to retard the reversal of a pancuronium neuromuscular block (Delisle and Bevan 1982) and the presence of isoflurane to similarly affect a vecuronium block (Baurain *et al.* 1991). The reversibility of atracurium or vecuronium appears to be less affected by the presence of a volatile agent than that of the longer acting relaxants (Engbaek *et al.* 1983; Swen 1984; Goudsouzian *et al.* 1986).

The mechanism by which the volatile agents potentiate the neuromuscular blocking agents is unknown. A number of mechanisms have been proposed. These include an increase in muscle blood flow and hence delivery of relaxant to the neuromuscular junction (Miller *et al.* 1976*a*), a decrease in release of acetylcholine from the nerve endings (Hughes and Payne 1979), and an action on the postjunctional membrane (Stanski *et al.* 1979). The muscle blood flow hypothesis seems unlikely because the volatile agents still show potentiation in an *in vitro* preparation and also when cardiovascular stability is carefully maintained (Knight *et al.* 1978). Although some alterations in the pharmacokinetics of muscle relaxants are caused by volatile agents — e.g. the clearance of pancuronium is decreased and elimination half-life increased following enflurane or halothane (Miller *et al.* 1979) — it seems unlikely that pharmacokinetic factors are the sole explanation. Waud and Waud (1979) demonstrated a greater effect on tetanic stimuli and on single twitches and advanced this as evidence in support of the interaction being prejunctional in origin. Subsequent *in vitro* studies did not, however, support this hypothesis (Waud 1979).

Actions on the postjunctional membrane have received the most attention. Waud and Waud (1975*a*) showed that the volatile agents depress carbachol-induced depolarization of the endplate. Young and Sigman (1981) and Young *et al.* (1981) were able to demonstrate interference with the acetylcholine receptor protein resulting from the presence of volatile anaesthetic agents. The conductance of the ion channels at the endplate is reduced in the presence of volatile anaesthetic agents (Kennedy and Galindo 1975; Waud and Waud 1975*b*; Gage and Hamill 1976; Bean *et al.* 1981), and, in view of the high lipid solubility of the volatile agents, these effects could be due to nonspecific actions upon the lipid component of the cell membrane. Other factors, including a direct action on the muscle contraction system (Komatsu *et al.* 1979; Clergue *et al.* 1986) or through the medium of calcium flux (Conahan and Blanck 1979; Rosenberg 1979; Diamond and Berman 1980) are also possible. In cases where there are a number of possibilities to consider, it must be remembered that it is very likely that more than one mechanism is involved simultaneously, and different volatile agents may not all be acting in exactly the same manner.

BENZODIAZEPINES

Reports concerning the effects of the benzodiazepines on neuromuscular transmission are conflicting. Studies in laboratory animals have generally demonstrated a potentiating effect of the benzodiazepines on the action of neuromuscular blocking agents (Sharma and Sharma 1978; Driessen *et al.* 1983, 1984, 1985*a*). This action may not be mediated through benzodiazepine receptors. Diazepam, desmethyldiazepan, and temazepam were examined in the rat diaphragm *in vitro* by Driessen *et al.* (1983, 1984), who found these agents to cause an increase in twitch tension at low concentrations followed by depression at higher concentrations. This action was not shared by oxazepam. Furthermore, low concentrations of diazepam antagonized a pancuronium neuromuscular block in that study.

These effects have not been demonstrated in the clinical situation and the benzodiazepines are usually regarded as having no effect on neuromuscular block (Tassonyi 1977, 1984; Bradshaw and Maddison 1979; Asbury *et al.* 1981; Lee *et al.* 1982; Cronnelly *et al.* 1983).

INTRAVENOUS AGENTS

Many studies, both clinical and in animals, have searched for any interaction between the intravenous anaesthetic agents and the neuromuscular blocking agents. Such an interaction could have considerable importance in the management of anaesthesia. It must be remembered that many of the intravenous induction agents are not water soluble and require to be formulated as emulsions (e.g. propofol), or with solubilizing agents (e.g. etomidate). Any possible effect of the vehicle must be considered. Appropriate control groups were included in the studies, and it seems likely that the vehicles presently in use do not have any measurable effect upon a neuromuscular block (Torda and Gage 1977; Torda and Murphy 1979; Gramstad *et al.* 1981).

The barbiturates are probably the most popular intravenous agents worldwide and these have been reported to potentiate the effects of muscle relaxants (Foldes 1959; Bonta *et al.* 1968; Kraunak *et al.* 1977; McIndewar and Marshall 1981; Cronnelly *et al.* 1983). However, no effect was reported by methohexitone on a pipecuronium neuromuscular block (Dutre *et al.* 1992).

Etomidate potentiates a pancuronium neuromuscular block (Booij and Crul 1979) and also a vecuronium block (Kreig *et al.* 1980; McIndewar and Marshall 1981). It was found, however, to have no effect upon a pipecuronium block (Dutre *et al.* 1992). Etomidate has also been shown to have no effect upon a suxamethonium block (Doenicke *et al.* 1980).

Ketamine has been examined in a number of studies and the overall conclusion lies in favour of a potentiation of neuromuscular block, although there is not universal agreement. Ketamine was shown to prolong the neuromuscular block resulting from tubocurarine (Johnston *et al.* 1974; Amaki *et al.* 1978; Tsai and Lee 1989), pancuronium (Kraunak *et al.* 1977; Amaki *et al.* 1978; Tsai and Lee 1989), suxamethonium (Kraunak *et al.* 1977; Nocite *et al.* 1977; Amaki *et al.* 1978), vecuronium (Cronnelly *et al.* 1973; Kreig *et al.* 1980; McIndewar and Marshall 1981; Durant *et al.* 1982, 1984*a*; Tsai and Lee 1989), and atracurium (Tsai and Lee 1989). There was no effect of ketamine reported on an atracurium block by Chapple *et al.* (1983) or on a block induced by pancuronium or vecuronium (Engbaek *et al.* 1984).

Propofol has been shown to potentiate a neuromuscular block resulting from atracurium (Robertson *et al.* 1983), vecuronium (Fragan *et al.* 1983; Robertson *et al.* 1983), pancuronium (Fragan *et al.* 1983), and suxamethonium (Fragan *et al.* 1983), but not by pipecuronium (Dutre *et al.* 1992).

The older agents althesin and propanidid demonstrated interactions with neuro-muscular blocking agents, principally potentiation (Kraunak *et al.* 1977; McIndewar and Marshall 1981). One interaction between propanidid and suxam-ethonium resulted from inhibition of plasma cholinesterase by propanidid. This could lead to awareness in a paralysed patient due to termination of the action of the propanidid before that of the suxamethonium (Doenicke *et al.* 1968, 1980; Torda and Gage 1977; Trotta *et al.* 1980).

The possible mechanism of these interactions between neuromuscular blocking agents and intravenous anaesthetic agents has been examined in a number of studies. In general, it appears that there is a reduction in the sensitivity of the postjunctional membrane to acetylcholine produced by most, if not all, intravenous agents (Ellis 1968; Giesecke *et al.* 1968; Cronnelly *et al.* 1973; Kraunak *et al.* 1977; Wali 1983). In further support of this view, Torda and Gage (1977) per-formed micro-electrode studies and demonstrated a reduction in the amplitude of endplate potentials. The exact mechanism of this effect on the postjunctional mem-brane is presently unclear, but it is possible that channel block might be involved (Adams 1976; Torda and Gage 1977; Sevcik 1980; Arnhem and Kristbjarnarson 1981; Maleque *et al.* 1981; Oswald 1983; Bowman 1985).

The contribution of channel block to any effects at drug concentrations within the clinical range is unproven, because channel block is usually a phenomenon taking place preferentially at higher drug concentrations. These effects on the postjunctional membrane are complicated by additional actions on the prejunctional nerve terminal. An increased release of acetylcholine has been described (Torda and Murphy 1979), although ketamine may conversely decrease acetylcholine release (Amaki *et al.* 1978). Finally, it must be noted that a direct effect on skeletal muscle is possible (Sirnes 1954; Kiraly and Hamilton 1978; Marwaha 1980).

LOCAL ANALGESICS

The local analgesics are all capable of producing neuromuscular block alone and also of potentiating a nondepolarizing neuromuscular block (Ellis *et al.* 1953; Usubiaga *et al.* 1967; Hall *et al.* 1972; Matsuo *et al.* 1978; Zukaitis and Hoech 1979; Morita *et al.* 1979; Chapple *et al.* 1983). Tetanic fade can be demonstrated in the presence of lignocaine alone (Suzuki *et al.* 1977) and the onset of a tubo-curarine block was faster following a dose of 2.5 mg/kg lignocaine (Zukaitis and Hoech 1979).

The mechanism of this interaction has been examined and it appears likely that it is due to a decrease in both responsiveness of the postjunctional membrane and acetylcholine release resulting from the presence of the local analgesic agent

(Matsuo *et al.* 1978; Prostan and Varagic 1981; Lee *et al.* 1983; Aracava *et al.* 1984; Ikeda *et al.* 1984; Wali 1984). Other mechanisms cannot, however, be discounted. The possibility exists that the local analgesics exert their effect on the neuromuscular junction through calcium actions (Trotta *et al.* 1980; Akaike *et al.* 1982; Marquis and Deschenes 1982; Saito *et al.* 1984), or directly on the contractile mechanism of the muscle (Huan 1981; Prostan and Varagic 1981). More than one site of action may be involved simultaneously.

An additional interaction may be seen with procaine due to its known action to inhibit plasma cholinesterase. The action of any other drug which is broken down by plasma cholinesterase (suxamethonium and mivacurium in the relaxant family) will therefore be prolonged (Zsigmond and Eldertton 1968), particularly in patients with an atypical cholinesterase.

OPIOID ANALGESICS

Opioid analgesics are commonly used during anaesthesia and are often administered concurrently with neuromuscular blocking agents. A number of studies have demonstrated that the opioids potentiate the nondepolarizing neuromuscular blocking agents but there is not universal agreement. Soteropoulos and Standaert (1973) found that morphine depressed twitch tension and also depressed post-tetanic facilitation. This was partly antagonized by naloxone, although naloxone alone had a similar qualitative effect to morphine. The suggestion was made that the action was taking place on the nerve terminals through a reduction in acetylcholine release. This view has been supported by other studies (Frederickson and Pinsky 1971; Pinsky and Frederickson 1971; Duke *et al.* 1979; Durham and Frank 1981). McIndewar and Marshall (1981) and Katz (1971*b*) were, however, unable to demonstrate any potentiation and Bellville *et al.* (1964) showed that morphine alone produced an increase in grip strength.

It is likely that the mechanism involved in any interaction is not simple. A biphasic effect has been reported by Boros *et al.* (1984) when they demonstrated in the rat diaphragm *in vitro* that pethidine in a concentration of 5 μg/ml augmented twitch height, whereas there was a slowly developing block at concentration higher than 40 μg/ml. These concentrations are considerably greater than are likely to be reached in general clinical use. Bell and Rees (1974) examined a series of opioid agonists and antagonists and confirmed that there was indeed a depressant action on neuromuscular transmission, but that the order of potency among the series did not correlate with the known order of potency for the opioid receptors. Their conclusion was that the effects of members of this family at the skeletal neuromuscular junction are not mediated through opioid receptors.

Meptazinol, the synthetic partial agonist, is capable of inhibiting neuromuscular transmission, although at low doses it paradoxically antagonizes a tubocurarine neuromuscular block. This latter effect is due to its additional anticholinesterase activity (Strahan *et al.* 1985).

DIURETICS

The diuretics are a broad family of drugs which include agents with widely differing actions, e.g. osmotic diuretics (mannitol), carbonic anhydrase inhibitors (acetazolamide), and loop diuretics (frusemide). It might therefore not be surprising to expect a variety of effects. Frusemide potentiates a tubocurarine block in humans (Miller *et al.* 1976*b*), and will also accelerate recovery from a pancuronium-induced neuromuscular block (Azar *et al.* 1980). *In vitro* studies with frusemide have shown a biphasic response with potentiation of both tubocurarine and suxamethonium at low concentration and antagonism at higher concentrations (Sappaticci *et al.* 1982).

Potentiation of a neuromuscular block was observed in animals following the administration of chlorthalidone, chlorothiazide, and acetazolamide (Gessa and Ferrari 1963). There have been no reports of an effect in humans with these agents or with mannitol (Miller *et al.* 1976*b*). The mechanism of all these actions is unknown.

ANTIBIOTICS

The existence of an interaction between certain antibiotics and the neuromuscular blocking agents was first suspected following a number of adverse incidents surrounding anaesthesia (Pridgen 1956; Engel and Denson 1957; Benz *et al.* 1961; Bodley and Brett 1962; Bush 1962; Foldes *et al.* 1962; Emery 1963; Pittinger *et al.* 1970; Eppens and Klein 1971). Since those preliminary observations a great many studies have been undertaken in an attempt to demonstrate which antibiotics exhibit these interactions and which do not. In addition, attempts have been made to unravel the mechanism underlying these interactions (Sokoll and Gergis 1981).

Aminoglycosides

Most interest has centred around the aminoglycoside antibiotics, possibly because they were principally implicated in the original reports. Most of the aminoglycosides are surprisingly potent in their potentiation of the neuromuscular blocking agents (Burkett *et al.* 1979). Indeed, a number of aminoglycoside antibiotics have been shown to produce neuromuscular block alone (de Rosayro and Healy 1978). Neomycin, streptomycin, dihydrostreptomycin, tobramycin, gentamycin, and kanamycin all exhibit this effect. There is evidence to support this action in potentiating a tubocurarine, pancuronium, gallamine, suxamethonium or vecuronium neuromuscular block (Barnett and Ackerman 1969; Chinyanga and Stoyka 1974; Lee *et al.* 1976; Wright and Collier 1977; Waterman and Smith 1977; Giala and Paradelis 1979; Lee and de Silva 1979*a, b*; Bruckner *et al.* 1980; Kreig *et al.* 1980; Durant *et al.* 1980; Potter *et al.* 1980; Torda 1980; Giala *et al.* 1982; Chapple *et al.* 1983). It does not appear to be necessary to receive a particularly large dose of the antibiotic for problems to arise. The anaesthetist may also be caught unawares. The rapidity of onset and intensity of effect vary according to the dose absorbed and the route of administration, but enough can be absorbed from irrigation of the intrapleural space, peritoneal cavity or even a wound. Sufficient neomycin has also been absorbed by mouth to result in a measurable effect (Benz *et al.* 1961; Argov and Mastaglia 1979; Kronenfeld *et al.* 1986). It is interesting to note that netilmicin has been reported to be devoid of any neuromuscular action (Bendtsen *et al.* 1983).

The mechanism of action of the aminoglycoside antibiotics on an neuromuscular block is presently unknown. There are similarities between the effect of the amino-glycosides and that of magnesium (Brazil and Prado-Franceschi 1969; Singh *et al.* 1978*a*, *b*; L'Hommedieu *et al.* 1983). Neomycin, streptomycin, and gentamicin have been reported to reduce the output of acetylcholine from the prejunctional nerve endings (Standaert and Riker 1967; Brazil and Prado-Franceschi 1969; Dretchen *et al.* 1973; Wright and Collier 1977; Lee *et al.* 1979*a*, *b*; Singh *et al.* 1979, 1982; Torda 1980; Fiekers 1983*a*). They may also reduce the sensitivity of the endplates on the postjunctional membrane (Standaert and Riker 1967; Dretchen *et al.* 1973; Singh *et al.* 1979, 1982; Fiekers 1983*b*). Streptomycin has also been reported to possess a local analgesic-like effect on nerves (Sokoll and Diecke 1969) and possibly to affect muscle contraction. Adams *et al.* (1976) studied several of the aminoglycoside antibiotics alone in the cat and concluded that there was both a prejunctional and a postjunctional mechanism, but that the proportions differed depending upon the muscle and the drug.

The block produced by the aminoglycoside antibiotics is not antagonized by the anticholinesterases (Stanley *et al.* 1969), although it is antagonized to a certain extent by calcium and 4-aminopyridine (Singh *et al.* 1978*c*; Sobek 1982).

Polymyxins and colistin

These classes of antibiotic also potentiate the actions of the neuromuscular block-ing agents (Lindesmith *et al.* 1968; Fogdall and Miller 1974*a*; McQuillen and Engbaek 1975; Wright and Collier 1976; Singh *et al.* 1982; Chapple *et al.* 1983; Kronenfeld *et al.* 1986). The combination of polymyxin with neomycin has been shown to be especially potent in this respect (Lee and de Silva 1979*b*). The mechan-ism of action of these agents is also not understood. Both a decrease in acetyl-choline output and a decrease in receptor sensitivity have been proposed (Wright and Collier 1976; Singh *et al.* 1982). This block may be difficult to antagonize, and an anticholinesterase may even make it worse (van Nyhuis *et al.* 1976; Lee *et al.* 1977). Antagonism may be produced by 4-aminopyridine (Lee *et al.* 1978).

Lincosamines

The principal agents in this family are lincomycin and clindamycin. Both have been reported to potentiate a neuromuscular block (Fogdall and Millar 1974*b*; Becker and Miller 1976; Rubbo *et al.* 1977; Singh *et al.* 1982). Once again, a mixture of prejunctional and postjunctional actions has been proposed (Rubbo *et al.* 1977; Tang and Schroeder 1978; Singh *et al.* 1982). This block is also difficult to reverse. Anticholinesterases either have a little effect or accentuate the block (Tang and Schroeder 1978; Singh *et al.* 1982) whereas the administration of 4-aminopyridine will produce antagonism (Singh *et al.* 1978c; Booij *et al.* 1978).

Penicillins, cephalosporins, and erythromycin

These families of drugs essentially have no effect on a neuromuscular block. Phenoxymethylpenicillin can decrease acetylcholine release (Futamachi and Prince 1975; Noebels and Prince 1977) although it is unlikely that this effect has any clinical importance.

Metronidazole

There has been one report suggesting that metronidazole may potentiate a vecuronium neuromuscular block (McIndewar and Marshall 1981). This has, however, been disputed (d'Hollander *et al.* 1985). It is likely that metronidazole has no significant effect on a neuromuscular block.

Tetracyclines

Members of this family of drugs have been reported to exhibit weak potentiation of a neuromuscular block (Bowen and McMullen 1975; Wright and Collier 1976; Singh *et al.* 1982). It is unlikely that this interaction has any clinical significance.

Chloramphenicol

The only study to examine any possible neuromuscular blocking potential of chloramphenicol has reported an effect on acetylcholine-operated ion channels (Henderson *et al.* 1986). The clinical significance of this, if any, has yet to be determined.

ANTICONVULSANTS

There are a number of interactions between the anticonvulsants and the neuromuscular blocking agents. Phenytoin interacts markedly with nondepolarizing neuromuscular blocking agents and resistance is seen in many patients receiving long-term treatment with phenytoin. This phenomenon has been observed with pancuronium (Messick *et al.* 1982; Chen *et al.* 1983; Hickey *et al.* 1988), vecuronium (Ornstein *et al.* 1987), tubocurarine (Harrah *et al.* 1970), and metocurine (Ornstein *et al.* 1985; Kim *et al.* 1992), although not with atracurium (Ornstein *et al.* 1987; Hickey *et al.* 1988). The resistance is manifest as an increase in requirements to achieve a given degree of block, an increase in the infusion rate requirements to maintain a steady-state block and reduction in the duration of action of a bolus dose. This interaction is not confined to phenytoin but has also been observed with the other anticonvulsants, carbamazepine (Blanc-Bimar *et al.* 1979; Hershkovitz *et al.* 1978; Roth and Ebrahim 1987) and sodium valproate (Blanc-Bimar *et al.* 1979).

It is well established that when a neuromuscular blocking agent is administered to a patient receiving chronic phenytoin therapy, resistance is seen. When phenytoin is administered acutely to a patient with a steady-state neuromuscular block, however, potentiation of the block results (Gray *et al.* 1989), although this effect is unlikely to be of clinical significance.

The mechanism underlying this effect of the anticonvulsants is not known. An increased binding of metocurine to plasma proteins has been demonstrated in the presence of phenytoin (Kim *et al.* 1992). Phenytoin therapy results in an increase in the metabolism of pancuronium (Haque *et al.* 1972). It is thought most likely, however, that the interactions are taking place at the level of the neuromuscular junction. Phenytoin and carbamazepine have both been shown to decrease acetylcholine release (Alderdice and Trommer 1980; Gage *et al.* 1980). Carbamazepine, phenobarbitone, and ethosuximide all decrease the sensitivity of the postjunctional membrane to acetylcholine (Alderdice and Trommer 1980). Phenytoin therapy has been reported to exacerbate pre-existing myasthenia gravis (Kornfeld 1976).

The mechanism of action may be more complex still, in view of the known effects of certain metabolites of the anticonvulsants. Primidone increases acetylcholine release and also decreases the sensitivity of the postjunctional membrane. There is a metabolite of primidone — phenylethylmalonamide — which decreases the sensitivity of the postjunctional membrane without any effect on prejunctional acetylcholine release (Talbot and Alderdice 1982, 1984). Trimethadione decreases the sensitivity of the postjunctional membrane without any effect on acetylcholine release, but dimethadione, a metabolite of trimethadione, decreases acetylcholine release with no effect on the postjunctional membrane (Alderdice and McMillan 1982).

BETA-ADRENERGIC BLOCKING AGENTS

An effect of catecholamines on the neuromuscular junction was first described some 70 years ago (Orbeli 1923) and since then many studies have been undertaken to examine these effects and also to elucidate the underlying mechanisms (Drury 1977). It should come as no surprise therefore that adrenergic antagonists might have an effect on neuromuscular transmission. The alpha-adrenergic antagonists have received very little attention. The beta-adrenergic antagonists, which have a widespread use in medicine have, however, been investigated.

The beta-adrenergic blocking agents potentiate a nondepolarizing neuromuscular block both clinically (Harrah *et al.* 1970; Rozen and Whan 1972) and in animals *in vivo* (Usubiaga 1968; Chiarandini 1980) and *in vitro* (Bowman and Nott 1969; Kuba 1970). There have also been reports of treatment with a beta-adrenergic blocker worsening the symptoms of myasthenia gravis (Weisman 1949; Herishanu and Rosenberg 1975; Hughes and Zacharias 1976). Despite all of these reports, it seems unlikely that beta blockers have any significant effects in normal clinical practice.

A particular interaction has been reported with suxamethonium, where its duration of action may be prolonged due to inhibition of breakdown by plasma cholinesterase. This effect has been reported with propranolol (Whittaker *et al.* 1981) and esmolol (Murthy *et al.* 1985), although its clinical significance is unclear (McCammon *et al.* 1985).

CALCIUM ANTAGONISTS

Calcium and calmodulin play an essential role in the release of neurotransmitters (Landers *et al.* 1989). Calcium is also involved in excitation–contraction coupling in muscle. It might seem surprising, therefore, if calcium antagonists did not have some effect on the neuromuscular transmission and the existence of such an effect has been confirmed. Verapamil has been shown to potentiate a nondepolarizing neuromuscular block *in vitro* and *in vivo* (Bikhazi *et al.* 1982*a*, *b*, 1983; Kraynak *et al.* 1983*a*, *b*; Lawson *et al.* 1983; Durant *et al.* 1984*b*; Anderson and Marshall 1985). Nifedipine has a similar effect. The potentiating effect is accentuated by antibiotics (Bikhazi *et al.* 1984; del Pozo and Baeyens 1984) and by enflurane (Williams *et al.* 1983). Verapamil has been reported to increase weakness in a patient with Duchenne muscular dystrophy (Zalman *et al.* 1983). A neuromuscular block has been reported to be easier to reverse with edrophonium than neostigmine in the presence of verapamil (van Poorten *et al.* 1984; Jones *et al.* 1985), and also to be effectively antagonized using 4-aminopyridine (Agoston *et al.* 1984).

The mechanism of action of the calcium antagonists on a neuromuscular block remains to be elucidated. Verapamil has been reported to possess a local analgesic-like effect (Kraynack *et al.* 1982*a*, *b*, *c*; Bikhazi *et al.* 1984). Verapamil has also been shown to block ion channels at the neuromuscular junction (Durant *et al.* 1984*b*; Wachtel 1985) and to have a direct effect on skeletal muscle (Foldes 1984; Anderson and Marshall 1985). Combined prejunctional and postjunctional mechanisms were favoured by Baraka (1985) who argued that the potentiating effect was unlikely to be due solely to an effect on muscular contraction. The only conclusion which can be drawn at present is that the calcium antagonists do potentiate neuromuscular blocking agents and that the exact mechanism is unknown.

GANGLIONIC BLOCKERS

The ganglionic blocking agents hexamethonium, pentolinium, and trimetaphan have been shown to have a neuromuscular blocking action alone *in vitro* (Pollard 1991). Ganglionic blocking agents also prolong the action of the nondepolarizing neuromuscular blocking agents. This has been shown to be true for hexamethonium (Barlow and

Ing 1948; Deacock and Davies 1958; Ferry and Marshall 1973; Rang and Rylett 1984; Pollard 1991) and trimetaphan (Deacock and Davies 1958; Aguilar and Boldrey 1960; Deacock and Hargrove 1962; Dale and Schroeder 1976; Wilson *et al.* 1976; Gergis *et al.* 1977; Nakamura *et al.* 1980; Pollard 1991) and pentolinium (Pollard 1991). This potentiation appears to hold true for all nondepolarizing neuromuscular blocking agents and also for suxamethonium. In the case of suxamethonium and trimetaphan *in vivo* the prolongation of effect is due at least in part to the reduction in the rate of breakdown of suxamethonium by the presence of trimetaphan (Tewfik 1957; Wilson *et al.* 1976; Dale and Schroeder 1976; Sklar and Lanks 1977; Poulton *et al.* 1979).

The mechanism underlying the interaction between the neuromuscular blocking agents and the ganglion blocking agents is not precisely clear. It has been suggested that the prejunctional receptors on the neuromuscular junction may resemble the nicotinic acetylcholine receptors on autonomic ganglia more than they do those on the postjunctional membrane at the neuromuscular junction (Bowman 1980). It is tempting, therefore, to suggest that herein lies the mechanism for the interaction, the ganglionic blocking agents reinforcing the action of a neuromuscular blocking agent by additionally blocking the prejunctional receptors. The addition of a prejunctional action from a ganglionic blocking agent might therefore be expected to potentiate a pancuronium block (principally postjunctional in action) more than it would a tubocurarine block (both prejunctional and postjunctional in action). This has not been borne out experimentally (Pollard 1991). Evidence has also been advanced to support a postjunctional action of hexamethonium (Rang and Rylett 1984). The interaction *in vitro* is also not as simple as expected because antagonism of the neuromuscular blocking agent is seen with lower concentrations of ganglionic blocker (Pollard 1991) followed by potentiation at higher concentrations. It is possible, however, that this observation could be explained by a dynamic interaction between two antagonists with different affinities (Ginsborg and Stephenson 1974).

ANTI-ARRHYTHMIC AGENTS

The anti-arrythmic agents include a variety of drugs belonging to several different families. Drugs grouped under this heading include the beta-adrenergic blockers, calcium channel blockers, phenytoin, lignocaine, disopyramide, bretylium, quinidine, and procainamide. The beta blockers and calcium channel blockers are covered individually above. Phenytoin is included with the anticonvulsants, and lignocaine with the local analgesics.

Quinidine and procainamide

These agents potentiate both depolarizing and a nondepolarizing neuromuscular blocks (Schmidt *et al.* 1963; Grogono 1963; Cuthbert 1966; Miller *et al.* 1967, Harrah *et al.* 1970). The mechanism behind this action is not known, but it seems likely that both a prejunctional (Thesleff 1980) and a postjunctional action are involved. Way *et al.* (1967) suggested that in the presence of quinidine recurarization is likely. Both quinidine and procainamide have also been reported to precipitate an episode of myasthenia gravis in susceptible patients (Weisman 1949; Drachman and Skou 1965; Kornfeld *et al.* 1976).

Disopyramide

Disopyramide potentiates a nondepolarizing neuromuscular block in animal studies *in vitro* (Healy *et al.* 1981). Despite this proven interaction no clinical effect has so far been reported. It seems likely therefore that any clinical effect is not important.

Bretylium

This drug also potentiates a nondepolarizing neuromuscular block in animal studies *in vitro* (Welch and Waud 1980, 1982). The mechanism is unknown. No interaction with neuromuscular blocking agents in the clinical situation has so far been reported.

STEROIDS

Certain of the neuromuscular blocking agents are steroids. It does not necessarily follow, however, that steroids all have an effect on neuromuscular transmission. Indeed, it is the presence of at least one positively charged nitrogen group that confers neuromuscular blocking activity in pancuronium, vecuronium, and allied compounds. The steroids comprise a large family of substances which have a common central structure but a variety of pharmacological actions from anaesthesia (alphaxolone) to electrolyte balance (aldosterone). There are a number of reports that steroids which are not muscle relaxants can affect neuromuscular transmission.

A tubocurarine neuromuscular block was antagonized by low concentrations of dexamethasone, but potentiated at higher concentrations *in vitro* (Leeuwin *et al.* 1981). The existence of this interaction was confirmed by Hall (1980), although Schwartz (1986) having examined the interactions of both dexamethasone and hydrocortisone with several neuromuscular blocking agents in the clinical situation was unable to demonstrate any effect.

Meyers (1977), Laflin (1977), and Azar *et al.* (1982) have all demonstrated antagonism between corticosteroids and pancuronium in clinical studies. A similar antagonism has also been demonstrated in animal experiments (Wilson *et al.* 1974; Arts and Oosterhuis 1975; Riker *et al.* 1975; Leeuwin and Walters 1977; van Wilgenberg 1979). Resistance to the effect of vecuronium was encountered in a patient receiving long-term testosterone therapy by Reddy *et al.* 1989.

The mechanism of any such interaction is not known. Theories include an increase in acetylcholine release (Arts and Oosterhuis 1975; Leeuwin *et al.* 1981; van Wilgenberg 1980), depression of the excitability of the postjunctional membrane (van Wilgenberg 1979), inhibition of phosphodiesterase (Liu 1984), an increase in prejunctional choline uptake (Veldsema-Currie and van Marle 1984; Leeuwin and Veldsema-Currie 1980) and the inhibition of cholinesterase (Robertson 1967; Bradamante *et al.* 1984). Whatever the mechanism, it appears that any interaction is not of undue clinical significance.

HYPOTENSIVE AGENTS

There are a number of drugs which belong to different families and which can be used as hypotensive agents. These include the ganglionic blockers and adrenergic blockers, both of which are covered separately. The two agents used most commonly in anaesthesia to reduce blood pressure are sodium nitroprusside and glyceryl trinitrate (and its derivatives).

Glyceryl trinitrate has been reported to increase the duration of action of pancuronium (Glisson *et al.* 1979). It has, however, also been reported to have no effect on a neuromuscular block produced by pancuronium, tubocurarine, gallamine, vecuronium or suxamethonium (Glisson *et al.* 1980; Schwartz *et al.* 1986). Sodium nitroprusside has no effect on a neuromuscular block (Gergis *et al.* 1977; Graham and Walts 1979).

IMMUNOSUPPRESSANTS

There have been reports which have suggested that the immunosuppressants may potentiate a nondepolarizing neuromuscular block (Bennett *et al.* 1977; Chung 1982). Cyclosporin potentiates an atracurium and vecuronium neuromuscular block (Gramstad *et al.* 1986). Azathioprine was shown to antagonize both a tubocurarine and a pancuronium neuromuscular block by Dretchen *et al.* (1976a) although Glidden *et al.* (1988) failed to demonstrate any interaction between azathioprine and tubocurarine. These drugs may also prolong the action of suxamethonium and this is thought to be due to an inhibitory effect on plasma cholinesterase (Zsigmond and Robbins 1972; Chung 1982).

PHOSPHODIESTERASE INHIBITORS

The presence of a phosphodiesterase inhibitor will lead to an increase in cyclic AMP concentrations. Cyclic AMP is one of the second messengers which may well be important with respect to acetylcholine release or mobilization (Dretchen *et al.* 1976b). An effect of the phosphodiesterase inhibitors on neuromuscular transmission might therefore be expected.

In the absence of a neuromuscular blocking agent, aminophylline has been shown to enhance diaphragmatic contractility (Aubier *et al.* 1981, 1983), and when aminophylline was administered in the presence of a pancuronium neuromuscular block antagonism was seen (Azar *et al.* 1982). Theophylline, caffeine, and certain other xanthines were seen to facilitate neuromuscular transmission *in vitro* (Giesecke *et al.* 1968) an action which might result in a reduction of the expected effect of a neuromuscular blocking agent.

The mechanism for these interactions may be related to cyclic AMP levels because adenosine depresses neuromuscular transmission (Varagic 1984), an effect which is counteracted by aminophylline. Evidence exists, however, to cast doubt upon this theory (Varagic *et al.* 1980). Kramer and Wells (1980) were unable to demonstrate a relationship between the degree of inhibition of phosphodiesterase and the increase in muscular contraction *in vitro*. Theophylline is a potent antagonist at adenosine receptors in lower concentrations than those at which it inhibits phosphodiesterase (Wells and Miller 1983). It is possible that the observed effects of phosphodiesterase inhibitors on neuromuscular transmission are not related to cyclic AMP effects but are mediated through adenosine receptors.

MISCELLANEOUS DRUGS

There are a number of drugs which do not belong to any of the above categories, yet have been shown to affect neuromuscular transmission. Many of these actions have been noticed in a serendipitous fashion, and then examined in greater detail.

Aprotinin

Aprotinin was shown by Chasapakis and Dinas (1966) to potentiate weakly a neuromuscular block. Aprotinin inhibits the activity of plasma cholinesterase and therefore may prolong a suxamethonium neuromuscular block (Doenicke *et al.* 1970).

Penicillamine

There have been no incidents described of an interaction between penicillamine and the neuromuscular blocking agents. Penicillamine has, however, been reported to worsen or precipitate a myasthenic episode (Vincent *et al.* 1978; Russell and Lindstrom 1978; Fried and Prothero 1986). This latter effect does not necessarily imply that there will be an effect on a neuromuscular block in an non-myasthenic patient.

Dantrolene

Potentiation of a tubocurarine (Flewellan *et al.* 1980), and a vecuronium (Driessen *et al.* 1985*b*) neuromuscular block have been reported with dantrolene. It is uncertain what mechanism is involved, because no other similar interactions have been described, nor has any effect of dantrolene been noted on the neuromuscular junction.

Phenothiazines

An increase in weakness in a myasthenic patient has been reported to be associated with chlorpromazine therapy (McQuillen *et al.* 1963). No direct affect on neuromuscular block has been described.

Cyclo-oxygenase inhibitors

Hill and Wong (1980) examined the effect of prostaglandins and indomethacin at the neuromuscular junction and could find no effect. This was confirmed by Madden and van der Koot (1985).

Ecothiopate

Eye drops containing the organophosphate anticholinesterase ecothiopate are used in the management of glaucoma. Sufficient may be absorbed for a parenteral effect to be seen, due to inhibition of plasma cholinesterase. The duration of action of suxamethonium is prolonged (Donati and Bevan 1981) and it is possible that mivacurium may be similarly affected.

ACID–BASE BALANCE

Changes in acid–base balance are not uncommon during anaesthesia or intensive care management. It is common practice to hyperventilate patients deliberately to a small extent, e.g. $PaCO_2$ approximately 4.5 kPa, and occasionally $PaCO_2$ between 3.5 and 4.0 kPa may be seen. This results in an acute respiratory alkalosis. At the termination of surgery, residual narcosis or paralysis may result in hypoventilation with a sudden change to an acute respiratory acidosis. There may already be an acidosis or alkalosis (metabolic or respiratory) resulting from a pre-existing medical condition upon which these acute changes will be superimposed. It is clearly important therefore to consider whether or not the action of a neuromuscular blocking agent is affected by changes in acid–base balance. It must of course be remembered that the pH in the arterial blood may not exactly reflect that in the muscle or at the neuromuscular junction.

It has been generally accepted that a neuromuscular block is potentiated by acidosis (Brooks and Feldman 1962; Hughes 1970). The neuromuscular blocking agent which has received the most attention in this respect is tubocurarine (Payne 1958, 1960; Utting 1963; Katz and Wolf 1964; Baraka 1964; Bush and Baraka 1964; Hughes 1970). All of those reports, except Payne (1960), describe the potentiation of a tubocurarine neuromuscular block by acidosis. The clear implication is that hypoventilation and hence respiratory acidosis in the early postoperative period may give rise to difficulties in reversal, or even to later reappearance of a block. Miller *et al.* (1975) described this problem with respect to neostigmine-induced reversal of a tubocurarine neuromuscular block. Not all neuromuscular blocking agents are similarly affected. A pancuronium or vecuronium neuromuscular block appears to be affected very little by changes in acid–base status (Norman *et al.* 1970; Dann 1971; Gencarelli *et al.* 1983, 1984). The neostigmine induced antagonism of a pancuronium neuromuscular block may, however, also be impaired by a coexistent acidosis (Miller and Roderick 1978; Wirtavuori *et al.* 1982). Metocurine, gallamine, and suxamethonium are also affected but to a lesser extent than tubocurarine.

POTASSIUM

The membrane potential is largely dependent upon the differences in potassium concentrations between the inside and outside of a cell and can be calculated from an application of the Nernst equation and its derivatives (Bowman and Rand 1980) Changes in the plasma (and hence extracellular) potassium concentrations will therefore affect the excitability of cells, and have also been shown to alter acetylcholine release. An increase in extracellular potassium concentration leads to an increase in acetylcholine release (Ginsberg and Jenkinson 1976). An increase in extracellular potassium has also been shown to decrease the sensitivity to a tubocurarine or pancuronium neuromuscular block *in vitro* (Waud and Waud 1980) which was reflected in an increased requirement for tubocurarine. This was evident within the range encountered clinically — an increase in potassium from 3.5 to 5.0 mmol/l increased the requirement by approximately one-third. Conversely, a decrease in plasma potassium concentration lead to a reduced requirement for nondepolarizing neuromuscular blocking agents (Hill *et al.* 1978). The amount of neostigmine required for reversal was found to be higher (Miller and Roderick 1978; Waud *et al.* 1982*a*) and the risk of recurarization was increased (Feldman 1963). Chronic potassium depletion also reduces the requirement for tubocurarine (Waud *et al.* 1982*a*).

There is a condition, familial periodic paralysis, where the potassium characteristically undergoes marked swings. Great care should be taken with the use of neuromuscular blocking agents in these patients.

LITHIUM

Lithium potentiates a neuromuscular block produced by tubocurarine (Basuray and Harris 1977; Hill *et al.* 1977), pancuronium (Borden *et al.* 1974), or suxamethonium (Hill *et al.* 1976). Lithium may produce muscular weakness when given alone in the absence of a neuromuscular blocking agent (Lynam *et al.* 1980). The mechanism underlying the effect of lithium on a neuromuscular block appears to be a decrease in acetylcholine release from the nerve endings (Vizi *et al.* 1972; Crawford 1975; Branisteanu and Volle 1975; Waud *et al.* 1982*b*).

CALCIUM

The release and mobilization of chemical transmitters and messengers and also excitation–contraction coupling are all dependent upon calcium ions. It should come as no surprise, therefore, that calcium ions and other divalent cations affect neuromuscular transmission. The actions of calcium at the neuromuscular junction, however, do not all affect a neuromuscular block in an identical fashion. Indeed, some of its actions oppose one another and it may therefore be difficult to predict the result. For example, an *in vitro* study has shown potentiation of a pancuronium or tubocurarine neuromuscular block in the presence of an increase in calcium concentration (Waud and Waud 1980). A clinical report, however, which described anaesthesia in a patient with a raised serum calcium secondary to hyperparathyroidism showed that the duration of action of suxamethonium was prolonged but that of atracurium was decreased (Al-Mohaya *et al.* 1986).

The mechanisms behind these actions are complex. An increase in calcium concentration will produce an increase in acetylcholine release (Katz and Miledi 1965; Hubbard *et al.* 1968; Miledi and Thies 1971). Calcium has been reported to produce a decrease in the sensitivity of the postjunctional membrane (Waud and Waud 1980) and also to enhance the excitation–contraction coupling process in skeletal muscle (Hanson 1974). An increase in calcium concentration may be expected partly to antagonize a nondepolarizing neuromuscular block; it may also help to antagonize a block which is partly due to antibiotics (Sokoll and Gergis 1981).

MAGNESIUM

Magnesium acts in the opposite way to calcium at the neuromuscular junction. It potentiates neuromuscular blocking agents both clinically and in animal studies (Giesecke *et al.* 1968; Morris and Giesecke 1968; Ghoneim and Long 1970; de Silva 1973; Skaredoff *et al.* 1982). When suxamethonium was administered in the presence of magnesium, potentiation of the block ensued and the suggestion has been made that the original phase I block may readily change in character to a phase II block (Crul *et al.* 1966). The existence of an interaction with magnesium is of clinical importance because magnesium has widespread uses in medicine. It is routinely used in pre-eclampsia and eclampsia in some centres and also during open heart surgery. Hypomagnesaemia may be seen in patients with malnutrition and also in patients on the critical care unit.

The mechanism by which magnesium affects neuromuscular transmission is in many respects related to an opposing effect on calcium actions. Magnesium and calcium are often regarded as being in direct competition (del Castillo and Engbaek 1954; Geisecke *et al.* 1968; Ghoneim and Long 1970). A reduction in acetylcholine release results from the presence of magnesium and it is likely that the main effect is prejunctional (Lee *et al.* 1979a).

There are a number of other divalent cations which behave in a manner very similar to magnesium. Manganese, beryllium, lead, and cadmium all share similar properties (Geisecke *et al.* 1968; Forshaw 1977; Schopp 1978; Haberman and Richard 1986).

COMBINATIONS OF NONDEPOLARIZING AGENTS

It was logical for the early investigators working with neuromuscular blocking agents to reach the conclusion that they all acted in the same way, namely by competitive antagonism of the action of acetylcholine at its receptors on the postjunctional membrane. The overall characteristics of their action were very similar and so there was no reason to doubt this assumption.

If two drugs act in exactly the same way on the same receptor system then, when they are given simultaneously, their effects should be additive. It would therefore be logical to assume that the nondepolarizing neuromuscular blocking agents were all additive in their actions. It was Riker and Wescoe (1951) who first examined combinations of two neuromuscular blocking agents using cats. They showed that consecutive doses of either gallamine or tubocurarine had the same effect whether the second dose followed the same agent, or the other agent. The implication was that their effects were additive.

Wong (1969) studied the same two agents, tubocurarine and gallamine. He reasoned that because they both had significant and different cardiovascular side-effects, mixing the two would allow the use of less of each, thereby reducing dose-dependant side-effects. He administered the mixture empirically to 11 patients and was surprised that less was needed for surgical relaxation than he had predicted. He therefore examined the combination in the rabbit and concluded that there existed 'a synergistic effect of tubocurarine and gallamine' (Wong and Jones 1971). He suggested that the reason might be that the two drugs acted in different ways at the neuromuscular junction. He called his mixture 'curadil', from *cura*re and flax*edil*, the latter being the trade name for gallamine.

A more extensive clinical study was undertaken by Ghoneim *et al.* (1972) also using tubocurarine and gallamine, and they reached the same conclusion. As new neuromuscular blocking agents were developed, their interactions were also investigated. Park *et al.* (1974) confirmed the synergistic interaction between tubocurarine and gallamine and reported a similar interaction between pancuronium and tubocurarine. The existence of synergism between neuromuscular blocking agents was then accepted, a situation which remained for about eight years. Matters then began to appear a little less straightforward.

Lebowitz *et al.* (1980) demonstrated synergism with pancuronium and tubocurarine and also with pancuronium and metocurine; tubocurarine and metocurine was, however, additive. Interest was immediately revived and the number of studies examining combinations multiplied. Figure 12.1 contains an overall summary: certain combinations are additive and others synergistic.

	Vecuronium	Atracurium	Gallamine	Metocurine	Alcuronium	Pancuronium
Atracurium	Addition					
Gallamine	Not studied	Not studied				
Metocurine	Not studied	Not studied	Potentation			
Alcuronium	Addition	Potentiation	Not studied	Not studied		
Pancuronium	Addition	Addition	Addition	Potentation	Addition	
Tubocurarine	Potentation	Addition	Addition	Addition	Potentation	Potentation

Fig.12.1 The results of mixing together nondepolarizing neuromuscular blocking agents in two-component combinations.

An explanation for these observations was required. There are many variables to be considered in the clinical situation, which include uptake, binding, metabolism, redistribution, and regional blood flow patterns. Most do not apply when using an *in vitro* preparation yet synergism is still seen, implying an action at the neuromuscular junction.

The reasons for the interaction between the nondepolarizing neuromuscular blocking agents are not yet clear. Possible mechanisms include differential actions upon the prejunctional and postjunctional acetylcholine receptors within the junction; differential sensitivity of the two alpha-subunit acetylcholine recognition sites; and effects on cholinesterase. It seems that pharmacokinetic effects outside the neuromuscular junction may not be the explanation (Martyn *et al.* 1983).

Tubocurarine and pancuronium

This has been the most extensively studied combination and the majority of the publications describe potentiation. This was demonstrated in clinical studies by Lebowitz *et al.* (1980), Mirakhur *et al.* (1984) and Jones *et al.* (1984). Three similar studies (Park *et al.* 1974; Duncalf *et al.* 1983; Foldes *et al.* 1984) all gave several doses of pancuronium on top of a partial block by tubocurarine and showed that there was a reduction in the ED_{50} of the pancuronium, i.e. the ED_{50} of one agent is reduced in the presence of another.

Assidao *et al.* (1984) examined the characteristics of two mixtures — tubocurarine 0.25 mg/kg with pancuronium 0.05 mg/kg, and tubocurarine 0.375 mg/kg with pancuronium 0.07 mg/kg. The first of these equates to 121% of an ED_{95} and the second to 180% of an ED_{95}. They were compared with each other and with suxamethonium 1.5 mg/kg. The second mixture gave a more profound block more rapidly, hardly surprising in view of the greater total number of relaxant molecules given. In a case report described by Balamoutsos *et al.* (1981), a patient incompletely relaxed despite 16 mg of pancuronium over the course of two hours became fully paralysed following a dose of 6 mg of tubocurarine.

Waud and Waud (1984, 1985) reported two studies using nerve stimulation of an *in vitro* preparation and recordings of carbachol-induced deploarizations. The first study showed weak potentiation and the second addition. Waud and Waud attribute the difference between the results of their two papers as being related to a difference in the concentration range of antagonist. A further *in vitro* study has also confirmed potentiation (Pollard and Jones 1983).

Two studies have described addition between pancuronium and tubocurarine (Schuh 1981; Booij *et al.* 1985). The first of these used rats *in vivo* and the second was a clinical study. The overall consensus favours potentiation.

Pancuronium and metocurine

There are six studies which have addressed this interaction, Lebowitz *et al.* (1980) used normal adult patients and Satwicz *et al.* (1984) examined a population composed entirely of children. Both found the combination to be more potent than was either component alone. The other four studies have used animals (Duncalf *et al.* 1983; Foldes *et al.* 1984; Waud and Waud 1984, 1985). One described addition and three potentiation.

It would appear therefore that the balance of evidence favours potentiation. Indeed, in view of the structural similarity between tubocurarine and metocurine, it might be surprising if metocurine did not behave in a manner similar to tubocurarine.

Tubocurarine and metocurine

Three studies have addressed this combination; two reported addition (Lebowitz *et al.* 1980; Waud and Waud 1985) and one reported very weak potentiation (Waud and Waud 1984). No consideration has been given to the rate of onset of this combination although Lebowitz *et al.* (1980) reported the duration of action not to be prolonged when compared with either component given alone. It is likely that these two agents are purely additive in effect. In view of the close structural similarity between them, it might be thought surprising if this were not the case.

Pancuronium and alcuronium

Three publications have addressed this combination. All reported simple addition of effect. Shanks (1982) conducted his investigations using anaesthetized patients. He gave pancuronium, alcuronium or their combination by infusion and constructed the relation between dose and response with respect to the total amount of drug administered against degree of block. The log dose–response line for the combination was midway between those for the two individual components, suggesting addition. Jones *et al.* (1984) and Pollard and Jones (1983) used the rat phrenic nerve hemidiaphragm *in vitro* and confirmed the existence of addition.

Tubocurarine and alcuronium

The only publication in which this combination has been considered is based on *in vitro* work in the rat (Pollard and Jones 1983). The conclusion was that this combination exhibits marked potentiation.

Gallamine and tubocurarine

Six published reports have considered this combination: three describe potentiation and three addition of effect.

Wong and Jones (1971) reported potentiation using the rabbit head drop test, and also the sciatic nerve–gastrocnemius preparation in anaesthetized rabbits. Although log concentration–response graphs were constructed, only two points were used to fix each line. Park *et al.* (1974) in a clinical study administered either gallamine or tubocurarine followed by an identical fixed increment of gallamine to both at a specific point of recovery. Although regarded as evidence of potentiation, the second increment was given at different levels of block. In a study by Ghoneim *et al.* (1972) tubocurarine, gallamine, or their combination were each administered in two doses to a series of patients and then the relation between log dose and response constructed. The conclusion was that the combination showed potentiation. The other three reports described addition of effect (Waud and Waud 1984, 1985; Schuh 1981). It is likely that the interaction is only additive.

Gallamine and pancuronium

The three reports in which this combination has been examined are all in agreement; the effects of gallamine and pancuronium are additive (Schuh 1981; Waud and Waud 1984, 1985).

Gallamine and metocurine

This combination has been considered in only two studies, both of which are from Waud and Waud (1984, 1985). They concern animal work *in vitro*. Both reach the conclusion that the combination is additive.

Atracurium and tubocurarine

There are three reports concerning this combination all of which are animal studies. The studies by Foldes *et al.* (1984) and Duncalf *et al.* (1983) both examined the effect of atracurium upon a subparalytic concentration of tubocurarine. They concluded that the ED_{50} of one agent is reduced in the presence of the other; i.e. potentiation exists. The third report, by Booij *et al.* (1985), suggested that these two agents are additive. The nature of the interaction between atracurium and tubocurarine is therefore not certain.

Atracurium and pancuronium

The two studies reported both concluded that this combination is additive (Jones *et al.* 1984; Booij *et al.* 1985).

Atracurium and metocurine

The only two reports on this combination are from Foldes *et al.* (1984) and from Duncalf *et al.* (1983). These studies used rats *in vivo* and *in vitro* respectively, and examined the effect of atracurium upon a subparalytic background concentration of metocurine. Potentiation was suggested.

Vecuronium and tubocurarine

There are four reports in the literature concerning this combination of relaxants. In the one clinical study, the relation between log dose and response was constructed for each component and their combination and the conclusion drawn that potentiation exists with this combination (Mirakhur *et al.* 1985). Foldes *et al.* (1984) and Duncalf *et al.* (1983) both reported that the ED_{50} for vecuronium was reduced in the presence of a subparalytic concentration of tubocurarine, which implies potentiation. Booij *et al.* (1985) using rats *in vivo* described addition between vecuronium and tubocurarine. The balance of evidence seems to favour potentiation.

Pancuronium and vecuronium

There are four publications in which this combination has been addressed. Ferres *et al.* (1984) reported addition. Pandit *et al.* (1986) confirmed this finding using a crude measure of intubating conditions at 60 seconds. Booij *et al.* (1985) reported additivity using rats *in vivo*.

Rashkowsky *et al.* (1985) did not consider the nature of the interaction between the two agents, but studied the action of each to continue a neuromuscular block which had been begun with either the same, or the other drug. All the reports agree that this combination is simply additive. This may not be surprising in view of the close structural similarity between the molecules.

Metocurine and vecuronium

The only two reports with respect to this combination are animal studies from Foldes *et al.* (1984) and Duncalf *et al.* (1983). Both reported potentiation.

Atracurium and vecuronium

Of the five studies which have examined this combination only four have examined characteristics of the degree of neuromuscular block; the fifth considered the onset and duration of the combination. Three reported addition (Booij *et al.* 1985; Esmaili *et al.* 1986; Van der Spek *et al.* 1988) and one reported potentiation (Black *et al.* 1985). The studies reporting addition were performed using rats, whereas that reporting potentiation was a clinical study. It is possible therefore that there is a species difference.

Extending a neuromuscular block

As the end of surgery approaches it is often necessary to administer a small dose of neuromuscular blocking agent to increase or extend the block in order to assist surgical closure. This can be achieved using small increments of the same neuromuscular blocking agent that has been used for the main part of the procedure. There may be certain advantages in using a second shorter-acting agent (Kay *et al.* 1987; Middleton *et al.* 1989; Eadsforth *et al.* 1990). It must be noted, however, that only a very small dose is required (atracurium 1–2 mg, or vecuronium 0.25 mg) in order to achieve a suitable extension of block. If much larger doses are administered there may be a profound block lasting much longer than anticipated.

SUXAMETHONIUM AND OTHER RELAXANTS

The depolarizing neuromuscular blocking agent suxamethonium has the fastest onset of any of the muscle relaxants in present use. It is therefore the drug of choice when the airway has to be secured without delay. It is not common practice to continue with the use of suxamethonium for longer procedures, but to subsequently administer a nondepolarizing neuromuscular blocking agent to maintain paralysis. Although it is good practice to await recovery from the suxamethonium before administering a second relaxant, this second agent is very likely to be given before the suxamethonium has completely worn off. The potential for interactions between suxamethonium and the nondepolarizing agents needs therefore to be considered.

Suxamethonium before a nondepolarizing agent

The prior administration of an intubating dose of suxamethonium has been shown to reduce the subsequent requirement for a pancuronium, atracurium, and vecuronium nondepolarizing neuromuscular block (Katz 1971*a*; Krieg *et al.* 1991; Stirt *et al.* 1983; d'Hollander *et al.* 1983). This observation has, however, been disputed. Walts and Rusin (1977) found no effect of a previous dose of suxamethonium on a pancuronium neuromuscular block and Fisher and Miller (1983) found the same for a vecuronium neuromuscular block. Swen *et al.* (1990) examined several nondepolarizing neuromuscular blocking agents and showed that prior administration of suxamethonium prolonged the duration of action of vecuronium but had no effect on the duration of action of atracurium, pancuronium, or pipecuronium. There is no clear reason for these differences. Although the evidence is conflicting it is believed by most clinicians that a prior dose of suxamethonium allows the use of a slightly smaller dose of nondepolarizing neuromuscular blocking agent for continuation of the block. It is possible that this simply reflects the fact that a more dense block is required for intubation than for surgical relaxation.

Precurarization before suxamethonium

A second situation where suxamethonium and a nondepolarizing neuromuscular blocking agent may be administered concurrently is when precurarization is employed. Suxamethonium has a number of unwanted and potentially hazardous side-effects. Many seem to be related to the muscular fasciculations resulting from the administration of suxamethonium. If a small dose of a nondepolarizing neuromuscular blocking agent is administered before the suxamethonium the fasciculations are lessened and this technique of precurarization has a widespread following in clinical anaesthesia.

The administration of a subparalysing dose of a nondepolarizing neuromuscular blocking agent delays the onset of the suxamethonium and shortens its duration of action (Cullen 1971; Blitt *et al.* 1981; Ferguson and Bevan 1981). It is therefore common practice to increase the dose of suxamethonium slightly if following a small dose of a nondepolarizing agent. The most commonly used agents for precurarization are probably tubocurarine in a dose of 3–5 mg (Cullen 1971), or gallamine in a dose of 5–20 mg (Cullen 1971; Virtue 1975; Jansen and Hanson 1979). Pancuronium is not as effective as tubocurarine or gallamine (Cullen 1971; Brodsky *et al.* 1979; Jansen and Howardy-Hanson 1979). It is likely that the mechanism behind the benefit of precurarization is a decrease in the side-effects of suxamethonium and the subsequent requirement for an increased dose of suxamethonium lies simply in the partial subclinical block which limits all of the responses to suxamethonium. In the presence of the partial block from the nondepolarizing agent it is not possible to achieve a maximum agonist effect from the suxamethonium, which therefore limits both the desired effects and the side-effects.

Suxamethonium after a nondepolarizing agent

It is not uncommon towards the end of a surgical procedure for the surgeon to notice the waning effect of a neuromuscular block. The block was adequate for surgery but a slightly deeper block is needed to facilitate closure of the surgical incision. Some anaesthetists have advocated the administration of a small dose of suxamethonium at this time. The majority of these reports are empirical and subjective. The effect of a dose of suxamethonium at that time may be quite unpredictable, depending upon the nondepolarizing agent in use, the exact degree of block present, total dose administered and the dose of suxamethonium. No written guidelines are available, possibly because they are not possible to construct. This technique is best avoided. The use of an additional dose of nondepolarizing agent (or even a different nondepolarizing agent) is more logical.

CONCLUSION

There are an enormous number of references on the subject of drug interactions which involve the neuromuscular blocking agents. As more drugs are released onto the market, the number of potential and actual interactions is likely to increase still further. Indeed, whole books are devoted to the subject of interactions between drugs. There are many possibilities, and interations may be difficult to predict. Some may be advantageous and some disadvantageous. If neuromuscular function is monitored every time a neuromuscular blocking agent is used, then much of the unpredictability is removed.

REFERENCES

Adams, R. (1976). Drug blockade of open end-plate channels. *Journal of Physiology*, **260**, 531–52.

Adams, H. R., Mathew, B. P., Teske, R. H., and Mercer, H. D. (1976). *Anesthesia and Analgesia*, **55**, 500–7.

Agoston, S., Maestrone, E., Van Hezik, E. J., Ket, J. M., Houwertjes, M. C., and Uges, D. R. A. (1984). Effective treatment of verapamil intoxication with 4-aminopyridine in the cat. *Journal of Clinical Investigation*, **73**, 1291–6.

Aguilar, J. A. and Boldrey, E. B. (1960). The effect of Arfonad on the monkey. *Anesthesiology*, **21**, 3–12.

Akaike, N., Ito, H., Nishi, K., and Oyama, Y. (1982). Further analysis of inhibitor effects of propranolol and local anaesthetics on the calcium current in helix. *British Journal of Pharmacology*, **76**, 37–43.

Al-Mohaya, S., Naguib, M., Abdelatif, M., and Farag, H. (1986). Abnormal responses to muscle relaxants in a patient with primary hyperparathyroidism. *Anesthesiology*, **65**, 554–6.

Alderdice, M. T. and McMillan, J. E. (1982). Comparison of the effects of trimethadione and its primary metabolite dimethadione on neuromuscular function and the effects of altered pH on the action of dimethadione. *Journal of Pharmacology and Experimental Therapeutics*, **221**, 547–51.

Alderdice, M. T. And Trommer, B. A. (1980). Differential effects of the anticovulsants phenobarbital etosuximide and carbamazepine on neuromuscular transmission. *Journal of Pharmacology and Experimental Therapeutics*, **215**, 92–6.

Amaki, Y., Nagashima, H., Radnay, P. A., and Foldes, F. F. (1978). Ketamine interaction with neuromuscular blocking agents in the phrenic nerve-hemidiaphragm preparation of the rat. *Anesthesia and Analgesia*, **57**, 238–43.

Anderson, K. A. and Marshall, R. J. (1985). Interactions between calcium entry blockers and vecuronium bromide in anaesthetized cats. *British Journal of Anaesthesia*, **57**, 775–81.

Aracava, Y., Ikeda, S. R., and Daly, J. W. (1984). Interactions of bupivacaine with ionic channels of the nicotinic receptor. Analysis of single channel currents. *Molecular Pharmacology*, **26**, 304–13.

Argov, Z., and Mastaglia, F. L. (1979). Disorders of neuromuscular transmission caused by drugs. *New England Journal of Medicine*, **301**, 409–13.

Arnhem, P. and Kristbjarnarson, H. (1981). A barbiturate-induced potassium permeability increase in the myelinated nerve membrane. *Acta Physiologica Scandinavica*, **113**, 387–92.

Arts, W. F. and Oosterhuis, H. (1975). Effects of prednisolone on neuromuscular blockade in mice in vivo. *Neurology*, **25**, 1088–90.

Asbury, A. J., Henderson, P. D., Brown, B. H., Turner, D. J., and Linkens, D. A. (1981). Effect of diazepam on pancuronium-induced neuromuscular blockade maintained by a feedback system. *British Journal of Anaesthesia*, **53**, 859–63.

Assidao, C. B., Burgos, L. G., and Gandhi, S. K. (1984). *d*-Tubocurarine and pancuronium combinations for rapid sequence intubation. *8th World Congress of Anaesthesiology, Book of Abstracts*, **2**, A296.

Aubier, M., de Troyer, A., Sampson, M., Macklem, P. T., and Roussos, C. (1981). Aminophylline improves diaphragmatic contractility. *New England Journal of Medicine*, **305**, 249–52.

Aubier, M., Murciano, D., Viires, N., Lecocquic, V., Palacios, S., and Pafiente, R. (1983). Increased ventilation caused by improved diaphragmatic efficiency during aminophylline infusion. *American Review of Respiratory Diseases*, **127**, 148–54.

Azar, I., Cottrell, J., Gupta, B., and Turndorf, H. (1980). Furosemide facilitates recovery of evoked twitch response after pancuronium. *Anesthesia and Analgesia*, **59**, 55–7.

Azar, I., Kumar, D., and Betcher, A. M. (1982). Resistance to pancuronium in an asthmatic patient treated with aminophylline and steroids. *Canadian Anaesthetists' Society Journal*, **29**, 280–2.

Balamoutsos, N. G., Papastephanou, C., and Skourtis, H. T. (1981). Potentiation and prolongation of neuromuscular blockade of pancuronium with *d*-tubocurarine. *Anesthesia and Analgesia*, **60**, 229.

Baraka, A. (1964). The influence of carbon dioxide on the neuromuscular block caused by tubocurarine chloride in the human subject. *British Journal of Anaesthesia*, **36**, 272–8.

Baraka, A. (1985). Action of verapamil at the neuromuscular junction: prejunctional or postjunctional? *Anesthesiology*, **63**, 234–6.

Barlow, R. B. and Ing, H. R. (1948). Curare-like action of polymethylene bis-quaternary ammonium salts. *Nature*, **161**, 718.

Barnett, A. and Ackerman, E. (1969). Neuromuscular blocking activity of gentamycin in cats and mice. *Archives Internationales de Pharmacodynamic*, **179**, 109–17.

Basuray, B. N. And Harris, C. A. (1977). Potentiation of *d*-tubocurarine neuromuscular blockade in cats by lithium chloride. *European Journal of Pharmacology*, **45**, 79–82.

Baurain, M. J., d'Hollander, A. A., Melot, C., Dernovoi, B. S., and Bervais, L. (1991). Effects of residual concentrations of isoflurane on the reversal of vecuronium-induced neuromuscular blockade. *Anesthesiology*, **74**, 474–8.

Bean, B. P., Shrager, P., and Goldstein, D. A. (1981). Modification of sodium and potassium channel gating kinetics by ether and halothane. *Journal of General Physiology*, **77**, 233–53.

Becker, L. D. and Miller, R. D. (1976). Clindamycin enhances a nondepolarizing neuromuscular blockade. *Anesthesiology*, **45**, 84–7.

Bell, K. M. and Rees, J. M. H. (1974). The depressant action of morphine on transmission at a skeletal neuromuscular junction is non-specific. *Journal of Pharmacy and Pharmacology*, **26**, 686–91.

Bellville, J. W., Cohen, E. N., and Hamilton, J. (1964). The interaction of morphine and *d*-tubocurarine on respiration and grip strength in man. *Clinical Pharmacology and Therapeutics*, **5**, 35–42.

Bendtsen, A., Engbaek, J., and Lehnsbo, J. (1983). The interaction between pancuronium and netilmicin on neuromuscular function. *Acta Anesthesiologica Scandinavica*, **27**, Suppl. 78, 83.

Bennett, E. J., Schmidt, G. B., Patel, K. P., and Grundy, E. M. (1977). Muscle relaxants, myasthenia and mustards? *Anesthesiology*, **46**, 220–1.

Bennett, M. J. and Hahn, J. F. (1985). Potentiation of the combination of pancuronium and metocurine by halothane and isoflurane in humans with and without renal failure. *Anesthesiology*, **62**, 759–64.

Benz, H. E., Lunn, J. N., and Foldes, F. F. (1961). Recurarization by intraperitoneal antibiotics. *British Medical Journal*, **ii**, 241–2.

Bikhazi, G. B., Leung, B. S., and Foldes, F. F. (1982*a*) Interaction of neuromuscular blocking agents with calcium channel blockers. *Anesthesiology*, **57**, A268.

Bikhazi, G. B., Leung, I., and Foldes, F. F. (1982*b*). Augmentation of the nueromuscular effect of tubocurarine by verapamil. In *Abstracts 6th European Congress of Anesthesia, London*, (ed. T. B. Boulton, R. S. Atkinson, J. N. Lunn, A. P. Adams, P. J. Horsey, M. Morgan, *et al.*), p. 315. Academic Press, London.

Bikhazi, G. B., Leung, B. S., and Foldes, F. F. (1983). Ca-channel blockers increase potency of neuromuscular blocking agents *in vivo*. *Anesthesiology*, **59**, A269.

Bikhazi, G. B., Foldes, F. F., and Flores, C. (1984). The *in vitro* neuromuscular effects of verapamil, gentamycin and polymyxin B combinations. *Anesthesiology*, **61**, A315.

Black, T. E., Healy, T. E. J., Pugh, N. D., Harper, N. J. N., Petts, H. V., and Sivalingham, T. (1985). Neuromuscular block: atracurium and vecuronium compared and combined. *European Journal of Anaesthesia*, **3**, 29–37.

Blanc-Bimar, M. C., Jadot, G., and Bruguerolle, B. (1979). Modifications of the curarizing action of two short acting curare like agents after the administration of two antiepileptic agents. *Annales Anesthesiologie Français*, **20**, 685–90.

Blitt, C. D., Carlson, G. L., Rolling, G. D., Hamenoff, S. R., and Otto, C. W. (1981). A comparative evaluation of pretreatment with nondepolarizing blockers prior to the administration of succinylcholine. *Anesthesiology*, **55**, 687–9.

Bodley, P. O. and Brett, J. E. (1962). Post-operative respiratory inadequacy and the part played by antibiotics. *Anaesthesia*, **17**, 438–43.

Bonta, I. L., Goorissen, E. M., and Derkx, F. H. (1968). Pharmacological interaction between pancuronium bromide and anaesthetics. *European Journal of Pharmacology*, **4**, 83–91.

Booij, L. H. D. J., Miller, R. D., and Cruyl, J. F. (1978). Neostigmine and 4-aminopyridine antagonism of lyncomycine–pancuronium neuromuscular blockade in man. *Anesthesia and analgesia*, **57**, 316–21.

Booij, L. H. D. J. and Crul, J. F. (1979). The comparative influence of gamma-hydroxy butyric acid, althesin and etomidate on the neuromuscular blocking potency of pancuronium in man. *Acta Anaesthesiologica Belgica*, **30**, 219–23.

Booij, L. H. D. J., Van Egmond, J., van de Pol, F., and Crul, J. F. (1985). Pharmacodynamics of vecuronium, atracurium, tubocurarine and their combinations in the rat *in vivo*. *European Journal of Anaesthesia*, **2**, 279–84.

Borden, H., Clarke, M. T., and Katz, H. (1974). The use of pancuronium bromide in patients receiving lithium carbonate. *Canadian Anaesthetists' Society Journal*, **21**, 79–82.

Boros, M., Chaudhry, I. A., Nagashima, H., Duncalf, R. M., Sherman E. H. and Foldes, F. F. (1984). Myoneural effects of pethidine and droperidol. *British Journal of Anaesthesia*, **56**, 195–201.

Bowen, J. M. and McMullen, W. C. (1975). Influence of induced hypermagnesemia and hypocalcemia on the neuromuscular blocking property of oxytetracycline in the horse. *American Journal of Veterinary Research*, **36**, 1025–8.

Bowman, W. C. (1980). Prejunctional and postjunctional cholinoceptors at the neuromuscular junction. *Anesthesia and Analgesia*, **59**, 935–43.

Bowman, W. C. (1985). The neuromuscular junction: recent developments. *European Journal of Anaesthesiology*, **2**, 59–93.

Bowman, W. C. and Nott, M. W. (1969). Actions of sympathomimetic amines and their antagonists on skeletal muscle. *Pharmacological Reviews*, **21**, 27–72.

Bowman, W. C. and Rand, M. J. (1980). *Textbook of Pharmacology* (2nd edn.) pp. 2.10–12. Blackwell Scientific Publications, Oxford.

Bradamante, V., Kunec-Vajic, E., and Dobric, I. (1984). Butyrilcholinesterase inhibition in patients on glucocorticoid therapy. In *Abstracts 9th IUPHAR Congress, London*, (ed. J. S Gillespie), p. 929P. Macmillan, London.

Bradshaw, E. G. and Maddison, S. (1979). Effect of diazepam at the neuromuscular junction. A clinical study. *British Journal of Anaesthesia*, **51**, 955–60.

Branisteanu, D. D. and Volle, R. L. (1975). Modification by lithium of transmitter release at the neuromuscular junction of the frog. *Journal of Pharmacology and Experimental Therapeutics*, **194**, 362–72.

Brazil, O. V. and Prado-Franceschi, L. (1969). The nature of neuromuscular block produced by neomycin and gentamicin. *Archives Internationales de Pharmacodynamie et Therapie*, **179**, 78–85.

Brodsky, J. B., Brock-Utne, J. G., and Samuels, S. I. (1979). Pancuronium pretreatment and post-succinylcholine myalgias. *Anesthesiology*, 259–61.

Brooks, D. K. and Feldman, S. A. (1962). Metabolic acidosis: A new approach to 'neostigmine resistant curarisation'. *Anaesthesia*, **17**, 161–9.

Bruckner, J., Thomas, K. C., Bikhazi, G. B., and Foldes, F. F. (1980). Neuromuscular drug interactions of clinical importance. *Anesthesia and Analgesia*, **59**, 678–2.

Burkett, L., Bikhazi, G. B., Thomas, K. C., Rosenthal, D. A., Wirda, M. A., and Foldes, F. F. (1979). Mutual potentiation of the neuromuscular effects of antibiotics and relaxants. *Anesthesia and Analgesia*, **58**, 107–15.

Bush, G. H. (1962). Antibiotic paralysis. *British Medical Journal*, **ii**, 1062–3.

Bush, G. H. and Baraka, A. (1964). Factors affecting the termination of curarization in the human subject. *British Journal of Anaesthesia*, **36**, 356–62.

Caldwell, J. E., Laster, M. J., Magorian, T., Heier, T., Yasuda, N., Lynam, D. P., *et al.* (1991). The neuromuscular effects of desflurane, alone and combined with pancuronium or succinylcholine in humans. *Anesthesiology*, **74**, 412–8.

Chapple, D. J., Clark, J. S., and Hughes, R. (1983). Interaction between atracurium and drugs used in anaesthesia. *British Journal of Anaesthesia*, **55**, 17S–22S.

Chasapakis, G. and Dinas, C. (1966). Possible interactions between muscle relaxants and the kallikrein-trypsin inactivator 'Trasylol'. *British Journal of Anaesthesia*, **38**, 838–9.

Chen, J., Kim, Y. D., Dubois, M., Kammerer, W., and MacNamara, T. E. (1983). The increased requirement of pancuronium in neurosurgical patients receiving dilantin chronically. *Anesthesiology*, **59**, A288.

Chiarandini, D. J. (1980). Curare-like effect of propranolol on rat extraocular muscles. *British Journal of Pharmacology*, **69**, 13–9.

Chinyanga, H. M. and Stoyka, W. W. (1974). The effect of colymycin M, gentamycin and kanamycin on depression of neuromuscular transmission induced by pancuronium bromide. *Canadian Anaesthetists Society Journal*, **21**, 569–79.

Chung, F. (1982). Cancer chemotherapy and anaesthesia. *Canadian Anaesthetists' Society Journal*, **29**, 364–71.

Clergue, F., Viires, N., Lemesle, P., Aubier, M., Viars, P., and Pariente, R. (1986). Effect of halothane on diaphragmatic muscle function in pentobarbital anesthetized dogs. *Anesthesiology*, **64**, 181–7.

Conahan, T. J. and Blanck, J. J. (1979). Sarcoplasmic reticulum: Enflurane effect on Ca^{++} dynamics. *Anesthesiology*, **51**, S146.

Crawford, A. C. (1975). Lithium ions and the release of transmitter at the frog neuromuscular junction. *Journal of Physiology*, **246**, 109–42.

Cronnelly, R., Dretchen, K. L., Sokoll, M. D., and Long, J. P. (1973). Ketamine: Myoneural activity and interaction with neuromuscular blocking agents. *European Journal of Pharmacology*, **22**, 17–22.

Cronnelly, R., Morris, R. B., and Miller, R. D. (1983). Comparison of thiopental and midazolam on the neuromscular responses to succinylcholine or pancuronium in humans. *Anesthesia and Analgesia*, **62**, 75–7.

Crul, J. F., Long, G. J., Brunner, E. A., and Coolen, J. M. W. (1966). The changing pattern of neuromuscular blockade caused by succinylcholone in man. *Anesthesiology*, **27**, 729–35.

Cullen, D.J. (1971). The effect of pretreatment with nondepolarizing muscle relaxants on the neuromuscular blocking action of succinylcholine. *Anesthesiology*, **35**, 572–8.

Cuthbert, M. F. (1966). The effect of quinidine and procainamide on the neuromuscular blocking action of suxamethonium. *British Journal of Anaesthesia*, **38**, 775–9.

d'Hollander. A. A., Agoston, S., Capouet, V., Barvais, L., Bomblet, J. P., and Esselen, M. (1985). Failure of metronidazole to alter a vecuronium neuromuscular blockade in humans. *Anesthesiology*, **63**, 99–102.

d'Hollander, A. A., Agoston, S., DeVille, A., and Cuvelier, F. (1983). Clinical and pharmacological actions of a bolus injection of suxamethonium: two phenomena of distinct duration. *British Journal of Anaesthesia*, **55**, 131–4.

Dale, R. C. and Schroeder, E. T. (1976). Respiratory paralysis during treatment of hypertension with trimethaphan camsylate. *Archives of Internal Medicine*, **136**, 816–8.

Dann, W. L. (1971). The effects of different levels of ventilation on the action of pancuronium in man. *British Journal of Anaesthesia*, **43**, 959–62.

Deacock, A. R. de C. and Davies, T. D. W. (1958). The influence of certain ganglionic blocking agents on neuromuscular transmission. B*ritish Journal of Anaesthesia*, **30**, 217–25.

Deacock, A. R. de C. and Hargrove, R. L. (1962). The influence of certain ganglionic blocking agents on neuromuscular transmission. *British Journal of Anaesthesia*, **34**, 357–62.

Del Castillo, J. and Engbaek, L. (1954). The nature of the neuromuscular block produced by magnesium. *Journal of Physiology*, **124**, 370–84.

Delisle, S. and Bevan, D. R. (1982). Impaired neostigmine antagonism of pancuronium during enflurane anaesthesia in man. *British Journal of Anaesthesia*, **54**, 441–5.

Del Pozo, E. and Baeyens, J. M. (1984). Neuromuscular blocking activity of calcium antagonists alone and with aminoglycoside antibiotics. In *Abstracts 9th IUPHAR Congress, London*, (ed. J.S. Gillespie), p. 206., Macmillan, London.

de Silva. A. J. C. (1973). Magnesium intoxication: An uncommon cause of prolonged curarization. Case report. *British Journal of Anaesthesia*, **45**, 1228–9.

de Rosayro, M. and Healy, T. E. J. (1978). Tobramycin and neuromuscular transmission in the rat isolated phrenic nerve–diaphragm preparation. *British Journal of Anaesthesia*, **50**, 251–4.

Diamond, E. M. and Berman, M. C. (1980). The effect of halothane on the stability of Ca transport activity of isolated fragmented sarcoplasmic reticulum. *Biochemistry and Pharmacology*, **29**, 375–81.

Doenicke, A. Dittmann-Kessler, I., Sramota, A., and Beyer, E. (1980). Etomidate and suxamethonium. The duration of relaxation and pseudocholinesterase activity. A clinical experimental study. *Anaesthesist*, **29**, 120–4.

Doenicke, A., Gesing, H., Krumey, I., and Schmidinger, St. (1970). Influence of aprotinin (Trasylol) on the action of suxamethonium. *British Journal of Anaesthesia*, **42**, 943–60.

Doenicke, A., Schmidinger, S., and Krumey, I. (1968). Suxamethonium and serum cholinesterase: comparative studies *in vitro* and *in vivo* on the catabolism of suxamethonium. *British Journal of Anaesthesia*, **40**, 834–44.

Donati, F. and Bevan, D. R. (1981). Controlled succinylcholine infusion in a patient receiving echothiophate eye drops. *Canadian Anaesthetists' Society Journal*, **28**, 488–90.

Donati, F. and Bevan, D. R. (1982). Effect of enflurane and fentanyl on the clinical characteristics of long-term succinylcholine infusion. *Canadian Anaesthetists' Society Journal*, **29**, 59–64.

Donati, R. and Bevan, D. R. (1983). Long-term succinylcholine infusion during isoflurane anesthesia. *Anesthesiology*, **58**, 6–10.

Drachman, D. A. and Skou, J. H. (1965). Procainamide — a hazard in myasthenia gravis. *Archives de Neurologie*, **13**, 316–20.

Dretchen, K. L., Sokoll, M. D., Gergis, S. D., and Long, J. P. (1973). Relative effects of streptomycin on motor nerve terminals and end-plate. *European Journal of Pharmacology*, **22**, 10–6.

Dretchen, K. L., Morgenroth, V. H., Standaert, F. G. and Walts, L. F. (1976*a*). Azathioprine: effects on neuromuscular transmission. *Anesthesiology*, **45**, 604–9.

Dretchen, K. L., Standaert, F. G., Skirbol, L. R., and Morgenroth, V. H. (1976*b*). Evidence for a prejunctional role of cyclic nucleotides in neuromuscular transmission. *Nature*, **264**, 79–81.

Driessen, J. J., Vree, T. B., Booij, L. H. D. J., Van der Pol, F. M., and Crul, J. F. (1983). Effects of some benzodiazepines on peripheral neuromuscular function in the rat *in vitro* hemidiaphragm preparation. *Journal of Pharmacy and Pharmacology*, **36**, 244–7.

Driessen, J. J., Vree, T. B., van Egmond, J., Booij, L. H. D. J.,and Crul, J. F. (1984). *In vitro* interaction of diazepam and oxazepam with pancuronium and suxamethonium. *British Journal of Anaesthesia*, **56**, 1131–7.

Driessen, J. J., Vree, T. B., van Egmont, J., Booij, L. H. D. J., and Crul, J. F. (1985*a*). Interaction of midazolam with two nondepolarizing neuromuscular blocking drugs in the rat '*in vivo*' sciatic nerve–tibialis anterior muscle preparation. *British Journal of Anaesthesia*, **57**, 1089–94.

Driessen, J. J., Wuis, E. W., and Gielen, M. J. M. (1985*b*). Prolonged vecuronium neuromuscular blockade in a patient receiving orally administered dantrolene. *Anesthesiology*, **62**, 523–4.

Drury, P. J. (1977). *The involvement of the adrenoreceptor in skeletal neuromuscular transmission*. PhD thesis, University of Nottingham.

Duke, P. C., Johns, C. H., Pinsky, C., and Goertzen, P. (1979). The effect of morphine on human neuromuscular transmission. *Canadian Anaesthetists' Society Journal*, **26**, 201–5.

Duncalf, D., Chaudhry, I., Aoki, T., Nagashima, H., and Foldes, F. F. (1983). Potentiation of pancuronium, vecuronium and atracurium by *d*-tubocurarine or metocurine. *Anesthesiology*, **59**, A292.

Durant, N. N., Lee, C., and Katz, R. L. (1980). Neuromuscular block with neomycin and tubocurarine. *Anesthesiology*, **53**, S287.

Durant, N. N., Lee, C., and Katz, R. L. (1981). Cumulation of neomycin and its residual potentiation of tubocurarine in the cat. *British Journal of Anaesthesia*, **53**, 571–6.

Durant, N. N., Nguyen, N., Lee, C., and Katz, R. L. (1982). The interaction between ketamine and the new muscle relaxant Norcuron. In: *Abstracts 6th European Congress of Anaesthesiology, London*. (ed. T. B. Boulton, R. S. Atkinson, J. N. Lunn, A. P. Adams, P. J. Horsey, M. Morgan, *et al.*), pp. 149–50. Academic Press, London.

Durant, N. N., Nguyen, N., and Katz, R. L. (1984*a*). Potentiation of vecuronium by ketamine. In *Abstracts 9th IUPHAR Congress, London*. (ed. J. S. Gillespie), pp. 394. Macmillan, London.

Durant, N. N., Nguyen, N., and Katz, R. L. (1984*b*). Potentiation of neuromuscular blockade by verapamil. *Anesthesiology*, **60**, 298–303.

Durham, H. D. and Frank, G. B. (1981). Dual action of meperidine on the frog neuromuscular junction: A prejunctional, opiate receptor-mediated depression of transmitter release and a postjunctional, nonopiate receptor effect on the endplate. *Archives Internationales de Pharmacodynamie et de Therapie* **251**, 150–65.

Dutre, P., Rolly, G., and Vermeulen, H. (1992). Effect of intravenous hypnotics on the actions of pipecuronium. *European Journal of Anaesthesiology*, **9**, 313–7.

Eadsforth, P., Hickmott, K. C., Pollard, B. J., and Kay, B. (1990). The use of atracurium and vecuronium to extend an existing alcuronium neuromuscular blockade. *European Journal of Anaesthesiology*, **7**, 153–7.

Ellis, C. H., Wnuck, A. L., de Beer, E. J., and Foldes, F. F. (1953). Modifying actions of procaine on the myoneural blocking actions of succinylcholine, decamethonium and *d*-tubocurarine in dogs and cats. *American Journal of Physiology*, **174**, 277–82.

Ellis, F. R. (1968). The neuromuscular interaction of propanidid with suxamethonium and tubocurarine. *British Journal of Anaesthesia*, **40**, 818–24.

Emery, E. R. J. (1963). Neuromuscular blocking properties of antibiotics as a cause of postoperative apnoea. *Anaesthesia*, **18**, 57–65.

Engbaek, J. Ording, H., Pedersen, T., and Viby-Mogensen, J. (1984). Dose–response relationship and neuromuscular blocking effects of vecuronium and pancuronium during ketamine anaesthesia. *British Journal of Anaesthesia*, **56**, 953–7.

Engbaek, J., Ording, H., and Viby-Mogensen, J. (1983). Neuromuscular blocking effects of vecuronium and pancuronium during halothane anaesthesia. *British Journal of Anaesthesia*, **55**, 497–500.

Engel, H. L. and Denson, J. S. (1957). Respiratory depression due to neomycin. *Surgery*, **42**, 862–4.

Eppens, H. and Klein, J. W. (1971). Antibiotics and muscle relaxants, a dangerous combination. *Archivum Chirurgicum Neerlandicum*, **23**, 241–8.

Esmaili, M. H., Pleuvry, B. J., and Healy, T. E. J. (1986). Interactions between atracurium and vecuronium on indirectly elicited muscle twitch *in vitro*. *European Journal of Anaesthesia*, **3**, 469–73.

Feldman, S. A. (1963). Effect of changes in electrolytes, hydration and pH upon the reactions to muscle relaxants. *British Journal of Anaesthesia*, **35**, 546–51.

Ferguson, A. and Bevan D. R. (1981). Mixed neuromuscular block: the effect of precurarization. *Anaesthesia*, **36**, 661–6.

Ferres, C. J., Mirakhur, R. K., Pandit, S. K., Clarke, R. S. J., and Gibson FM. (1984). Dose–response studies with pancuronium, vecuronium and their combination. *British Journal of Clinical Pharmacology*, **18**, 947–50.

Ferry, C. B. and Marshall, A. R. (1973). An anti-curare affect of hexamethonium at the mammalian neuromuscular junction. *British Journal of Pharmacology*, **47**, 353–62.

Fiekers, J. F. (1983*a*). Effects of the aminoglycoside antibiotics, streptomycin and neomycin, on neuromuscular transmission, I. Presynaptic considerations. *Journal of Pharmacology and Experimental Therapeutics*, **225**, 487–95.

Fiekers, J. F. (1983*b*). Effects of the aminoglycoside antibiotics, streptomycin and neomycin, on neuromuscular transmission, II. Postsynaptic considerations. *Journal of Pharmacology and Experimental Therapeutics*, **225**, 496–502.

Fisher, D. M. and Miller, R. D. (1983). Interaction of succinylcholine and vecuronium during N_2O-halothane anaesthesia. *Anesthesiology*, **59**, A278.

Flewellen, E. H., Nelson, T. E., and Bee, D. E. (1980). Effect of dantrolene on neuromuscular block by d-tubocurarine and subsequent antagonism by neostigmine in the rabbit. *Anesthesiology*, **52**, 126–30.

Fogdall, R. P. and Miller, R. D. (1974*a*). Prolongation of a pancuronium-induced neuromuscular blockade by polymyxin B. *Anesthesiology*, **40**, 84–7.

Fogdall, R. P. and Miller, R. D. (1974*b*). Prolongation of a pancuronium-induced neuromuscular blockade by clindamycin. *Anesthesiology*, **41**, 407–9.

Fogdall, R. P. and Miller, R. D. (1975). Neuromuscular effects of enflurane, along and combined with *d*-tubocurarine, pancuronium and succinylcholine, in man. *Anesthesiology*, **42**, 173–8.

Foldes, F. F. (1959). Factors which alter the effects of muscle relaxants. *Anesthesiology*, **20**, 464–504.

Foldes, F. F. (1984). Concerning the site of action of verapamil on skeletal muscle *Anesthesiology*, **61**, 783–5.

Foldes, F. F., Bencini, A., and Newton, D. E. F. (1980). Influence of halothane and enflurane on the neuromuscular effects of Org NC45 in man. *British Journal of Anaesthesia*, **52**, 64–5S.

Foldes, F. F., Aoki, T., Ono, K., Duncalf, D., and Nagashima, H. (1984). Potentiation of pancuronium, vecuronium and atracurium by *d*-tubocurarine and metocurine. *Anesthesia and Analgesia*, **63**, 211.

Foldes, F. F., Lunn, J. N. and Benz, H. G. (1962). Respiratory depression from drug combinations. *Journal of the American Medical Association*, **183**, 672–3.

Forshaw, P. J. (1977). The inhibitory effect of cadmium on neuromuscular transmission in the rat. *European Journal of Pharmacology*, **42**, 371–7.

Fragan, R. J., Booij, L. H. D. J., van der Pol, F., Robertson, E. N., and Crul, J. F. (1983). Interactions of diisopropyl phenol (ICI35868) with suxamethonium, vecuronium and pancuronium *in vitro*. *British Journal of Anaesthesia*, **55**, 433–5.

Frederickson, R. C. A., and Pinsky, C. (1971). Morphine impairs acetylcholine release but facilitates acetylcholine action at a skeletal neuromuscular junction. *Nature*, **231**, 93–4.

Fried, M. J. and Protheroe, D. T. (1986). D-penicillamine-induced myasthenia gravis: its relevance for the anaesthetist. *British Journal of Anaesthesia*, **58**, 1191–3.

Futamachi, K. J. and Prince, D. A. (1975). Effect of penicillin on an excitatory synapse. *Brain Research*, **100**, 589–97.

Gage, P. W. and Hamill, P. O. (1976). Effects of several inhalation anaesthetics on the kinetics of postsynaptic conductance in mouse diaphragm. *British Journal of Pharmacology*, **57**, 263–72.

Gage, P. W., Lonergan, M., and Torda, T. A. (1980). Presynaptic and postsynaptic depressant effects of phenytoin sodium at the neuromuscular junction. *British Journal of Pharmacology*, **69**, 119–21.

Gencarelli, P. J., Swen, J., Koot, H. W. J., and Miller, R. D. (1983). The effects of hypercarbia and hypocarbia on pancuronium and vecuronium neuromuscular blockades in anesthetized humans. *Anesthesiology*, **59**, 376–80.

Gencarelli, P. J., Swen, J., Koot, H. W. J., and Miller, R. D. (1984). Hypocarbia and spontaneous recovery from vecuronium neuromuscular blockade in anesthetized patients. *Anesthesia and Analgesia*, **63**, 608–10.

Gergis, S. D., Sokoll, M. D., and Rubbo, J. T. (1977). Effect of sodium nitroprusside and trimethaphan on neuromuscular transmission in frog. *Canadian Anaesthetists' Society Journal*, **24**, 220–7.

Gessa, G. L. and Ferrari, W. (1963). Influence of chlorothiazide, hydrochlorothiazide, and acetazolamide on neuromuscular transmission in mammals. *Archives Internationales de Pharmacodynamie et Therapie*, **144**, 258–68.

Ghoneim, M. M. and Long, J. P. (1970). The interaction between magnesium and other neuromuscular blocking agents. *Anesthesiology*, **32**, 23–7.

Ghoneim, M. M., Urgena, R. B., Dretchen, K., and Long, J. P. (1972). The interaction between *d*-tubocurarine and gallamine during halothane anaesthesia. *Canadian Anaesthetists' Society Journal*, **19**, 66–74.

Giala, M. M. and Paradelis, A. G. (1979). Two cases of prolonged respiratory depression due to interaction of pancuronium with colistin and streptomycin. *Journal of Antimicrobial Chemotherapy*, **5**, 234–5.

Giala, M., Sareyiannis, E., Cortsaris, N., Paradelis, A., and Lappas, D. G. (1982). Possible interaction of pancuronium and tubocurarine with oral neomycin. *Anaesthesia*, **37**, 776.

Giesecke, A. H., Morris, R. A., and Dalton, M. D. (1968). Of magnesium, muscle relaxants, toxemic parturients and cats. *Anesthesia and Analgesia*, **47**, 689–95.

Giesecke, A. H., Morris, R. E., Dalton, M. D. and Stephen C. R. (1968). Of magnesium, muscle relaxants, toxemic parturients, and cats. *Anesthesia and analgesia*, **47**, 689–95.

Ginsborg, B. C. and Stephenson, R. P. (1974). On the simultaneous action of two competitive antagonists. *British Journal of Pharmacology*, **51**, 287–300.

Ginsberg, B. L. and Jenkinson, D. H. (1976). Transmission of impulses from nerves to muscle. In *Neuromuscular junction: handbook of experimental pharmacology*, (ed. E. Zaimis), p. 229. Springer-Verlag, Berlin.

Glidden, R. S., Martyn, J. A. J., and Tomera, J. F. (1988). Azathioprine fails to alter the dose–response curve of *d*-tubocurarine in rats. *Anesthesiology*, **68**, 595–8.

Glisson, S. N., El-Etr, A. A., and Lim, R. (1979). Prolongation of pancuronium-induced neuromuscular blockade by intravenous infusion of nitroglycerin. *Anesthesiology*, **51**, 47–9.

Glisson, S. N., Sanchez, M. M., El-Etr, A. A., and Lim, R. A. (1980). Nitroglycerin and the neuromuscular blockade produced by gallamine, succinylcholine, *d*-tubocurarine, and pancuronium. *Anesthesia and Analgesia*, **59**, 117–22.

Goudsouzian, N., Martyn, J., Rudd, G. D., Liu, L. M. P., and Lineberry, C. G. (1986). Continuous infusion of atracurium in children. *Anesthesiology*, **64**, 171–4.

Graham, C. W. and Walts, L. F. (1979). Nitroprusside and the duration of tubocurarine and pancuronium. *Anaesthesia*, **34**, 1005–9.

Gramstad, L., Lilleaasen, P., and Minsaas, B. (1981). Onset time for alcuronium and pancuronium after cremophor-containing anaesthetics. *Acta Anaesthesiologica Scandinavica*, **25**, 484–6.

Gramstad, L., Gjerlow, J. A., Hysing, E. S, and Rugstad, H. E. (1986). Interaction of cyclosporin and its solvent, cremophor, with atracurium and vecuronium. *British Journal of Anaesthesia*, **58**, 1149–55.

Gray, H. St. J., Slater, R. M., and Pollard, B. J. (1989). The effect of acutely administered phenytoin on vecuronium-induced neuromuscular blockade. *Anaesthesia*, **44**, 379–81.

Grogono, A. W. (1963). Anaesthesia for atrial defibrillation: Effect of quinidine on muscular relaxation. *Lancet*, **II**, 1039–40.

Haberman, E. and Richard, T. (1986). Intracellular calcium binding proteins as targets for heavy metal ions. *Trends in Pharmacological Sciences*, **7**, 298–9.

Hall, D. R., McGibbon, D. H., Evans, C. C., and Meadows, G. A. (1972). Gentamicin, tubocurarine, lignocaine and neuromuscular blockade: a case report. *British Journal of Anaesthesia*, **44**, 1329–32.

Hall, E. D. (1980). Glucocorticoid modification of the responsiveness of fast (type 2) neuromuscular system to edrophonium and *d*-tubocurarine. *Experimental Neurology*, **69**, 349–59.

Hanson, J. (1974). Effects of repetitive stimulation on membrane potentials and twitches in humans and rat intercostal muscle fibres. *Acta Physiologica Scandinavica*, **92**, 238–48.

Haque, N., Thrasher, K., Werk, E. E., Knowles, H. C., and Sholiton, L. J. (1972). Studies on dexamethasone metabolism in man: effect of diphenylhydantoin. *Journal of Clinical Endocrinology and Metabolism*, **34**, 44–50.

Harrah, M. D., Way, W. L., and Katzung, B. G. (1970). The interaction of *d*-tubocurarine with anti-arrhythmic drugs. *Anesthesiology*, **33**, 406–10.

Healy, T. E. J., O'Shea, M., and Massey, J. (1981). Disopyramide and neuromuscular transmission. *British Journal of Anaesthesia*, **53**, 495–8.

Henderson, F., Prior, C., Dempster, J., and Marshall, I. G. (1986). The effects of chloramphenicol isomers on the motor end plate nicotinic receptor-ion channel complex. *Molecular Pharmacology*, **29**, 52–64.

Herishanu, Y. and Rosenberg, P. (1975). Beta blockers and myasthenia gravis. *Annals of Internal Medicine*, **83**, 834–5.

Hershkowitz, N., Dretchen, K. L., and Raines, A. (1978). Carbamazepin suppression of posttetanic potentiation at the neuromuscular junction. *Journal of Pharmacology and Experimental Therapeutics*, **207**, 810–6.

Hickey, D. R., Sangwan, S., and Bevan, J. C. (1988). Phenytoin-induced resistance to pancuronium. *Anaesthesia*, **43**, 757–9.

Hilgenberg, J. C. and Stoelting, R. K. (1981). Characteristics of succinylcholine-produced phase II neuromuscular block during enflurane, halothane and fentanyl anesthesia. *Anesthesia and Analgesia*, **60**, 192–6.

Hill, G. E. and Wong, K. C. (1980). Effects of prostaglandins and indomethacin on neuromuscular blocking agents. *Canadian Anaesthetists Society Journal*, **27**, 146–9.

Hill, G. E., Wong, K. C., and Hodges, M. R. (1976). Potentiation of succinylcholine neuromuscular blockade by lithium carbonate. *Anesthesiology*, **44**, 439–42.

Hill, G. E., Wong, K. C., and Hodges, M. R. (1977). Lithium carbonate and neuromuscular blocking agents. *Anesthesiology*, **46**, 122–6.

Hill, G. E., Wong, K. C., Shaw, C. L., and Blatnick, R. A. (1978). Acute and chronic changes in intra- and extracellular potassium and responses to neuromuscular blocking agents. *Anesthesia and Analgesia*, **57**, 417–21.

Huan, C. L. H. (1981). Effects of local anaesthetics on the relationship between charge movements and the contractile threshold in frog skeletal muscle. *Journal of Physiology*, **320**, 381–91.

Hubbard, J. I., Jones, S. F., and Landon, E. M. (1968). On the mechanism by which calcium and magnesium affect the release of transmitter by nerve impulses. *Journal of Physiology*, **196**, 75–86.

Hughes, R. (1970). The influence of changes in acid–base balance on neuromuscular blockade in cats. *British Journal of Anaesthesia*, **42**, 658–68.

Hughes, R. and Payne, J. P. (1979). Interactions of halothane with nondepolarizing neuromuscular blocking drugs in man. *British Journal of Clinical Pharmacology*, **7**, 485–90.

Hughes, R. and Zacharias, F. J. (1976). Myasthenic syndrome during treatment with practolol. *British Medical Journal*, **i**, 460–1.

Ikeda, S. R., Aronstam, R. S., and Daly, J. W. (1984). Interactions of bupivacaine with ionic channels of the nicotinic receptor. Electrophysiological and biochemical studies. *Molecular Pharmacology*, **26**, 293–303.

Jansen, E. C. and Howardy-Hansen, P. (1979). Objective measurement of succinylochline-induced fasciculations and the effect of pretreatment with pancuronium and gallamine. *Anesthesiology*, **51**, 159–60.

Johnston, R. R., Miller, R. D., and Way, W. L. (1974). Interaction of ketamine with neuro-muscular blocking drugs. *Anesthesia and Analgesia*, **53**, 496–9.

Jones, R. M., Cashman, J. N., Casson, W. R., and Broadbent, M. P. (1985). Verapamil potentiation of neuromuscular blockade: Failure of reversal with neostigmine but prompt reversal with edrophonium. *Anesthesia and Analgesia*, **64**, 1021–5.

Jones, R. M., Pearce, A. C., and Adams, A. P. (1984). Muscle relaxant synergy: relation to multiple sites of action within the neuromuscular junction. *8th World Congress of Anaesthesiology, Book of Abstracts*, **2**, A309.

Katz, R. L. (1971). Clinical neuromuscular pharmacology of pancuronium. *Anesthesiology*, **34**, 550–8.

Katz, B. and Miledi, R. (1965). The effect of calcium on acetylcholine release from motor nerve terminals. *Proceedings of The Royal Society London*, **161**, 496–502.

Katz, R. L. (1971a). Modification of the action of pancuronium by succinylcholine and halothane. *Anesthesiology*, **35**, 602–6.

Katz, R. L. (1971b). Clinical neuromuscular pharmacology of pancuronium. *Anesthesiology*, **34**, 550–6.

Katz, R. L. and Gissen, A. J. (1967). Neuromuscular and electromyographic effects of halothane and its interaction with *d*-tubocurarine in man. *Anesthesiology*, **28**, 564–7.

Katz, R. L. and Wolf, C. E. (1964). Neuromuscular and electromyographic studies in man: Effects of hyperventilation, carbon dioxide inhalation and *d*-tubocurarine. *Anesthesiology*, **25**, 781–7.

Kay, B., Chestnut, R. J., Sum Ping, J. S. T., and Healy, T. E. J. (1987). Economy in the use of muscle relaxants. Vecuronium after pancuronium. *Anaesthesia*, **42**, 277–80.

Kennedy, R. and Gallindo, A. (1975). Neuromuscular transmission in a mammalian prepara-tion during exposure to enflurane. *Anesthesiology*, **42**, 432–42.

Kim, C. S., Arnold, F. J., Itani, M. S. and Martyn, J. A. J. (1992). Decreased sensitivity to metocurine during long-term phenytoin therapy may be attributable to protein binding and acetylcholine receptor changes. *Anesthesiology*, **77**, 500–6.

Kiraly, S. J. and Hamilton, J. T. (1978). Ketamine and the neuromuscular junction. Interpretation of the mechanism of some clinical peripheral side effects. *Progress in Neuropsychopharmacology*, **2**, 179–89.

Knight, C. L., Barnes, P. K., and Feldman, S. A. (1978). The interaction of halothane and pancuronium bromide. *Anaesthesia*, **33**, 139–42.

Komatsu, T., Mori, K., Uchida, M., and Seukane, K. (1979). The effects of halothane on the contractile properties of human skeletal muscles. *Hiroshima Journal of Anaesthesia*, **15**, S81–7.

Kornfeld, P., Horowitz, S. H., and Genkins, G. (1976). Myasthenia gravis unmasked by antiarrhythmic agents. *Mount Sinai Journal of Medicine, NY*, **43**, 10–4.

Kramer, G. L. and Wells, J. N. (1980). Xanthines and skeletal muscles: lack of relationship between phosphiodiesterase inhibition and increased twitch tension in rat diaphragm. *Molecular Pharmacology*, **17**, 73–8.

Kraunak, P., Pleuvry, B. J., and Rees, J. M. H. (1977). *In vitro* study of interactions between i.v. anaesthetics and neuromuscular blocking agents. *British Journal of Anaesthesia*, **49**, 765–70.

Kraynack, B. J., Lawson, N. W., and Gintautas, J. (1982a). Local anaesthetic effect of verapamil *in vitro*. *Regional Anaesthesia*, **7**, 76–7.

Kraynack, B. J., Lawson, N. W., and Gintautas, J. (1982b). Local anesthetic effect of verapamil *in vitro*. *Regional Anaesthesia*, **7**, 114–7.

Kraynack, B. J., Lawson, N. W., and Gintautas, J. (1982c). Verapamil reduces indirect muscle twitch amplitude and potentiates pancuronium *in vitro*. *Anesthesiology*, **57**, A265.

Kraynack, B. J., Lawson, N. W., and Gintautas, J. (1983*a*). Neuromuscular blocking action of verapamil in cats. *Canadian Anaesthetists' Society Journal*, **30**, 242–7.

Kraynack, B. J., Lawson, N. W., and Gintautas, J. (1983*b*). Effects of verapamil on indirect muscle twitch responses. *Anesthesia and Analgesia*, **62**, 827–30.

Krieg, N., Rutten, J. M. J., Crul, J. F., and Booij, L. H. D. J. (1980). Preliminary review of the interactions of Org NC45 with anaesthetics and antibiotics in animals. *British Journal of Anaesthesia*, **52**, 33S–36S.

Krieg, N., Hendrickx, H. H. L., and Crul, J. F. (1981). Influence of suxamethonium on the potency of Org NC45 in anaesthetized patients. *British Journal of Anaesthesia*, **53**, 259–62.

Kronenfeld, M. A., Thomas, S. J., and Turndorf, H. (1986). Recurrence of neuromuscular blockade after reversal of vecuronium in a patient receiving polymyxin/amikacin sternal irrigation. *Anesthesiology*, **65**, 93–4.

Kuba, K. (1970). Effects of catecholamines on the neuromuscular junction in the rat diaphragm. *Journal of Physiology*, **211**, 551–70.

Laflin, M. J. (1977). Interaction of pancuronium and corticosteroids. *Anesthesiology*, **47**, 471–2.

Landers, D. F., Becker G. L., and Wong, K. C. (1989). Calcium, calmodulin, and anesthesiology. *Anesthesia and Analgesia*, **69**, 100–12.

Lawson, N. W., Kraynack, B. J. and Gintautas, J. (1983). Neuromuscular and electrocardiographic responses to verapamil in dogs. *Anesthesia and Analgesia*, **62**, 50–4.

Lebowitz, H. M., Blitt, C. D., and Walts, L. F. (1970). Depression of twitch response to stimulation of the ulnar nerve during ethrane anesthesia in man. *Anesthesiology*, **33**, 52–7.

Lebowitz, P. W., Ramsey, F. M., Savarese, J. J., and Ali, H. H. (1980). Potentiation of neuromuscular blockade in man produced by combinations of pancuronium and metocurine or pancuronium and *d*-tubocurarine. *Anesthesia and Analgesia*, **59**, 604–9.

Lee, C. and de Silva, A. J. C. (1979*a*). Acute and subchronic neuromuscular blocking characteristics of streptomycin: a comparison with neomycin. *British Journal of Anaesthesia*, **51**, 431–4.

Lee, C. and de Silva, A. J. C. (1979*b*). Interaction of neuromuscular blocking effects of neomycin and polymyxin B. *Anesthesiology*, **50**, 218–20.

Lee, C., Chen, D., Barnes, A., and Katz, R. L. (1976). Neuromuscular block by neomycin in the cat. *Canadian Anaesthetists' Society Journal*, **23**, 527–33.

Lee, C., Chen, D., and Nagel, E. L. (1977). Neuromuscular block by antibiotics: polymyxin B. *Anesthesia and Analgesia*, **56**, 373–7.

Lee, C., Chen, D., and Engel, E. L. (1977). Neuromuscular block by antibiotics: polymyxin B. *Anesthesia and Analgesia*, **56**, 373–7.

Lee, C., de Silva, A. J..C., and Katz, R. L. (1978). Antagonism of polymyxin B-induced neuromuscular and cardiovascular depression by 4-aminopyridine in the anaesthetized cat. *Anesthesiology*, **49**, 256–9.

Lee, C., Durant, N., Heng, A., and Katz, R. L. (1979*a*). Prejunctional neuromuscular block 'in vivo'. *Anesthesiology*, **51**, S273.

Lee, C., Durant, N. N., and Katz, R. L. (1979*b*). Mechanism of neomycin-induced neuromuscular block. *Anesthesiology*, **51**, S285.

Lee, C., Yang, E., and Katz, R. L., (1982). Norcuron: neuromuscular effects and absence of interaction with diazepam. In *Abstracts 6th European Congress of Anaesthesiology, London*. (ed. T. B. Boulton *et al.*), p. 306. Academic Press, London.

Lee, D. C., Liu, H. H., and John, T. R. (1983). Presynaptic and postsynaptic actions of procainamide on neuromuscular transmission. *Muscle and Nerve*, **6**, 442–7.

Leeuwin, R. S. and Veldsema-Currie, R. D. (1980). Direct effects of glucocorticoids at the neuromuscular junction. *British Journal of Pharmacology*, **68**, 144p–5p.

Leeuwin, R. S., Veldsema-Currie, R. D., Van Wilgenburg, H., and Ottenhof, M. (1981). Effects of corticosteroids on neuromuscular blocking actions of d-tubocurarine. *European Journal of Pharmacology*, **69**, 165–73.

Leeuwin, R. S. and Walters, E. C. M. J. (1977). Effects of corticosteroids on sciatic nerve-tibialis anterior muscle of rats treated with hemicholinium-3. *Neurology*, **27**, 171–7.

Lindesmith, L. A., Baines, R. O., Bigelow, D. B., and Petty, T. L. (1968). Reversible respiratory paralysis associated with polymyxin therapy. *Annals of Internal Medicine*, **68**, 318–27.

Liu, A. Y. C. (1984). Modulation of the function and activity of CAMP dependent protein kinase by steroid hormones. *Trends in Pharmacological Sciences*, **5**, 107–8.

L'Hommedieu, C. S., Nicholas, D., Armes, D. A., Jones, P., Nelson, T., and Pickering, L. K. (1983). Potentiation of magnesium sulphate-induced neuromuscular weakness by gentamicin, tobramycin and amikacin. *Journal of Pediatrics*, **102**, 629–31.

Lynam, G. H., Williams, C. C., and Preston, D. (1980). The use of lithium carbonate to reduce infection and leukopenia during systemic chemotherapy. *New England Journal of Medicine*, **302**, 257–60.

Madden, K. S. and Van der Koot, W. (1985). Indomethacin, prostaglandin E, and transmission at the frog neuromuscular junction. *Journal of Pharmacology and Experimental Therapeutics*, **232**, 305–14.

Maleque, M. A., Warnick, J. E., and Albuquerque, E. X. (1981). The mechanism and site of action of ketamine on skeletal muscle. *Journal of Pharmacology and Experimental Therapeutics*, **219**, 638–45.

Marquis, J. K. and Deschenes, R. J. (1982). A reevaluation of calcium-local anesthetic antagonism. *Experimental Neurology*, **76**, 547–52.

Martyn, J. A. J., Leibel, W. S., and Matteo, R. S. (1983). Competitive nonspecific binding does not explain the potentiating effects of muscle relaxant combinations. *Anesthesia and Analgesia*, **62**, 160–3.

Marwaha, J. (1980). Some mechanisms underlying actions of ketamine on electromechanical coupling in skeletal muscle. *Journal of Neuroscience Research*, **5**, 43–50.

Matsuo, S., Rao, D. B. S., Chaudry, I. and Foldes, F. F. (1978). Interaction of muscle relaxants and local anesthetics at the neuromuscular junction. *Anesthesia and Analglesia*, **57**, 580–7.

McCammon, R. L., Hilgenberg, J. C., Sandage, B. W., and Stoelting, R. K. (1985). The effect of esmolol on the onset and duration of succinylcholine induced neuromuscular blockade. *Anesthesiology*, **63**, A317.

McIndewar, I. C. and Marshall, R. J. (1981). Interactions between the neuromuscular blocking drug ORG NC 45 and some anaesthetic, analgesic and antimicrobial agents. *British Journal of Anaesthesia*, **53**, 785–92.

McQuillen, M. P. and Engbaek, L. (1975). Mechanism of colistin-induced neuromuscular depression. *Archives of Neurology*, **32**, 235–8.

McQuillen, M. P., Gross, M., and Johns, R. J. (1963). Chlorpromazine induced weakness in myasthenia gravis. *Archives of Neurology*, **8**, 286–90.

Messick, J. M., Maas, L., Faust, R. J., and Cucchiara, R. F. (1982). Duration of pancuronium neuromuscular blockade in patients taking anticonvulsant medication. *Anesthesia and Analgesia*, **61**, 203–4.

Meyers, E. F. (1977). Partial recovery from pancuronium neuromuscular blockade following hydrocortisone administration. *Anesthesiology*, **46**, 148–50.

Middleton, C. M., Pollard, B. J., Kay, B., and Healy, T. E. J. (1988). Use of atracurium or vecuronium to prolong the action of tubocurarine. *British Journal or Anaesthesia*, **62**, 659–63.

Miledi, R. and Thies, R. (1971). Tetanic and post-tetanic rise in frequency of miniature end-plate potentials in low calcium solutions. *Journal of Physiology*, **212**, 245–57.

Miller, R. D. and Roderick, L. L. (1977). Pancuronium-induced neuromuscular blockade. *Anesthesiology*, **46**, 333–5.

Miller, R. D. and Roderick, L. L. (1978). Diuretic induced hypokalaemia, pancuronium neuromuscular blockade and its antagonism by neostigmine. *British Journal of Anaesthesia*, **50**, 541–4.

Miller, R. D., Way, W. L., and Katzung, B. G. (1967). The potentiation of neuromuscular blocking agents by quinidine. *Anesthesiology*, **28**, 1036–41.

Miller, R. D., Way, W. L., Dolan, W. M., Stevens, W. C., and Eger, E. I. (1971*a*). Comparative neuromuscular effects of pancuronium, gallamine and succinylcholine during forane and halothane anesthesia in man. *Anesthesiology*, **35**, 509–14.

Miller, R. D., Eger, E. I., Way, W. L., Stevens, W. C., and Dolan, W. M. (1971*b*). Comparative neuromuscular effects of forane and halothane alone and in combination with *d*-tubocurarine in man. *Anesthesiology*, **35**, 38–42.

Miller, R. D., Way, W. L., Dolan, W. M., Stevens W. C., and Eger, E. I. (1972). The dependence of pancuronium and *d*-tubocurarine-induced neuromuscular blockades on alveolar concentrations of halothane and forane. *Anesthesiology*, **37**, 573–81.

Miller, R. D., Van Nyhuis, L. S., Eger, II, E. I., and Way, W. L. (1975). The effect of acid–base balance on neostigmine antagonism of *d*-tubocurarine-induced neuromuscular block. *Anesthesiology*, **42**, 377–383.

Miller, R. D., Crique, M., and Eger, E. I. (1976*a*). Duration of halothane anesthesia and neuromuscular blockade with *d*-tubocurarine. *Anesthesiology*, **44**, 206–10.

Miller, R. D., Sohn, Y. J., and Matteo, R. S. (1976*b*). Enhancement of *d*-tubocurarine neuromuscular blockade by diuretics in man. *Anesthesiology*, **45**, 442–5.

Miller, R. D., Agoston, S., Van der Pol, F., Booij, L. H. D. J., and Crul, J. F. (1979). Effect of different anesthetics on the pharmacokinetics and pharmacodynamics of pancuronium in the cat. *Acta Anesthesiologica Scandinavica*, **23**, 285–90.

Mirakhur, R. K., Gibson, F. M., and Ferres, C. J. (1985). Vecuronium and *d*-tubocurarine combination: potentiation of effect. *Anesthesia and Analgesia*, **64**, 711–4.

Mirakhur, R. K., Pandit, S. K., Ferres, C. J., and Gibson, F. M. (1984). Time course of muscle relaxation with a combination of pancuronium and tubocurarine. *Anesthesia and Analgesia*, **63**, 437–40.

Morita, K., Matsuo, S., Nagashima, H., Kanarek, B., Duncalf, D. and Foldes, F. F. (1979). *In vivo* muscle relaxant–local anesthetic interactions. *Anesthesiology*, **51**, S282.

Morris, R. E. and Giesecke, A. (1968). Potentiation of muscle relaxants by magnesium sulphate therapy in toxemia of pregnancy. *Southern Medical Journal*, **61**, 25–8.

Murthy, V. S., Patel, K. D., Elangovan, R. G., Hwang, T. F., Solochek, S. M., Steck, J. D., and Laddu, A. R. (1985). Effects of esmolol on circulatory response to intubation and succinylocholine-induced neuromuscular blockade in man. *Anesthesiology*, **63**, A361.

Nakamura, K., Koide, M., Imanaga, T., Ogasawara, H., Takahashi, M., and Yoshikana, M. (1980). Prolonged neuromuscular blockade following trimethaphan infusion. A case report and *in vitro* study of cholinesterase inhibition. *Anaesthesia*, **35**, 1202–7.

Nocite, J. R., Zuccolotto, S. N., De Vasconcelo, R. A., and Pereira, I. T. (1977). Influence of ketamine on duration of action of suxamethonium. *Revista Brasileira Anestesiologia*, **27**, 619–24.

Noebels, J. L. and Prince, D. A. (1977). Presynaptic origin of penicillin afterdischarges at mammalian nerve terminals. *Brain Research*, **138**, 59–75.

Norman, J., Katz, R. L., and Seed, R. F. (1970). The neuromuscular blocking action of pancuronium in man during anaesthesia. *British Journal of Anaesthesia*, **42**, 702–10.

Orbeli, L. A. (1923). Die sympathetische innervation der Skelettmuskeln. *Bulletin Institut Science Leshaft*, **6**, 194–7.

Ornstein, E., Matteo, R. S., Schwartz, A. E., Silverberg, P. A., Young, W. L., and Diaz, J. (1987). The effect of phenytoin on the magnitude and duration of neuromuscular block following atracurium and vecuronium. *Anesthesiology*, **67**, 191–6

Ornstein, E., Matteo, R. S., Young, W. L., and Diaz, J. (1985). Resistance to metocurine-induced neuromuscular blockade in patients receiving phenytoin. *Anesthesiology*, **63**, 294–8.

Oswald, R. E. (1983). Binding of phencyclidine to the detergent solubilized acethlcholine receptor from *Torpedo marmorata*. *Life Sciences*, **32**, 1143–9.

Pandit, S. K., Ferres, C. J., Gibson, F. M., and Mirakhur, R. K. (1986). Time course of action of combinations of vecuronium and pancuronium. *Anaesthesia*, **41**, 151–4.

Payne, J. P. (1958). The influence of carbon dioxide on neuromuscular blocking activity of relaxant drugs in the cat. *British Journal of Anaesthesia*, **30**, 206–14.

Payne, J. P. (1960). The influence of changes in blood pH on the neuromuscular blocking properties of tubocurarine and dimethyl tubocurarine in the cat. *Acta Anaesthesiologica Scandinavica*, **4**, 83–90.

Park, W. Y., Balingit, P. E., and MacNamara, T. E. (1974). Interactions of gallamine and pancuronium with tubocurarine under morp-nine–nitrous oxide–oxygen anesthesia in man. *Anesthesia and Analgesia*, **53**, 723–9.

Pinsky, C., and Frederickson, R. C. A. (1971). Morphine and nalorphine impair neuromuscular transmission. *Nature*, **231**, 94–6.

Pittinger, C. B., Eryasa, Y., and Adamson, R. (1970). Antibiotic induced paralysis. *Anesthesia and Analgesia*, **49**, 487–501.

Pollard, B. J. (1991). *Studies concerning the interactions between nondepolarising neuromuscular blocking agents*. MD Thesis, University of Sheffield, pp. 211–50.

Pollard, B. J. and Jones, R. M. (1983). Interactions between tubocurarine, pancuronium and alcuronium demonstrated in the rat phrenic nerve–hemidiaphragm preparation. *British Journal of Anaesthesia*, **55**, 1127–31.

Pollard, B. J. and Miller, R. A. (1973). Potentiating and depressant effects of inhalational anaesthetics on the rat phrenic nerve-diaphragm preparation. *British Journal of Anaesthesia*, **45**, 404–15.

Potter, J. M., Edeson, R. O., Campbell, R. J., and Forbes, A. M. (1980). Potentiation by gentamicin of nondepolarizing neuromuscular block in the cat. *Anaesthesia and Intensive Care*, **8**, 20–5.

Poulton, T. J., James, F. M., and Lockridge, O. (1979). Prolonged apnea following trimethapan and succinylcholine. *Anesthesiology*, **50**, 54–6.

Pridgen, J. E. (1956). Respiratory arrest thought to be due to intraperitoneal neomycin. *Surgery*, **40**, 571–4.

Prostan, M. and Varagic, V. M. (1981). The effect of local anaesthetics on the isometric contraction of the isolated hemidiaphragm of the rat. *Archives Internationales de Pharmacodynamie*, **250**, 30–9.

Rang, H. P. and Rylett, R. J. (1984). The interaction between hexamaethonium and tubocurarine on the rat neuromuscular junction. *British Journal of Pharmacology*, **81**, 519–31.

Rashkovsky, O. M., Agoston, S., and Ket, J. M. (1985). Interaction between pancuronium bromide and vecuronium bromide. *British Journal of Anaesthesia*, **57**, 1063–6.

Reddy, P., Guzman, A, Robalino, J., and Shevde, K. (1989). Resistance to muscle relaxants in a patient receiving prolonged testosterone therapy. *Anesthesiology*, **70**, 871–3.

Riker, W. F., and Wescoe, W. C. (1951). The pharmacology of Flaxedil with observations on certain analogs. *Annals of New York Academy of Science*, **54**, 373–94.

Riker, W. F., Baker, T., and Okamato, M. (1975). Glucocorticoids and mammalian nerve excitability. *Archives of Neurology*, **32**, 688–94.

Robertson, E. N., Fragen, R. J., Booij, L. H. D. J., Van Egmond, J., and Crul, J. F. (1983). Some effects of diisopropyl phenol (ICI 35868) on the pharmacodynamics of atracurium and vecuronium in anaesthetized man. *British Journal of Anaesthesia*, **55**, 723–8.

Robertson, G. S. (1967). Serum protein and cholinesterase changes in association with oral contraceptive pills. *Lancet*, **i**, 232–3.

Rosenberg, H. (1979). Sites and mechanisms of action of halothane on skeletal muscle function *in vitro*. *Anesthesiology*, **50**, 331–5.

Roth, S. and Ebrahim, Z. Y. (1987). Resistance to pancuronium in patients receiving carbamezepine. *Anesthesiology*, **66**, 691–3.

Rozen, M. S. and Whan, F. McK. (1972). Prolonged curarization associated with propranolol. *Medical Journal of Australia*, **1**, 467–9.

Rubbo, J. T., Sokoll, M. D., and Gergis, S. D. (1977). Comparative neuromuscular effects of lincomycin and clindamycin. *Anesthesia and Analgesia*, **56**, 329–32.

Rupp, S. M., Fahey, M. R., and Miller, R. D. (1983). Neuromuscular and cardiovascular effects of attracurium during nitrous oxide–fentanyl and nitrous oxide–isoflurane anaesthesia. *British Journal of Anaesthesia*, **55**, 67S–70S.

Rupp, S. M., Miller, R. D., and Gencarelli, P. J. (1984a). Vecuronium induced neuromuscular blockade during enflurane, isoflurane and halothane anesthesia in humans. *Anesthesiology*, **60**, 102–5.

Rupp, S. M., McChristian, J. W., and Miller, R. D. (1984b). Atracurium neuromuscular blockade during halothane/N$_2$O and enflurane/N$_2$O anesthesia in humans. *Anesthesiology*, **61**, A288.

Rupp, S. M., McChristian, J. W., and Miller, R. D. (1985). Neuromuscular effects of atracurium during halothane–nitrous oxide and enflurane–nitrous oxide anesthesia in humans. *Anesthesiology*, **63**, 16–9.

Russell, A. S. and Lindstrom, J. M. (1978). Penicillamine-induced myasthenia gravis associated with antibodies to acetylcholine receptors. *Neurology*, **28**, 847–9.

Sabawala, P. B. and Dillon, J. B. (1958). Action of volatile anesthetics on human muscle preparations. *Anesthesiology*, **19**, 587–94.

Saito, H., Akutagawa, T., Kitahata, L. M., Stagg, P., Collins, J. G., and Scurlock, J. E. (1984). Interactions of lidocaine and calcium in blocking the compound action potential of frog sciatic nerve. *Anesthesiology*, **60**, 205–8.

Sappaticci, K. A., Ham, J. A., Sohn, Y. J., Miller, R. D., and Dretchen, K. L. (1982). Effects of furosemide on the neuromuscular junction. *Anesthesiology*, **57**, 381–8.

Satwicz, P. R., Martyn, J. A. J., Szyfelbein, S. K., and Firestone, S. (1984). Potentiation of neuromuscular blockade using a combination of pancuronium and dimethyltubocurarine. *British Journal of Anaesthesia*, **56**, 479–84.

Schmidt, L., Vick, N. A., and Sadove, N. S. (1963). The effect of quinidine on the action of muscle relaxants. *Journal of the American Medical Association*, **183**, 669–72.

Schopp, R. T. (1978). Paralytic action of manganese in the dog. *Archives Internationales de Pharmacodynamie et de Therapie*, **232**, 235–45.

Schuh, F. T. (1981). Über den synergismus bei der kombination von nichtdepolarisierenden muskelrelaxantien. *Anesthesist*, **30**, 537–42.

Schwartz, A. E., Matteo, R. S., Ornstein, E., and Silverberg, P. A. (1986). Acute steroid therapy does not alter nondepolarizing muscle relaxant effects in humans. *Anesthesiology*, **65**, 326–7.

Schwarz, S., Agoston, S., and Houwertjes, M. C. (1986). Does intravenous infusion of nitroglycerin potentiate pancuronium and vecuronium induced neuromuscular blockade? *Anesthesia and Analgesia*, **65**, 156–60.

Sevcik, C. (1980). Differences between the actions of thiopental and pentobarbital in squid giant axons. *Journal of Pharmacology and Experimental Therapeutics*, **214**, 657–63.

Shanks, C. A. (1982). Dose–response curves for alcuronium and pancuronium alone and in combination. *Anaesthesia and Intensive Care*, **10**, 248–51.

Sharma, K. K. and Sharman, U. C. (1978). Influence of diazepam on the effect of neuromuscular blocking agents. *Journal of Pharmacy and Pharmacology*, **30**, 64.

Singh, Y. N. Marshall, I. G., and Harvey, A. L. (1978*a*). Some effects of the aminoglycoside antibiotic amikacin on neuromuscular and autonomic transmission. *British Journal of Anaesthesia*, **50**, 109–17.

Singh, Y. N., Harvey, A. L., and Marshall, I. G. (1978*b*). Antibiotic-induced paralysis of the mouse phrenic nerve–hemidiaphragm preparation, and reversibility by calcium and by neostigmine. *Anesthesiology*, **48**, 418–24.

Singh, Y. N., Marshall, I. G., and Harvey, A. L. (1978*c*). Reversal of antibiotic induced muscle paralysis by 3,4-aminopyridine. *Journal of Pharmacy and Pharmacology*, **30**, 249–50.

Singh, Y. N., Marshall, I. G., and Harvey, A. L. (1979). Depression of transmitter release and post-junctional sensitivity during neuromuscular block produced by antibiotics. *British Journal of Anaesthesia*, **51**, 1027–33.

Singh, Y. N., Marshall, I. G., and Harvey, A. L. (1982). Pre- and postjuncitonal blocking effects of aminoglycoside, polymyxin, tetracycline and lincosamide antibiotics. *British Journal of Anaesthesia*, **54**, 1295–1306.

Sirnes, T. B. (1954). Some effects of barbituric acid and derivatives on function of mammalian skeletal muscles. *Acta Pharmacologica Toxocologica*, **10**, 1–12.

Skaredoff, M. N., Roaf, E. R., and Datta, S. (1982). Hypermagnesaemia and anaesthetic management. *Canadian Anaesthetists' Society Journal*, **29**, 35–41.

Sklar, G. S. and Lanks, K. W. (1977). Effects of trimethaphan and sodium nitroprusside on hydrolysis of succinylcholine *in vitro*. *Anesthesiology*, **47**, 31–3.

Sobek, V. (1982). The effect of calcium, neostigmine and 4-aminopyridine upon respiratory arrest and depression of cardiovascular functions after aminoglycosidic antibiotics. *Arzneimittelforschung Drug Research*, **32**, 222–4.

Sokoll, M. D. and Diecke, F. P. J. (1969). Some effects of streptomycin on frog nerve in vitro. *Archives International de Pharmacodynamie et Therapie*, **177**, 332–9.

Sokoll, M. D. and Gergis, S. D. (1981). Antibiotics and neuromuscular function. *Anesthesiology*, **55**, 148–59.

Soterpoulos, G. C. and Standaert, F. G. (1973). Neuromuscular effects of morphine and naloxone. *Journal of Pharmacology and Experimental Therapeutics*, **184**, 136–84.

Standaert, F. G. and Riker, W. F. (1967). The consequences of cholinergic drug actions on motor nerve terminals. *Annals of the New York Academy of Science*, **144**, 517–33.

Stanley, V. G., Giesecke, A. H., and Jenkins, M. T. (1969). Neomycin-curare neuromuscular block and reversal in cats. *Anesthesiology*, **31**, 228–32.

Stanski, D. R., Ham, J., Miller, R. D., and Sheiner, L. B. (1979). Pharmacokinetics and pharmacodynamics of *d*-tubocurarine during nitrous oxide–narcotic and halothane anesthesia in man. *Anesthesiology*, **51**, 235–41.

Stanski, D. R., Ham, J., Miller, R. D., and Sheiner, L. B. (1980). Time-dependent increase in sensitivity of *d*-tubocurarine during enflurane anesthesia in man. *Anesthesiology*, **52**, 483–7.

Stirt, J. A., Katz, R. L., Murray, A. L., Schehl, D. L. and Lee, C. (1983). Modification of atracurium blockade by halothane and by suxamethonium. A review of clinical experience. *British Journal of Anaesthesia*, **55**, 71–5S.

Strahan, S. K., Pleuvry, B. J., and Modla, C. Y. (1985). Effect of meptazinol on neuromuscular transmission in the isolated rat phrenic nerve-diaphragm preparation. *British Journal of Anaesthesia*, **57**, 1095–9.

Suzuki, H., Yazaki, S., Kanayama, T., Nahagawa, H., Ogawa, S., Kuniyoshi, K., and Tai, K. (1977). Neuromuscular effects of i.a. infusion of lignocaine in man. *British Journal of Anaesthesia*, **49**, 1117–22.

Swen, J. (1984). Vecuronium, pipecuronium and pancuronium in inhalation anaesthesia. In *Abstracts 6th European Congress of Anaesthesiology London*, (ed. S. Agoston, H. Bergmann, S. Schwarz, and K. Steinbereithner), pp. 160–9. Wilhelm Maudrich, Vienna.

Swen, J., Gencarelli, P. J., and Koot, H. W. J. (1985). Vecuronium infusion dose requirements during fentanyl and halothane anesthesia in humans. *Anesthesia and Analgesia*, **64**, 411–4.

Swen, J., Koot, H. W. J., Bencini, A., Ket, J. M., Hermans, J., and Agoston, S. (1990). The interaction between suxamethonium and the succeeding non-depolarizing neuromuscular blocking agent. *European Journal of Anaesthesiology*, **7**, 203–9.

Talbot, P. A. and Alderdice, M. T. (1982). Primidone but not phenylethylmalonamide, a major metabolite, increases nerve evoked transmitter release at the frog neuromuscular junction. *Journal of Pharmacology and Experimental Therapeutics*, **222**, 87–93.

Talbot, P. A. and Alderdice, M. T. (1984). Effects of primidone, phenobarbital and phenylethylmalonamide in the stimulated frog neuromuscular junction. *Journal of Pharmacology and Experimental Therapeutics*, **228**, 121–7.

Tang, A. H. and Schroeder, L. A. (1968). The effect of lincomycin on neuromuscular transmission. *Toxicology and Applied Pharmacology*, **12**, 44–7.

Tassonyi, E. (1977). A clinical study on the effects of flunitrazepam (rohypnol) in neuromuscular blockade. *Annales Anesthesiologie Francais*, **18**, 740–6.

Tassonyi, E. (1984). Effects of midazolam (Ro 21-3981) on neuromuscular block. *Pharmatherapeutica*, **3**, 678–81.

Tewfik, G. I. (1957). Trimethaphan — its effect on the pseudocholinesterase level of man. *Anaesthesia*, **12**, 326–9.

Thesleff, S. (1980). Aminopyridines and synaptic transmission. *Neurosciences*, **6**, 1413–9.

Torda, T. (1980). The nature of gentamicin-induced neuromuscular block. *British Journal of Anaesthesia*, **52**, 325–9.

Torda, T. A. and Gage, P. W. (1977). Postsynaptic effect of i.v. anaesthetic agents at the neuromuscular junction. *British Journal of Anaesthesia*, **49**, 771–6.

Torda, T. A. and Murphy, E. C. (1979). Presynaptic effect of i.v. anaesthetic agents at the neuromuscular junction. *British Journal of Anaesthesia*, **51**, 353–6.

Trotta, E. E., Freire, G. L., and Godinho, C. S. (1980). The mode of action of local anaesthetics on the calcium pump of brain. *Journal of Pharmacology and Experimental Therapeutics*, **214**, 670–4.

Tsai, S. K. and Lee, C. (1989). Ketamine potentiates nondepolarizing neuromuscular relaxants in a primate. *Anesthesia and Analgesia*, **68**, 5–8.

Usubiaga, J. E. (1968). Neuromuscular effects of beta-adrenergic blockers and their interaction with skeletal muscle relaxants. *Anesthesiology*, **29**, 485–92.

Usubiaga, J. E., Wikinski, J. A., and Morales, R. L. (1967). Interaction of intravenously administered procaine, lidocaine and succinylcholine in anesthetized subjects. *Anesthesia and Analgesia*, **46**, 39–45.

Utting, J. (1963). pH as a factor influencing plasma concentrations of *d*-tubocurarine. *British Journal of Anaesthesia*, **35**, 706–10.

Van Nyhuis, L. S., Miller, R. D., and Fogdall, R. P. (1976). The interaction between *d*-tubocurarine, pancuronium, polymyxin B, and neostigmine on neuromuscular function. *Anesthesia and Analgesia*, **55**, 224–8.

van der Spek, A. F. L., Zupan, J. T., Pollard, B. J., and Shork, M. A. (1988). Interactions of vecuronium and atracurium in an *in vitro* nerve muscle preparation. *Anesthesia and Analgesia*, **67**, 240–6.

van Poorten, J. F., Dhasmana, K. M., Kuypers, R. S. M., and Erdmann, W. (1984). Verapamil and reversal of vecuronium neuromuscular blockade. *Anesthesia and Analgesia*, **63**, 155–7.

Van Wilgenburg, H. (1979). The effect of prednisolone on neuromuscular transmission in the rat diaphragm. *European Journal of Pharmacology*, **55**, 355–61.

van Wilgenburg, H. (1980). Effects of glucocorticoid on acetylcholine release at the neuro-muscular junction. *British Journal of Pharmacology*, **68**, 144.

Varagic, V. M. (1984). Opposite effects of adenosine on the isolated diaphragm of the rat. Direct and indirect electrical stimulation. In *Abstracts 9th IUPHAR Congress, London*, (ed. J. S. Gillespie), p. 386. Macmillan, London.

Varagic, V. M., Prostran, M., and Kentera, D. (1980). Interaction of halothane and amino-phylline on the isolated hemidiaphragm of the rat. *European Journal of Pharmacology*, **61**, 35–45.

Veldsema-Currie, R. D. and Van Marle, J. (1984). Depletion of acetylcholine by hemicholin-ium 3 in rat diaphragm is less with dexamethasone. In *Abstracts 9th IUPHAR Congress, London*, (ed. J. S. Gillespie), p. 2059P. Macmillan, London.

Vincent, A., Newsom-Davis, J., and Martin, V. (1978). Anti-acetylcholine receptor anti-bodies in *d*-penicillamine associated with myasthenia gravis. *Lancet*, **i**, 1254.

Virtue, R. W. (1975). Comparison of gallamine and *d*-tubocurarine effects on fasciculations after succinylcholine. *Anesthesia and analgesia*, **54**, 81–2.

Vitez, T. S., Miller, R. D., Eger, E. I., van Nyhuis, L. S., and Way, W. L. (1974). Comparison in vitro of isoflurane and halothane potentiation of *d*-tubocurarine and suc-cinylcholine neuromuscular blocks. *Anesthesiology*, **41**, 53–6.

Vizi, E. S., Illes, P., Ronai, A., and Knoll, J. (1972). The effect of lithium on acetylcholine release and synthesis. *Neuropharmacology*, **11**, 521–30.

Wachtel, R. E. (1985). Calcium channel antagonists shorten the lifetime of endplate channels activated by acetylcholine. *Anesthesiology*, **63**, A326.

Wali, F. A. (1983). Interactions between i.v. anaesthetics and depolarization agents at chick neuromuscular junction. *British Journal of Anaesthesia*, **55**, 240P.

Wali, F. A. (1984). The neuromuscular effects of lignocaine. *General Pharmacology*, **15**, 197–200.

Walts, L. F. and Dillon, J. (1970). The influence of the anesthetic agent on the action of curare in man. *Anesthesia and Analgesia*, **49**, 17–21.

Walts, L. F. and Rusin, W. D. (1977). The influence of succinylcholine on the duration of pancuronium neuromusuclar blockade. *Anesthesia and Analgesia*, **56**, 22–5.

Waterman, P. M. and Smith, R. B. (1977). Tobramycin-curare interactions. *Anesthesia and Analgesia*, **56**, 587–8.

Watland, D. C., Long, J. P., Pittinger, C. B., and Cullen, S. C. (1957). Neuromuscular effects of ether, cyclopropane, chloroform and fluothane. *Anesthesiology*, **18**, 883–90.

Waud, B. E. (1979). Decrease in dose requirement of *d*-tubocurarine by volatile anesthetics. *Anesthesiology*, **51**, 298–302.

Waud, B. E., Farrell, L., and Waud, D. R. (1982*b*). Lithium and neuromuscular transmission. *Anesthesia and Analgesia*, **61**, 399–402.

Waud, B. E. and Waud, D. R. (1975*a*). Comparison of the effects of general anesthetics on the end plate of skeletal muscle. *Anesthesiology*, **43**, 540–7.

Waud, B. E. and Waud, D. R. (1975*b*). The effects of diethyl ether, enflurane and isoflurane at the neuromuscular junction. *Anesthesiology*, **42**, 275–80.

Waud, B. E. and Waud, D. R. (1979). Effects of volatile anesthetics on directly and indirectly stimulate skeletal muscle. *Anesthesiology*, **50**, 103–10.

Waud, B. E. and Waud, D. R. (1980). Interaction of calcium and potassium with neuromuscular blocking agents. *British Journal of Anaesthesia*, **52**, 863–6.

Waud, B. E. and Waud, D. R. (1984). Quantitative examination of the interation of competitive neuromuscular blocking agents on the indirectly elicited muscle twitch. *Anesthesiology*, **61**, 420–27.

Waud, B. E. and Waud, D. R. (1985). Interaction among agents that block end-plate depolarization competitively. *Anesthesiology*, **63**, 4–15.

Waud, B. E., Mookerjee, A., and Waud, D. R. (1982). Chronic potassium depletion and sensitivity to tubocurarine. *Anesthesiology*, **57**, 111–5.

Way, W. L., Katzung, B. G., and Larson, Jr, C. P. (1967). Recurarization with quinidine. *Journal of the American Medical Association*, **200**, 163–4.

Weisman, S. J. (1949). Masked myasthenia gravis. *Journal of the American Medical Association*, **141**, 917–9.

Welch, G. W. and Waud, B. E. (1980). Bretylium tosylate and neuromuscular transmission. *Anesthesiology*, **53**, S285.

Welch, G. W. and Waud, B. E. (1982). Effect of bretylium on neuromuscular transmission. *Anesthesia and Analgesia*, **61**, 442–4.

Wells, J. N. and Miller, J. R. (1983). Inhibition of cyclic nucleotide phosphodiesterase in muscles. *Trends in Pharmacological Sciences*, **4**, 385–7.

Whittaker, M., Britten, J. J., and Wicks, R. J. (1981). Inhibition of the plasma cholinesterase variants by propranolol. *British Journal of Anaesthesia*, **53**, 511–6.

Williams, J. P., Broadbent, M. P., Pearce, A. C., and Jones, R. M. (1983). Verapamil potentiates the neuromuscular blocking effects of enflurane *in vitro*. *Anesthesiology*, **59**, A276.

Wilson, R. W., Ward, M. D., and Johns, T. R. (1974). Corticosteroids: a direct effect at the neuromuscular junction. *Neurology*, **24**, 1091–5.

Wilson, S. L., Miller, R. D., Wright, C., and Hasse, D. (1976). Prolonged neuromuscular blockade associated with trimethaphan. A case report. *Anesthesia and Analgesia*, **55**, 353–6.

Wirtavuori, K., Salmenpera, M., and Tammisto, T. (1982). Effect of hypocarbia and hypercarbia on the antagonism of pancuronium induced neuromuscular blockade with neostigmine in man. *British Journal of Anaesthesia*, **54**, 57–61.

Wong, K. C. (1969). Some synergistic effects of curare and gallamine. *Federation Proceedings* **28**, 420.

Wong, K. C. and Jones, J. R. (1971). Some synergistic effects of *d*-tubocurarine and gallamine. *Anesthesia and Analgesia*, **50**, 285–90.

Wright, J. M. and Collier, B. (1976). The site of neuromuscular block produced by polymyxin B and rolitetracycline. *Canadian Journal of Physiology and Pharmacology*, **54**, 926–36.

Wright, J. M. and Collier, B. (1977). The effect of neomycin upon transmitter release and action. *Journal of Pharmacology and Experimental Therapeutics*, **200**, 576–87.

Young, A. P. and Sigman, D. S. (1981). Allosteric effects of volatile anesthetics on the membrane-bound acetylcholine receptor protein, Part 1. *Molecular Pharmacology*, **20**, 498–505.

Young, A. P., Oshiki, J. R., and Sigman, D. S. (1981). Allosteric effects of volatile anesthetics on the membrane-bound acetylcholine receptor protein, Part 2. *Molecular Pharmacology*, **20**, 506–10.

Zalman, F., Perloff, J. K., Durant, N. N., and Campion, D. S. (1983). Acutre respiratory failure following intravenous verapamil in Duchenne's muscular dystrophy. *American Heart Journal*, **105**, 510–11.

Zsigmond, K. L. and Robbins, G. (1972). The effect of a series of anticancer drugs on plasma cholinesterase activity. *Canadian Anaesthetists' Society Journal*, **19**, 75–82.

Zsigmond, E. and Eldertton, T. E. (1968). Abnormal reaction to procaine and succinylcholine in a patient with inherited atypical plasma cholinesterase. *Canadian Anaesthetists' Society Journal*, **15**, 498–500.

Zukaitis, M. G. and Hoech, G. P. (1979). Train of 4 measurement of potentiation of curare by lidocaine. *Anesthesiology*, **51**, S288.

13

What the relaxant does to the patient

B. J. Pollard

It is probably true that all drugs have some effects which are additional to their principal action. Drugs used in anaesthesia are no exception. Some of these side-effects can be turned to the anaesthetists' advantage; the majority, however, are unwanted. It is important to be aware of these additional effects in order to make a more logical choice of drug for each patient. In fact, the more aware the anaesthetist is of these potential side-effects, the more safely should the drug be used. The principal unwanted effects are those on the cardiovascular system and the potential for histamine release. A number of other considerations are important however, which include effects on the central nervous system, autonomic nervous system, muscles, plasma electrolytes, and cholinesterase, as well as potential effects of the metabolic breakdown products of the relaxants.

CARDIOVASCULAR EFFECTS

Most of the older neuromuscular blocking agents possess unwanted actions on the cardiovascular system. Indeed, the demise of some agents has been brought about by the presence of cardiovascular side-effects and yet more potential neuromuscular blocking agents have been found to have considerable effect on the cardiovascular system which have prevented their further development. The cardiovascular system is one of the most important systems in the body, so any adverse effects on this system are potentially serious, in particular in patients who are critically ill or who already have significant cardiovascular disease. One of the criteria for the ideal neuromuscular blocking agent is that it should be devoid of adverse cardiovascular side-effects (see Chapter 1). The new neuromuscular blocking agents, although not all completely devoid of adverse effects, have must less effect on the cardiovascular system.

Tubocurarine

The original neuromuscular blocking agent, tubocurarine, is probably the agent with the most severe unwanted effects on the cardiovascular system. Hypotension commonly follows the injection of tubocurarine even in normal clinical doses. There may be a small compensatory tachycardia, but this does not always happen and the heart rate may even fall slightly. There is usually a decrease in systemic vascular resistance with very little effect on cardiac output, although an increase in systemic vascular resistance and a decrease in cardiac output have been reported (Stoelting 1972). The reduction in blood pressure following tubocurarine depends upon the anaesthetic agents in use and their doses (Munger *et al.* 1974). The time course of the fall in blood pressure parallels the onset of neuromuscular block, reaching a maximum in approximately four to five minutes.

There seem to be two main mechanisms underlying the cardiovascular effects of tubocurarine — block of autonomic ganglia and histamine release. Tubocurarine is a surprisingly potent blocking agent at autonomic ganglia in doses very similar to those producing neuromuscular block (McCullough *et al.* 1970; Hughes and Chapple 1976*a*; Lee Son and Waud 1980). This was well demonstrated by Hughes and Chapple (1976*a*), who constructed dose–response curves to neuromuscular block and ganglionic block which were very similar (Fig. 13.1). It is interesting that the heart rate changes little and may even fall, despite a reduction in the blood pressure which would be expected to be accompanied by a compensatory tachycardia. It is likely that this is due to a simultaneous blocking action at both parasympathetic and sympathetic ganglia which are similarly affected by tubocurarine (Guyton and Reeder 1950). It must be noted that other potential mechanisms have been identified which may contribute to the hypotensive effect of tubocurarine. The preservative agent chlorbutanol is included in some formulations and this may have a hypotensive effect (Stoelting 1971). A direct myocardial depressant action of

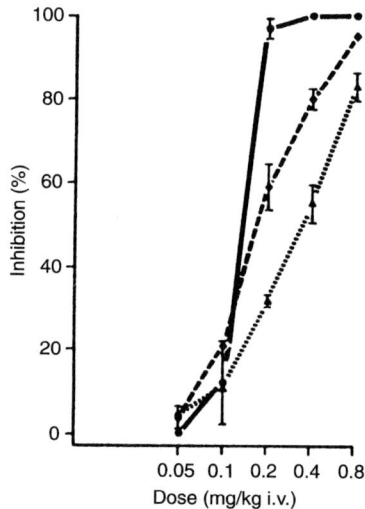

Fig. 13.1 Log dose–response curves with respect to inhibition of neuromuscular transmission (solid line), vagal activity (dashed line) and sympathetic ganglionic activity (dotted line) of tubocurarine in the cat. (From Hughes and Chapple 1976.)

tubocurarine has been described (Johnstone *et al.* 1978) and tubocurarine may have effect on dopaminergic systems (Nelson and Steinsland 1983).

When tubocurarine is used, clinically the cardiovascular actions must be constantly remembered. They may not be particularly important in the fit healthy patient. If the patient is hypovolaemic or has a reduction in cardiovascular reserve, however, the use of tubocurarine may be associated with potentially serious falls in blood pressure.

Alcuronium

The cardiovascular side-effects of alcuronium are considerably less than those of tubocurarine (Baraka 1967). There may be a fall in blood pressure accompanied by an increase in heart rate at normal clinical doses, although this is not usually of any clinical significance in the fit healthy patient (Foldes *et al.* 1963; Kennedy and Kelman 1970). In higher doses or in a patient with pre-existing cardiovascular disease, a decrease in blood pressure, cardiac output, and systemic vascular resistance may occur (Hunter 1964; Coleman *et al.* 1972; Harrison 1972; Blanloeil *et al.* 1982).

The mechanism for the cardiovascular effects is not precisely known. Histamine release may be involved. A weak vagal blocking action and weak antagonism at autonomic ganglia have also been reported (Kennedy and Kelman 1970; Hughes and Chapple 1976*a*; Karhunen *et al.* 1985).

Metocurine

Metocurine was developed in an attempt to reduce the unwanted side-effects seen with tubocurarine. The cardiovascular side-effects are certainly less (Stoelting 1974; Savarese *et al.* 1977; Antonio *et al.* 1979; Zaidan and Kaplan 1982), and haemodynamically metocurine is reported to be approximately eight times safer than tubocurarine (Hughes and Chapple 1976*a*, *b*). The only significant cardiovascular effects are a small decrease in blood pressure with associated increase in heart rate which occur at doses over about 0.4 mg/kg. The capacity for ganglion block from metocurine is very much less than that with tubocurarine (Hughes and Chapple 1976*a*, *b*) and it is possible that the cardiovascular effects are the results of histamine release.

Gallamine

Tachycardia is a characteristic of the use of gallamine. Doses as small as 20 mg may result in an increase in heart rate, and rates above 120 beats per minute are occasionally seen (Eisele *et al.* 1971). The tachycardia begins with a similar time-course to the onset of neuromuscular block but outlasts the block. In addition to the tachycardia there may also be an increase in arterial pressure and cardiac output (Kennedy and Farman 1968; Stoelting 1973). Gallamine is not a wise choice of relaxant in patients where a tachycardia might be hazardous, e.g. many patients with ischaemic heart disease.

The mechanism underlying the tachycardia caused by gallamine is principally a block of the cardiac vagus nerve. This has been conclusively demonstrated in laboratory animals and takes place at the muscarinic receptors on the heart (Riker and Wescoe 1951; Hughes and Chapple 1976a; Lee Son and Waud 1980). The administration of atropine in the presence of gallamine may cause a further increase in heart rate, suggesting that gallamine does not maximally block the vagus. Gallamine has also been reported to increase noradrenalin release from sympathetic nerve endings and also to inhibit re-uptake of released noradrenalin, both of which could contribute to the tachycardia (Brown and Crout 1970; Vercruysse et al. 1979). The significance of the effects on noradrenalin is uncertain (Reitan et al. 1973).

Pancuronium

The administration of a normal clinical dose of pancuronium is frequently accompanied by a tachycardia together with an increase in blood pressure and cardiac output (Loh 1970; Kelman and Kennedy 1971; Stoelting 1972; Coleman et al. 1972). These effects are often only present to a small degree, which possibly reflects the cardiovascular depressant effect of the anaesthetic agents which are effectively antagonizing these side-effects of pancuronium. The sympathomimetic side-effects of pancuronium are usually to the advantage of the patient. They can, however, be troublesome if pancuronium is administered to patients with pre-existing tachyarrhythmias or who are receiving other drugs which may themselves have a sympathomimetic action, e.g. tricyclic antidepressants (Edwards et al. 1979) or aminophylline (Belani et al. 1982). In the presence of medical conditions which may be associated with an increase in circulating catecholamines, e.g. phaeochromocytoma, pancuronium has been reported to be able to produce a potentially hazardous increase in heart rate and blood pressure (Jones and Hill 1981; Hirano et al. 1984). Abnormal heart rhythms, e.g. nodal rhythm or ventricular extrasystoles, may occasionally be encountered (Saemund and Dalenius 1981). Pancuronium is regarded by many anaesthetists as the relaxant of choice for cardiac anaesthesia.

The mechanism behind the cardiovascular actions of pancuronium appears to be partly due to an inhibitory action on the cardiac vagus (Saxena and Bonta 1970; Hughes and Chapple 1976a; Lee Son and Waud 1980). Pancuronium also appears to exert an inhibitory action on muscarinic receptors at a number of other sites, which include blood vessels (Vercruysse et al. 1978, 1979) and sympathetic ganglia (Gardiner et al. 1978). Pancuronium also increases noradrenalin release from sympathetic nerve endings and inhibits the re-uptake of noradrenalin at these sites (Domenech et al. 1976; Quintana 1977; Docherty and McGrath 1978). The existance of a direct myocardial effect of pancuronium is uncertain because it has been reported both to produce no effect on myocardial contractility (Duke et al. 1975) and also to increase myocardial contractility (Seed and Chamberlain 1977; Iwatsuki et al. 1980). Pancuronium inhibits cholinesterase in clinical doses, the significance of which is unclear (Barzu et al. 1974; Stovner et al. 1975; Cardan et al. 1976; Cardan 1978; Schuh 1977; Foldes and Deery 1983).

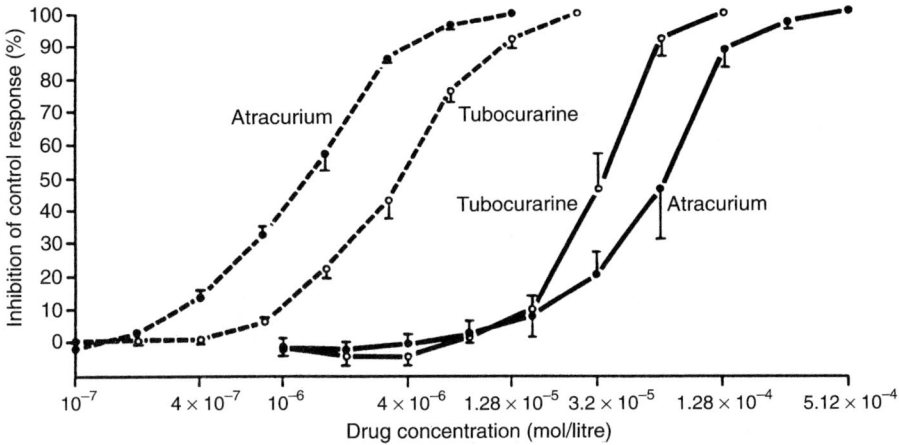

Fig. 13.2 Log dose–response curves for tubocurarine and atracurium *in vitro* at the neuromuscular junction (phrenic nerve–diaphragm, dashed lines) and at the autonomic ganglia (hypogastric nerve–vas deferens, solid lines). (From Healy and Palmer 1982.)

Atracurium

One of the key factors which promoted the development of atracurium was its favourable cardiovascular profile (Stenlake 1982). There is a wide separation between the dose which produces neuromuscular block and that at which significant cardiovascular effects appear (Hughes and Chapple 1981; Healy and Palmer 1982). The ratio of potency for vagal inhibition to neuromuscular block may be as high as 1:25 (Hughes and Chapple 1981). The ganglionic blocking capacity of atracurium was compared with that of tubocurarine by Healy and Palmer (1982) who showed that the dose ratio of atracurium for neuromuscular block: ganglion block was approximately 48:1 (Fig. 13.2).

The excellent cardiovascular profile has been noted in many studies (Katz *et al.* 1982; Moyers *et al.* 1982; Sokoll *et al.* 1983; Robertson *et al.* 1983; Hilgenberg and Stoelting 1986). No changes were observed in cardiac output, systemic vascular resistance or pulmonary vascular resistance in dogs in doses up to 0.4 mg/kg (Moyers *et al.* 1982), although a small decrease in blood pressure with associated increase in heart rate has been reported, especially when using higher doses. It is thought that this effect may be caused by released histamine (Basta *et al.* 1982; Guggiari *et al.* 1985). One interesting effect which has been associated with the use of atracurium is sudden profound bradycardia developing during the anaesthetic (Carter 1983; Hunter 1983). It seems likely that this is not caused by atracurium but rather reflects a lack of vagolytic action of atracurium allowing the unmasking of bradycardias due to surgical stimulation. It would seem that the older neuromuscular blocking agents possessed a greater degree of vagolytic action than we realized at the time. These bradycardias can be profound (asystole has been observed) and are more often seen when a high dose narcotic technique is in use.

Vecuronium

Vecuronium is very similar to atracurium in its lack of cardiovascular side-effects (Marshall *et al.* 1980; Gregoretti *et al.* 1982; Saxena *et al.* 1983; Fitzal *et al.* 1983; Morris *et al.* 1983; Mirakhur *et al.* 1983). The dose ratio for neuromuscular block to vagal block has been estimated as between 1:60 (Durant *et al.* 1979) and 1:96 (Sutherland *et al.* 1983). Vecuronium has negligible action on autonomic ganglia even at higher doses (Barnes *et al.* 1982). The clean cardiovascular profile of vecuronium gives it the same propensity for unmasking bradycardias as atracurium (Ferres *et al.* 1983; Salmanpera *et al.* 1983; Starr *et al.* 1986), a problem which is most noticeable when a narcotic technique is employed.

Pipecuronium

One of the principal features of pipecuronium is its lack of cardiovascular side-effects. Following an intubating dose of pipecuronium there are negligible changes in heart rate, mean arterial pressure, cardiac index, or rate pressure product (Tassonyi *et al.* 1988; Stanley *et al.* 1991). A small reduction in both cardiac output and mean arterial pressure of less than 10% with no change in heart rate was reported following a dose of four times the ED_{95} by Wierda *et al.* (1990). Bradycardia was reported following pipecuronium by Dubois *et al.* (1991).

Doxacurium

The cardiostability when using doxacurium is as impressive as that following pipecuronium. A number of studies have examined the cardiovascular effects of doxacurium and no changes were seen except for a small decrease in heart rate in a few patients (Stoops *et al.* 1988; Reich *et al.* 1989; Emmott *et al.* 1990).

Rocuronium

This neuromuscular blocking agent has been noted to be devoid of cardiovascular effects within the normal dose range (Cason *et al.* 1990). When the dose was increased to 2.5–5 times the ED_{95}, an increase in heart rate was observed in some patients (Booij and Knape 1991; Mellinghoff *et al.* 1991). Vagal block has been noted in laboratory animals at high doses (Muir *et al.* 1989). The drug is relatively new and the amount of data on this subject is presently limited.

Mivacurium

Initial studies in patients scheduled to undergo coronary artery surgery showed no important changes in mean arterial pressure, systemic vascular resistance or cardiac index (Stoops *et al.* 1989). Further studies have, however, shown that when the dose is increased above 0.2 mg/kg a decrease in blood pressure is seen with an accompanying tachycardia (Choi *et al.* 1989; Savarese *et al.* 1989; From *et al.* 1990). This effect is more pronounced if the mivacurium is given rapidly (Savarese *et al.* 1989). Many of these cardiovascular changes appear to be the result of histamine release by the mivacurium.

Suxamethonium

A commonly seen cardiovascular side-effect of suxamethonium is bradycardia. This may occur after the initial intubating dose of suxamethonium, especially in patients who have received a prior dose of fentanyl (Sorensen *et al.* 1984) and also not uncommonly in children. It is more commonly seen following a second or subsequent dose of suxamethonium and it is good anaesthetic practice to administer a prophylactic dose of atropine (or similar) if repeated doses of suxamethonium are being considered. The bradycardia may be extreme, leading to asystole.

The mechanism underlying this effect is thought to be due to a direct stimulation of the vagus by the suxamethonium molecules which structurally closely resemble acetylcholine. A possible alternative mechanism involving noradrenalin release triggered by suxamethonium (Nigrovic *et al.* 1983*a*) leading to an imbalance between autonomic mechanisms has been proposed (Nigrovic 1984). This hypothesis remains unproven.

HISTAMINE RELEASE

The release of histamine is not an uncommon sequel to the administration of a drug. The higher the dose administered, the more likely is there to be a significant release of histamine, which may manifest itself clinically. It must be remembered that although histamine release is associated with allergic and anaphylactic reactions, where it is one of the principal mediators, drugs may release histamine by a direct action upon mast cells without invoking any form of immunological response (Assem 1984). Certain families of drugs are particularly troublesome in this respect, and the neuromuscular blocking agents are one of these groups. It has been suggested that the presence of a charged quaternary nitrogen moiety is the important factor (Baldo *et al.* 1985; Harle *et al.* 1985) and it is also possible that drug-specific IgE antibodies might be involved (Fisher and Munro 1983; Vervloet *et al.* 1983; Vervloet 1985) in some of these 'anaphylactoid' reactions. It is certain, however, that many drugs can release histamine through a direct action on mast cells. It is only necessary to produce plasma levels above approximately 3 ng/ml for clinical manifestations of flushing to appear. Further increases in the plasma concentration progressively cause hypotension, tachycardia, and urticaria. When the plasma concentration is higher than 10 ng/ml severe bronchospasm and cardiac arrest may be seen (Lorenz *et al.* 1982).

The neuromuscular blocking agent which possesses the greatest potential for histamine release is tubocurarine. Histamine release is often seen in clinical doses, manifest as cutaneous flushing, particularly of the upper part of the body (McCullough *et al*. 1970). The histamine release from tubocurarine is dose-related (Moss *et al*. 1981) which limits the dose of tubocurarine which can be given as a single bolus to about 0.5 mg/kg. Hypotension is a common feature following the administration of tubocurarine and, although block of autonomic ganglia is an important mechanism, histamine release also contributes to the hypotension (Stoelting and Longnecker 1972).

Metocurine is a safer drug than tubocurarine with respect to histamine-releasing potential (McCullough *et al*. 1972; Basta *et al*. 1983*a*). Savarese (1979) produced what he called the 'autonomic margin of safety' of metocurine and tubocurarine in the cat, one parameter of which he defined as the ED_{50} for histamine release divided by the ED_{95} for neuromuscular block. This ratio was 1.14 for tubocurarine but 35.2 for metocurine, suggesting that metocurine has an approximately 30 times less propensity to release histamine than does tubocurarine.

Gallamine appears to be associated with serious histamine release in a number of cases (Fisher and Munro 1983; Hatton *et al*. 1983; Galletly and Treuren 1985; Laxenaire *et al*. 1985). There has been one case of a profound histamine-releasing reaction following a small precurarizing dose of gallamine (Harrison and Bird 1986) but it is possible that the reaction described in that report may have been anaphylactic rather than anaphylactoid in view of the small dose of gallamine administered.

Alcuronium appears to have a low capacity for inducing histamine release by a direct action. Its capacity to precipitate a more serious anaphylactic action appears to be no less than the other relaxants and might even be higher (Chan and Yeung 1972; Fadel *et al*. 1982; Fisher and Munro 1983; Panning *et al*. 1985).

The steroid-based neuromuscular blocking agents pancuronium vecuronium, rocuronium, and pipecuronium appear to have a very low propensity to release histamine. There are very few reports in the literature of histamine release resulting from pancuronium and these were not serious (Brauer and Ananthanarayan 1978; Buckland and Avery 1973; Fisher and Munro 1983; Heath 1973; Mishima and Yamamura 1984). Vecuronium has a similar safety profile to pancuronium. Basta *et al*. (1983*b*) could not detect histamine release in doses up to 0.2 mg/kg. Sporadic reports of adverse reactions to vecuronium do exist (Clayton and Watkins 1984; Spence and Barnetson 1985; Lavery *et al*. 1985) and there is one case report of a serious reaction involving cross-sensitivity to pancuronium (Conil *et al*. 1985). No significant histamine release was observed following the administration of four times the ED_{95} of rocuronium (Davis *et al*. 1991).

The relaxants in the benzylisoquinolinium series (atracurium, mivacurium, doxacurium) do appear to have some tendency to release histamine, although this is usually only a problem in doses greater than the normal clinical range (Hughes and Chapple 1981). As the dose of atracurium is increased, there is a dose-dependent decrease in blood pressure with an associated tachycardia. These changes are associated with a measurable increase in the plasma concentration of histamine (Basta *et al*. 1983*a*; Mirakahur *et al*. 1985). The hypotension resulting from these higher doses of atracurium can be attenuated with pretreatment, using H_1 and H_2 receptor antagonists (Basta *et al.* 1982; Savarese *et al.* 1982; Stirt *et al.* 1983; Hughes and Payne 1983; Barnes *et al.* 1983). Skin flushing is common following an intravenous injection of atracurium, particularly along the course of vein, occasionally spreading to the whole arm and to the chest and neck (Basta *et al.* 1983*a*; Philbin *et al.* 1983; Lavery and Mirakhur 1984; Barnes *et al.* 1986; Goudsouzian *et al.* 1986; Watkins 1986). The more rapid the injection, the greater the likelihood of problems. If atracurium is allowed to mix with thiopentone in the cannula or vein, the incidence of adverse effects is said to be increased (Moss and Rosen 1983). More serious adverse events have been described which are likely to be related to histamine liberation, including bronchospasm, angioneurotic oedema, and serious hypotension (Sale 1982; Srivastave 1984; Siler *et al.* 1985).

Doxacurium appears to have very little capacity for histamine release. Following the administration of approximately twice the ED_{95}, Basta *et al.* (1988) found plasma histamine levels not to be increased. Mivacurium, however, may release histamine, the amount depending upon the dose and speed of injection (Savarese *et al.* 1989). The transient hypotension which may be seen after the administration of mivacurium is probably principally related to histamine release.

Suxamethonium is the only depolarizing agent in regular clinical use and is the most frequent relaxant indicated in adverse reactions ranging from minor skin flushing to profound bronchospasm and cardiovascular collapse (Smith 1957; Ravindran and Klemm 1980; Assem *et al.* 1981; Moss *et al.* 1981; Cohen *et al.* 1982; Laxenaire *et al.* 1982; Youngman *et al.* 1983).

CENTRAL NERVOUS SYSTEM EFFECTS

The neuromuscular blocking agents are all polar molecules. Being highly ionized, they do not easily cross the blood–brain barrier. The nondepolarizing agents have no direct effect on intracranial pressure, even if the intracranial pressure is raised (Stullken and Sokoll 1975; Giffin *et al.* 1985; Minton *et al.* 1985; Rosa *et al.* 1986; Haigh *et al.* 1986). Intracranial pressure may be reduced secondary to any fall in systemic blood pressure. Following a dose of suxamethonium there is often a transient small increase in intracranial pressure (Marsh *et al.* 1980; Cottrell *et al.* 1983). The rise in intracranial pressure may be marked and could be hazardous in patients with pre-existing raised intracranial pressure or impaired intracranial compliance (McLeskey *et al.* 1974; Marsh *et al.* 1980) and suxamethonium is therefore best avoided in these patients.

The nondepolarizing neuromuscular blocking agents generally have no effect on intra-ocular pressure (Tattersall *et al.* 1985; Schneider *et al.* 1986). A reduction in intra-ocular pressure has been reported following alcuronium (Balamoutsos *et al.* 1983). Suxamethonium leads to an increase in intra-ocular pressure (Cook 1981). This rise is usually approximately 8 mmHg and may persist for up to fifteen minutes (Taylor *et al.* 1968; Pandey *et al.* 1972). The mechanism is thought to be related to suxamethonium-induced contraction of the extra-ocular muscles (Kornblueth *et al.*

1960; Wislicki 1977). In the normal eye, this rise in intra-ocular pressure is not of any significance. If there is pre-existing raised intra-ocular pressure, suxamethonium may produce a hazardous further rise in pressure. When the integrity of the globe of the eye has been breached, any rise in intra-ocular pressure may result in extrusion of some of the contents of the eye, leading to permanent damage.

In emergency cases requiring a rapid control of the airway, suxamethonium is the relaxant of choice. Various pharmacological manoeuvres have been used to prevent the suxamethonium-induced rise in intra-ocular pressure. They include precurarizing doses of nondepolarizing neuromuscular blocking agent, a very small dose of suxamethonium itself ('self-taming'), diazepam, acetazolamide, and lignocaine. None of these measures will prevent the rise but most will attenuate it to some degree.

ACTIONS ON CHOLINESTERASE

A number of studies have examined a possible action of the nondepolarizing neuromuscular blocking agents on cholinesterase. The variety of responses is large and depends upon the tissue source of the cholinesterase. All the nondepolarizing neuromuscular blocking agents tested thus far inhibit cholinesterase, with two exceptions, namely gallamine and metocurine (Table 13.1). Gallamine weakly potentiates the activity of bovine erythrocyte cholinesterase, and metocurine has no effect on rat diaphragm cholinesterase. The cholinesterase in the neuromuscular junction differs from that in plasma, although it is similar to the cholinesterase in red cells. Mivacurium and suxamethonium are metabolized by plasma cholinesterase and therefore the presence of either of these will retard the metabolism by cholinesterase of any other drug due to simple competition.

EFFECTS ON ELECTROLYTES

Alterations in the plasma electrolyte concentrations may have a profound effect on the action of a neuromuscular blocking agent (see Chapter 12). The neuromuscular blocking agents in general, however, have no effect on the electrolytes, with one exception — suxamethonium. A recognized side-effect of suxamethonium is an almost immediate increase in the plasma potassium concentration of 0.5–1.0 mmol/l in normal patients (Weintraub *et al.* 1969). This acute rise may be considerably greater in certain pathological states, and cardiac arrest may result. These pathological disorders include burns, trauma, denervation disorders, tetanus, encephalitis, and certain muscle-wasting conditions.

The time-course in the rise in plasma potassium concentration is fairly constant, a peak being reached after approximately three minutes, after which the concentration

Table 13.1 The effects of the neuromuscular blocking agents on the activity of cholinesterase

Source of cholinesterase	Observation
Human red cell (Foldes and Deery 1983)	Atracurium — weak inhibition Vecuronium — weak inhibition Pancuronium — weak inhibition Tubocurarine — weak inhibition
Human red cell (Laget *et al.* 1974)	Gallamine — weak inhibition
Human plasma (Foldes and Deery 1983)	Vecuronium — strong inhibition Pancuronium — strong inhibition Atracurium — weak inhibition Tubocurarine — weak inhibition
Human plasma (Laget *et al.* 1974)	Pancuronium — strong inhibition
Human serum (Cardan 1978)	Pancuronium — strong inhibition
Human serum (Cardan 1976)	Pancuronium — weak inhibition
Bovine red cells (Desire *et al.* 1975)	Tubocurarine — strong inhibition Gallamine — weak potentiation
Bovine red cells (Barzu *et al.* 1974)	Pancuronium — weak inhibition
Horse serum (Barzu *et al.* 1974)	Pancuronium — strong inhibition
Electric organ of *Torpedo marmorata* (Wins *et al.* 1970)	Tubocurarine — strong inhibition
Electric organ of *Torpedo marmorata* (Changeux 1966)	Tubocurarine — strong inhibition Gallamine — strong inhibition
Electric organ of *Electrophorus electricus* (Robari and Kato 1975)	Tubocurarine — weak inhibition
Human red cells (Wembacher and Wolf 1971)	Tubocurarine — strong inhibition Gallamine — strong inhibition

slowly declines to the previous baseline. Various techniques have been proposed to lessen the hyperkalaemic response, which include precurarization with a non-depolarizing agent, diazepam, lignocaine, and thiopentone, none of which reliably works (Bali *et al*. 1975).

The source of the potassium which leads to the increase in plasma potassium appears to be the muscle cells. There may be transient damage to muscle fibre membranes, possibly associated with the fasciculations, which may allow leakage of potassium into the extracellular fluid. The exact mechanism, including why the potassium is not immediately taken up again into the cells, remains unclear.

EFFECTS ON MUSCLES

The nondepolarizing neuromuscular blocking agents have no direct effect on muscles except that of paralysis by an action at the neuromuscular junction. Suxamethonium, however, possesses a number of actions which affect skeletal muscles. These include myalgia, biochemical evidence of muscular damage, and triggering of a malignant hyperpyrexia crisis.

During the onset of action of a dose of suxamethonium there is a generalized asynchronous contraction of skeletal muscle fibres which produces visible fasciculations. This is presumably caused by the random activation of individual motor units or nerve fibres. Myalgia commonly follows the use of suxamethonium and is manifest as a dull ache. It predominantly affects the muscles of posture but may affect any muscle of the body. It can be most severe, with the patient being extremely uncomfortable for up to three to four days post-operatively. The severity of the pain does not seem to be related to the intensity of the fasciculations. It is worse in female patients than in male patients and worse in ambulatory patients than in those confined to bed.

The mechanism behind the production of suxamethonium myalgia is unclear, but reversible damage to muscle fibres caused by shearing stresses from the uncoordinated activation of individual muscle fibres is a likely explanation (Waters and Mapelson 1971). There may be an associated increase in plasma creatine phosphokinase concentration and a measurable myoglobinaemia following suxamethonium, which would lend support to the existence of mild muscle damage (Laurence 1985).

There have been many suggestions on ways to reduce or prevent the fasciculations, the myalgia, and the muscle damage. These include pretreatment with a nondepolarizing agent (Lamoreaux and Urbach 1960; Bennetts and Khalil 1981; Erkola *et al*. 1983), a small dose (10 mg) of suxamethonium (Baraka 1977), diazepam (Eisenberg *et al*. 1979; Davis 1983), lignocaine (Miller and Way 1971), fentanyl (Lindgren and Saarnivaara 1983), magnesium sulphate (James *et al*. 1986), thiopentone (Manani *et al*. 1981), dantrolene (Collier 1979), vitamin C (Gupta and Savant 1971), and calcium gluconate (Shrivastava *et al*. 1983). No method is fully effective. Precurarization with a nondepolarizing neuromuscular blocking agent is probably the most reliable, but may lead to partial paralysis in susceptible patients (Jones 1989).

ACTION AT THE NEUROMUSCULAR JUNCTION

The neuromuscular blocking agents are all agents which by definition exert an inhibitory effect at the neuromuscular junction. The structure and function of the neuromuscular junction is described in Chapter 2 and the physiochemical characteristics of the drugs in Chapter 3. It is appropriate here to consider in a broad clinical sense the actions at the neuromuscular junction.

Suxamethonium

Traditional beliefs regard the action of suxamethonium as being wholly on the postjunctional membrane. It is, however, quite likely that suxamethonium also has a prejunctional action and it is possible that fasciculations may be attributable to effects on prejunctional receptors (Standaert and Adams 1965; Hubbard *et al.* 1965; Hartman *et al.* 1986). If, immediately following the injection of a dose of suxamethonium, a motor nerve is stimulated, an enhancement of the height of contraction will be seen (Donati and Bevan 1984). This is rapidly followed by neuromuscular block, characterized by a lack of fade to tetanus or a train of four. This is a phase I block, and is the classical depolarizing block. If repeated doses of suxamethonium are given, then the characteristics of the block change. Fade to the train of four begins to appear and the block takes on the superficial appearance of a nondepolarizing block. This is now a phase II block. Although resembling a nondepolarizing block it should not be regarded as such, but as a desensitization phenomenon. The rate of development of a phase II block is dose dependent, i.e. it develops more rapidly as more suxamethonium is given. It is also dependent upon other drugs present, in particular the anaesthetic agents (Hilgenberg and Stoelting 1981; Donati and Bevan 1983*a*, *b*). It is possible that a phase II block begins to develop immediately following the initial dose of suxamethonium. Although not immediately obvious, it becomes more noticeable with time. The rate of recovery from a phase II block also depends upon the total dose of suxamethonium administered and upon the anaesthetic agent. Rapid recovery from the phase II block has been reported following an anticholinesterase agent (Lee 1976; Futter *et al.* 1983) but great care must be taken otherwise the block may be accentuated and not antagonized. Patience is probably a better treatment than an anticholinesterase.

Suxamethonium requirements increase with time if a constant infusion is used. The extent of this tachyphylaxis varies widely between patients (Donati and Bevan 1983*a*; Futter *et al.* 1983). The onset of tachyphylaxis appears with a similar time-course to the appearance of a phase II block. The exact relationship (if any) between these is unclear.

The nondepolarizing agents

All the nondepolarizing relaxants exhibit a similar pattern of action. Following a bolus injection, there is a lag period which depends upon the drug and the dose.

Table 13.2   Comparative potencies of the nondepolarizing neuromuscular blocking agents

DMS	ED_{95} (mg/kg)
Alcuronium	0.23
Atracurium	0.25
Doxacurium	0.03
Gallamine	2.3
Metacurine	0.28
Mivacurium	0.08
Pancuronium	0.06
Pipecuronium	0.045
Rocuronium	0.3
Tubocurarine	0.5
Vecuronium	0.05

This is followed by a steadily progressive block of transmission, which is characterized by fade to the train of four. Provided that an adequate dose has been administered, 100% block of transmission is achieved. Recovery begins after a delay which depends upon a number of factors, most important being the drug, the dose administered, other drugs, and the patient's response. The first response of the train of four is the first to recover, followed by the second, third, and fourth. Recovery can be accelerated by the use of an anticholinesterase agent.

There does not appear to be any tachyphylaxis or change of the characteristics of the block with time when the nondepolarizing agents are in use. An increase in requirement has been described when a neuromuscular blocking agent is administered by continuous infusion for several days to patients on the intensive care unit, but it is not clear whether or not this is true tachyphylaxis.

The relative potencies between the nondepolarizing relaxants are shown in Table 13.2. Doxacurium is the most potent and rocuronium the least potent. Doxacurium has the slowest onset and rocuronium the fastest, and these factors may be related (see Chapter 4).

EFFECTS ON AUTONOMIC SYSTEMS

A number of the neuromuscular agents have an effect on autonomic ganglia. Tubocurarine is the most potent in this regard and the ganglionic blocking capacity of other neuromuscular blocking agents is not really of undue clinical importance.

It would be logical to expect the muscle relaxants to exert an effect on autonomic ganglia because the acetylcholine receptors at ganglia are also nicotinic. They are, however, of a different nicotinic subtype as evidenced from the different effects of hexamethonium and decamethonium (Paton and Zaimis 1949). It is likely that all of the muscle relaxants do block autonomic ganglia but that the potency ratio of ganglionic block to neuromuscular block is so low in many muscle relaxants that ganglion block is negligible.

The ganglionic blocking agents do themselves affect neuromuscular transmission both alone and by potentiating the muscle relaxants (see Chapter 12). Evidence exists, however, to suggest that their action on the autonomic ganglia may be caused by effects at the ion channel rather than the receptor site alone (Rang 1982). It is possible that the muscle relaxants also operate in this manner.

Certain of neuromuscular blocking agents have an effect at the other variety of acetylcholine receptors — the muscarinic receptor. Gallamine is the most potent at blocking the cardiac muscarinic receptors and does so at doses close to those which block the neuromuscular junction. This results in a tachycardia.

There are a number of different subtypes of muscarinic receptors, for example M_1 in brain, M_2 in heart and M_3 in smooth muscle and glands (Mitchelson 1988). Gallamine appears to act at only the cardiac muscarinic receptors. It appears that the neuromuscular blocking agents may be devoid of actions at the M_1 and the M_3 receptors.

THE EFFECTS OF METABOLITES

The neuromuscular blocking agents have a number of effects as well as inhibiting transmission at the neuromuscular junction. The action of each is terminated by excretion of the parent drug, metabolism and excretion of metabolites, or a combination of these two. In the cases of drugs which undergo metabolism it is appropriate to consider whether or not the metabolities also have a neuromuscular blocking action or any other pharmacological effect.

Alcuronium and gallamine appear to undergo no metabolic change in the body and are excreted unchanged in the urine. It is this fact which makes them unwise choices in the patient with impaired renal function. Metocurine and tubocurarine also appear to undergo negligible metabolic change (Meijer *et al.* 1979). They are, however, eliminated in both bile and urine. The biliary excretion of tubocurarine is much greater than that of metocurine and increases in renal failure. That of metocurine does not increase by a great deal, however, making metocurine also an unwise choice in the patient with renal failure.

Pancuronium and vecuronium show close similarities in their metabolism in that both are broken down to the 3-hydroxy, 17-hydroxy, and 3,17 di-hydroxy metabolites, although the 17-hydroxy and the 3,17 di-hydroxy derivatives of pancuronium have not so far been detected in humans. In both cases, the 3-hydroxy metabolite possesses neuromuscular blocking activity but with a potency of between 50 and 60%

of that of the parent compound. The 17-hydroxy and 3,17 di-hydroxy metabolites have less than 2% of the activity of the parent compound (Agoston *et al.* 1973; Miller *et al.* 1978; Marshall *et al.* 1983). The metabolites appear to be excreted in the urine and it has been suggested that accumulation of the 3-hydroxy metabolite of vecuronium might account for the prolongation of effect which is sometimes seen after large doses of vecuronium in patients with impaired renal function (Segredo *et al.* 1990).

Atracurium breaks down by two separate processes, ester hydrolysis in the liver, and Hofmann elimination in the plasma. There are a number of metabolites, which include laudanosine and various quaternary acrylates and quaternary alcohols. The quaternary acrylates and quaternary alcohols are capable of producing neuromuscular block at high doses in laboratory animals. The acrylates are also highly active molecules and may produce hypertension (Chapple and Clark 1983) and direct tissue damage (Nigrovic 1983*b*, 1984). Much attention has been focused on laudanosine because it is capable of inducing cerebral arousal in laboratory animals (Lanier *et al.* 1985; Shi *et al.* 1985; Ingram *et al.* 1986). Because laudanosine is renally excreted there is the potential for accumulation of laudanosine when atracurium is given by continuous infusion to a patient with absent renal function (Fahey *et al.* 1985). It is not known if laudanosine is toxic in humans. Various isolated reports have described apparently epileptiform movements in patients who have received a prolonged infusion of atracurium in renal failure (Duncan 1983). These are, however, more than evenly balanced by many reports where no problems were encountered even in the presence of laudanosine concentrations in excess of 8 μg/ml (Gwinnutt *et al.* 1990). The balance of evidence appears to favour laudanosine being a theoretical disadvantage but not a problem in clinical practice.

The four newer drugs doxacurium, pipecuronium, mivacurium, and rocuronium appear to be metabolized solely to compounds with no pharmacological activity.

Suxamethonium is hydrolysed rapidly by plasma cholinesterase to succinylmonocholine and subsequently to succinic acid and choline. Succinylmonocholine is also a depolarizing neuromuscular blocking agent with a potency approximately 15–20% of that of suxamethonium.

REFERENCE

Agoston, S., Vermeer, G. A., Kersten, U. W., and Meijer, D. K. F. (1973). The fate of pancuronium bromide in man. *Acta Anaesthesiologica Scandinavica*, **17**, 267–75.

Antonio, R. P., Philbin, D. M., and Savarese, J. J. (1979). Comparative haemodynamic effects of tubocurarine and metocurine in the dog. *British Journal of Anaesthesia*, **51**, 1007–10.

Assem, E. S. K. (1984). Characteristics of basophil histamine release by neuromuscular blocking drugs in patients with anaphylactoid reactions. *Agents Actions*, **14**, 435–40.

Assem, E. S. K., Frost, P. J., and Levis, R. D. (1981). Anaphylactic-like reaction to suxamethonium. *Anaesthesia*, **36**, 405–10.

Balamoutsos, N. G., Tsakona, H., Kanakoudes, P. S., Iliadelis, E., and Georgiades, C. G. (1983). Alcuronium and intraocular pressure. *Anesthesia and Analgesia*, **62**, 521–3.

Baldo, B. A., Harle, D. G., and Fisher, M. M. (1985). *In vitro* diagnosis and studies on the mechanism(s) of anaphylactoid reactions to muscle relaxant drugs. *Annales Francais Anesthesie et Reanimation*, **4**, 139–45.

Bali, I. M., Dundee, J. W., and Doggart, J. R. (1975). The source of increased plasma potassium following succinylcholine. *Anesthesia and Analgesia*, **54**, 680–6.

Baraka, A. (1967). A comparative study between diallyl-nortoxiferine and tubocurarine. *British Journal of Anaesthesia*, **39**, 624–8.

Baraka, A. (1977). Self-taming of succinylcholine-induced fasciculations. *Anesthesiology*, **46**, 292.

Barnes, P. K., Brindle-Smith, G., White, W. D., and Tennant, R. (1982). Comparison of the effects of ORG NC45 and pancuronium bromide on heart rate and arterial pressure in anaesthetized man. *British Journal of Anaesthesia*, **54**, 435–9.

Barnes, P. K., Thomas, V. J. E., Boyd, I., and Hollway, T. (1983). Comparison of the effects of atracurium and tubocurariane on heart rate and arterial pressure in anaesthetised man. *British Journal of Anaesthesia*, **55**, 91–4S.

Barnes, P. K., de Renzy-Martin, N., Thomas, V. J. E., and Watkins, J. (1986). Plasma histamine levels following atracurium. *Anaesthesia*, **41**, 821–4.

Barzu, T., Cuparencu, B., and Cardan, E. (1974). The anticholinesterase activity of pancuronium bromide (Pavulon). *Biochemistry and Pharmacology*, **23**, 166–8.

Basta, S. J., Ali, H. H., Savarese, J. J., Sunder, N., Gionfriddo, M., Cloutier, G., *et al.* (1982). Clinical pharmacology of atracurium besylate (BW33A): A new nondepolarising muscle relaxant. *Anesthesia and Analgelsia*, **61**, 723–9.

Basta, S. J., Savarese, J. J., Ali, H. H., Moss, J., and Gionfriddo, M. (1983*a*). Histamine-releasing potencies of atracurium, dimenthyl tubocurarine and tubocurarine. *British Journal of Anaesthesia*, **55**, 105S–6S

Basta, S. J., Savarese, J. J., Ali, H. H., Sunder, N., Moss J., Gionfriddo, M., and Embree, P. (1983*b*). Vecuronium does not alter serum histamine within the clinical dose range. *Anesthesiology*, **59**, A273.

Basta, S. J., Savarese, J. J., Ali, H. H., Embee, P. B., Schwarz, A. F., Rudd, G. D., *et al.* (1988). Clinical pharmacology of doxacurium chloride. *Anesthesiology*, **69**, 478–86.

Belani, K. G., Anderson, W. W., and Buckley, J. J. (1982). Adverse drug interaction involving pancuronium and aminophylline. *Anesthesia and Analgesia*, **61**, 473–4.

Bennetts, F. E. and Khalil, K. I. (1981). Reduction of post-suxamethonium pain by pretreatment with four nondepolarising agents. *British Journal of Anaesthesia*, **53**, 531–6.

Blanloeil, Y., Pinaud, M., Rochedreux, A., and Arnould, F. (1982). Comparison des effets hemodynamiques du fazadinium, du pancuronium et de l'alcuronium chez l'insuffisant coronaire. *Annales Francais Anesthesie et Reanimation*, **1**, 313–8.

Booij, L. H. D. J. and Knape, H. D. A. (1991). The neuromuscular blocking effect of Org 9426, a new intermediately acting nondepolarising muscle relaxant in man. *Anaesthesia*, **46**, 341–3.

Brauer, F. S. and Ananthanarayan, C. R. (1987). Histamine release by pancuroniu. *Anesthesiology*, **49**, 434–5.

Brown, B. B. and Crout, J. R. (1970). The sympathomimetic effect of gallamine on the heart. *Journal of Pharmacology and Experimental Therapeutics*, **172**, 266–73.

Buckland, R. W. and Avery, A. F. (1973). Histamine release following pancuronium. *British Journal of Anaesthesia*. **45**, 518–21.

Cardan, E. (1978). Anticholinesterase action of pancuronium. *Anaesthesia*, **33**, 277.

Cardan, E., Ruckert, I., and Urcan, S. (1976). Modificarile acetilcolinesterazei serice dupa pancuronium. *Revue de Chirurgie*, **25**, 297–301.

Carter, M. L. (1983). Bradycardia after the use of atracurium. *British Medical Journal*, **287**, 247–8.

Cason, B., Baker, D. G., Hickey, R. F., Miller, R. D., and Agoston, S. (1990). Cardiovascular and neuromuscular effects of three steroidal neuromuscular blocking drugs in dogs (ORG 9616, ORG 9426, ORG 9991). *Anesthesia and Analgesia*, **70**, 382–8.

Chan, C. S. and Yeung, M. L. (1972). Anaphylactic reaction to alcuronium. *British Journal of Anaesthesia*, **44**, 103–5.

Changeux, J. P. (1966). Responses of acetylcholinesterase from Torpedo marmorata to salts and curarising drugs. *Molecular Pharmacology*, **2**, 369–92.

Chapple, D. J. and Clark, J. S. (1983). Pharmacological action of breakdown products of atracurium and related substances. *British Journal of Anaesthesia*, **55**, 11–6S.

Choi, W. W., Mehta, M. P., Murray, D. J., Sokoll, M. D., Forbes, R. B., Gergis, S. D., *et al.* (1989). Neuromuscular and cardiovascular effects of mivacurium chloride in surgical patients receiving nitrous oxide–narcotic or nitrous oxide–isoflurance anaesthesia. *Canadian Journal of Anaesthesia*, **36**, 641–50.

Clayton, D. G. and Watkins, J. (1984). Histamine release with vecuronium. *Anaesthesia*, **39**, 1143–4.

Cohen, S., Liu, K. H. and Marx, G. F. (1982). Upper airway edema-an anaphylactoid reaction to succinylcholine? *Anesthesiology*, **56**, 467–8.

Coleman, A. J., Downing, J. W., Leary, W. P., Moyes, D. G., and Styles, M. (1972). The immediate cardiovascular effects of pancuronium, alcuronium and tubocurarine in man. *Anaesthesia*, **27**, 414–22.

Collier, D. B. (1979). Dantrolene and suxamethonium: The effect of pre-operative dantrolene on the action of suxamethonium. *Anesthesiology*, **34**, 152–8.

Conil, C., Bornet, J. L., Jean-Noel, M., Conil, J. M., and Brouchet, A. (1985). Choc anaphylactique au pancuronium et au vecuronium. *Annales Francais Anesthesie et Reanimation*, **4**, 241–3.

Cook, J. H. (1981). The effect of suxamethonium on intraocular pressure. *Anaesthesia*, **35**, 359–65.

Cottrell, J. E., Hartung, J., Giffin, J. P., and Shwiry, B. (1983). Intracranial and hemodynamic changes after succinylcholine administration in cats. *Anesthesia and Analgesia*, **62**, 1006–9.

Davis, G. K., Szlam, F., Lowdon, J. D., and Levy, J. H. (1991). Evaluation of histamine release following Org 9426 administration using a new radioimmunoassay. *Anesthesiology*, **75**, A818.

Davis, A. O. (1983). Oral diazepam premedication reduces the incidence of post-succinylcholine muscle pains. *Canadian Anaesthetists Society Journal*, **30**, 603–6.

Desire, B., Blanchet, G., Definod, G., and Arnaud, R. (1975). Acétylcholinestérase II — Aspects expérimentaux de l'interaction avec les effecteurs reversibles en milieu de force ionique élevée. *Biochimie*, **57**, 1359–70.

Docherty, J. R. and McGrath, J. C. (1978). Sympathomimetic effects of pancuronium bromide on the cardiovascular system of the pitted rat: A comparison with the effects of drugs blocking the neural uptake of noradrenaline. *British Journal of Pharmacology*, **64**, 589–99.

Domenech, J. S., Garcia, R. C., Sasian, J. M. R., Loyola, A. Q., and Oroz, J. S. (1976). Pancuronium bromide: an indirect sympathomimetic agent. *British Journal of Anaesthesia*, **48**, 1143–48.

Donati, F. and Bevan, D. R. (1983*a*). Long-term succinycholine infusion during isoflurane anesthesia. *Anesthesiology*, **58**, 6–10.

Donati, F. and Bevan, D. R. (1983*b*). Potentiation of succinylcholine phase II block with isoflurane. *Anesthesiology*, **58**, 552–5.

Donati, F. and Bevan, D. R. (1984). Muscle electromechanical correlations during succinyl-choline infusion. *Anesthesia and Analgesia*, **63**, 891–4.

Dubois, R., Fleming, N. W. and Lee, E. (1991). Effects of succinylcholine on the pharmaco-dynamics of pipecuronium and pancuronium. *Anesthesia and Analgesia*, **72**, 364–8.

Duke, P. C., Fung, H., and Gartner, J. (1975). The myocardial effect sof pancuronium. *Canadian Anaesthetists Society Journal*, **22**, 680–6.

Duncan, P. W. (1983). A problem with atracurium. *Anesthesia*, **38**, 597.

Durant, N. N., Marshall, I. G., Savage, D. S., Nelson, D. J., Sleigh, T. and Carlyle, I. C. (1979). The neuromuscular and autonomic blocking activities of pancuronium. Org NC 45, and other pancuronium analogues in the cat. *Journal of Pharmacy and Pharmacology*, **31**, 831–6.

Edwards, R. P., Miller, R. D., Roizen, M. F., Ham, J., Way, W. L., Lake, C. R., *et al.* (1979). Cardiac responses to imipramine and pancuronium during anesthesia with halothane or ethrane. *Anesthesiology*, **50**, 421–5.

Eisele, J. H., Marta, J. A., and Davis, H. S. (1971). Quantitative aspects of the chronotropic and neuromuscular effects of gallamine in anesthetised man. *Anesthesiology*, **35**, 630–3.

Eisenberg, M., Balsley, S., and Kartz, R. L. (1979). Effects of diazepam on succinylcholine-induced myalgia, potassium increase, creatine phosphokinase elevation, and relaxation. *Anesthesia and Analgesia*, **58**, 314–7.

Emmott, R. S., Bracey, B. J., Goldhill, D. R., Yate, P. M., and Flynn, P. J. (1990). Cardiovascular effects of doxacurium, pancuronium and vecuronium in anaesthetised patients presenting for coronary artery bypass surgery. *British Journal of Anaesthesia*, **65**, 480–6.

Erkola, O., Salmenpera, A., and Kuoppamaki, R. (1983). Five nondepolarizing muscle relaxants in precurarisation. *Acta Anaesthesiologica Scandinavica*, **27**, 427–432.

Fadel, R., Herpin-Richard, N., Rassemont, R., Salomon, J., David, B., Laurent, M., and Henocq, E. (1982). Choc anaphylactique a la diallyl-nortoxiferine. Etude clinique et immunolgique. *Annales Français Anesthesie et Reanimation*, **1**, 531–4.

Fahey, M. R., Rupp, S. M., Canfell, C., Fisher, D. M., Miller, R. D., Sharma, M., *et al.* (1985). Effect of renal failure on laudanosine excretion in man. *British Journal of Anaesthesia*, **57**, 1049–51.

Foldes, F. F. and Deery, A. (1983). Protein binding of atracurium and other short acting neuromuscular blocking agents and their interaction with human cholinesterase. *British Journal of Anaesthesia*, **55**, 31–4S.

Foldes, F. F., Brown, I. M., Lunn, J. N., Moore, J., and Duncalf, D. (1963). The neuromuscular effects of diallylnortoxiferine in anaesthetised subjects. *Anesthesia and Analgesia*, **42**, 177–81.

From, R. P., Pearson, K. S., Choi, W. W., Abou-Donia, M., and Sokoll, M. D. (1990). Neuromuscular and cardiovascular effects of mivacurium chloride (BW B1090U) during nitrous oxide–fentanyl–thiopentone and nitrous oxide–halothane anaesthesia. *British Journal of Anaesthesia*, **64**, 193–8.

Futter, M. E., Donati, F., Sadikot, A. S., and Bevan, D. R. (1983). Neostigmine antagonism of succinylcholine phase II block: A comparison with pancuronium. *Canadian Anaesthetists' Society Journal*, **30**, 575–80.

Galletly, D. C. and Treuren, B. C. (1985). Anaphylactoid reactions during anaesthesia. *Anaesthesia*, **40**, 329–33.

Gardiner, R. W., Tserdos, E. J., and Jackson, D. B. (1978). Effect of gallamine and pancuronium on inhibitory transmission in cat sympathetic ganglia. *Journal of Pharmacology and Experimental Therapeutics*, **204**, 46–53.

Giffin, J. P., Litwak, B., and Cottrell, J. E. (1985). Intracranial pressure, mean arterial pressure and heart rate after rapid paralysis with atracurium in cats. *Canadian Anaesthetists' Society Journal*, **32**, 618–21.

Goudsouzian, N. G., Young, E. T., Moss, J., and Liu, L. M. P. (1986). Histamine release during the administration of atracurium or vecuronium in children. *British Journal of Anaesthesia*, **58**, 1229–33.

Gregoretti, S. M., Sohn, T. J., and Sia, R. L. (1982). Heart rate and blood pressure changes after ORG NC45 (vecuronium) and pancuronium during halothane and enflurane anaesthesia. *Anesthesiology*, **56**, 392–5.

Guggiari, M., Gallais, S., Bianchi, A., Guillaume, A., and Viars, P. (1985). Effects hemodynamiques de l'atracurium chez l'homme. *Annales Francais Anesthesie et Reanimation*, **4**, 484–8.

Gupta, S. R. and Savant, N. S. (1971). Post suxamethonium pains and vitamin C. *Anaesthesia*, **26**, 436–40.

Guyton, A. C. and Reeder, R. C. (1950). Quantitative studies on the autonomic action of curare. *Journal of Pharmacology and Experimental Therapeutics*, **98**, 188–94.

Gwinnutt, C. L., Eddleston, J. M., Edwards, D., and Pollard, B. J. (1990). Concentrations of atracurium and laudanosine in cerebrospinal fluid and plasma in 3 intensive care patients. *British Journal of Anaesthesia*, **65**, 829–32.

Haigh, J. K., Nemato, E. M., and Bleyaerst, A. L., (1986). Comparison of the effects of succinylcholine and atracurium on intracranial pressure in monkeys with intracranial hypertension. *Canadian Anaesthetists' Society Journal*, **33**, 421–6.

Harle, D. G., Baldo., B. A., and Fisher, M. M. (1985). Cross-reactivity of metocurine, atracurium, vecuronium and fazadinium with IgE antibodies from patients unexposed to these drugs but allergic to other myoneural blocking drugs. *British Journal of Anaesthesia*, **57**, 1073–6.

Harrison, J. F. and Bird, A. G. (1986). Anaphylaxis to precurarising doses of gallamine triethiodide. *Anaesthesia*, **41**, 600–4.

Harrison, G. A. (1972). The cardiovascular effects and some relaxant properties of four relaxants in patients about to undergo cardiac surgery. *British Journal of Anaesthesia*, **44**, 485–9.

Hartmann, G. S., Flamengo, S. A., and Riker, W. F. (1986). Succinyllcholine: Mechanism of fasciculations and their prevention by *d*-tubocurarine or diphenylhydantoin. *Anesthesiology*, 65, 405–13.

Hatton, F., Tiret, L., Maujol, L., N'Dove, P., Vourc'h, G., Desmonts, J. M., *et al.* (1983). Enquete epidemiologique sur les anesthesies. *Annales Français Anesthesia et Reanimation*, **2**, 333–85.

Healy, T. E. J. and Palmer, J. P. (1982). *In vitro* comparison between the neuromuscular and ganglion blocking potency ratios of atracurium and tubocurarine. *British Journal of Anaesthesia*, **54**, 1307–11.

Heath, M. L. (1973). Bronchospasm in an asthmatic patient following pancuronium. *Anaesthesia*, **28**, 4370–40.

Hilgenberg, J. C. and Stoelting, R. K. (1981). Characteristics of succinylcholine-produced phase II neuromuscular block during enflurnae, halothane, and fentanyl anesthesia. *Anesthesia and Analgesia*, **60**, 182–6.

Hilgenberg, J. C. and Stoelting, R. K. (1986). Haemodynamic effects of atracurium in the presence of potent inhalational agents. *British Journal of Anaestheisa*, **58**, 70–4S.

Hirano, S., Ueki, O., Misaki, T., and Hisazumi, H. (1984). Severe hypertension and tachycardia associated with pancuronium bromide in a patient with asymptomatic pheochromocytoma. *Acta Urologica Japanica*, **30**, 709–12.

Hubbard, J. I., Schmidt, R. F., and Yokota, T. (1965). The effect of acetylcholine upon mammalian motor nerve terminals. *Journal of Physiology*, **181**, 810–29.

Hughes, R. and Chapple, D. J. (1976*a*). Effects of non-depolarising and neuromuscular blocking agents on peripheral autonomic mechanisms in cats. *British Journal of Anesthesia*, **48**, 59–68.

Hughes, R. and Chapple, D. J. (1981). The pharmacology of atracurium: a new competitive neuromuscular blocking agent. *British Journal of Anaesthesia*, **53**, 31–43.

Hughes, R. and Chapple, D. J. (1976*b*). Cardiovascular and neuromuscular effects of dimethyl tubocurarine in anaesthetised cats and rhesus monkeys. *British Journal of Anaesthesia*, **48**, 847–51.

Hughes, R. and Payne, J. P. (1983). Clinical assessment of atracurium using the single twitch and tetanic responses of the adductor pollicis. *British Journal of Anaesthesia*, **55**, 47–52S.

Hunter, A. R. (1964). Diallyl toxiferine. *British Journal of Anaesthesia*, **36**, 466–9.

Hunter, J. M. (1983). Bradycardia after the use of atracurium. *British Medical Journal*, **287**, 759.

Ingram, M. D. M., Sclabassi, R. J., Cooke, D. R., Stiller, R. L., and Bennett, M. H. (1986). Cardiovascular and electroencephalographic effect of laudanosine in 'nephrectomized' cats. *British Journal of Anaesthesia*, **58**, 14–8S.

Iwatsuki, N., Hashimoto, Y., Amaha, K., Obara, S., and Iwatsuki, K. (1980). Inotropic effects of non-depolarising muscle relaxants in isolated canine heart muscle. *Anesthesia and Analgesia*, **59**, 717–21.

James, M. F. M., Cock, R. C., and Dennett, J. E. (1986). Succinylcholine pretreatment with magnesium sulfate. *Anesthesia and Analgesia*, **65**, 373–6.

Johnstone, M., Mahmoud, A. A., and Mrozinski, R. A. (1978). Cardiovascular effects of tubocurarine in man. *Anaesthesia*, **33**, 587–93.

Jones, R. M. (1989). The priming principle: how does it work and should we be using it? *British Journal of Anaesthesia*, **63**, 1–3.

Jones, R. M. and Hill, A. B. (1981). Severe hypertension associated with pancuronium in a patient with a phaeochromocytoma. *Canadian Anaesthetists' Society Journal*, **28**, 394–6.

Karhunen, U., Nilsson, E., and Brander, P. (1985). Comparison of four nondepolarising neuromuscular blocking drugs in the suppression of the oculocardiac reflex during strabismus surgery in children. *British Journal of Anaesthesia*, **57**, 1209–12.

Katz, R. L., Stirt, J., Murray, A. L., and Lee, C. (1982). Neuromuscular effects of atracurium in man. *Anesthesia and Analgesia*, **61**, 730–4.

Kelman, G. R. and Kennedy, B. R. (1971). Cardiovascular effects of pancuronium in man. *British Journal of Anaesthesia*, **43**, 335–8.

Kennedy, B. R. and Farman, J. V. (1968). Cardiovascular effects of gallamine triethiodide in man. *British Journal of Anaesthesia*, **40**, 773–80.

Kennedy, B. R. and Kelman, G. R. (1970). Cardiovascular effects of alcuronium in man. *British Journal of Anaesthesia*, **42**, 625–9.

Kornblueth, W., Jampolsky, A., Tamler, E., and Marg, E. (1960). Contraction of the oculorotatory muscles and intraocular pressure. *American Journal of Ophthalmology*, **49**, 1381–7.

Laget, P., Chomel, A., and Pieri, J. (1974). Etude du mode d'action de la choline, du tetramethylammonium, de la gallamine, du tetraethylammonium et du calcium sur l'acetylcholinesterase des membranes d'erythrocytes humains. *Biochimie*, **56**, 1119–27.

Lamoreaux, L. F. and Urbach, K. F. (1960). Incidence and prevention of muscle pain following the administration of succinylcholine. *Anesthesiology*, **21**, 394–6.

Lanier, W. L., Milde, J. H., and Michenfelder, J. D. (1985). The cerebral effects of pancuronium and atracurium in halothane-anesthetised dogs. *Anesthesiology*, **63**, 589–97.

Laurence, A. S. (1985). Biochemical changes following suxamethonium: serum myoglobin, potassium and creatinine kinase changes before commencement of surgery. *Anaesthesia*, **40**, 854–59.

Lavery, G. G. and Mirakhur, R. K. (1984). Atracurium besylate in paediatric anaesthesia. *Anaesthesia*, **39**, 1243–6.

Lavery, G. G. Hewitt, A. J., and Kenny, N. T. (1985). Possible histamine release after vecuronium. *Anaesthesia*, **40**, 389–90.

Laxenaire, M.-C., Moneret-Vautrin, D. A., and Boileau, S. (1982). Choc anaphylactique au suxamethonium a propos de 18 cas. *Annales Francis Anesthesie et Reanimation*, **1**, 29–36.

Laxenaire, M.-C., Moneret-Vautrin, D. A., Vervloet, D., Alazia, M., and Francois, G. (1985). Accidents anaphylactoides graves peranesthesiques. *Annales Francais Anesthesie et Reanimation*, **4**, 30–46.

Lee, C. (1976). Train-of-four fade and edrophonium antagonism of neuromuscular block by succinylcholine in man. *Anesthesia and Analgesia*, **55**, 663–7.

Lee Son S. and Waud, D. R. (1980). Effects of non-depolarising neuromuscular blocking agents on the cardiac vagus nerve in the guinea pig. *British Journal of Anaesthesia*, **52**, 981–7.

Lindgren, L. and Saarnivaara, L. (1983). Effect of competitive myoneural blockade and fentanyl on muscle fasciculations caused by suxamethonium in children. *British Journal of Anaesthesia*, **55**, 747–51.

Loh, L. (1970). The cardiovascular effect of pancuronium bromide. *Anaesthesia*, **25**, 356–63.

Lorenz, W., Doenicke, A., Schoring, B., Ohmann, C., Grote, B., and Neugebaur, E. (1982). Definition and classification of the histamine release response to drugs in anaesthesia and surgery. Studies in the conscious human subject. *Klinische Wochenschrift*, **60**, 896–913.

Manani, G., Valenti, S., Segatto, A., Angel, A, Meroni, M., and Giron, G. P. (1981). The influence of thiopentone and alfathesin on succinylcholine-induced fasciculations and myalgias, *Canadian Anaesthetists' Society Journal*, **28**, 253–8.

Marsh, M. L., Dunlop, B. J., Shapiro, H. M., Gagnor, R. L., and Rockoff, M. A. (1980). Succinylcholine-intracranial pressure effecs in neurosurgical patients. *Anesthesia and Analgesia*, **59**, 550–1.

Marshall, I. G., Gibb, A. J., and Durant, N. N. (1983). Neuromuscular and vagal blocking actions of pancuronium bromide, its metabolites, and vecuronium bromide (ORG NC45) and its potential metabolites in anaesthetized cat. *British Journal of Anesthesia*, **55**, 703–14.

Marshall, R. J., McGrath, J. C., Miller, R. D., Docherty, J. R., and Lamar, J. C. (1980). Comparison of the cardiovascular actions of Org NC 45 with those produced by other non-depolarising neuromuscular blocking agents in experimental animals. *British Journal of Anaesthesia*, **52**, 21–32S.

McCullough, L. S., Stone, W. A., Delaunois, A. L., Reier, C. E., and Hamelberg, W. (1972). The effect of dimenthyl tubocurarine iodide on cardiovascular parameters, postganglionic sympathetic activity and histamine release. *Anesthesia and Analgesia*, **51**, 554–9.

McCullough, L. S., Reier, C. E., Delaunois, A. J., Gardier, R. W., and Hamelberg, W. (1970). The effects of *d*-tubocurarine on spontaneous post-ganglionic sympathetic activity and histamine release. *Anesthesiology*, **33**, 328–34.

McLeskey, C. H., Cullen, B. F., Kennedy, R. D., and Galindo, A. (1974). Control of cerebral perfusion pressure during induction of anaesthesia in high-risk neurosurgical patients. *Anesthesia and Analgesia*, **53**, 985–92.

Meijer, D. K. F., Weitering, J. G., Vermeer, G. A., and Scaf, A. H. J. (1979). Comparative pharmacokinetics of *d*-tubocurarine and metocurine in man. *Anesthesiology*, **51**, 402–7.

Mellinghoff, H., Diefenbach, C., and Buzello, W. (1991). Neuromuscular and cardiovascular properties of Org 9426. *Anesthesiology*, **75**, A807.

Miller, R. D. and Way, W. L. (1971). Inhibition of succinylcholine-induced increased intragastric pressure by nondepolarising muscle relaxants and lidocaine. *Anesthesiology*, **34**, 185–8.

Miller, R. D., Agoston, S., Booij, L. H. D. J., Kersten-Kleef, U. W., Crul, J. F., and Ham, J. (1978). The comparative potency and Pharmacokinetics of pancuronium and its metabolites in anesthetized man. *Journal of Pharmacology and Experimental Therapeutics*, **207**, 539–43.

Minton, M. D., Stirt, J. A., Bedford, R. F., and Haworth, C. (1985). Intracranial pressure after atracurium in neurosurgical patients. *Anesthesia and Analgesia*, **64**, 1113–6.

Mirakhur, R. K., Ferres, C. J., Clarke, R. S. J., Bali, I. M., and Dundee, J. W. (1983). Clinical evaluation of Org NC 45. *British Journal of Anaesthesia*, **55**, 119–24.

Mirakhur, R. K., Lavery, G. G., Clarke, R. S. J., Gibson, F. M., and McAteer, E. (1985). Atracurium in clinical anaesthesia: Effect of dosage on onset, duration and conditions for tracheal intubation. *Anaesthesia*, **40**, 801–5.

Mishima, S. and Yamamura, T. (1984). Anaphylactoid reaction to pancuronium. *Anesthesia and Analgesia*, **63**, 865–6.

Mitchelson, F. (1988). Muscarinic receptor differentiation. *Pharmacology and Therapeutics*, **37**, 357–423.

Morris, R. B., Cahalan, M. K., Miller R. D., Wilkinson, P. L., Quasha, A. L., and Robinson, S. L. (1983). The cardiovascular effects of vecuronium (ORG NC45) and pancuronium in patients undergoing coronary artery bypass grafting. *Anesthesiology*, **58**, 438–40.

Moss, J. and Roson, C. E. (1983). Histamine release by narcotics and muscle relaxants in humans. *Anesthesiology*, **59**, 330–9.

Moss, J., Roscow, C. E., Savarese, J. J., Philbin, D. M., and Kniffen, K. J. (1981). Role of histamine in the hypotensive action of *d*-tubocurarine in humans. *Anesthesiology*, **55**, 19–25.

Moyers, J. R., Carter, J. G., Davies, L. R., Carter, A. L., and Shimosata, S. (1982). Circulatory effects of BW33A in the dog. *Anesthesiology*, **57**, A285.

Muir, A. W., Houston, J., Marshall, R. J., Bowman, W. C., and Marshall, I. G. (1989). A comparison of neuromuscular blocking and autonomic effects of two new short-acting muscle relaxants with those of succinylcholine in the anaesthetised cat and pig. *Anesthesiology*, **70**, 533–40.

Munger, M. L., Miller, R. D., and Stevens, W. C. (1974). The dependence of *d*-tubocurarine-induced hypotension on the alveolar concentration of halothane and the presence of nitrous oxide. *Anesthesiology*, **40**, 442–8.

Nelson, S. H. and Steinsland, O. S. (1983). *d*-Tubocurarine as a dopaminergic antagonist in the rabbit ear artery. *Anesthesiology*, **59**, 98–101.

Nigrovic, V. (1984). Succinylcholine, cholinoceptors and catecholamines: proposed mechanism of early adverse haemodynamic reactions. *Canadian Anaesthetists' Society Journal*, **31**, 381–94.

Nigrovic, V. and Koechel, D. A. (1984). Atracurium — more information needed. *Anesthesiology*, **60**, 606–7.

Nigrovic, V., McCullough, L. S., Wajskol, A., Levin, J. A., and Martin, J. T. (1983*a*). Succinylcholine-induced increases in plasma catecholamine levels in humans. *Anesthesia and Analgesia*, **62**, 627–32.

Nigrovic, V., Klaunig, J. E., Smith, S. L., Schultz, N. E., and Wajskol, A. (1983*b*). Comparative toxicity of atracurium and metocurine in isolated rat hepatocytes. *Anesthesia and Analgesia*, **65**, 1107–11.

Pandey, K., Badola, R. P., and Kumar, S. (1972). Time course of intraocular hypertension produced by suxamethonium. *British Journal of Anaesthesia*, **44**, 191–5.

Panning, B., Peest, D., Kirchner, E., and Schedel, I. (1985). Anaphylaktoider Schock nach Alloferin. *Anaesthesists*, **34**, 211–4.

Paton, W. D. M. and Zaimis, E. J. (1949). The pharmacological action of polymethylene bistrimethylammonium salts. *British Journal of Pharmacology*, **4**, 381–400.

Philbin, D. M., Machaj, V. R., Tomichek, R. C., Schneider, R. C., Alban, J. C., Lowenstein, E., *et al.* (1983). Haemodynamic effects of bolus injections of atracurium in patients with coronary artery disease. *British Journal of Anaesthesia*, **55**, 131–4S.

Quintana, A. (1977). Effect of pancuronium bromide on the adrenergic reactivity of the isolated rate vas deferens. *European Journal of Pharmacology*, **46**, 275–7.

Rang, H. P. (1982). The action of ganglion blocking drugs on the synaptic responses of rate submandibular ganglion cells. *British Journal of Pharmacology*, **75**, 151–68.

Ravindran, R. S. and Klemm, J. E. (1980). Anaphylaxis to succinylcholine in a patient allergic to penicillin. *Anesthesia and Analgesia*, **59**, 944–5.

Reich, D. L., Constadt, S. N., Thys, D. M., Hillel, Z. (1989). Effects of doxacurium chloride on biventricular cardiac function in patients with cardiac disease. *British Journal of Anaesthesia*, **63**, 675–81.

Reitan, J. A., Fraser, A. I., and Eisele, J. H. (1973). Lack of cardiac inotropic effects of gallamine in anaesthetised man. *Anesthesia and Analgesia*, **52**, 974–9.

Riker, W. F. and Wescoe, W. C. (1951). The pharmacology of Flaxedil with observations on certain analogs. *Annals of the New York Academy of Sciences*, **54**, 373–92

Robari, B. and Kato, g. (1975). Effects of edrophonium eserine, decamethonium, *d*-tubocurarine and gallamine on the kinetics of membrane bound and solubilised eel acetylcholinesterase. *Molecular Pharmacology*, **11**, 722–34.

Robertson, E. N., Booij, L. H. D. J., Fragen, R. J., Crul, J. F. (1983). Clinical comparison of atracurium and vecurorium (Org NC45). *British Journal of Anaesthesia*, **55**, 125–9.

Rosa, G., Orfei, P., Sanfilippo, M., and Gasparetto, A. (1986). The effects of atracurium besylate (Tracrium) on intracranial pressure and cerebral perfusion rophonium eserine, decamethonium, *d*-tubocurarine and gallamine on the kinetics of membrane bound and solubilised eel acetylcholinesterase. *Molecular Pharmacology*, **11**, 722–34.

Robertson, E. N., Booij, L. H. D. J., Fragen, R. J., Crul, J. F. (1983). Clinical comparison of atracurium and vecurorium (Org NC45). *British Journal of Anaesthesia*, **55**, 125–9.

Rosa, G., Orfei, P., Sanfilippo, M., and Gasparetto, A. (1986). The effects of atracurium besylate (Tracrium) on intracranial pressure and cerebral perfusion pressure. *Anesthesia and Analgesia*, **65**, 381-4.

Saemund, O and Dalenius, E. (1981). Pancuronium and nodal rythm (Letter). *British Journal of Anaesthesia*, **53**, 780.

Sale, J. P. (1982). Bronchospasm following the use of atracurium. *Anaesthesia*, **38**, 511–2.

Salmanpera, M., Peltola, K., Takkunen, O., and Heinonen, J.(1983). Cardiovascular effects of pancuronium and vecuronium during high-dose fentanyl anesthesia. *Anesthesia and Analgesia*, **62**, 1059–64.

Savarese, J. J. (1979). The automatic margin of safety of metocurine and *d*-tubocurarine in the cat. *Anesthesiology*, **50**, 40–6.

Savarese, J. J., Basta, S. J., Ali, H. H., Sunder, N., and Moss, J. (1982). Neuromuscular and cardiovascular effects of BW33A (atracurium) in patients under halothane anesthesia. *Anesthesiology*, **57**, A262.

Savarese, J. J., Ali, H. H., Basta, S. J., Scott, R. P., Embree, P. B., Wastila, W. B., *et al.* (1989). The cardiovascular effects of mivacurium chloride (BW B1090U) in patients receiving nitrous oxide–opiate–barbiturate anesthesia. *Anesthesiology*, **70**, 386–94.

Saxena, P. R., Dhasmana, K. M., and Prakash, O. (1983). A comparison of systemic and regional hemodynamic effects of *d*-tubocurarine, pancuronium, and vecurorium. *Anesthesiology*, **59**, 102–8.

Saxena, P. R. and Bonta, F. L. (1970). Mechanism of selective cardiac vagolytic action of pancuronium bromide: specific blockade of cardiac muscarinic receptors. *European Journal of Pharmacology*, **11**, 332–41.

Schneider, M. J., Stirt, J. A., and Finholt, D. A. (1986). Atracurium, vecuronium and intraocular pressure in humans. *Anesthesia and Analgesia*, **65**, 877–82.

Schuh, F. T. (1977). Zur cholinesterase-Hemmung durch pancuronium. *Anesthesist*, **26**, 125–9.

Seed, R. F. and Chamberlain, J. H. (1977). Myocardial stimulation by pancuronium bromide. *British Journal of Anaesthesia*, **49**, 401–7.

Segredo, V., Matthay, M. M., Sharma, M. L., Gruenke, L. D., Caldwell, J. E., and Miller, R. D. (1990). Prolonged neuromuscular blockade after long-term administration of vecuronium in two critically ill patients. *Anesthesiology*, **72**, 566–70.

Shi, W. Z., Fahey, M. R., Fisher, D. M., Miller, R. D., Canfell, C. and Eger, E. I. (1985). Laudanosine (a metabolite of atracurium) increases the minimal alveolar concentration of halothane in rabbits. *Anesthesiology*, **63**, 584–8.

Shrivastava, O. P., Chatterji, S., Kachhawa, S., and Daga, S. R. (1983). Calcium gluconate pretreatment for prevention of succinylcholine-induced myalgia. *Anesthesia and Analgesia*, **62**, 59–62.

Siler, J. N., Mager, J. G., and Wyche, M. Q. (1985). Atracurium: hypotension, tachycardia and bronchospasm. *Anesthesiology*, **62**, 645–6.

Smith, K. L. (1957). Histamine release by suxamethonium. *Anaesthesia*, **12**, 293–8.

Sokoll, M. D., Gergis, S. D., Mehta, M., Ali, N. M., and Lineberry, C. (1983). Safety and efficacy of atracurium (BW33A) in patients receiving balanced or isoflurane anesthesia. *Anesthesiology*, **58**, 450–5.

Sorensen, M., Engbaek, J., Viby-Mogensen, J., Guldager, H., and Molke Jensen, F. (1984). Bradycardia and cardiac asystole following a single injection of suxamethonium. *Acta Anaethesiological Scandinavica*, **28**, 232–5.

Spence, A. A. and Barnetson, R. S. (1985). Reaction to vecuronium bromide. *Lancet*, **1**, 979–80.

Srivastava, S. (1984). Angioneurotic oedema following atracurium. *British Journal of Anaesthesia*, **56**, 932–3.

Standaert, F. G. and Adams, J. E. (1965). The actions of succinylcholine on the mammalian motor nerve terminal. *Journal of Pharmacology and Experimental Therapeutics*, **149**, 113–21.

Stanley, J. C., Lyons, S. M., Mirakhur, R. K., Carson, I. W., Gibson, F. M., McMurray, T. J., *et al.* (1991). Comparison of the haemodynamic effects of pipecuronium and pancuronium during fentanyl anaesthesia. *Acta Anaesthesiologica Scandinavica*, **35**, 262–6.

Starr, N. J., Sethna, D. H., and Estafanous, F. G. (1986). Bradycardia and asystole following the rapid administration of sufentanil with vecuronium. *Anesthesiology*, **64**, 521–3.

Stenlake, J. B. (1982). Atracurium: a contribution to anaesthetic practice. *Pharmacology Journal*, **229**, 116–20.

Stirt, J.A., Murray, A. L., Katz, R. L., Schehl, R. N., and Lee, C. (1983). Atracurium during halothane anesthesia in humans. *Anesthesia and Analgesia*, **62**, 207–10.

Stoelting, R. K. (1974). Hemodynamic effects of dimethyl tubocurarine during nitrous oxide-halothane anesthesia. *Anesthesia and Analgesia*, **53**, 513–5.

Stoeling, R. K. (1973). Hemodynamic effects of gaamine during halothane-nitrous oxide anesthesia. *Anesthesiology*, **39**, 645–7.

Stoeling, R. K. (1972). The hemodynamic effects of pancuronium and *d*-tubocurarine in anesthetized patients. *Anesthesiology*, **36**, 615–5.

Stoeling, R. K. (1971). Blood pressure response to *d*-tubocurarine and its preservatives in anesthetized patients. *Anesthesiology*, **35**, 315–7.

Stoeling, R. K and Longnecker, D. E. (1972). Effect of promethazine on hypotension following *d*-tubocurarine use in anesthetized man. *Anesthesia and Analgesia*, **51**, 509–13.

Stoops, C. M., curtis, C. A., kovach. D. A., McCammon, R. L.,Stoeing, R. K., Warren, T. M., *et al.* (1989). Hemodynamic effects of mivacurium choride administered to patients during oxygen-sufentanil anesthesia for coronary artery bypass grafting of valve replacement. *Anesthesia and Analgesia*, **68**, 333–9.

Stoops, C. M., Curtis, C. A., Kovach, D. A., McCammon, R. L., Steling, R. K. Warren, T. M., *et al.* (1988). Hemodynamic effects of doxacurium choride in patients receiving oxygen-sufentanil anesthesia for coronary artery bypass grafting or valve replacement. *Anesthesiology*, **69**, 365–70.

Stovner, J., Oftedal, N., and Holmboe, J. (1975). The inhibition of cholinesterases by pancuronium. *British Journal of Anaesthesia*, **47**, 949–54.

Stullken, E. H. and Sokoll, M. D. (1975). Anesthesia and subarachnoid intracranial pressure. *Anesthesia and Analgesia*, **54**, 494–8.

Sutherland, G. A., Squire, I. B., Gibb, A. J., and Marshal, I. G. (1983). Neuromuscular blocking and autonomic effects of vecuronium and atracurium in the anaesthised cat. *British Journal of Anaesthesia*, **55**, 1119–26.

Tassonyi E., Neidhard, E., Pittet, J. F., Morel, D. R., and Gemperle, M. (1988). Cardiovascular effects of pipecuronium and pancuronium in patients undergoing coronary artery bypass grafting. *Anesthesiology*, **69**, 793–6.

Tattersall, M. P., Manus, N. J., and Jackson, D. M. (1985). The effect of atracurium or fazadinium on intraocular pressure. A comparative study during induction of general anaesthesia. *Anaesthesia*, **40**, 805–7.

Taylor, T. H., Mulcahy, M., and Nightingale, D. (1968). Suxamethonum chloride in intraocular surgery. *British Journal of Anaesthesia*, **40**, 113–8.

Vercruysse, P., Hanegreefs, G., and Vanhoutte, P. M. (1978). Influence of skeletal muscle relaxants on the prejunctional effects of acetylcholine in adrenergically-innervated blood vessels. *Archives Internationales de Pharmacodynamie*, **232**, 350–2.

Vercruysse, P., Bossuyt, P., Hanegreefs, G., Verbeuren, T. J., and Vanhoutte, P. M. (1979). Gallamine and pancuronium inhibit prejunctional and postjunctional muscarinic receptors in canine saphenous veins. *Journal of Pharmacology and Experimental Therapeutics*, **209**, 225–30.

Vervloet, D. (1985). Allergy to muscle relaxants and related compounds. *Clinical Allergy*, **15**, 501–8.

Vervloet, D., Nizankowska, E., Arnaud, A., Senft, M., Alazia, M., and Charpin, J. (1983). Adverse reactions to suxamethonium and other muscle relaxants under general anaesthesia. *Journal of Allergy and Clinical Immunology*, **71**, 552–9.

Waters, D. J. and Mapleson, W. W. (1971). Suxamethonium pains; hypothesis and observation. *Anaesthesia*, **26**, 127–41.

Watkins, J. (1986). Histamine release and atracurium. *British Journal of Anaesthesia*, **58**, 19–22S.

Weintraub, H. D., Heisterkamp, D. V., and Cooperman, L. H. (1969). Changes in plasma potassium concentration after depolarising blockers in anaesthetised man. *British Journal of Anaesthesia*, **41**, 1048–52.

Wembacher, H. and Wolf, H. H. (1971). Regulation of membrane bound acetylcholinesterase activity by bisquaternary nitrogen compounds. *Molecular Pharmacology*, **7**, 554–66.

Wierda, J. M. K. H., Karliczek, G. F., Vandenbrom, R. H. G., Pinto, I., Kersten-Kleef, U. E., Meijer, D. K. F., *et al.* (1990). Pharmacokinetics and cardiovascular dynamics of pipecuronium bromide during coronary artery surgery. *Canadian Journal of Anaesthesia*, **37**, 183–91.

Wins, P., Schoffeniels, E., and Foidart, J. M. (1970). Inhibition of membrane-bound acetylcholinesterase by *d*-tubocurarine and its reversal by bivalent cations. *Life Sciences*, **9**, 259–67.

Wislicki, L. (1977). Factors affecting intraocular pressure. *Proceedings of the Royal Society of Medicine*, **70**, 372.

Youngman, P. R., Taylor, K. M., and Wilson, J. D. (1983). Anaphylactoid reactions to neuromuscular blocking agents: a commonly undiagnosed condition? *Lancet*, **ii**, 597–9.

Zaidan, J. R. and Kaplan, J. A. (1982). Cardiovascular effects of metocurine in patients with aortic stenosis. *Anesthesiology*, **56**, 395–7.

14

What the patient does to the relaxant

P. Duvaldestin and E. Baubillier

Drug action may be modified by alteration of either pharmacodynamics or pharmacokinetics. Most of the factors which alter the duration or intensity of action of the muscle relaxants have a pharmacokinetic origin. One of the best examples is the enhanced duration of action of pancuronium in patients with kidney failure, where there is a reduced plasma drug clearance (Wood 1986). A few alterations have a pharmacodynamic origin, for example in burned patients the response to muscle relaxants may be altered due to changes in the drug–acetylcholine receptor interaction (Dwersteg *et al.* 1986), and in patients with neuromuscular disease like myasthenia sensitivity to muscle relaxants is increased (Agoston *et al.* 1978).

In this chapter, the influence of a number of different conditions on the action of muscle relaxants will be discussed. These include the effects of renal failure, liver failure, obesity, and age.

RENAL FAILURE

Use of muscle relaxants in renal failure

Muscle relaxants are very hydrophilic compounds and most are excreted predominantly in urine. As a result, renal failure is a main cause of prolongation of the neuromuscular blocking effects of pancuronium, gallamine, and tubocurarine.

Until atracurium and vecuronium became available, suxamethonium was the only muscle relaxant where drug elimination was not primarily dependent upon renal function. However, despite their prolonged effects in patients with renal failure, nondepolarizing muscle relaxants are often preferred to suxamethonium because of the significant side-effects of the latter in the anuric patient. The widespread use today of atracurium and vecuronium as the muscle relaxants of choice in patients with renal failure reflects their relatively large systemic clearance and short duration of action.

Renal elimination of muscle relaxants

Muscle relaxants are very hydrophilic because they contain one to three quaternary ammonium groups. They are, therefore, usually completely ionized at body pH.

They are also poorly bound to plasma proteins, although some controversies over drug binding do exist (Wood 1986). The magnitude of binding varies between 20% and 50%. As a result, muscle relaxants are excreted via the kidneys by ultrafiltration. Once filtered at the glomeruli, the muscle relaxants cannot be re-absorbed in the tubular regions because of the high degree of ionization at the pH of the ultrafiltrate. Urinary excretion of muscle relaxants occurs with all the different agents. However, this pathway is the predominant pathway for gallamine (Agoston *et al.* 1978), pancuronium (Agoston *et al.* 1973), alcuronium (Raaflaub and Frey 1972), metocurine (Meijer *et al.* 1979), and tubocurarine (Meijer *et al.* 1979). For the latter four relaxants, it accounts for 50–80% of the dose eliminated in 24 hours; for gallamine, renal elimination accounts for 80–90% (Agoston *et al.* 1978). Urinary elimination of unchanged atracurium and suxamethonium probably represents an additional rather than the major route of drug excretion (Kalow 1959; Goedde *et al.* 1968). The importance of the urinary elimination of vecuronium is still unclear but it may account for 30–50% of the total dose (Bencini *et al.* 1983). The new long-lasting muscle relaxants pipecuronium and doxacurium are also mainly eliminated unchanged by the kidneys. Mivacurium is hydrolysed by plasma cholinesterase at about 70–88% of the rate of suxamethonium. The new compound rocuronium (Org 9426) is probably partly eliminated in urine since its elimination is delayed in animals with renal pedicle ligation (Khuenl-Brady *et al.* 1990).

Pharmacodynamic properties of muscle relaxants in renal failure

Depolarizing agents

As a result of its hydrolysis by the enzyme plasma pseudocholinesterase, the elimination of suxamethonium is largely independent of kidney function. Studies in patients with chronic renal failure, however, suggest that they may have reduced plasma cholinesterase activity (Robertson 1966; Lee and Atkinson 1973). The decrease in cholinesterase activity observed in patients with chronic renal failure may be explained by both haemodilution and decreased liver synthesis. Conflicting data is available concerning the effect of dialysis on plasma cholinesterase activity. Thomas and Holmes (1970), comparing pre- and post-dialysis values found both an increase and a decrease in cholinesterase activity after dialysis. Desmonds and Gordon (1969), however, reported no change while Ryan (1977) observed no significant difference in the cholinesterase activity in patients with chronic renal failure whether they were predialysis or being treated by peritoneal dialysis or haemodialysis. Except in these patients with an atypical cholinesterase enzyme, it seems unlikely that the moderate decrease in plasma cholinesterase activity (30%) seen in patients with chronic renal failure will result in significant prolongation of suxamethonium-induced neuromuscular block.

The risk of hyperkalaemia causing cardiac arrest is also low in adequately treated renal failure patients. The transient increase in the plasma potassium concentration following a single dose of suxamethonium averages 0.3 mmol/l in patients with renal failure and does not differ from that seen in healthy control subjects (Miller *et al.* 1972). As a result, there is little risk of life-threatening hyperkalaemia in patients with renal failure provided there are no coexisting factors predisposing to hyperkalaemia, for example burns, prolonged immobilization or the denervation syndrome (Gronert and Theye 1975).

Nondepolarizing agents

Tubocurarine   Reports on the influence of renal failure on the duration of action of tubocurarine are controversial. Riordan and Gilbertson (1971) have described a patient with chronic renal failure in whom there was prolonged neuromuscular block following repeated doses of tubocurarine. On the other hand, Churchill Davidson *et al.* (1967) found the duration of action of this drug to be unchanged in patients with terminal renal failure. Miller and Gillen (1976) have described three patients with end-stage renal failure who where successfully antagonized by neostigmine following a large dose (48–54 mg) of tubocurarine but who later became recurarized.

In dogs with ligated renal pedicles, there was a reduction in the rate of decline of the plasma concentration of tubocurarine; Gilbaldi *et al.* (1972) have predicted the dose–duration relationship of tubocurarine in the presence of altered renal function. They concluded that the duration of effect of small single doses of tubocurarine would be unaltered by renal failure, whereas larger doses may have a prolonged action due to the exponential relationship between dose and duration of effect. This observation may help to explain some of the controversial results found with tubocurarine. It will also apply to some of the other muscle relaxants. With a small single dose, the duration of effect is influenced mainly by drug redistribution. The duration of effect becomes more dependant on the rate of elimination as the dose increases. Because the main pathophysiological change in renal failure is a decrease in drug clearance in the absence of marked alteration of drug distribution, it can be predicted that the duration of action of tubocurarine will be prolonged especially when large initial doses or incremental doses are administered to the patient with renal failure. Miller *et al.* (1977) reported a longer elimination half-life tubocurarine in patients with renal dysfunction (Table 14.1), coupled with a prolonged effect following a single dose of 0.5 mg/kg. The combined analysis of the plasma decay curve and of evolution of the effect led to a simultaneous modelling of the pharmacokinetics and pharmacodynamics of tubocurarine (Sheiner *et al.* 1979). The prolonged effect of tubocurarine in patients without renal function was shown to be due to pharmacokinetic alterations as the sensitivity of the neuromuscular junction to tubocurarine remained unchanged (Sheiner *et al.* 1979). The plasma concentration at steady-state corresponding to a 50% recovery level was of 0.38 μg/ml in patients with renal failure and this was similar to that observed in the healthy subjects.

Metocurine

In a comparison of the urinary excretion of tubocurarine and metocurine in normal patients, Meijer *et al.* (1979) showed metocurine to be more dependent on renal excretion than tubocurarine. Brotherton and Matteo (1980) found an increased elimination half-life of 10.7 h for metocurine in patients with renal failure, instead of 5.3 h in controls. This change was caused by a decrease in plasma drug clearance.

P. Duvaldestin and E. Baubillier

Table 14.1   Pharmacokinetics of muscle relaxants in patients with renal failure

	Elimination half-life $T^{1}\!/_{2\beta}$ (min)	Total apparent volume of distribution V_d (1/kg)	Plasma clearance Cl (ml/min/kg)
Tubocurarine			
Miller *et al.* 1977			
Controls	152	–	–
Renal failure	256	–	–
Metocurine			
Brotherton and Matteo 1980			
Controls	315	–	1.1
Renal failure	640*	–	0.4
Gallamine			
Ramzan *et al.* 1981			
Controls	131	0.23	1.2
Renal failure	752***	0.29	0.2
Fazadinium			
Duvaldestin *et al.* 1979			
Controls	85	0.29	2.1
Renal failure	140***	0.31	1.5*
Pancuronium			
McLeod *et al.* 1976			
Controls	104	0.15	1.1
Renal failure	489**	0.24	0.3**
Somogyi *et al* 1977*a*			
Controls	133	0.34	1.8
Renal failure	257**	0.33	0.6**
Vecuronium			
Fahey *et al.* 1981			
Controls	80	0.19	3.0
Renal failure	97	0.24	2.5
Bencini *et al.* 1986*a*			
Controls	117	0.51	3.2
Renal failure	149	0.47	2.6
Lynam *et al.* 1988			
Controls	53	0.20	5.3
Renal failure	83*	0.24	3.2*
Atracurium			
Fahey *et al.* 1984			
Controls	21	0.19	6.1
Renal failure	24	0.26	6.7

Table 14.1 (*cont.*)

	Elimination half-life $T_{1/2\beta}$ (min)	Total apparent volume of distribution V_d (1/kg)	Plasma clearance Cl (ml/min/kg)
De Bros *et al.* 1986			
Controls	17	0.14	5.9
Renal failure	21	0.21	6.9
Rocuronium			
Szenohradzky *et al.* 1991			
Controls	203	0.28	2.8
Renal failure	112	0.31	4.6
Pipecuronium			
Caldwell *et al.* 1989			
Controls	137	0.31	2.4
Renal failure	263*	0.44	1.6*
Doxacurium			
Cook *et al.* 1991			
Controls	99	0.2	2.7
Renal failure	221	0.27	1.2*

* $p < 0.05$; ** $p < 0.01$; *** $p < 0.001$, versus controls.

Alcuronium

Signs of neuromuscular block were evident more than 2 h after the administration of alcuronium to a patient with acute renal failure. This was reversed by haemodialysis (Cozanitis and Haapenen 1979). The same study found that the dialysis clearance rates of alcuronium, gallamine, and metocurine are all similar (20–25 ml/min). In a single patient with renal failure, Raaflaub and Frey (1972) observed the half-life of alcuronium was 16 h, compared with 3.6 h in healthy subjects.

Gallamine

Several cases have been reported of prolonged neuromuscular block following the administration of gallamine to patients with renal failure (Feldman and Levy 1963; Lee and Atkinson 1973). Administration of gallamine will result in prolonged paralysis lasting several days in patients with renal failure. It is readily reversed by haemodialysis or peritoneal dialysis (Lowenstein *et al.* 1970; Singer *et al.* 1971). Gallamine is almost exclusively eliminated by the kidney in animals (Feldman *et al.* 1969) as well as in humans (Agoston *et al.* 1978) and therefore this drug is clearly contraindicated in patients with renal failure. In a single case report, however, the successful use of low doses of gallamine in patients with renal failure has been cited (White *et al.* 1971). This is not surprising as the duration of effect with low doses will be limited by redistribution. Ramzan *et al.* (1981*b*) showed the elimination half-life of gallamine to be greatly prolonged from 2.2 h in healthy patients to 12.5 h in patients with renal failure. Again, this change was due primarily to a decrease in plasma clearance.

Pancuronium

Pancuronium has been used successfully in patients with renal failure without any apparent prolonged effect. Delayed recovery was, however, observed by Miller *et al.* (1973) in patients with renal failure and this has been confirmed by d'Hollander *et al.* (1978). McLeod *et al.* (1976) found the elimination half-life of pancuronium to be increased by 500% in patients with renal failure, in whom it averaged 8.3 h instead of 1.7 h in controls. This change reflected a decreased plasma clearance. An increase in the volume of the central compartment was also observed in patients with renal failure (McLeod *et al.* 1976). Delayed elimination of pancuronium was also observed in two other pharmacokinetic studies with the relaxant (Buzello and Ruthven-Murray 1976; Somogyi *et al.* 1977*a*). In practice, the same rules can apply for pancuronium, alcuronium, tubocurarine, and metocurine. After a single dose in the patient with renal failure, the initial degree of paralysis will be either similar to that in a healthy subject, or less because of the increased volume of distribution. The duration of effect will be unchanged provided a relatively small dose has been administered. After a larger bolus dose or incremental doses, a prolonged effect may be expected in renal failure. This effect was described by d'Hollander *et al.* (1978).

Fazadinium

Fazadinium is a relatively short-acting nondepolarizing neuromuscular blocking agent which is excreted mainly unchanged in urine (Duvaldestin *et al.* 1979). The clinical use of this drug was limited owing to its vagolytic properties and to the development of newer short-acting agents with fewer cardiovascular effects. Camu and d'Hollander (1979) reported that, at doses of 0.25 or 0.50 mg/kg, there was no prolongation of the neuromuscular blocking effect of fazadinium in patients with end-stage renal failure. An increased elimination half-life of fazadinium from 1.4 h to 2.3 h was observed in patients with renal failure (Duvaldestin *et al.* 1979).

Vecuronium

In contrast to its bisquaternary analogue pancuronium, vecuronium has a relatively short duration of action, and less cumulative effect in both healthy patients and in patients with renal failure (Lebrault *et al.* 1985). These characteristics can be explained by a plasma clearance of vecuronium double that of pancuronium. Urinary elimination contributes little to the total plasma clearance. Fahey *et al.* (1981) studied the pharmacokinetics of vecuronium in patients with end-stage renal failure following a bolus dose of 0.28 mg/kg. Using a high-pressure liquid chromatographic method for measurement of the plasma drug concentration, they showed the pharmacokinetics of vecuronium to be unaltered in patients with renal failure. In a subsequent pharmacokinetic study, however, Bencini *et al.* (1986*a*), using a more sensitive fluorometric method, observed prolongation of the elimination half-life from 2 h in controls to 2.5 h in patients with renal failure. In those patients with renal failure, an increased onset time was observed after 0.1 mg/kg vecuronium. The plasma vecuronium concentrations corresponding to fixed levels of paralysis were higher in patients with renal failure. This suggests that patients with renal failure may be less sensitive to vecuronium than healthy patients with normal renal function. Another hypothesis is that there is retention of vecuronium metabolites in patients with renal failure due to their decreased rate of elimination. However, since the fluorometric assay does not discriminate unchanged vecuronium from its metabolites, the apparent increase in plasma concentration of vecuronium in patients with renal failure may be related to the presence of metabolites. More recently, Lynam *et al.* (1988) have studied the pharmacokinetics and pharmacodynamics of vecuronium in patients with renal failure using a specific gas chromatographic assay. After a dose of 0.1 mg/kg, they observed an elimination half-life of 83 min in patients with renal failure and 53 min in healthy subjects. Despite large inter-individual variability, the interval from drug administration to recovery to 25% of twitch height was longer (99 min) in renal failure patients than in controls (54 min). Using repeated doses, Bevan *et al.* (1984) have shown vecuronium to have a cumulative effect in patients with renal failure.

Atracurium

Several pharmacokinetic and pharmacodynamic studies with atracurium in patients with renal failure have shown no significant changes compared to normal patients (Fahey *et al.* 1984; Lebrault *et al.* 1984; de Bros *et al.* 1986; Mongin-Long *et al.* 1986). The dose needed to maintain neuromuscular block below a given degree of paralysis was also similar in renal failure and healthy individuals. Recovery from paralysis has, however, been found to be prolonged following repeated dose administration to patients in renal failure (Nguyen *et al.* 1985). Atracurium undergoes spontaneous or enzyme-catalysed hydrolysis. One of the metabolites, laudanosine, may accumulate in patients with renal failure as 2–12% of laudanosine is eliminated unchanged in urine (Hennis *et al.* 1986). Following the administration of atracurium 0.5 mg/kg in patients with renal failure undergoing cadaver kidney transplantation, plasma concentrations of laudanosine were higher than those found in normal patients (Fahey *et al.* 1984). The risk of laudanosine concentrations above the plasma level associated with convulsions (17 μg/ml in the dog) appears, however, to be low in patients with renal failure (Ward *et al.* 1985). Using pharmacokinetic data for laudanosine following administration of atracurium, Ward *et al.* (1985) calculated that the steady-state plasma concentration attained after a continuous infusion of atracurium (0.6 mg/kg/h) will be 10 times less than toxic plasma level observed in the dog. Thus, atracurium appears to be the neuromuscular blocking agent best suited for use in the patient with renal failure.

Mivacurium

This agent is a new short-acting neuromuscular relaxant. It is rapidly metabolized by plasma cholinesterase (Savarese *et al.* 1988*a*, *b*) and presumably this accounts for its short and non-cumulative duration of action. Savarese (1989) found that the duration of action of mivacurium is slightly prolonged by 20% in renal failure. It might therefore be expected that the pharmacokinetics of mivacurium would be minimally altered in renal failure patients although additional studies are needed.

Rocuronium (Org 9426)

Preliminary studies in animals have shown that rocuronium is eliminated unchanged, primarily via the bile; urinary elimination is a minor pathway. Indirect evidence for a similar pattern of elimination in humans has been presented by Szenohradszky *et al.* (1991) who reported that there were no differences between the pharmaco-kinetics and pharmacodynamics of rocuronium in patients with normal or absent renal function. In fact, it seemed that rocuronium followed a pattern of both renal and hepatic elimination without significant metabolism.

Doxacurium

This new nondepolarizing neuromuscular blocking agent is a long-acting relaxant with a duration of action similar to that of tubocurarine or pancuronium (Agoston *et al.* 1992). Pharmacokinetic data concerning doxacurium are consistent with a predominantly renal route of elimination of unchanged drug, and with little or no metabolism. Savarese *et al.* (1988*b*) found that 40–50% of an injected dose could be recovered from the urine within 12 hours. Cashman *et al.* (1990) evaluated the characteristics of the neuromuscular block induced by doxacurium in patients with end-stage chronic renal failure, and in a group of healthy patients. No differences between the two groups were found with respect to onset and duration of action. A wide inter-individual variation in the duration of action of doxacurium was, however, observed in patients with renal failure. In contrast, Cook *et al.* (1991) found that patients with renal dysfunction tend to clear doxacurium at a slower rate than normal patients. A prolonged duration of action of doxacurium can therefore be expected in some patients with renal dysfunction at least and neuromuscular monitoring is advisable.

Pipecuronium

This new long-acting relaxant is predominantly eliminated unchanged by the kidney and its excretion characteristics resemble those of pancuronium. In patients with renal failure, there is a prolonged elimination half-life of 263 min (compared with 137 min in control patients), which is due to a decreased clearance (Caldwell *et al.* 1989). At a dose of 70 μg/kg pipecuronium produced a long-lasting effect. The recovery of twitch to 25% of control varied between 55 and 198 min in controls and was even more variable in renal failure, from 30 to 267 min.

Protein binding in patients with renal failure

Protein binding of drugs is frequently altered in the patient with renal failure. For acidic compounds a decreased albumin-binding capacity is the main abnormality observed during end-stage renal failure (Reidenberg and Drayer 1984). Alterations in the binding of basic compounds, which bind to both albumin and alpha-glyco-protein acid, may also occur during renal failure (Piafsky 1980; Wood 1986). Ghoneim *et al.* (1973) showed the protein binding of tubocurarine to be unchanged in patients with renal failure, while Wood *et al.* (1985) found that chronic renal failure did not modify the binding of pancuronium to plasma proteins.

LIVER FAILURE

General considerations

Increased resistance and prolonged effect are the two main abnormalities reported in patients with hepatic dysfunction (Duvaldestin *et al.* 1985). Resistance to tubocurarine was first reported in patients with liver dysfunction (Dundee and Gray 1953; Haselhuhn 1957). A prolonged effect following the administration of pan-curonium to patients with liver disease has also been reported (Ward *et al.* 1975). It was originally thought that the resistance to muscle relaxants was due to increased binding of the relaxants to gammaglobulins (Stovner *et al.* 1971; see Arden *et al.* 1988) with a decreased free fraction. Since the initial reports, however, it has been shown that muscle relaxants are not significantly bound to plasma proteins in either healthy patients or in patients with liver disease (Stovner 1975; Duvaldestin and Henzel 1982; Wood 1986; Arden *et al.* 1988). Another suggestion was that tubocu-rarine may be stored in the enlarged liver and spleen sometimes found in patients with chronic liver disease (Feldman 1973).

Hepatic disposition of muscle relaxants

The role of the liver in the elimination of muscle relaxants in humans is less import-ant than renal excretion. The percentages of a dose of relaxant excreted in bile are much lower than those excreted in urine (Table 14.2). Biliary excretion accounts for about 10% of the dose for pancuronium (Agoston *et al.* 1973), tubocurarine (Meijer *et al.* 1979), and alcuronium (Raaflaub and Frey 1972) and is less for metocurine (Meijer *et al.* 1979). Gallamine does not appear to be excreted in bile (Arden *et al.* 1988).

The biliary excretion of vecuronium may represent an important pathway in humans (Bencini *et al.* 1986*b*). Biliary excretion of muscle relaxants in man is, however, probably underestimated for several reasons. Firstly, the volume of bile flow collected via a T-tube does not necessarily account for the total bile flow. Secondly, in patients requiring biliary drainage the processes involved in biliary excretion of muscle relaxants may be altered. Thirdly, because the drainage tube is

Table 14.2 Pharmacokinetics of muscle relaxants in patients with hepatic diseases

	Terminal elimination half-life $T_{1/2\beta}$ (min)	Total apparent volume V_d (l/kg)	Total body clearance Cl (ml/min/kg)
Pancuronium			
Somogyi *et al.* 1977*b*			
Controls	133	0.34	1.8
Cholestasis		0.38	0.8**
Duvaldestin *et al.* 1978			
Controls	114	0.28	1.9
Cirrhosis	208**	0.42*	1.4*
Westra *et al.* 1981			
Controls	141	0.27	1.8
Cholestasis	224*	0.43	1.5
Ward *et al.* 1982			
Controls	94	0.19	1.4
Hepatitis	303*	0.19	0.6***
Gallamine			
Westra *et al.* 1981			
Controls	162	0.24	1.2
Cholestasis	220	0.26	0.9
Ramzan *et al.* 1981b			
Controls	135	0.21	1.2
Cholestasis	160	0.25	1.2
Fazadinium			
Duvaldestin *et al.* 1980			
Controls	82	0.29	2.3
Cirrhosis	153*	0.45***	1.9
Cholestasis	103*	0.5	2.0
Vecuronium			
Lebrault *et al.* 1985, 1986			
Controls	55	0.27	5.1
Cirrhosis	73*	0.23	2.7**
Cholestasis	98*	0.21	2.4**
Atracurium			
Ward and Neill 1983			
Controls	21	0.16	5.3
Hepatitis	22	0.21	6.5
Doxacurium			
Cook *et al.* 1991			
Controls	99	0.22	2.7
End-stage liver disease	115	0.29	2.3

Table 14.2   (*cont.*)

	Terminal elimination half-life $T^1/_{2\beta}$ (min)	Total apparent volume $V_{\rm d}$ (l/kg)	Total body clearance Cl (ml/min/kg)
Rocuronium			
Magorian *et al.* 1991			
Controls	79	0.174	3.4
Hepatic dysfunction	173	0.322	3

$^* p < 0.05$; $^{**} p < 0.01$; $^{***} p < 0.001$, versus controls.

placed *in situ* towards the end of surgery, some excreted drug may not be collected. Fourthly, since biliary excretion is proportional to plasma concentration, the fraction excreted in bile during the first few hours probably accounts for a large fraction of the total dose eliminated.

Mechanism of biliary secretion of muscle relaxants

Studies using radiolabelled muscle relaxants indicate that most of the drugs are present in high concentration in the liver (Waser 1973; Shindo *et al.* 1974). Although the highest concentrations are found in the kidneys and in cartilage, a recent study with ^{14}C-labelled vecuronium in the rat suggested that the highest activity was present in the liver (Waser *et al.* 1987).

Using the isolated perfused rat liver, it was shown that tubocurarine enters the hepatocyte by passive diffusion, which is limited by the unbound plasma fraction (Vonk *et al.* 1978; Wood *et al.* 1985). Tubocurarine is then concentrated in the lysosomes and biliary excretion occurs through breakdown of these lysosomes into the lumen of the biliary canaliculi (Meijer *et al.* 1976; Vonk *et al.* 1978). Active transport systems involved in biliary secretion of other drugs do not seem to be involved in the secretion of the muscle relaxants, since neither inhibition of the sodium–potassium ATPase by cardiac glycosides (Meijer and Scaf 1968) nor stimulation of the biliary secretion by bile acids modify the biliary excretion of tubocurarine (Vonk *et al.* 1978; Westra *et al.* 1981*a*, *b*). The biliary excretion of the tubocurarine is increased by 300% in dogs made anephric. The increased biliary excretion of tubocurarine may be passive and related to the higher plasma concentrations of tubocurarine in anephric animals. Similar studies with gallamine have shown no increase in biliary excretion in anephric dogs (Feldman *et al.* 1969). In an experimental cat model, exclusion of the liver increased the intensity and duration of the neuromuscular block caused by vecuronium, which still had a shorter duration of action than pancuronium (Durant *et al.* 1979). The dose of steroidal relaxants recovered in urine and bile in animal and human studies is often incomplete, suggesting that the muscle relaxant may be stored in the liver and secondarily excreted into the bile (Blom *et al.* 1982). Liver uptake of pancuronium in the cat resulted in 28% of the dose appearing in bile with a further 24% remaining in the liver 8 h after its administration (Nagashima *et al.* 1983). The shorter duration of effect of vecuronium is believed to be caused by a more rapid hepatic handling of muscle relaxants (Savage *et al.* 1980; Upton *et al.* 1982; Nagashima *et al.* 1983; Bencini *et al.* 1985).

Biotransformation of muscle relaxants

Steroidal neuromuscular blocking agents are metabolized by hydrolysis of the acetyl group at the 3 and 17 positions. This biotransformation has been presumed to occur mainly in the liver since appreciable amounts of pancuronium metabolites are found in hepatic tissues (Agoston *et al.* 1978). The amount of the dose which is metabolized varies from 10% to 20%. Vecuronium is de-acetylated into 3-hydroxy, 17-hydroxy, or 3,17-dihydroxy derivatives (Savage *et al.* 1980). The main metabolite, the 3-hydroxy metabolite, accounts for one-third of the dose recovered in urine (Bencini *et al.* 1983). Fazadinium is partly metabolized in the liver but this pathway of elimination is negligible since only 5% of the dose undergoes such biotransformation (Duvaldestin *et al.* 1980). The other muscle relaxants are not metabolized by the liver to any significant extent.

Pharmacokinetics of muscle relaxants in patients with liver disease

There are three types of liver failure which may affect the pharmacokinetics of muscle relaxants during anaesthesia. The first is liver cirrhosis in which hepatocyte function and hepatic blood flow are disturbed. Cirrhosis is associated with hypoproteinaemia, ascites, oedema and often kidney dysfunction. The second is cholestasis where a selective insufficiency of biliary excretion appears without notable liver parenchymatous failure. The third is acute hepatic failure which may occur in patients with viral or toxic hepatitis. The influence of these three different types of liver disease on the pharmacokinetics of most of the currently available muscle relaxants has been investigated.

Pancuronium

Cholestasis The pharmacokinetics of pancuronium in patients with complete biliary obstruction due to cancer or gallstones and the degree of neuromuscular block were investigated by Somogyi *et al.* (1977*b*). They found that cholestasis caused a 50% decrease in the plasma clearance of pancuronium (Table 14.2) leading to a prolonged elimination half-life of 270 min as compared with 132 min. Cholestasis resulted in an increased volume of distribution but had no effect on plasma clearance. Under experimental conditions in the laboratory, cholestasis increased the duration of effect of the short-acting steroidal relaxants (Vonk *et al.* 1978), and it has been suggested that liver uptake and biliary excretion of these short-acting compounds may be inhibited by a high plasma concentration of bile salts. The delayed elimination of some relaxants in patients with cholestasis may be explained by the same mechanism.

Cirrhosis Prolongation of both distribution and elimination half-lives of pancuronium in anaesthetized patients with cirrhosis were reported by Duvaldestin *et al.* (1978). The increase in the elimination half-life was due to a decreased plasma clearance as well as an increased volume of distribution (see Table 14.2). The volumes of both central and peripheral compartments were greater in patients with cirrhosis. This may be due to an increased extracellular fluid volume, despite the absence of overt signs of overhydration such as ascites or oedema (Duvaldestin *et al.* 1978). An alternative hypothesis is that pancuronium and some other relaxants have a high affinity for chondroitin sulfate (Olsen *et al.* 1975), and hence the increased mass of collagen due to hepatic fibrosis may prolong both the distribution and elimination half-lives (Stovner 1975). The enlarged volume of distribution may provide one explanation for the resistance to muscle relaxants seen in patients with cirrhosis (Duvaldestin *et al.* 1978). The greater dilution of relaxant will prevent plasma drug concentrations adequate for muscle relaxation being attained. The increased volume of distribution will also delay the onset of action.

Hepatitis Ward *et al.* (1982) studied the kinetics of pancuronium in patients with severe acute hepatic failure caused by paracetamol overdosage. All patients had severe hepatic failure with grade IV coma but had no renal failure. The mean elimination half-life was increased to 310 min (see Table 14.2), but associated with considerable inter-individual variability. This change was due to a reduced plasma clearance. The volumes of distribution were unchanged in patients with acute liver failure, but the dose of drug required to produce adequate muscle paralysis was much greater than in controls.

Gallamine

Several separate studies have investigated gallamine pharmacokinetics in patients with extrahepatic biliary obstruction. Cholestasis had no effect on the elimination of gallamine (Ramzan *et al.* 1981*a*). A small but significant increase in the total apparent volume of distribution of gallamine was reported by Ramzan *et al.* (1981*a, b*). The absence of any pharmacokinetic alteration in patients with cholestasis is not surprising since gallamine is almost exclusively excreted by the kidneys in humans (Bell *et al.* 1985).

Fazadinium

The pharmacokinetics of fazadinium are unaltered in patients with complete renal failure (Duvaldestin *et al.* 1979) and it was, therefore, believed that the drug was primarily eliminated by the liver. In patients with cholestasis a slight prolongation of the elimination half-life (103 min instead of 82 min) was reported by Duvaldestin *et al.* (1980). However, in patients with cirrhosis the elimination half-life was significantly prolonged (153 min compared with 82 min). Cirrhosis, therefore, caused changes in the pharmacokinetics of fazadinium which were similar to those previously observed for pancuronium. The total apparent volume of distribution of fazadinium was increased by 50% in cirrhotics while plasma clearance remained unchanged (see Table 14.2).

Vecuronium

Cirrhosis   The elimination half-life of vecuronium was increased from 55 to 73 min in patients with mildly decompensated cirrhosis as the result of a decrease in clearance, while the volume of distribution remained unchanged (Lebrault *et al.* 1985). The response of cirrhotics to vecuronium varies according to the dose. After a dose of 0.1 mg/kg, vecuronium was shorter acting in patients with cirrhosis than in healthy individuals (Bell *et al.* 1985; Hunter *et al.* 1985). After larger doses (0.2 mg/kg), however, cirrhosis increased the duration of action of vecuronium (Lebrault *et al.* 1985; Hunter *et al.* 1985). These differences in results can be explained by the influences of distribution and elimination upon the duration of action of vecuronium. After low doses the duration of action is limited by the distribution half-life, while after larger doses metabolism is the rate-limiting step. In a more recent study, Arden *et al.* (1988) observed that the pharmacokinetics of vecuronium were unchanged in patients with alcoholic liver disease, in which half of the patients were in Child's class C.

Cholestasis   In patients with cholestasis undergoing biliary surgery, Lebrault *et al.* (1986) observed similar findings to patients with cirrhosis, with an increased elimination half-life (70% higher) which was explained by a decrease in plasma clearance (Table 14.2). These changes were associated with a prolonged duration of effect following a dose of 0.2 mg/kg. The recovery of twitch height to 75% of control was increased from 74 min in healthy patients to 111 min in patients with cholestasis. Because of the wide inter-individual variation seen in the response to vecuronium in patients with biliary obstruction, the monitoring of neuromuscular function in these patients is desirable, with titration of dose to effect.

Atracurium

Atracurium has been used successfully in patients with liver disease. The duration of action of atracurium was unaltered in patients with cirrhosis and also when administered to infants with biliary atresia (Bell *et al.* 1985; Simpson and Green 1986). The pharmacokinetics of atracurium have also been studied by Ward and Neill (1983) in patients with fulminant hepatic failure, most of whom also had accompanying renal failure. The elimination half-life of atracurium was unchanged (20 min in controls and 23 min in patients with liver failure) while the volume of distribution was significantly increased in patients with liver failure (Table 14.2). Similarly Cook *et al.* (1984) observed no alteration in the kinetics of atracurium in children with severe chronic liver disease. Atracurium therefore seems to be the muscle relaxant of choice in cases of hepatic dysfunction.

Mivacurium

Mivacurium is hydrolysed by plasma cholinesterase at about 70–88% of the rate of suxamethonium and seems to be subject to the same alterations of duration in the presence of disorders of the enzyme as does suxamethonium. This drug is also metabolized by the liver. Its duration of effect is slightly prolonged in severe liver disease (Savarese 1989).

Rocuronium

Metabolic studies have shown rocuronium to be mainly excreted into the bile. In a cat model, with hepatic exclusion, rocuronium showed marked prolongation of effect (Khuenl-Brady *et al.* 1989). Magorian *et al.* (1991) investigated the effect of hepatic dysfunction in humans on the pharmacokinetics of rocuronium. They found that the duration of action was prolonged (114 min vs 47 min in healthy patients) with a larger volume of distribution but that hepatic dysfunction had no influence on the onset of action.

Doxacurium

Basta *et al.* (1988) found that doxacurium, like pancuronium, had prolonged effects in cases of hepatic dysfunction. Cook *et al.* (1991) in an other study found no differences between patients with liver disease and patients without. They concluded that liver disease appeared to have no significant impact on the pharmacokinetics of doxacurium.

Pipecuronium

Pipecuronium follows a similar pattern of renal elimination to pancuronium with little or no metabolism and only a minor secondary biliary pathway. Agoston *et al.* (1988) found that in cats, there was hepatic metabolism of pipecuronium bromide to the inactive 17-hydroxy and 3,17-dihydroxy metabolites. In rats, Badragi *et al.* (1980) found only a minimal hepatic elimination. In humans, in the presence of cholestasis neither the pharmacokinetics nor the time-course of action of pipecuronium were significantly different form those in normal patients (Wierda *et al.* 1991).

Protein binding of muscle relaxants in patients with liver disease

An increase in the binding of muscle relaxant to plasma proteins, especially gamma globulins, has been suggested as being responsible for resistance to muscle relaxants in patients with liver disease. This theory is supported by indirect arguments (Thompson 1976) and has not been confirmed by clinical studies (Table 14.3) (Ghoneim *et al.* 1973; Duvaldestin and Henzel 1982; Wood *et al.* 1985). It is accepted that small variations in the degree of binding do not produce a significant change in free concentration because muscle relaxants are poorly bound to plasma proteins anyway. Changes in plasma protein binding should not therefore affect the potency and duration of effect of neuromuscular blocking agents.

Table 14.3 Plasma protein binding of muscle relaxants, influence of liver disease (values are mean values determined by equilibrium dialysis)

Muscle relaxant	Fraction bound to plasma protein (%)		
	controls	cirrhosis	reference
Tubocurarine	44	37	39
	56	44	28
Fazadinium	51	57	28
Pancuronium	29	38	28
Vecuronium	30	24	28

ELDERLY PATIENTS

The distribution and elimination of drugs in the elderly may be altered by any of the multitude of physiological changes that accompany the ageing process. These changes include decreases in lean body mass, in total body water, in glomerular filtration, in renal blood flow, in splanchnic blood flow, and in serum albumin levels, together with an increase in fat content of the body. The long-acting non-depolarizing muscle relaxants pancuronium (McLeod *et al.* 1979; Duvaldestin *et al.* 1982), metocurine (Matteo *et al.* 1985), and tubocurarine (Matteo *et al.* 1985) have prolonged durations of action in the elderly, related to decreased elimination of these drugs through the kidneys. For vecuronium, in a study comparing patients older than 60 years with two groups of younger patients, d'Hollander *et al.* (1982) found that spontaneous recovery of the twitch height from 10% to 25% and from 25% to 75% were significantly longer in the older patients. In a recent study, Lien *et al.* (1991) found the action of vecuronium to be secondary to a decrease in drug elimination in older patients which was consistent with age-associated decreases in hepatic and renal blood flow.

There are few data concerning atracurium and elderly patients but it seems that the duration of its action is similar in older or younger patients (Agoston *et al.* 1992). The half-life may, however, be longer and the volume of distribution larger (Kent *et al.* 1989; Kitts *et al.* 1990) than in young adults, which could prolong recovery from neuromuscular block after multiple or large doses in the elderly. Basta *et al.* (1989) showed that neither the neuromuscular effects nor the pharmacokinetics of mivacurium were affected by the normal physiological changes in organ function seen in elderly patients. Matteo *et al.* (1991) studied elderly patients who received rocuronium and found a prolonged recovery time, a prolonged elimination half-life and a decreased plasma clearance. Dresner *et al.* (1990) showed that doxacurium had a longer duration of action in elderly patients.

OBESITY

Obesity usually tends to increase the clearance of renally cleared drugs (Abernathy and Greenblatt 1986). It does not, however, cause prolonged neuromuscular block except when dosage has been calculated on the basis of total body weight. Tsueda *et al.* (1978) investigated the amount of pancuronium necessary to maintain a constant depression of 90% of twitch height in obese and non-obese patients. They found the mean dose of pancuronium to be greater in the obese subjects. However, when dose was corrected for body surface area, there was no difference between the amounts of pancuronium needed in the two groups. Since pancuronium is highly water soluble, it will not distribute widely in the fat tissue, and hence the increased dose requirement in obesity probably relates to the increase in the extracellular fluid volume (Morse and Soeldner 1965).

REFERENCES

Abernathy, D. R. and Greenblatt, D. J. (1986). Drug disposition in obese humans: an update. *Clinical Pharmacokinetics*, **11**, 199–213.

Agoston, S., Vermeer, G. A., Kersten, U. W., Meijer, D. K. F. (1973). The fate of pancuronium bromide in man. *Acta Anaesthiologica Scandinavica*, **17**, 267–75.

Agoston, S., Vermeer, G. A., Kersten, U. W., and Scaf, A. H. J. (1978). A preliminary investigation of the renal and hepatic excretion of gallamine triethiodide in man. *British Journal of Anaesthesia*, *50*, 345–51.

Agoston, S., Vandenhom, R. H. G., Wierda, J. M. K. H., Houvertjes, M. C., and Kersten U. W. (1988). Pharmacokinetics and disposition of pipecuronium bromide in the cat. *European Journal of Anaesthesiology*, *5*, 233–42.

Agoston, S., Vandenbrom, R. H. G., and Wierda, J. M. K. H. (1992). Clinical pharmacokinetics of neuromuscular blocking drugs. *Clinical Pharmacokinetics*, **22**, 94–115.

Arden, J. R., Lynam, D. P., Castagnoli, K. P., Canfell, C., Cannon, J. C., and Miller, R. D. (1988). Vecuronium in alcoholic liver disease: a pharmacokinetic and pharmacodynamic analysis. *Anesthesiology*, **68**, 771–6.

Badragi, L., Feher, T., Varadi, A., and Vereczkey, L. (1980). Pharmacokinetics of pipecuronium bromide in the rat. *Arzneimittel Forschung*, **30**, 366–70.

Basta, S. J., Savarese, J. J., and Ali, H. H. (1988). Clinical pharmacology of doxacurium chloride (BW A938U): a new long acting depolarizing muscle relaxant. *Anesthesiology*, **69**, 472–86.

Basta, S. J., Dresner, D. L., Shaff, L. P., Lai, A. A., and Welch, R. (1989). Neuromuscular effects and pharmacokinetics of mivacurium in elderly patients under isoflurane anesthesia. *Anesthesia and Analgesia*, **68**, 518.

Bell, C. F., Hunter, J. M., Jones, R. S., and Utting, J. E. (1985). Use of atracurium and vecuronium in patients with oesophageal varices. *British Journal of Anaesthesia*, **57**, 160–8.

Bencini, A., Scaf, A. H. J., Sohn, Y. L., Keisten, U., and Agoston, S. (1983). Clinical pharmacokinetics of vecuronium. In *Clinical experience with Norcuron*, (ed. S. Agoston, W. C. Bowman, R. D. Miller, and J. Viby-Mogensen), pp. 115-123 Elsevier, Amsterdam.

Bencini, A. F., Houwwertjes, M. C., and Agoston, S. (1985). Effects of hepatic uptake of vecuronium bromide and its putative metabolites on their neuromuscular blocking actions in the cat. *British Journal of Anaesthesia*, **57**, 789–95.

Bencini, A. F., Scaf, A. H. J., Sohn, Y. J., Meistelman, C., Lienhart, A., Kersten, U. W., *et al.* (1986*a*). Disposition and urinary excretion of vecuronium bromide in anesthetized patients with normal renal function or renal failure. *Anesthesia and Analgesia*, **65**, 245–51.

Bencini, A. F., Scaf, A. H. J., Sohn, Y. J., Kersten Kleef, U. W., and Agoston, S. (1986*b*). Hepatobiliary disposition of vecuronium in patients with cholestasis. *British Journal of Anaesthesia*, **58**, 988–95.

Bevan, D. R., Donati, F., Gyasi, H., and Williams, A. (1984). Cumulation of vecuronium in renal failure. *Anesthesiology*, **61**, A296.

Blom, A., Scaf, A. H. J., and Meijer, D. K. F. (1982). Hepatic drug transport in the rat. *Biochemical Pharmacology*, **31**, 1553–65.

Brotherton, W. P. and Matteo, R. S. (1980). Pharmacokinetics of metocurine in man with renal failure. *Anesthesiology*, **53**, S268.

Buzello, W. and Ruthven-Murray, J. (1976). Der Konzentrationsverlauf von Pancuronium im serum anurischer Patienten. *Anaesthesist*, **25**, 440–3.

Caldwell, J. E., Canfell, P. C., Castagnoli, K. P., Lynam, D. P., Fahey M. R., Fisher, D. M., *et al.* (1989). The influence of renal failure on the pharmacokinetics and duration of action of pipecuronium bromide in patients anesthetized with halothane and nitrous oxide. *Anesthesiology*, **70**, 7–12.

Camu, F. and D'Hollander, A. (1979). Neuromuscular blockade of fazadinium bromide (AH 8165) in renal failure patients. *Acta Anesthesiologica Scandinavica*, **22**, 221.

Cashman, J. N., Luke, J. J., and Jones, R. M. (1990). Neuromuscular block with doxacurium (BW A 938U) in patients with normal or absent renal function. *British Journal of Anaesthesia*, **64**, 186–92.

Churchill Davidson, H. C., Way, W. L., and De Jones, R. H. (1967). The muscle relaxants and renal excretion. *Anesthesiology*, **28**, 540.

Cook, D. R., Brandom, B. W., Stiller, R. L., Woelel, S., Lair, A., and Slater, J. (1984). Pharmacokinetics of atracurium in normal and liver failure patients. *Anesthesiology*, **61**, A433.

Cook, D. R., Freeman, J. A., Lai, A. A., Robertson, K. A., Kang Y., Stiller, R. L., *et al.* (1991). Pharmacokinetics and pharmacodynamics of doxacurium in normal patients and in those with hepatic or renal failure. *Anaesthesia and Analgesia*, **72**, 145–50.

Cozanitis, D. and Haapanen, E. (1979). Studies on muscle relaxants during haemodialysis. *Acta Anaesthesiologica Scandinavica*, **23**, 225–34.

De Bros, F., Lai, A., Scott, R., de Bros, J., Goudsouzian, N., and Ali, H. H. (1986). Pharmacokinetics and pharmacodynamics of atracurium during isoflurane anesthesia in normal and anephric patients. *Anesthesia and Analgesia*, **65**, 743–6.

Desmonds, J. W. and Gordon, R. A. (1969). The effect of haemodialysis on blood volume and plasma cholinesterase levels. *Canadian Anaesthetists' Society Journal*, **16**, 292–301.

d'Hollander, A. A., Camu, F., and Sanders, M. (1978). Comparative evaluation of neuromuscular blockade after pancuronium administration in patients with and without renal failure. *Acta Anaesthesiologica Scandinavica*, **22**, 21–26.

d'Hollander, A. A., Massause, F., Nevelsteen, M., and Agoston, S. (1982). Age dependent dose–response relationship of ORG NC45 in anaesthetized patients. *British Journal of Anaesthesia*, **54**, 653–7.

Dresner, D. C., Basta, S. J., Ali, H. H., Schwartz, A. F., and Embree, P. B. (1990). Pharmacokinetics and pharmacodynamicss of atracurium in young and elderly patients during isolufane anesthesia. *Anesthesia and Analgesia*, **71**, 498–502.

Dundee, J. W. and Gray, T. C. (1953). Resistance to *d*-tubocuranine chloride in the presence of liver drainage. *Lancet*, **ii**, 16–17.

Durant, N. N., Houwerjes, M. C., and Agoston, S. (1979). Hepatic elimination of ORG NC 45 and pancuronium. *Anesthesiology*, **51**, S267.

Duvaldestin, P. and Henzel, D. (1982). Binding of tubocuranine, fazadinium, pancuronium and ORG NC45 to serum proteins in normal man and in patients with cirrhosis. *British Journal of Anaesthesia*, **54**, 513–6.

Duvaldestin, P., Agoston, S., Henzel, D., Kersten, U. W., and Desmonts, J. M. (1978). Pancuronium pharmacokinetics in patients with liver cirrhosis. *British Journal of Anaesthesia*, **50**, 1131–6.

Duvaldestin, P., Bertrand, P., Concina, D., Henzel, D., Lareng, L., and Desmonts, J. M. (1979). Pharmacokinetics of fazadinium in patients with renal failure. *British Journal of Anaesthesia*, **51**, 943–7.

Duvaldestin, P., Saada, J., Henzel, D., and Saumon, G. (1980). Fazadinium pharmacokinetics in patients with liver disease. *British Journal of Anaesthesia*, **52**, 789–94.

Duvaldestin, P., Saada, J., Berger, J. L., D'Hollander, A., and Desmonts, J. M. (1982). Pharmacokinetics, pharmacodynamics and dose response relationships of pancuronium in control and elderly subjects. *Anesthesiology*, **56**, 36–40.

Duvaldestin, P., Lehautt, C., and Chauvin, M. (1985). Pharmacokinetics of muscle relaxants in patients with liver disease. *Clinics in Anaesthesiology*, **3**, 293–306.

Dwersteg, J. F., Pavlin, E. G., and Heimbach, D. M. (1986). Patients with burns are resistant to atracurium. *Anesthesiology*, **65**, 517–20.

Fahey, M. R., Maris, R. B., Miller, R. D., Nguygen, T. L., and Upton, R. A. (1981). Pharmacokinetics of ORG NC 45 (Norcuron) in patients with and without renal failure. *British Journal of Anaesthesia*, **53**, 1049–52.

Fahey, M. R., Rupp, S. M., Fischer, D. M., Miller, R. D., Sharma, M., Canfell, C., *et al.* (1984). The pharmacokinetics and pharmacodynamics of atracurium in patients with and without renal failure. *Anesthesiology*, **61**, 699–702.

Feldman, S. A. (1973). Muscle relaxants in pathological states. In *Muscle relaxants*, p. 129. Saunders, London.

Feldman, S. A. and Levy, J. Z. (1963). Prolonged paresis following gallamine. *British Journal of Anaesthesia*, **35**, 804–6.

Feldman, S. A., Cohen, E. N., and Golling, R. C. (1969). The excretion of gallamine in dog. *Anesthesiology*, **30**, 593–8.

Gilbaldi, M., Levy, G., and Hayton, W. L. (1972). Tubocurarine and renal failure. *British Journal of Anaesthesia*, **44**, 163–5.

Goedde, H. W., Held, K. R., and Altland, K. (1968). Hydrolysis of succinylcholine and succinylmonocholine in human serum. *Molecular Pharmacology*, **4**, 274–87.

Ghoneim, M. M., Kramer, S. E., and Barrow, R. (1973). Binding of *d*-tubocurarine to plasma proteins in normal man and in patients with hepatic or renal disease. *Anesthesiology*, **39**, 410–15.

Gronert, G. A. and Theye, R. A. (1975). Pathophysiology of hyperkalaemia induced by succinylcholine. *Anesthesiology*, **43**, 89–99.

Haselhuhn, D. H. (1957). The use of pentothal in the presence of severe hepatic disease. *Anesthesia and Analgesia*, **36**, 73–5.

Hennis, P. J., Fahey, M. R., Canfell, P. C., Shi, W. Z., and Miller, R. D. (1986). Pharmacology of laudanosine in dogs. *Anesthesiology*, **65**, 56–60.

Hunter, J. M., Parker, C. J. R., Bell, C. F., Jones, R. S., and Utting, J. E. (1985). The use of different doses of vecuronium impatients with liver dysfunction. *British Journal of Anaesthesia*, **57**, 758–64.

Kalow, W. (1959). The distribution, destruction and elimination of muscle relaxants. *Anesthesiology*, **20**, 505–18.

Kent, A. P., Parker, C. J. R., and Hunter, J. M. (1989). Pharmacokinetics of atracurium and laudanosine in the elderly. *British Journal of Anaesthesia*, **63**, 661–6.

Khuenl-Brady, K., Canfell, P. C., Miller, R. D., Castagnoli, K. P., and Agoston S. (1989). Pharmacokinetics and disposition of ORG 9416 and ORG 9426 in cat. *British Journal of Anaesthesia*, **62**, 225–6.

Khuenl-Brady, K., Castagnoli, K. P., Canfell, P. C., Caldwell, J. E., Agoston, S., and Miller, R. D. (1990). The neuromuscular blocking effects and pharmacokinetics of ORG 9426 and ORG 9616 in the cat. *Anesthesiology*, **72**, 669–74.

Kitts, J. B., Fisher, D. M., Canfell, C. P., Spellman, B. A., and Caldwell, J. E. (1990). Pharmacokinetics and pharmacodynamics of atracurium in the elderly. *Anesthesiology*, **72**, 272–5.

Lebrault, C., Lavaud, E., Strumza, P., Nebout, T., and Duvaldestin, P. (1984). Effet myorelaxant de L'atracurium chez les patients insuffisants rénaux chroniques. *Annales Français Anesthesie et Reanimation* **3**, 273–6.

Lebrault, C., Berger, J. L., D'Hollander, A. A., Gomeni, R., Henzel, D., and Duvaldestin, P. (1985). Pharmacokinetics and pharmacodynamics of vecuronium (ORG NC 45) in patients with cirrhosis. *Anesthesiology*, **62**, 601–5.

Lebrault, C., Duvaldestin, P., Henzel, D., Chauvin, M., and Guesnon, P. (1986). Pharmacokinetics and pharmacodynamics of vecuronium in patients with cholestasis. *British Journal of Anaesthesia*, **58**, 983–7.

Lee, J. A. and Atkinson, R. S. (1973). In *Synopsis of anaesthesia*, 7th edn. (ed. J. A. Lee and R. E. Atkinson), p. 312. John Wright and Sons, Bristol.

Lien, C. A., Matteo, R. S., Ornstein, E., Schwartz, A. E., and Diaz, J. (1991). Distribution, elimination and action of vecuronium in the elderly. *Anesthesia and Analgesia*, **73**, 39–42.

Lowenstein, E., Goldfine, C., and Flacke, W. E. (1970). Administration of gallamine in the presence of renal failure, reversal of neuromuscular blockade by peritoneal dialysis. *Anesthesiology*, **33**, 556–8.

Lynam, D. P., Cronnelly, R., Castagnoli, K. P., Canfell, C., Caldwell, J., and Arden, J. (1988). The pharmacodynamics, pharmacokinetics of vecuronium in patients anesthetized with isoflurane with normal renal function or with renal failure. *Anesthesiology*, **69**, 227–31.

Magorian, T., Wood, P., Caldwell, J. E., Szenohradszky, J., Segredo, V., Sharma, H., *et al.* (1991). Pharmacokinetics, onset, duration of action of rocuronium in humans: normal vs hepatic dysfunction. *Anesthesiology*, **75**, A1069.

Matteo, R. S., Backers, W. W., and McDaniel, D. D. (1985). Pharmacokinetics, pharmacodynamics of *d*-tubocurarine and metocurine in the elderly. *Anesthesia and Analgesia*, **64**, 22–8.

Matteo, R. S., Ornstein, E., Schwartz, A. E., Stone, J. G., Ostapkovich, N., Spencer, H. K., *et al.* (1991). Pharmacokinetics, pharmacodynamics of ORG 9426 in elderly surgical patients. *Anesthesiology*, **75**, A1065.

McLeod, K., Watson, M. J., and Rawlins, M. D. (1976). Pharmacokinetics of pancuronium in patients with normal and impaired renal function. *British Journal of Anaesthesia*, **48**, 341–5.

McLeod, K., Hull, C. J., and Watson, M. J. (1979). Effects of aging on the pharmacokinetics of pancuronium. *British Journal of Anaesthesia*, **51**, 435–8.

Meijer, D. K. F., Waitering, J. G., and Vonk, R. J. (1976). Hepatic uptake, biliary excretion of *d*-tubocuranine and trimethyl-tubocuranine in the rat *in vivo*, and in isolated perfused rat livers. *Journal of Pharmacology and Experimental Therapeutics*, **198**, 229–39.

Meijer, D. K. F. and Scaf, A. H. J. (1968). Inhibition of the transport of *d*-tubocurarine from blood to the bile by strophanthoside-K in the isolated perfused rat liver. *European Journal of Pharmacology*, **4**, 343–6.

Meijer, D. K. F., Weitering, J. G., Vermeer, G. A., and Scaf, A. H. I. (1979). Comparative pharmacokinetics of *d*-tubocurarine, metocurine in man. *Anesthesiology*, **51**, 402–7.

Miller, R. D. and Gillen, D. J. (1976). Renal failure and post-operative respiratory failure: recurarization. *British Journal of Anaesthesia*, **48**, 253–6.

Miller, R. D., Way, W. L., Hamilton, W. K., and Layzer, R. B. (1972). Succinylcholine induced hyperkalaemia in patients with renal failure. *Anesthesiology*, **36**, 138–41.

Miller, R. D., Stevens, W. C., and Way, W. L. (1973). The effect of renal failure and hyperkalaemia on the duration of pancuronium neuromuscular blockade in man. *Anesthesia and Analgesia*, **52**, 661–6.

Miller, R. D., Matteo, R. S., Benet, L. Z., and Sohn, Y. J. (1977). The pharmacokinetics of *d*-tubocurarine in man with and without renal failure. *Journal of Pharmacology and Experimental Therapeutics*, **202**, 1–7.

Mongin-Long, D., Chabrol, B., Baude, C., Ville, D., Renaudie, M., Dubernard, J. M., *et al.* (1986). Atracurium in patients with renal failure. *British Journal of Anaesthesia*, **58**, 449.

Morse, W. I., and Soeldner, J. S. (1965). The measurement of human adipose tissue mass. In *Handbook of physiology, Section 5, Adipose tissue*, pp. 653–9. American Physiological Society, Washington.

Nagashima, H., Khilkin, A., Ono, K., Fu, S., Duncalf, D., and Foldes, F. F. (1983). Effect of portocaval shunt and/or renal vessel ligation on disposition of muscle relaxants. *Anesthesiology*, **59**, A264.

Nguyen, H. D., Kaplan, R., Nagashima, H., Duncalf, D., and Foldes, F. F. (1985). The neuromuscular effect of atracurium in anephric patients. *Anesthesiology*, **63**, A335.

Olsen, G. D., Chan, E. M., and Riker, W. K. (1975). Binding of *d*-tubocurarine dimethyl-^{14}C-ether iodide and other amines to cartilage, chondroitin sulfate, and human plasma protein. *Journal of Pharmacology and Experimental Therapeutics*, 195, 242–50.

Piafsky, K. M. (1980). Disease induced changes in plasma binding of basic drugs. *Clinical Pharmacokinetics*, **5**, 246–62.

Raaflaub, J. and Frey, P. (1972). Zur Pharmacokinetik von Diallylnortoxiferin beim Menschen. *Arzneimittel Forschung Drug Research*, **22**, 73–8.

Ramzan, M. I., Shanks, C. A., and Triggs, E. J. (1981*a*). Pharmacokinetics and pharmacodynamics of gallamine triethiodide in patients with total biliary obstruction. *Anesthesia and Analgesia*, **60**, 289–96.

Ramzan, M. I., Shanks, C. A., and Triggs, E. J. (1981*b*). Gallamine disposition in surgical patients with chronic renal failure. *British Journal of Clinical Pharmacology*, **12**, 141–7.

Reidenberg, M. M. and Drayer, D. E. (1984). Alteration of drug–protein binding in renal disease. *Clinical Pharmacokinetics*, **9**, 18–26.

Riordan, D. D. and Gilbertson, A. A. (1971). Prolonged curarization in a patient with renal failure. *British Journal of Anaesthesia*, **43**, 506–7.

Robertson, G. S. (1966). Serum cholinesterase deficiency, I: disease, inheritance. *British Journal of Anaesthesia*, **38**, 355–60.

Ryan, D. W. (1977). Preoperative serum cholinesterase concentration in chronic renal failure. *British Journal of Anaesthesia*, **46**, 945–9.

Savage, D. S., Sleigh, T., and Carlyle, J. (1980). The emergence of ORG NC 45, 1-((2B, 3x, 5x, 16B, 17B)-3, 17bis (acetyloxy)-2-(1-piperidnyl)-androstan-1 6yl)-1–methylpiperidinium bromide from the pancuronium series. *British Journal of Anaesthesia*, **52**, 3–10S.

Savarese, J. J., Ali, H. H., Basta, S. J., Embree, P. B., Scott, R. P. F., Seinder, W., *et al.* (1988*a*). The clinical neuromuscular pharmacology of mivacurium chloride (BW B1090 U). *Anesthesiology*, **68**, 723–32.

Savarese, J. J., Wastila, W. B., El Sayad, H. A., Ali, H. H., Basta, S. J., and Embree, P. B. (1988*b*). Some preliminary aspects of the basic clinical pharmacology of mivacurium

(BW 1090U) and doxacurium (BW A 938U), a preliminary report. In *Recent developments in muscle relaxation: atracurium in perspective*, (ed. R. M. Jones and J. P. Payne), pp. 55–60. Royal Society of Medicine, London.

Savarese, J. J. (1989). Clinical properties of the new relaxants: update. *Acta Anaesthesiologica Scandinavica*, **33**, Suppl. 91, 97–8.

Sheiner, L. B., Stanski, D. R., Vozeh, S., Miller, R. D., and Ham, J. (1979). Simultaneous modeling of pharmacokinetics, pharmacodynamics application to *d*-tubocurarine. *Clinical Pharmacology and Therapeutics* **25**, 358–71.

Shindo, H., Nakajima, E., Miyakoshi, N., and Shigehara, E. (1974). Autoradiographic studies on the distribution of quaternary ammonium compounds, III: distribution, excretion, and metabolism of ^{14}C-labelled pancuronium bromide in rats. *Chemical and Pharmaceutical Bulletin*, **22**, 2502–10.

Simpson, D. A. and Green, D. W. (1986). Use of atracurium during major abdominal surgery in infants with hepatic dysfunction from biliary atresia. *British Journal of Anaesthesia*, **58**, 1214–17.

Singer, M. M., Eutton, R., and Way W. L. (1971). Untoward results of gallamine administration during bilateral nephrectomy: treatment with haemodialysis. *British Journal of Anaesthesia*, **43**, 404–5.

Somogyi, A. A., Shanks, C. A., and Triggs, E. J. (1977*a*). The effect of renal failure on the disposition and neuromuscular blocking action of pancuronium bromide. *European Journal of Clinical Pharmacology*, **12**, 23–9.

Somogyi, A. A., Shanks, C. A., and Triggs, E. J. (1977*b*). Disposition kinetics of pancuronium bromide in patients with total biliary obstruction. *British Journal of Anaesthesia*, **49**, 1103–8.

Stovner, J. (1975). Protein binding. In *Recent progress in anaesthesiology and resuscitation*, (ed. I. M. Arias), pp. 238–40. Elsevier, Amsterdam.

Stovner, J., Theodorsen, L., and Bjelke, E. (1971). Sensitivity to tubocuranine and alcuronium with special reference to plasma protein pattern. *British Journal of Anaesthesia*, **43**, 385–91.

Szenohradszky, J., Segredo, V., Caldwell, J. E., Sharma, M., Gruenke, L. D., and Miller, R. D. (1991). Pharmacokinetics, onset, and duration of action of ORG 9426 in humans: normal vs absent renal function. *Anesthesia and Analgesia*, **72**, S290.

Thomas, J. L. and Holmes, J. H. (1970). Effect of hemodialysis on plasma cholinesterase. *Anesthesia and Analgesia*, **49**, 323–5.

Thompson, J. M. (1976). Pancuronium binding by serum proteins. *Anesthesiology*, **31**, 219–27.

Tsueda, K., Warren, J. E., McCafferty, L. A., and Nagle, J. P. (1978). Pancuronium bromide requirement during anesthesia for the morbidly obese. *Anesthesiology*, **78**, 438–9.

Upton, R. A., Nguyen, T. L., Miller, R. D., and Castagnoli, N. (1982). Renal and biliary elimination of vecuronium (ORG NC 45) and pancuronium in rats. *Anesthesia and Analgesia*, **61**, 313–6.

Vonk, R. J., Scholtens, E., Keulemans, G. T. P., and Meijer, D. K. F. (1978). Choleresis and transport mechanisms, IV. Influence of bile salt choleresis on the hepatic transport of the organic cations *d*-tubocuranine, and *N*-acetylprocaine ethobromide. *Naunyn-Schmiedebergs Archives of Experimental Pharmacology*, **302**, 1–7.

Ward, M. E., Adu-Gyamfi, Y., and Strunin, L. (1975). Althesin and pancuronium in chronic liver disease. *British Journal of Anaesthesia*, **47**, 1199–204.

Ward, S., Judge, S., and Corall, I. (1982). Pharmacokinetics of pancuronium bromide in liver failure. *British Journal of Anaesthesia*, **54**, 277.

Ward, S. and Neill, E. A. M. (1983). Pharmacokinetics of atracurium in acute hepatic failure (with acute renal failure). *British Journal of Anaesthesia*, **55**, 1169–72.

Ward, S., Boheimer, N., Weatherley, B. C., and Williams, S. G. (1985). The effect of renal impairment on the disposition of atracurium and its breakdown products. *Anesthesiology*, **63**, A337.

Waser, P. G. (1973). Localization of ^{14}C-pancuronium by histology and whole body autoradiography in normal and pregnant mice. *Naunyn-Schmiedebergs Archives of Experimental Pharmacology*, **279**, 399–412.

Waser, P. G., Wiederkehr, H., Chang Sin Ren, A., and Kaiser-Schonenberg, E. (1987). Distribution and kinetics of ^{14}C-vecuronium in rats and mice. *British Journal of Anaesthesia*, **59**, 1044–51.

Westra, P., Keulemans, G. T. P., Houwertjes, M. C., Harrdonk, M. J., and Meijer, D. K. F. (1981*a*). Mechanisms underlying the prolonged duration of action of muscle relaxants caused by extrahepatic cholestasis. *British Journal of Anaesthesia*, **53**, 217–26.

Westra, P., Vermeer, G. A., De Lange, A. R., Scaf, A. H. J., Meijer, D. K. F., and Wesseling, H. (1981*b*). Hepatic and renal disposition of pancuronium and gallamine in patients with extrahepatic cholestasis. *British Journal of Anaesthesia*, **53**, 331–8.

White, R. D., de Weerd, J. H., and Dawson, B. (1971). Gallamine in anesthesia for patients with chronic renal failure undergoing bilateral nephrectomy. *Anesthesia and Analgesia*, **50**, 11–16.

Wierda, J. M. K. H., Szenohradszky, J., de Wit, A. P. M., Zentai, G., Agoston, S., Kakas, M., *et al.* (1991). The pharmacokinetics urinary and biliary excretion of pipecuronium bromide (Arduan). *European Journal of Anaesthesiology*, **8**, 451–7.

Wood, M. (1986). Plasma drug binding: implications for anesthesiologist. *Anesthesia and Analgesia*, **65**, 786–804.

Wood, M., Stone, W. J., and Wood, A. J. J. (1985). Plasma binding of pancuronium: effects of age, sex and disease. *Clinics in Anaesthesiology* **3**, 293–306.

15

Neuromuscular block in children and neonates

Nishan G. Goudsouzian

The judicious use of muscle relaxants in infants and children requires a knowledge of the drugs themselves as well as an understanding of how pharmacokinetic and pharmacodynamic factors differ in neonates, infants, children, and adults. Notice must be given to the volume of distribution, the pathways of elimination, the sensitivity of the neuromuscular junction to the muscle relaxant, and the structure and function of the muscle itself. In addition, a better understanding of the neonate's distinctive behavioural response to neuromuscular blocking agents requires some knowledge of the development of the myoneural junction and receptors.

DEVELOPMENT OF THE NEUROMUSCULAR JUNCTION

The neuromuscular junction undergoes several changes during embryogenesis. In the early stages the motor neuron, which at first lies in apposition to the developing muscle, starts growing into it. At this early point the acetylcholine (ACh) receptors are uniformly distributed along the surface of the muscle fibre, albeit at low concentrations (Schuetze and Role 1987). Thereafter, morphological specialization, evidenced by clustering of ACh receptors in the post-synaptic region, can be detected. These irregular post-synaptic receptor clusters continue to develop into well-defined plaques juxtaposed to the nerve terminal (Bloch and Pumplin 1988). Further remodelling occurs with an increase in receptor density at the sites associated with nerve endings and gradual elimination of sites away from the nerve endings (Dennis *et al.* 1981). It is possible at this stage to detect deep secondary folds at the tips of which the receptors are condensed (Taxt *et al.* 1983).

The ACh receptors are one of the first membrane proteins to appear during formation of skeletal muscles. During myogenesis, they are found on the entire surface of the uninnervated myotubes. Once a nerve contacts the muscle fibre, a cluster of ACh receptors develops beneath the nerve terminal. These embryonic synaptic receptors are metabolically unstable; like extrajunctional receptors, they have a lower conductance and a longer channel open time than do junctional or mature receptors when activated by ACh (Vicini and Schuetze 1985). Further, their

synaptic currents take much longer to decay. In fact, these embryonic low conductance channels have a mean channel open time which is three-fold that of
the mature receptors.

Almost all of the extrajunctional receptors disappear within days to weeks of
muscle innervation, while the synaptic receptors become metabolically stable and
their ion channels begin to demonstrate adult properties (Schuetze and Role 1987).
Part of this developmental acceleration in synaptic current decay can be attributed
to the appearance of cholinesterase; this cannot, however, account for the entire
change (Brehm and Henderson 1988). Recent evidence indicates, in fact, that junctional and extrajunctional receptors are of separate molecular types, rather than
junctional states of a single type. It is speculated that the changes in channel function result from a substitution of the epsilon subunit for the gamma subunit at the
molecular level (Mishina *et al.* 1986; Leonard *et al.* 1988). Of interest here is the
fact that the channel types are not fixed but are labile and are altered during embryonic development or by innervation or denervation (Brenner and Sakman 1983;
Siegelbaum *et al.* 1984; Allen and Albuquerque 1986).

Acetylcholine released by nerve activity in the embryonic muscle generates long-
duration synaptic currents by opening low-conductance (long open time) channels.
With maturation, this channel activity diminishes and high-conductance fast-gated
channels predominate, producing the brisk synaptic response characteristic of adult
fast twitch muscle. Nerve function mediates this developmental change by preferentially modulating the expression of low-conductance ACh receptors. Moreover
nerve-induced activity in muscle cells seems to be a controlling factor in suppress-
ing the production of extrajunctional receptors (Brehm and Henderson 1988).

The functional significance of high-conductance channels lies in the fact that
they mediate synaptic transmission and are thus well-suited to the task of initiating
fine discriminate movements. By contrast, the significance of low-conductance
channels is more speculative. Their role could be one of activity detection and they
might or might not play a part in the proper development of muscle function.
Because of their long open times, these channels could act as very sensitive trans-
ducers, allowing for the passage of many ions per opening. Sodium and calcium ion
entry would be localized to the region of the muscle surface where a nerve fibre is
approaching with its growth cone secreting ACh. The local build-up of ions could
thus provide a spatial clue for the quick transformation of the region to a mature
endplate (Leonard *et al.* 1988).

Regardless of the function of low-conductance channels, the non-synaptic membrane in the embyronic muscle is highly sensitive to ACh whenever contact with
the nerve occurs; in this, it is similar to the adult muscle in which an increased sensitivity to ACh follows denervation (Henderson *et al.* 1987). This characteristic of
early sensitivity diminishes as the density of low-conductance channels decreases
secondary to neural influences.

The nerve is very important in the development and maturation of the receptors.
Initially the nerve leaves an imprint in the muscle at the basal lamina; the resultant
synaptic aggregates are maintained throughout the life of the muscle cell. Following

the aggregation of receptors at the synapses, the nerve terminal induces a decrease in the density of receptors in the non-contacted muscle membrane (Smith and Slater 1983). Neural influence induces changes in the receptors as well, there being a slower rate of receptor degradation subsequent to innervation (Brehm 1986). The clustering of ACh receptors at the postsynaptic membrane of newly innervated muscle fibres occurs because of the release of a trophic factor by the neuron, or by contact and adhesion of the nerve to the muscle (Bloch and Pumplin 1988). A further localization of receptors occurs at the postjunctional membrane with the development of complex junctional folds and the accumulation of receptors at the crests of these folds.

In addition to ultramicroscopic modifications in the myoneural junction, the pattern of innervation in striated muscle changes markedly over the first two weeks of life (Redfern 1970; Brown *et al*. 1976). Initially, each muscle fibre is innervated by many branches of more than one motor axon and each motor axon innervates many muscle fibres. By maturity, this generality is lost. With the exception of the extraocular muscles, each muscle fibre typically receives branches from only one motor axon (focal innervation). The number of muscle fibres innervated by each axon depends on the precision of the movement performed. In human limb muscle, for example, where precision is not as important each axon innervates about 2000 muscle fibres, whereas in extrinsic eye muscles, where precision is crucial, each axon innervates fewer than five muscle fibres.

Clinical correlations

Indirect evidence implies that less ACh is released from the neonatal nerve terminal in very young infants than in older ones. Both tetanic (50 Hz for 5 s) and train-of-four (TOF) fade may be demonstrated in human infants (but not in children or adults) in the absence of neuromuscular blocking agents (Churchill-Davidson and Wise 1963; Koenigsberger *et al*. 1973; Goudsouzian 1980). Theoretically, fade may represent a presynaptic effect (Bowman 1990). Functionally, the presence of fade indicates that infants have less reserve of neuromuscular function than do more mature individuals. The kinetics of this presynaptic effect may account for the greater sensitivity of the neuromuscular junction to nondepolarizing muscle relaxants in infants less than two months old. In such patients, for example, the steady-state plasma concentration necessary to produce 50% twitch depression for vecuronium and tubocurarine is about half that required in older children (Fisher *et al*. 1982; Fisher *et al*. 1985).

Clinicians and investigators have observed an occasional but marked resistance to nondepolarizing relaxants in the neonate (Goudsouzian *et al*. 1975; Goudsouzian *et al*. 1978; Matteo *et al*. 1984; Meretoja and Luosto 1990). This circumstance cannot be explained by pharmacokinetic factors; it probably occurs in infants who are born with an unusually large number of fetal receptor channels sensitive to ACh (and hence resistant to nondepolarizing relaxants). That this resistance is seen only in the first few weeks of life is an indication that healthy infants rid themselves of these fetal receptors in a very short time (Goudsouzian and Standaert 1986).

Striated muscle fibres also undergo important changes during infancy. In animals, a conversion of type I (slow-twitch oxidative) to type II (fast-twitch glycolytic) has been studied and described (Curless 1977). The opposite observation has been made on autopsy diaphragm specimens using histochemical techniques; here an increase in the percentage of slow-twitch fibres (from 25% in newborns to 55% at eight months of age) has been noted (Keens *et al.* 1978). Anaesthetized infants, however, show slower contraction times than do older children (Goudsouzian 1980).

An additional method for indirect evaluation of muscle development is the tetanus: twitch ratio. This parameter has a strong correlation with age in infants when frequencies of 20 and 50 Hz are employed. At 20 Hz (5 s duration), tetanic height is 3.5 times greater than single twitch height in infants less than one month old, whereas in older children it is 5.5 times greater (Goudsouzian 1980).

PHARMACOKINETIC FACTORS

Volume of distribution

The volume of distribution (V_d) denotes a proportionally constant value that relates the total amount of drug in the body to the concentration at a site where the drug is measurable. It does not refer to an anatomical compartment. Since muscle relaxants are poorly lipid-soluble ionized molecules, they tend to distribute within the extracellular compartment; the lipid bilayer of cell membranes thus constitutes a barrier to intracellular distribution. The changes in extracellular fluid volume (ECF) that are noticed with growth and ageing will therefore produce comparable changes in the volume of distribution. This has been clearly demonstrated with tubocurarine (Fisher *et al.* 1982; Matteo *et al.* 1984); with this drug the volume of distribution in the neonate (per kilogram body weight) is twice that observed in older children. V_d decreases further as the individual matures; in fact adult ECF percentages are reached at mid-adolescence (approximately 20%).

Two studies (Fisher *et al.* 1982; Matteo *et al.* 1984) have evaluated the pharmacokinetic properties of tubocurarine in neonates, infants, and children. Both remarked an increase distribution volume of the drug in neonates and infants as compared to that in children. Fisher *et al.* (1982) noted that the plasma concentration necessary for 50% depression of the twitch response in infants was about half that in children, whereas Matteo *et al.* (1984) found no such trend. The reason for these varying results may lie in part with the differences in investigative protocols. The earlier study was carried out with general surgical patients who were probably well hydrated while the latter included mostly neurosurgical patients who probably were on fluid restriction. The methodologies were also different. The first used a continuous infusion technique and a two-compartment pharmacokinetic model, whereas the second used bolus dosing and a three-compartment pharmacokinetic model. Further, neither study took into account the plasma binding of tubocurarine. In fact, further research has shown that tubocurarine (like metocurine) binds less to plasma protein in neonates than in children due to lower alpha₁-acid glycoprotein levels in the younger patients (Ledez *et al*. 1986). This means that the free fraction of the muscle relaxant will be higher in neonatal blood than in that of the adult (Wood and Wood 1981); consequently these drugs may in fact be more effective in neonates at a lower plasma concentration.

The pharmacokinetic profile of vecuronium in infants has some similarity to that of long-acting nondepolarizing muscle relaxants. In this patient group the plasma concentration necessary to elicit 50% twitch depression is about half that in children (57 vs 110 ng/ml, respectively), whereas the steady-state volume of distribution of vecuronium in the very young is greater than in children (357 vs 204 ml/kg). These factors are likely to partially counteract one another when it comes to determining effective bolus dose requirements. The lower plasma concentration of vecuronium in combination with the larger distribution volume leads to a relatively slow decrease in the plasma concentration during recovery, which is expressed as the drug's prolonged mean residence time in the very young patients (66 vs 34 min) (Fisher *et al*. 1985). Consequently, the dose of vecuronium (especially with repetitive dosing) needs to be more carefully titrated in infants than in children. The same precaution needs to be applied with tubocurarine and probably with any other long-acting agent, since the elimination half-life is so prolonged.

A recent pharmacokinetic study on atracurium (Fisher 1990) has shown that the volume of distribution is in fact larger and the clearance faster in infants than in children. Because the age-related changes in these two parameters are parallel, however, the elimination half-life of atracurium does not change as the patient grows; this confirms earlier findings that atracurium-induced neuromuscular block changes minimally with age (Fisher *et al*. 1990).

In general, the enzymes responsible for hepatic metabolism of drugs are already present in neonates. They are, however, immature, are present in lower concentrations, and have lower activity than those in adults. Understandably, this results in reduced hepatic clearance (Morselli *et al*. 1980). Vecuronium is metabolized by O-dealkylation and hydroxylation by liver enzymes, so this is probably the factor that makes it a long-acting neuromuscular blocking agent in neonates and infants. Unlike small infants, children demonstrate a greater capacity to metabolize drugs than do adults. This may be due to the fact that the size of the liver relative to whole body weight is greater in children than in adults.

Glomerular filtration rate

The glomerular filtration rate (GFR) is lower in preterm infants (especially those less than 34 weeks) than in the full-term neonate. In full-term neonates, glomerular filtration rate increases rapidly over the first few days of life (from 2–4 ml/min to 8–20 ml/min); in pre-term infants increases are much slower (Arant 1978). Since GFR is an important determinant in the clearance of long-acting muscle relaxants (particularly that of tubocurarine), it is not surprising that the effect of such drugs is prolonged in infants (Matteo *et al*., 1984).

NEUROMUSCULAR BLOCKING AGENTS

In this section the neuromuscular blocking agents commonly used in infants and children will be discussed in alphabetical order, emphasizing features pertinent to infants and children. Of these suxamethonium is the only depolarizing agent and has the fastest onset and the shortest duration of action. The newly developed agent mivacurium has a shorter duration of action than atracurium and vecuronium (which are generally acknowledged to be of intermediate duration). The others — tubocurarine, pancuronium, metocurine, alcuronium, gallamine, pipecuronium, and doxacurium — are long-acting agents.

Alcuronium

Alcuronium, a long-acting relaxant frequently used in Europe, has not yet been marketed in the US. Its ED_{95} in children is 270 μg/kg and in infants is about 200 μg/kg; the latter is comparable to that reported for adults (Meretoja and Brown 1990). An impression has grown that alcuronium should be thought of as a shorter-acting agent than pancuronium; however, the hourly maintenance dose of this drug in children is 0.4 times the individual ED_{95}, a figure that is quite similar to that for any long-acting agent. A simple explanation lies in dosing regimens, for alcuronium is usually given in smaller amounts than is pancuronium, the standard dose for adults being 250 μg/kg (93% of ED_{95}) as opposed to the standard pancuronium dose of 100 μg/kg (approximately 130% of ED_{95}).

Atracurium

Atracurium is one of the two intermediate-acting muscle relaxants used frequently in infants and children. The ED_{95} determined in children has varied from 170–280 μg/kg (Goudsouzian 1986; Meakin *et al.* 1988). The higher values are usually those reported from evaluations made during $N_2O:O_2$ anaesthesia. The reported ED_{95} values in infants are 156–230 μg/kg (Brandom *et al.* 1984; Goudsouzian *et al.* 1985). In addition, neonates seem to exhibit slightly lower values than infants (ED_{50} 82 μg/kg and ED_{95} 119 μg/kg) (Meakin *et al.* 1988). Interestingly, the studies that noted lower drug requirements in infants than in children also reported shorter duration of action (Brandom *et al.* 1984). This shorter duration is explained by the greater plasma clearance of atracurium in the very young patient and the fact that atracurium undergoes non-enzymatic hydrolysis in body fluids (Hofmann elimination). That infants have a relatively larger extracellular fluid volume than do children implies that atracurium will have a shorter duration of action.

Atracurium's rapid degradation and its non-cumulative properties have made it a drug of choice for continuous infusion. The average infusion requirement during $N_2O:O_2$ anaesthesia is 9 μg/kg/min; during halothane anaesthesia it is 7 μg/kg/min, with isoflurane it is 6 μg/kg/min and with enflurane it is 5 μg/kg/min (Brandom *et al.* 1985; Goudsouzian *et al.* 1986*b*; Kalli and Meretoja 1988). Studies using continuous infusion of atracurium in infants have reported that the dose requirement is similar to that in children, but that individual variations are more apparent and more extensive (Goudsouzian 1988). As in children during balanced anaesthesia, the infant's requirement was slightly higher (approximately 9 μg/kg/min) while the neonate's was about 25% less than that of older infants and children (Kalli and Meretoja 1988).

With atracurium as with other neuromuscular blocking agents, a standard dose two to three times the ED_{95} (0.3–0.6 mg/kg) is administered to produce rapid neuromuscular block for the facilitation of endotracheal intubation in infants or children. Such doses provide satisfactory conditions for intubation in children within two minutes, and in an even shorter time in infants. Though a smaller dose (by about 25%) might theoretically be indicated for infants than for children, the difference is offset by the fact that metabolism is somewhat faster in infants (Meretoja and Kalli 1986); for practical purposes, then, the same dose (mg/kg) of atracurium can be safely used in both infants and children, with a predictable clinical effect and duration of action within the normal clinical variation. In addition the histamine-related side-effects (which are sometimes seen with adult patients) are practically absent in this young age group (Goudsouzian *et al.* 1986*a*).

An exception to this general indication might be the very young neonate who is hypothermic (with central body temperature less than 36°C); in such a patient a standard dose of 0.5 mg/kg atracurium has been shown to have a longer clinical duration of 47 min (Nightingale 1986). It remains to be determined whether the prolongation of action is specifically due to the hypothermia, or whether the small and weak neonate who becomes hypothermic for any reason is more sensitive to the effects of the drug.

The side-effects of atracurium are minimal. Doses up to 0.6 mg/kg in infants or children do not alter the heart rate or blood pressure. Cutaneous flushes around the neck or face are occasionally seen in adolescents (Goudsouzian and Gelb 1991). In a study focusing on children histamine release was less frequent than in adults; and even in the presence of high plasma histamine levels, children did not develop cardiovascular signs or symptoms (Goudsouzian *et al.* 1986*a*).

One of the metabolites of atracurium is laudanosine, high levels of which (above 17 μg/ml in animals) may induce convulsions. It is almost impossible to achieve such high levels in clinical situations (Brandom *et al.* 1986). Even after the inadvertent administration of 37 mg of the drug in a 2.7 kg infant (Charlton *et al.* 1989), a dose of over 14 mg/kg, the highest plasma laudanosine level observed was 0.59 μg/ml. In another situation, a six-month-old infant was kept paralysed by atracurium for seven days with infusion requirements of up to 30 μg/kg/min; under this extreme circumstance the highest plasma laudanosine level was one-tenth of the toxic level, about 1.5 μg/ml (Tabardel *et al.* 1990).

Doxacurium

The newly available agent doxacurium is presently the most potent long-acting nondepolarizing muscle relaxant; it is approximately twice as potent as pancuronium or pipecuronium. In children as in adults it is devoid of any side-effects. The ED_{95}

in children is 30 μg/kg, about one and one-half times that in adults (Sarner *et al.* 1988; Goudsouzian *et al.* 1989*b*). As with other long-acting agents, the duration of action of an effective clinical dose is shorter in children than in adults. So far no recommendations of the clinical dosage range have been made for infants.

Gallamine

This agent was one quite popular with some paediatric anaesthesiologists because of its marked tachycardic (vagolytic) effects. With the introduction and general availability of pancuronium, however, its usage lapsed, due mostly to the fact that its cardiovascular effects outlast its neuromuscular effects. With an ED_{95} of 3.4 mg/kg during $N_2O:O_2$ narcotic anaesthesia (Goudsouzian *et al.* 1984), it remains the least potent of the currently available relaxants.

Metocurine

At equipotent doses, metocurine tends to exhibit fewer histaminergic properties than does tubocurarine (in particular it causes only minimal changes in blood pressure), and hence maintains a slight advantage in the clinical situation. Further, it is approximately twice as potent as tubocurarine. In infants and children, an effective dose of 0.5 mg/kg generally provides excellent to satisfactory conditions for endotracheal intubation. Following such a dose tetanic fade and post-tetanic facilitation can be elicited (and hence drug-mediated reversal can be attempted) in about 19 min in the presence of $N_2O:O_2$ anaesthesia and in 38 min in the presence of halothane anaesthesia. These recovery rates are shorter than those reported in adults. Clinical studies have found the ED_{95} to be about 0.2 mg/kg during halothane anaesthesia with no differences noted in neonates, infants, and children (Goudsouzian *et al.* 1978).

Mivacurium

Mivacurium is the shortest-acting nondepolarizing neuromuscular blocking agent. Its duration of action is about one third that of atracurium but two to three times as long as suxamethonium. The ED_{95} during halothane anaesthesia is about 0.1 mg/kg. An intubating dose of 0.2 mg/kg in children will cause complete twitch suppression in 1.8 min with recovery to 25% and 95% in 11 min and 19 min, respectively (Goudsouzian *et al.* 1989*a*).

The main degradation pathway of mivacurium is through the action of plasma cholinesterase, which for the most part explains its short duration of action. Like atracurium, mivacurium has the potential to cause histamine release; this usually occurs with a large initial dose and manifests as flushing of the skin around the neck and upper chest. The main advantage of mivacurium is its use in continuous infusion. Even after prolonged infusion (up to four hours) the spontaneous recovery rate holds steady at about 15 min for 5–95% return of twitch response (Alifimoff and Goudsouzian 1989; Brandom *et al.* 1990).

Pancuronium

Dose–response studies of pancuronium in both children and adults have shown it to be about five times more potent than tubocurarine. During $N_2O:O_2$ narcotic anaesthesia, the observed ED_{95} in younger children is about 93 μg/kg, somewhat higher than the figure of 77 μg/kg than has been reported for adolescents (Meretoja and Luosto 1990). In neonates and infants the ED_{95} is 66–72 μg/kg, significantly lower (30%) than the value in children but similar to that in adolescents (Meretoja and Luosto 1990). During halothane anaesthesia the same trend is seen: the ED_{90} for infants is 42 μg/kg while that of children is 62 μg/kg (Laycock *et al.* 1988). In infants and children (rather like adults) the dosage required to block the diaphragm is 1.6 times more than the dose needed to depress the adductor of the thumb (Laycock *et al.* 1988).

Before the intermediate-acting relaxants became routinely available, pancuronium was the most commonly used agent in infants and children. The predictable rise in heart rate and blood pressure (presumably from vagal block and release of noradrenalin from adrenergic nerve endings) would produce an increase in cardiac output (Nightingale and Bush 1973; Cabal *et al.* 1985). This is desirable effect in infants and children, as it counteracts the vagotonic effects of fentanyl and halothane and results in cardiovascular stability. Because of this, pancuronium is still advocated for a variety of cardiac surgical procedures. Infants requiring ligation of the patent ductus arteriosus, for example, tolerate the anaesthetic technique of fentanyl–air–oxygen pancuronium satisfactorily (Robinson and Gregory 1981). Here, the use of a potent inhalational agent is avoided; further the vagolytic effect of pancuronium effectively counteracts the bradycardic effect of fentanyl, and its neuromuscular blocking properties counteract fentanyl-induced stiffness. Pancuronium is also useful for correction of cyanotic and acyanotic congenital cardiac anomalies. Large doses of fentanyl (75 μg/kg) or sufentanil (10 μg/kg) can be used with standard doses of pancuronium (Hickey and Hansen 1984).

The onset and recovery from pancuronium seems to occur faster in children than in adults. A dose of 70 μg/kg causes 90% twitch suppression in 2.4 min in children and in 4.3 min in adults (Bevan *et al.* 1985); recovery to 10% of control twitch height occurs in 25 min in children and 46 min in adults. A pharmacokinetic study in children three to six years old has, however, demonstrated a distribution volume of 20 ml/kg in children and a plasma clearance of 1.7 ml/min/kg, values comparable to those seen in adults (Meistelman *et al.* 1986*b*).

Pancuronium has recently been used to achieve temporary fetal paralysis in order to allow for intra-uterine surgery. Under these very special circumstances this agent has been administered directly into the fetal umbilical cord by funipuncture (Moise *et al.* 1989) at an initial dose of 0.2 mg/kg of the estimated (by ultrasound) fetal weight. An alternative to fetal intravascular pancuronium is intramuscular pancuronium (or tubocurarine) in the fetal thigh. This latter route is technically simpler but requires an additional needle insertion, and the onset of paralysis takes several minutes, during which time the fetal movements an obscure the cord insertion site.

Pipecuronium

Pipecuronium, one of the two new long-acting neuromuscular blocking agents, has an ED_{95} of 47 μg/kg in infants during nitrous oxide — fentanyl anaesthesia and approximately 37 μg/kg during halothane anaesthesia (Pittet *et al*. 1989, 1990*a*; Sarner *et al*. 1990). The ED_{95} during narcotic $N_2O:O_2$ anaesthesia is about 80 μg/kg (vs 60 μg/kg in adults) (Pittet *et al*. 1989, 1990a) and is about 50 μg/kg during halothane anaesthesia. Isoflurane markedly potentiates the action of pipecuronium whereas halothane's effect is less pronounced. As with other long-acting muscle relaxants, children seem to require more of pipecuronium than adults to achieve the same degree of neuromuscular relaxation and they recover faster from its effects.

Suxamethonium

It has been repeatedly demonstrated that on a mass of drug per kilogram basis, infants require more suxamethonium than do older children or adults (Cook 1981). Echoing earlier findings, a recent investigation has reported an ED_{95} of 620 μg/kg in newborns, 729 μg/kg in infants, 423 μg/kg in children, and 290 μg/kg in adults, all in the presence of thiopentone–narcotic anaesthesia (Meakin *et al*. 1989).

These high requirements in the very young are also observed when the drug is administered by continuous infusion. Investigators have reported that the initial average dose requirement to produce more than 90% depression of the twitch response is about 250 μg/kg/min (Goudsouzian and Liu 1984) in infants and 100 μg/kg/min in children (DeCook and Goudsouzian 1980). In addition, the infusion study in infants highlighted wide individual variations, some patients requiring as little as 125 μg/kg/min and others requiring up to 580 μg/kg/min; the younger infants in the series required the larger amounts.

Lately, it has been noted that the infants' high initial requirement (230 μg/kg/min in the first 20 min, peaking to 300 μg/kg/min in 40 min), decreases gradually due to development of phase II block (Bevan *et al*. 1986). As is commonly seen in adults, in fact, infants and children generally develop tachyphylaxis and phase II block following a prolonged infusion of suxamethonium. Research has demonstrated tachyphylaxis in infants after a dose of 4 mg/kg when the drug is administered in a 20 min period and phase II block after about 5 mg/kg. Of interest here is the fact that infants who required more of the drug during their infusion were the fastest to recover; further, prolongation of the infusion for more than 90 min resulted in a decrease in dose requirement (bradyphylaxis).

It has been postulated that suxamethonium undergoes a first-order pharmacokinetic elimination (Cook and Fisher 1975). Since the extracellular volume occupies a higher percentage of body weight in infants (45% of body weight in the neonate, 30% at the age of two months, and 16–18% in adulthood), it has been suggested that the drug's smaller molecular size allows it to distribute into the larger volume, with the result that a lower concentration reaches the myoneural junction. Because the extracellular space and body surface area are related throughout childhood, a correlation between dosage (per square metre of body surface area) and neuromuscular response is to be expected (Cook 1981).

Infants appear to recover more rapidly from suxamethonium-induced paralysis than do children. The effect of the drug is normally terminated by diffusion away from the neuromuscular junction. The relatively small muscle mass and large extracellular fluid space in infants tends to facilitate this diffusion, thus terminating relaxation more rapidly. This effect more than offsets the slow rate of enzyme hydrolysis caused by the low concentration of plasma pseudocholinesterase typical of small infants (Zsigmond and Downs 1971).

Muscle fasciculations following suxamethonium tend to be mild or practically non-existent in infants. Such occurrences are usually described as gross muscle movement. Fasciculations are more frequently seen in older patients. Given the fact that fasciculations are absent in infants, or are present only as uncoordinated muscle movements (Cozanitis *et al.* 1987), it is usually unnecessary and generally ill-advised to make any effort to abolish them by the prior administration of small doses of nondepolarizing relaxants. Furthermore, should the infant be unusually sensitive to the nondepolarizer, the possibility exists that a fast paralysis will unexpectedly occur.

Clinically the usual recommended dose of suxamethonium is 2 mg/kg i.v. in infants; a larger dose of 3 mg/kg has recently been suggested (Meakin *et al.* 1989). Since suxamethonium is water soluble it can be absorbed from intramuscular sites; in fact, it is the only muscle relaxant whose efficacy has been demonstrated with intramuscular injection. In this instance, the clinician must make allowances for the greater dose requirements and slower onset of action. An i.m. dose of 3 mg/kg usually produces a mean twitch depression of 85%; 4 mg/kg produces profound relaxation in all children (Liu *et al.* 1981). Typically, however, the very youngest patients require doses as high as 5 mg/kg (Liu and Goudsouzian 1982).

Suxamethonium administration is almost always associated with varying degrees of jaw stiffness, a circumstance that occurs in children as well as adults. This increase in muscle tone is usually mild and can be overcome manually by opening the mouth; on rare occasions it is severe enough to prevent this. Whether this occasional increased masseter spasm in children is related to the trismus observed in patients at risk for malignant hyperthermia remains a controversial matter (Ellis and Halsall 1984; Brandom 1990; Berry 1991). In prospective evaluations in which masseter muscle tension has been monitored (in patients presenting for strabismus surgery as well as in others) a marked increase in jaw muscle tone has never led to malignant hyperthermia (Plumley *et al.* 1989; Meakin *et al.* 1990; Saddler *et al.* 1990). Several retrospective case reports, however, have identified some patients with trismus who do go on to develop malignant hyperthermia. Under the circumstances, some investigators have come to advocate cancelling surgery for all patients who develop trismus following suxamethonium, and recommend muscle biopsy preparatory to rescheduling (Rosenberg 1987). Others, however, continue the anaesthetic but avoid exposure to triggering agents while observing the patient closely for signs of the full-blown syndrome. Given the fact that most patients do not develop signs and symptoms of the syndrome, careful management with either course seems reasonable when suxamethonium use is indicated. Given, however, that the incidence of malignant hyperthermia is higher in children than in adults (Britt and Kalow 1970), the lack of a clear consensus of opinion has led many practitioners to limit the drug's use in children to cases specifically calling for it (as, for example, in the presence of laryngospasm, or when there is need for rapid intubation for i.m. use).

Arrhythmias frequently occur in children after a single clinical dose of suxamethonium. These are more common in the presence of halothane (about 50%) than with other anaesthetic agents (Goudsouzian 1981; Lerman *et al.* 1983). These arrhythmias, which are usually mild, last only for a few beats and resolve spontaneously. Prior administration of atropine markedly decreases their incidence.

Myoglobinemia and myoglobinurea seem to be specific complications of suxamethonium in children; the former occurs in 40% of those anaesthetized with halothane, the latter in about 8% (Ryan *et al.* 1971). Myoglobinurea is less frequent in children anaesthetized with enflurane (Laurence 1988) and does not occur with intramuscular administration. Such changes in serum myoglobin levels can be attenuated by small doses of a nondepolarizing relaxant (Blanc *et al.* 1986) given just before suxamethonium use.

Serum phosphocreatine kinase levels may rise following suxamethonium in children, especially in the presence of halothane. A recent study has established that this finding is true both for children requiring strabismus surgery and those undergoing tonsillectomy (McLaughlin 1991).

Perioperative dreaming, a side-effect that seems to be unique to children, has been reported following suxamethonium use; 19% of patients report such an occurrence. This anomaly is unrelated to awareness and can be prevented with pretreatment with tubocurarine. It is thought that cerebral arousal and hence the dream experience occur secondary to an increase in muscle discharge following suxamethonium administration (Hobbs *et al.* 1988; O'Sullivan *et al.* 1988).

Other-side effects of suxamethonium (e.g. hyperkalaemia and a rise in intraocular pressure), do not significantly differ in quality or quantity in adults and children.

Tubocurarine

Early studies demonstrated that infants required less tubocurarine than did children (Bush and Stead 1962). The initial dose for full control of respiration and adequate clinical relaxation was lowest on the first day of life (0.3 mg/kg), increased to 0.44 mg/kg by the ninth day and subsequently rose slightly to 0.53 mg/kg. A later trial series of 50 neonates (Bennett *et al.* 1976) confirmed this observation. Improved neuromuscular monitoring techniques have allowed a more careful analysis and better insight into this and other dosing practices. The ED_{95} during halothane anaesthesia, for example, appears to be about 0.3 mg/kg in neonates and infants as well as in children (Goudsouzian *et al.* 1975). The range in values for different patient groups does vary markedly, however. For infants less than 10 days old, the ED_{95} has ranged between 0.16 and 0.64 mg/kg whereas older children demonstrate a range of only 0.23–0.46 mg/kg. Recent data suggest that infants in fact require 21% less tubocurarine to establish 95% neuromuscular block than do other children, and that the onset time is much shorter in infants than in children (1.6 and 5.2 min) following a dose of 0.4 mg/kg (Meretoja *et al.* 1990).

Indirect evidence of histamine release has been seen in children following the intravenous administration of tubocurarine. This usually manifests as an erythema along the tract of the injected vein or a mild hypotension; such effects are more frequent in adolescents than in children (Nightingale and Bush 1973).

A recent report has indicated that children with abdominal, bone or cerebral tumours are resistant to the effect of tubocurarine, as evidenced by a longer time to onset time (3 times the control) and the need of more frequent doses. Interestingly, once such children are treated effectively by chemotherapy and/or surgery their response reverts to normal (Brown *et al.* 1990).

In normal paediatric practice the usual initial dose of tubocurarine varies between 0.25–0.8 mg/kg. Lower doses are usually used in infants or children already anaesthetized and intubated, whereas larger doses are used to facilitate endotracheal intubation itself. The duration of effective relaxation varies with the amount of drug given, the dose of 0.25 mg/kg providing adequate surgical relaxation for about 25 minutes and 0.8 mg/kg giving about an hour's relaxation (Goudsouzian *et al.* 1981*b*).

Vecuronium

In children during halothane anaesthesia the reported ED_{95} of vecuronium has varied between 56 and 64 μg/kg — values higher than those reported in adolescents and adults (Fisher and Miller 1983, Goudsouzian *et al.* 1983; Meistelman *et al.* 1986*a*). In general children recover faster from the neuromuscular effects of vecuronium than do their older counterparts. Infants, by contrast, are markedly more sensitive to the drug's effects. During $N_2O:O_2$ anaesthesia in infants an ED_{95} of 47 μg/kg has been suggested whereas a dose of 81 μg/kg seems to obtain in children 3–10 years old (Meretoja *et al.* 1988). The same tendency has been seen in a milder form during halothane anaesthesia (Fisher and Miller 1983). It is interesting to note that infants are generally more sensitive to most of the long-acting relaxants; with vecuronium, however, this characteristic sensitivity extends to about one year of age whereas sensitivity to other relaxants is generally limited to the immediate neonatal period.

In general satisfactory to excellent conditions of intubation can be achieved by 70–120 μg/kg vecuronium, complete paralysis thereafter occurring in 2–3 min. Time to onset is generally faster in infants than in children (Ferres *et al.* 1985), but the duration of action is longer, nearly twice that observed in older patients. During halothane anaesthesia 90% recovery following 70 μg/kg vecuronium occurs in 73 min in infants and 35 min in children (Motsch *et al.* 1985). In infants during balanced anaesthesia, 100 μg/kg of the drug produces 42 min of surgical relaxation (10% of control); recovery to 90% of control occurs in about 55 min. These intervals are 1.7–2.9 times those of older patients (Kalli and Meretoja 1989). Such observations have also been made in studies employing constant infusion techniques. The dose requirement is generally highest in children about four years old, and declines thereafter throughout adolescence. Maintenance of 90–95% neuromuscular block during balanced anaesthesia requires a rate of about 1 μg/kg/min in infants and neonates and 1.5 μg/kg/min in children. This fact has led some investigators to suggest that vecuronium should be considered a long-acting neuromuscular blocking agent in infants less than one year old (Meretoja 1989).

The main advantage of vecuronium is a complete absence of side-effects even at larger doses; hence it is frequently used for rapid intubation is situations where suxamethonium is undesirable. Increasing the dose of vecuronium from 0.1 mg/kg to 0.4 mg/kg shortens the onset time from 83 to 39 sec in children (Sloan *et al.* 1991). Here, as expected, the larger dose will result in a more prolonged duration of effect; recovery to 25% at 0.4 mg/kg occurs in about 75 min while a dose of 0.1 mg/kg will last only 25 min. Since nondepolarizing muscle relaxants have practically no effect on intraocular pressure, a large dose of vecuronium is considered a good choice for rapid intubation in the patient with an open eye injury.

Evidence of cumulative effects (a decreased requirement following prolonged administration), is generally not observed when vecuronium is administered by continuous infusion during narcotic $N_2O:O_2$ anaesthesia or in paediatric intensive care unit (Eldadah and Newth 1989). During halothane anaesthesia (and even more so with isoflurane) a decreased requirement can be seen after about 30 min of continuous infusion (Dong *et al.* 1989; Pittet *et al.* 1990*b*). Occasional instances of prolonged effect have also been reported in infants with impaired renal function (Haynes and Morton 1990).

Since the cardiovascular profile of vecuronium is remarkably stable, the drug can be used as the relaxant of choice for endotracheal intubation, especially for surgical procedures of longer than one hour duration. Here a dose of 70–100 μg/kg can safely be used. In infants there is the added advantage of a rapid onset of action (1.2 min to effective clinical relaxation vs 2.5 min in children) (Motsch *et al.* 1985; Kalli and Meretoja 1989); here it is thought that the greater cardiac output (mg/kg) in infants may deliver the vecuronium to its site of action more quickly.

GENERAL CONSIDERATIONS

A review of the literature on neuromuscular blocking agents in children reveals a number of characteristic features.

First, the distribution volume of muscle relaxants (relative to body weight) is greater in infants than in children and is more pronounced in neonates than in older children (Cook and Fisher 1975; Fisher *et al.* 1982; Matteo *et al.* 1984; Fisher *et al.* 1985). This observation correlates well with the fact that neonates have a larger extracellular volume (40% of body weight vs 18% in adults), which implies that a given relaxant will be distributed in a larger pool and hence the concentration of the drug reaching the myoneural junction is less. This is initially counterbalanced by an increased sensitivity in the myoneural junction ($CPss_{50}$), the outcome being that the newborn at first requires approximately the same dose of a nondepolarizing relaxant as does the older child. However, these compensating factors do not occur in all infants in a parallel fashion, so we find a marked variation in this select population especially in the neonatal period.

Full neuromuscular paralysis is not clinically needed in all neonates and small infants presenting for surgery. In the very young, and especially in neonates, muscles are quite weak, with a high water content and the capacity to stretch very easily. Further, the muscles' ability to sustain prolonged tone is less, as evidenced by more marked fade and poorer sustained tetanus. An able paediatric surgeon will therefore usually be satisfied with less relaxation in neonates than is needed for older infants and children.

Most of the long-acting relaxants are excreted by the kidneys. Since renal function is relatively immature in small infants, the elimination half-life of long-acting relaxants tends to be prolonged. This factor would have only limited effect with one or two small doses of a relaxant, where termination of action depends mostly on redistribution. After repeated doses, however, excretion plays a large role, so there is always the possibility of a prolonged duration as surgery proceeds. This is especially true in the infant with impaired renal function (Haynes and Morton 1990). Atracurium is a unique exception in this regard. Since it undergoes spontaneous non-enzymatic degradation in body fluids, its duration of action is practically the same in all age groups (though there is some evidence to suggest that it might be faster in infants). Vecuronium is different in another regard. It is mostly metabolized by the liver and the metabolites are eventually excreted by the kidneys. As noted earlier, the prolonged duration typical of infants lasts with this drug almost throughout the first year of life; again, by contrast, the prolongation of clearance with the long-acting agents is mostly limited to the first few weeks. The clinician must always remember that as infants mature and become more active, their clinical response to relaxants changes, dose requirement and duration of action quickly approaching the values observed in older children and adults.

Durations of action of the seven long-acting muscle relaxants are comparable; in infants, depending on the measurement technique used, the recovery index (25–75% of control twitch response) is about 25 min, with full recovery of an ED_{95} dose occurring in about one hour. These tend to be lower values than those seen in adults, but are on the whole similar to those in children. Therefore a second dose is needed within about 30–45 min of the first for adequate maintenance of muscle relaxation with follow-up doses similarly timed. As a general rule the hourly requirement is about 50% of the initial dose. The exception is the neonate, in whom clinical doses of long-acting relaxants seem to last for longer, especially after repeated doses; this is probably due to the immaturity of renal function. An important additional concern in infants is hypothermia; during hypothermia the duration of action of nondepolarizing relaxants is markedly prolonged, especially in premature infants (Nightingale 1986; Heier *et al.* 1990).

REVERSAL OF NEUROMUSCULAR BLOCK

In general the dose requirement of neostigmine is lower in children than in adults. If the twitch response is present a dose of 20 μg/kg of neostigmine with 10 μg/kg of atropine is more than satisfactory (Fisher *et al*. 1983). Although edrophonium has the theoretical advantage of a faster onset, the dose requirement is higher: at least 0.3 mg/kg. More frequently doses of 0.5–1 mg/kg, will be needed (Fisher *et al*. 1984). Because heart changes seem to occur earlier with this agent, its administration is usually delayed until the vagolytic effect (tachycardia) is evident. In children as in adults, though, it is the degree of neuromuscular block rather than the particular reversal agent that is the prime determinant in the success of reversal. Generally speaking, the lesser the block, the faster the antagonism (Meistelman *et al*. 1988).

REFERENCES

Alifimoff, J. K. and Goudsouzian, N. G. (1989). Continuous infusion of mivacurium in children. *British Journal of Anaesthesia*, **63**, 520–4.

Allen, C. N. and Albuquerque, E. Y. (1986). Characteristics of acetylcholine activated channels of innervated and chronically denervated skeletal muscles. *Experimental Neurology*, **91**, 532–45.

Arant, B. S. (1978). Developmental patterns of renal functional maturation compared in the human neonate. *Journal of Pediatrics*, **92**, 705–12.

Bennett, E. J., Ignacio, A., Patel, K., Grundy, E. M., and Salem, M. R. (1976). Tubocurarine and the neonate. *British Journal of Anaesthesia*, **48**, 687–9.

Berry, F. A. (1991). Masseter spasm in perspective (editorial). *Paediatric Anaesthesia*, **1**, 61–3.

Bevan, J. C., Donati, F., and Bevan D. R. (1985). Attempted acceleration of the onset of action of pancuronium. Effect of divided doses in infants and children. *British Journal of Anaesthesia*, **57**, 1204–8.

Bevan, J. C., Donati, F., and Bevan D. R. (1986). Prolonged infusion of suxamethonium in infants and children. *British Journal of Anaesthesia*, **58**, 839–43.

Blanc, V. F., Vaillancourt, G., and Brisson, G. (1986). Succinylcholine fasciculations and myoglobinemia. *Canadian Anaesthetists' Society Journal*, **33**, 178–84.

Bloch, R. J. and Pumplin, D. W. (1988). Molecular events in synaptogenesis: nerve muscle adhesion and postsynaptic differentiation. *American Journal of Physiology*, **254**, C345–64.

Bowman, W. C. (1990). *Pharmacology of neuromuscular function*. 2nd edn, p. 87. Wright, London.

Brandom, B. W. (1990). Atracurium and succinylcholine on the masseter muscle (editorial). *Canadian Journal of Anaesthesia* **37**, 7–11.

Brandom, B. W., Woelfel, S. K., Cook, D. R., Fehr, B. L., and Rudd, D. G. (1984). Clinical pharmacology of atracurium in infants. *Anesthesia and Analgesia*, **63**, 309–12.

Brandom, B. W., Cook, D. R., Woelfel, S. K., Rudd, G. D., Fehr, B., and Lineberry, C. G. (1985). Atracurium infusion requirements in children during halothane, isoflurane, and narcotic anesthesia. *Anesthesia and Analgesia*, **64**, 471–6.

Brandom, B. W., Stiller, R. L., Cook, D. R., Woelfel, S. K., Chakravorti, S., and Lai, A. (1986) Pharmacokinetics of atracurium in anaesthetized infants and children. *British Journal Anaesthesia* **58**, 1210–3.

Brandom, B. W., Sarner, J. B., Woelfel, S. K., Dong, M. L., Horn, M. C., Borland, L. M., *et al.* (1990). Mivacurium infusion requirements in pediatric surgical patients during nitrous oxide–halothane and during nitrous oxide–narcotic anesthesia. *Anesthesia and Analgesia*, **71**, 16–22.

Brehm, P. (1986). Alteration in the rate of receptor degradation during development of Xenopus myotomal muscle. *Biophysics Journal*, **49**, 362.

Brehm, P. and Henderson, L. (1988). Regulation of acetylcholine receptor channel function during development of skeletal muscle. *Developmental Biology*, **129**, 1–11.

Brenner, H. R. and Sakman, B. (1983), Neurotrophic control of channel properties at neuromuscular synapses of rat muscle. *Journal of Physiology* (London), **337**, 159–71.

Britt, B. A. and Kalow, W. (1970). Malignant hyperthermia, a statistical review. *Canadian Anaesthetists Society Journal*, **17**, 293–315.

Brown, M. C., Jansen, J. K. S., and Van Essen, D. (1976). Polyneuronal innervation of skeletal muscles in newborn rats and its elimination during maturation. *Journal of Physiology*, **261**, 387–422.

Brown, T. C. K., Gregory, M., Bell, B., and Clare, D. (1990). Response to non-depolarizing muscle relaxants in children with tumours. *Anaesthesia and Intensive Care*, **18**, 460–5.

Bush, G. H. and Stead, A. L. (1962). The use of *d*-tubocurarine in neonatal anaesthesia. *British Journal of Anaesthesia*, **34**, 721–8.

Cabal, L. A., Siassi, B., Artal, R., Gonzalez, F., Hodqman, J., and Plajstek, C. (1985). Cardiovascular and catecholamine changes after administration of pancuronium in distressed neonates. *Pediatrics*, **75**, 284–7.

Charlton, A. J., Harper, N. J. N., Edwards, D., and Wilson, A. C. (1989). Atracurium overdose in a small infant. *Anaesthesia*, **44**, 485–6.

Churchill-Davidson, H. C. and Wise, R. P. (1963). Neuromuscular transmission in the newborn infant. *Anesthesiology*, **24**, 271–8.

Cook, D. R. (1981). Muscle relaxants in infants and children. *Anesthesia and Analgesia*, **60**, 335–43.

Cook, D. R. and Fisher, C. G. (1975). Neuromuscular blocking effects of succinylcholine in infants and children. *Anesthesiology*, **42**, 662–5.

Cozanitis, D. A., Erkola, O., Klemola, U. M., and Makela, V. (1987). Precurarisation in infants and children less than three years of age. *Canadian Anaesthetists' Society Journal*, **34**, 17–20.

Curless, R. G. (1977). Developmental patterns of peripheral nerve, myoneural junction and muscle. A review. *Progress in Neurobiology*, **9**, 197–209.

DeCook, T. H. and Goudsouzian, N. G. (1980). Tachyphylaxis and phase II block development during infusion of succinylcholine in children. *Anesthesia and Analgesia*, **59**, 639–43.

Dennis, M. J., Ziskind-Conhaim, L. S., and Harris, A. J. (1981). Development of neuromuscular junction in rat embryos. *Developmental Biology* **81**, 266–79.

Dong, M. L., Woelfel, S. K., Brandom, B. W., Sarner, J. B., and Cook, D. R. (1989). Vecuronium infusion requirements in children during halothane N20, isoflurane N20 and fentanyl N20 anesthesia. *Anesthesiology*, **71**, A1039.

Eldadah, M. K. and Newth, C. J. (1989). Vecuronium by continuous infusion for neuromuscular blockade in infants and children. *Critical Care Medicine*, **10**, 989–92.

Ellis, F. R. and Halsall, P. J. (1984). Suxamethonium spasm. A differential diagnostic conundrum. *British Journal of Anaesthesia*, **56**, 381–3.

Ferres, C. J., Cream, P. M., and Mirakhur, R. K. (1985). An evaluation of ORG NC45 (vecuronium) in paediatric anaesthesia. *Anaesthesia*, **18**, 943–7.

Fisher, D. M., and Miller, R. D. (1983). Neuromuscular effects of vecuronium (ORG NC45) in infants and children during N20 halothane anesthesia. *Anesthesiology*, **58**, 519–23.

Fisher, D. M., O'Keeffe, C., Stanski, D. R., Cronelly, R., Miller, R. D., and Gregory, G. A. (1982). Pharmacokinetics and pharmacodynamics of *d*-tubocurarine in infants, children and adults. *Anesthesiology*, **57**, 203–8.

Fisher, D. M., Cronnelly, R., Miller, R. D., and Sharma, M. (1983). The neuromuscular pharmacology of neostigmine in infants and children. *Anesthesiology*, **59**, 220–5.

Fisher, D. M., Cronnelly, R., Sharma, M., and Miller, R. D. (1984). Clinical pharmacology of edrophonium in infants and children. *Anesthesiology*, **61**, 428–33.

Fisher, D. M., Castagnoli, K., and Miller, R. D. (1985). Vecuronium kinetics and dynamics in anesthetized infants and children. *Clinical Pharmacology and Therapeutics*, **37**, 402–6.

Fisher, D. M., Canfell, P. C., Spellman, M. J., and Miller, R. D. (1990). Pharmacokinetics and pharmacodynamics of atracurium in infants and children. *Anesthesiology*, **73**, 33–7.

Goudsouzian, N. G. (1980). Maturation of neuromuscular transmission in the infant. *British Journal of Anaesthesia*, **52**, 205–14.

Goudsouzian, N. G. (1981). Turbe del ritmo cardiaco durante intubazione tracheale nei banbini. *Acta Anaesthetica Italica*, **32**, 293–9.

Goudsouzian, N. G. (1986). Atracurium in infants and children. *British Journal of Anaesthesia*, **58**, 23–28S.

Goudsouzian, N. G. (1988). Atracurium infusion in infants. *Anesthesiology*, **68**, 267–9.

Goudsouzian, N. G. and Gelb, C. (1991). Histamine release from succinylcholine and atracurium in adolescents. *Paediatric Anaesthesia*, **1**, 41–5.

Goudsouzian, N. G. and Liu, I. M. P. (1984). The neuromuscular response of infants to a continuous infusion of succinylcholine. *Anesthesiology*, **60**, 97–101.

Goudsouzian, N. G. and Standaert, F. G. (1986). The infant and the myoneural junction. *Anesthesia and Analgesia*, **65**, 1208–17.

Goudsouzian, N. G., Donlon, J. V., Savarese, J. J. and Ryan, J. F. (1975). Re-evaluation of dosage and duration of action of *d*-tubocurarine in the pediatric age group. *Anesthesiology*, **43**, 416–25.

Goudsouzian, N. G., Liu, L. M. P., and Savarese, J. J. (1978). Metocurine in infants and children: Neuromuscular and clinical effects. *Anesthesiology*, **49**, 266–9.

Goudsouzian, N. G., Liu, L. M. P., and Cote, C. J. (1981). Comparison of equipotent doses of non-depolarizing muscle relaxants in children. *Anesthesia and Analgesia*, **60**, 862–6.

Goudsouzian, N. G., Martyn, J. A. J., Liu, L. M. P., and Gionfriddo, M. (1983) Safety and efficacy of vecuronium in adolescents and children. *Anesthesia and Analgesia*, **62**, 1083–8.

Goudsouzian, N. G., Martyn, J. J. A., Liu, L. M. P., and Gionfriddo, M. (1984). The dose response effect of long acting nondepolarizing neuromuscular blocking agents in children. *Canadian Anaesthetists Society Journal*, **31**, 246–50.

Goudsouzian, N. G., Liu, L. M. P., Gionfriddo, M., and Rudd, G. D. (1985). Neuromuscular effects of atracurium in infants and children. *Anesthesiology*, **62**, 75–9.

Goudsouzian, N. G., Young, E. T., Moss, J., and Liu, L. M. P. (1986*a*). Histamine release during the administration of atracurium or vecuronium in children. *British Journal of Anaesthesia*, **58**, 1229–33.

Goudsouzian, N. G., Martyn, J. J., Rudd, G. D., and Gionfriddo, M. (1986*b*). Continuous infusion of atracurium in children. *Anesthesiology*, **64**, 171–4.

Goudsouzian, N. G., Alifimoff, J. K., Eberly, C., Smeets, R., Griswold, J., Miler, V., *et al.* (1989*a*). Neuromuscular and cardiovascular effects of mivacurium in children. *Anesthesiology*, **70**, 237–42.

Goudsouzian, N. G., Alifimoff, J. K., Liu, L. M. P., Foster, V., McNulty, B., and Savarese, J. J. (1989*b*). Neuromuscular and cardiovascular effects of doxacurium in children anaesthetized with halothane. *British Journal of Anaesthesia*, **62**, 263–8.

Haynes, S. R. and Morton, N. S. (1990). Prolonged neuromuscular blockade with vecuronium in a neonate with renal failure. *Anaesthesia*, **45**, 743–5.

Heier, T., Caldwell, J. E., Sessler, D. I., and Miller, R. D. (1990). Mild intra-operative hypothermia increases duration of action and recovery time of vecuronium. *Anesthesia and Analgesia*, **70**, S153.

Henderson, L. P., Lechleiter, J. D., and Brehm, P. (1987). Single channel properties of newly synthesized acetylcholine receptors following denervation of mammalian skeletal muscles. *Journal of General Physiology*, **89**, 999–1014.

Hickey, P. R. and Hansen, D. D. (1984). Fentanyl and sufentanil–oxygen–pancuronium anesthesia for cardiac surgery in infants. *Anesthesia and Analgesia*, **63**, 117–24.

Hobbs, A. J., Bush, G. H. and Downham, D. Y. (1988). Perioperative dreaming and awareness in children. *Anaesthesia*, **43**, 560–2.

Kalli, I. and Meretoja, O. A. (1988). Infusion of atracurium in neonates, infants, and children. A study of dose requirements. *British Journal of Anaesthesia*, **60**, 651–4.

Kalli, I. and Meretoja, O. A. (1989). Duration of action of vecuronium in infants and children anaesthetized without potent inhalational agents. *Acta Anaesthesiologica Scandinavica*, **33**, 29–33.

Keens, T. G., Bryan, A. C., Levison, H., and Ianuzzo, C. D. (1978). Developmental pattern of muscle fiber type in human ventilatory muscles. *Journal of Applied Physiology*, **44**, 909–13.

Koenigsberger, M. R., Patten, B., and Lovelace, R. E. (1973). Studies of neuromuscular function in the newborn: A comparison of myoneural function in the full term and premature infant. *Neuropediatrie*, **4**, 350–61.

Laurence, A. S. (1988). Serum myoglobin release following suxamethonium administration to children. *European Journal of Anaesthesiology*, **5**, 31–8.

Laycock, J. R. D., Baxter, M. K., Bevan, J. C., Sangwan, S., Donati, F., and Bevan, D. R. (1988). The potency of pancuronium at the adductor pollicis and diaphragm in infants and children. *Anesthesiology*, **68**, 908–11.

Ledez, K. M., Swartz, J., Strong, A., Burrows, F. A., and Lerman, J. (1986). The effect of age on the serum concentration of alpha-1-acid glycoprotein in newborns, infants and children. *Anesthesiology*, **65**, A421.

Leonard, R. J., Nakajima, S., Nakajima, Y., and Carlson, C. G. (1988). Early development of two types of nicotinic acetylcholine receptors. *Journal of Neuroscience*, **8**, 4038–48.

Lerman, J., Robinson, S., and Willis, M. M. (1983). Succinylcholine-induced heart rate changes in children during isoflurane and halothane anesthesia. *Anesthesiology*, **59**, A443.

Liu, L. M. P., DeCook, T. H., Goudsouzian, N. G., Ryan, J. F., and Liu P. L. (1981). Dose response to intramuscular succinylcholine in children. *Anesthesiology*, **55**, 599–602.

Liu, L. M. P. and Goudsouzian, N. G. (1982). Neuromuscular effects of intramuscular succinylcholine in infants. *Anesthesiology*, **57**, A413.

Matteo, R. S., Lieberman, I. G., Salanitre, E., McDaniel, D. D., and Diaz, J. (1984). Distribution, elimination, and action of *d*-tubocurarine in neonates, infants and children. *Anesthesia and Analgesia*, **63**, 799–804.

McLaughlin, C. J., Mirakhur, R. K., Elliott, P., Craig, H. J. L., Trimble, E. R., and Elliott, P. (1991). Changes in serum potassium, calcium and creatin kinase following suxamethonium administration in children with and without strabismus. *Paediatric Anaesthesia*, **1**, 101–6.

Meakin, G., Shaw, E. A., Baker, R. D., and Morris, P. (1988). Comparison of atracurium-induced neuromuscular blockade in neonates, infants and children. *British Journal of Anaesthesia*, **60**, 171–5.

Meakin, G., McKiernan, E. P., Morris, P., and Baker, R. D. (1989). Dose response curves for suxamethonium in neonates, infants and children. *British Journal of Anaesthesia*, **62**, 655–8.

Meakin, G., Walker, R. W. M., and Dearlove, O. R. (1990). Myotonic and neuromuscular blocking effects of increased dose of suxamethonium in infants and children. *British Journal of Anaesthesia*, **65**, 816–8.

Meistelman, C., Loose, J. P., Saint-Maurice, C., Delleur, M. M., and DaSilva, G. L. (1986a). Clinical pharmacology of vecuronium in children. Studies during nitrous oxide and halothane in oxygen anesthesia. *British Journal of Anaesthesia*, **58**, 996–1000.

Meistelman, C., Agoston, S., Kersten, U. W., Saint-Maurice, C., Bencini, A. F., and Loose, J. P. (1986b). Pharmacokinetics and pharmacodynamics of vecuronium and pancuronium in anesthetized children. *Anesthesia and Analgesia*, **65**, 1319–23.

Meistelman, C., Debaene, B., D'Hollander, A., Donati, F., and Saint-Maurice, C. (1988). Importance of the level of paralysis recovery for a rapid antagonism of vecuronium with neostigmine in children during halothane anesthesia. *Anesthesiology*, **69**, 97–9.

Meretoja, O. A. (1989). Is vecuronium a long-acting neuromuscular blocking agent in neonates and infants? *British Journal of Anaesthesia*, **62**, 184–7.

Meretoja, O. A., and Brown, T. C. K. (1990). Maintenance requirement of alcuronium in pediatric patients. *Anaesthesia and Intensive Care*, **18**, 452–4.

Meretoja, O. A. and Kalli, I. (1986). Spontaneous recovery of neuromuscular function after atracurium in pediatric patients. *Anesthesia and Analgesia*, **65**, 1042–46.

Meretoja, O. A. and Luosto, T. (1990). Dose response characteristics of pancuronium in neonates infants and children. *Anaesthesia Intensive Care*, **18**, 445–59.

Meretoja, O. A., Wirtavuori, K., and Neuvonen, P. J. (1988). Age-dependence of the dose–response curve of vecuronium in pediatric patients during balanced anaesthesia. *Anesthesia and Analgesia*, **67**, 21–6.

Meretoja, O. A., Brown, T. C. K., and Clare, D. (1990). Dose response to a alcuronium and d-tubocurarine in infants children and adolescents. *Anaesthesia Intensive Care*, **18**, 449–51.

Mishina, M., Takai, T., Imoto, K., Noda, M., Takahashi, T., Numa, S., et al. (1986). Molecular distinction between fetal and adult form of muscle acetylcholine receptors. *Nature*, **321**, 406–11.

Moise, K. J., Deter, L. D., Kirshon, B., Adam, K., Patton, D. E., and Carpenter, R. J. (1989). Intravenous pancuronium bromide for fetal neuromuscular blockade during intrauterine transfusion for red-cell alloimmunization. *Obstetric Gynecology*, **74**, 905–8.

Morselli, P. L., Franco-Morselli, R., and Bossi, L. (1980). Clinical pharmacokinetics in new-borns and infants. *Clinical Pharmacokinetics*, **5**, 485–527.

Motsch, J., Hutschenreuter, K., Ismaily, A. J., and von Blohn, K. (1985). Vecuronium in infants and children. Clinical and neuromuscular effects. *Anaesthesist*, **34**, 382–7.

Nightingale, D. A. (1986). Use of atracurium in neonatal anaesthesia. *British Journal of Anaesthesia*, **58**, 32–6S.

Nightingale, D. A. and Bush, G. H. (1973). A clinical comparison between tubocurarine and pancuronium in children. *British Journal of Anaesthesia*, **45**, 63–70.

O'Sullivan, E. P., Childs, D., and Bush, G. H. (1988). Perioperative dreaming in paediatric patients who receive suxamethonium. *Anaesthesia*, **43**, 104–6.

Pittet, J. F., Tassonyi, E., Morel, D. R., Gemperle, G., Richter, M., and Rouge, J. C. (1989). Pipecuronium induced neuromuscular blockade during nitrous oxide fentanyl, isoflurane and halothane anaesthesia. *Anesthesiology*, **71**, 210–13.

Pittet, J. F., Tassonyi, E., Morel, D. R., Gemperle, G., and Rouge, J. C. (1990a). Neuromuscular effects of pipecuronium bromide in infants and children during nitrous oxide–alfentanyl anesthesia. *Anesthesiology*, **72**, 432–5.

Pittet, J. F., Melis, A., Rouge, J. C., Morrel, D. R., Gemperle, G., and Tassonyi, E. (1990b). Effect of volatile anesthetics on vecuronium-induced neuromuscular blockade in children. *Anesthesia and Analgesia*, **70**, 248–52.

Plumley, M. H., Bevan, J. C., Saddler, J. M., Donati, F., and Bevan, D. R. (1989). Dose related effects of succinylcholine on the adductor pollicis and masseter muscle in children. *Canadian Journal of Anaesthesia*, **37**, 15–20.

Redfern, P. A. (1970). Neuromuscular transmission in newborn rats. *Journal of Physiology*, **109**, 701–9.

Robinson, S. and Gregory, G. A. (1981). Fentanyl–air–oxygen for ligation of patent ductus arteriosus in preterm infants. *Anesthesia and Analgesia*, **60**, 331–4.

Rosenberg, H. (1987). Trismus is not trivial (editorial). *Anesthesiology*, **67**, 453–5.

Ryan, J. F., Kagen, L. J., and Hyman, A. I. (1971). Myoglobinemia after a single dose of succinylcholine. *New England Journal of Medicine*, **285**, 824–7.

Saddler, J. M., Bevan, J. C., Plumley, M. H., Polomeno, R. C., Donati, F., and Bevan, D. R. (1990). Jaw muscle tension after succinylcholine in children undergoing strabismus surgery. *Canadian Anaesthetists' Society Journal*, **37**, 21–5.

Sarner, J. B., Brandom, B. W., Cook, D. R., Dong, M. L., Horn, M. C., and Woelfel, S. K. (1988). Clinical pharmacology of doxacurium chloride (BW A938U) in children. *Anesthesia and Analgesia*, **67**, 303–6.

Sarner, J. B., Brandom, B. W., Dong, M. L., Pickle, D., Cook, D. R., and Weinberger, M. J. (1990). Clinical pharmacology of pipecuronium in infants and children during halothane anesthesia. *Anesthesia and Analgesia*, **71**, 362–6.

Schuetze, S. M. and Role, L. W. (1987). Developmental regulation of nicotinic acetylcholine receptors. *Annual Review of Neurosciences*, **10**, 403–57.

Siegelbaum, S. A., Trautmann, A., and Koenig, J. (1984). Single acetylcholine activated channel currents in developing muscle cells. *Developmental Biology*, **104**, 366–79.

Sloan, M. H., Lerman, J., and Bissonnette, B. (1991). Pharmacodynamics of high-dose vecuronium in children during balanced anesthesia. *Anesthesiology*, **74**, 656–9.

Smith, M. A. and Slater, C. R. (1983). Spatial distribution of acetylcholine receptors at developing chick neuromuscular junctions. *Journal of Neurocytology*, **12**, 993–1005.

Tabardel, Y., Paquay, T., and Senterre, J. (1990). Prolonged infusion of atracurium in an infant. *Developmental Pharmacology and Therapeutics*, **15**, 52–6.

Taxt, T., Ding, R., and Jansen, J. K. S. (1983). A note on the elimination of polyneuronal innervation of skeletal muscles in neonatal rats. *Acta Physiologica Scandinavica*, **117**, 557–60.

Vicini, S. and Schuetze, M. (1985). Gating properties of acetylcholine receptors at developing rat endplates. *Journal of Neuroscience*, **5**, 2212–24.

Wood, M. and Wood, A. J. J. (1981). Changes in plasma drug binding and alpha$_1$-acid glycoprotein in mother and newborn infant. *Clinical Pharmacology and Therapeutics*, **4**, 522–6.

Zsigmond, E. K. and Downs, J. R. (1971). Plasma cholinesterase activity in newborns and infants. *Canadian Anaesthetists' Society Journal*, **18**, 278–85.

16

Neuromuscular blockade: measurement and monitoring

N. J. N. Harper

It is common practice to monitor the end-organ response to the administration of any drugs. Monitoring the action of each drug is desirable during anaesthesia. Although it is not possible to monitor accurately certain responses, e.g. depth of anaesthesia, monitoring of neuromuscular block is relatively straightforward. The first part of this chapter discusses the indications for monitoring neuromuscular transmission and the second part considers how the process of monitoring is best performed.

MANAGEMENT OF NEUROMUSCULAR BLOCK DURING SURGERY

Suxamethonium

The duration of action of suxamethonium varies considerably even when the plasma cholinesterase activity falls within normal limits. The use of a nerve stimulator is therefore highly desirable. A peripheral nerve stimulator is mandatory in measuring the duration of action of suxamethonium in a patient in whom a deficiency of plasma cholinesterase is suspected. It is important to be able to differentiate between central and peripheral respiratory depression; prolonged apnoea during an anaesthetic technique incorporating suxamethonium and an opioid can be fully elucidated only with a nerve stimulator. A prolonged infusion of suxamethonium may be complicated by the development of phase II block and it is generally accepted that neuromuscular monitoring is desirable in avoiding this complication.

Nondepolarizing muscle relaxants

There is considerable variation between patients in their sensitivity to a given dose of a nondepolarizing muscle relaxant. An indication of the typical variability in response is given by the duration to 25% recovery of a small (ED_{95}) bolus dose of atracurium (0.23 mg/kg) which ranges from 11.5 minutes to 28.0 minutes (Harper *et al.* 1993). Setting aside differences between patients in the rate of drug elimination, it is not surprising that there is a considerable variation in the duration of an intubating dose of relaxant drug. Many factors influence the relation between the plasma concentration of drug and the response of the patient and the management of neuromuscular block is facilitated by neuromuscular monitoring in these situations.

Although continuous infusions of muscle relaxants have been given without neuromuscular monitoring, accurate assessment of neuromuscular transmission enables block to be maintained at the ideal level during prolonged surgery. The management of reversal begins well in advance of the administration of the anticholinesterase drug. The timing of the last dose of relaxant or the cessation of a continuous infusion is critical in determining the plasma concentration of the drug and hence its reversibility. A simple nerve stimulator is valuable in deciding whether spontaneous recovery of neuromuscular transmission has progressed to the stage when antagonism with an anticholinesterase will be accomplished satisfactorily.

The safe level of spontaneous recovery at which to reverse depends principally upon the neuromuscular blocking drug and also the dose of anticholinesterase, although there are other factors. Assuming that neostigmine 40 μg/kg is given, satisfactory reversal can be confidently predicted if a nerve stimulator is used to ensure that neuromuscular transmission has recovered spontaneously to an acceptable, minimum level. The reappearance of the second twitch response of the train-of-four or the second twitch response to double burst stimulation indicates that reversal with neostigmine is likely to be satisfactory.

MEASUREMENT OF RESIDUAL BLOCK IN THE RECOVERY ROOM

Clinically significant residual neuromuscular block in the recovery room is considerably more frequent than is generally realized (Viby-Mogenson *et al.* 1979). Routine neuromuscular monitoring during surgery significantly reduces the incidence of residual curarization in the recovery room after pancuronium but the advantage appears to be less marked after atracurium or vecuronium. The postoperative sequelae of the neuromuscular blocking drugs are discussed in Chapter 8.

MONITORING NEUROMUSCULAR TRANSMISSION IN THE INTENSIVE CARE UNIT

Anecdotal evidence suggests that neuromuscular monitoring is used infrequently when neuromuscular blocking drugs are used in the intensive care unit (ICU). The reason for this practice is unclear. Individual pharmacokinetic and pharmacodynamic differences are considerably greater in the ICU population in comparison with a general surgical population and it is difficult to imagine how the administration of muscle relaxant drugs in the ICU can be optimized without routine monitoring of the depth of neuromuscular block. It is the author's practice to monitor the train-of-four count at regular intervals when a muscle relaxant drug is being administered as a continuous infusion. It is especially important to avoid 'over-paralysing' patients in the ICU and excessively high infusion rates of muscle relaxants are associated with considerable cost.

MONITORING TECHNIQUES

When the membrane of a single muscle fibre has been depolarized sufficiently to reach threshold, the contractile process is activated and the muscle fibre responds in an all-or-none fashion. The force of contraction of the muscle as a whole depends predominantly on the number of individual muscle fibres contracting and the frequency with which they are activated. In the normal physiological situation repeated depolarization of the nerve results in graded muscle contraction. The majority of monitoring techniques depend upon stimulating a peripheral motor nerve and measuring a response from the muscle. The muscles and their nerves which may be used to monitor neuromuscular block during anaesthesia are shown in Table 16.1.

Table 16.1 Muscles (and their nerves) which may be used to monitor neuromuscular block during anaesthesia

---

Muscles of the hand (ulnar nerve)
    adductor pollicis
    first dorsal interosseous
    abductor digiti minimi and other hypothenar muscles
    abductor and flexor policis brevis and opponens (median nerve)

Muscles of the face (facial nerve)
    orbicularis oculi
    orbicularis oris
    frontalis

Muscles of the leg and foot (posterior tibial nerve)
    gastrocnemius (posterior tibial nerve)
    soleus (posterior and medial tibial nerves)
    long flexors of the foot (posterior tibial nerve)
    short flexors of the foot (medial plantar nerve)

Abdominal muscles (intercostal nerve T7–T12)
    external oblique
    rectus abdominis

Diaphragm (phrenic nerve)
    crural fibres
    costal fibres

Laryngeal adductors (recurrent laryngeal nerve)

THE RESPONSE OF THE MUSCLE: FADE AND FACILITATION

Monitoring is dependent upon measuring the response of a muscle to stimulation of its motor nerve. The response of the muscle — whether an index of the force of contraction, or the evoked electrical activity — comprises the cumulative responses of all the individual muscle fibres, each of which is an all-or-none phenomenon. When a muscle relaxant is given, increasing numbers of individual muscle fibres 'drop out', starting with the most sensitive, as depolarization of successive fibres fails to reach the threshold for contraction. This is the result of, but is not numerically proportional to, the extent to which cholinceptors are occupied by the drug. The contraction of a muscle in response to a single stimulus applied to its nerve is not demonstrably reduced until approximately 70% of its receptors (as distinct from 70% of its muscle fibres) are blocked (Paton and Waud 1967).

If neuromuscular transmission is stressed by administering trains of several stimuli at specified frequencies, neuromuscular block may be measured not only quantitatively, but also qualitatively. Depolarizing block is classically associated with little or no fade in the responses of the muscle to repetitive stimuli — train-of-four (TOF), double burst, or tetanic. If phase II block intervenes, fade will develop progressively. The nondepolarizing muscle relaxants are associated with significant fade which is greater during the offset of action than during the onset. The degree to which fade becomes evident varies between the nondepolarizing drugs, and the fade characteristics of a particular drug are probably one manifestation of the relative preponderance of prejunctional or postjunctional receptor occupancy (Chapter 2). Fade is normally quantified by comparing the amplitude of the final response of the muscle to the train of stimuli with that of the first response, and expressing the proportion as a ratio or as a percentage.

If, during partial nondepolarizing neuromuscular block, the nerve is subjected to a burst of stimuli at a high frequency (e.g. 50 Hz) for a few seconds, the response of the muscle to subsequent low frequency stimulation (e.g. 1 Hz) is enhanced. This phenomenon is post-tetanic facilitation. Slight post-tetanic facilitation can be observed even in the absence of a muscle relaxant if the force of muscle contraction is measured, but not if electromyography is the method of measurement (Katz 1973).

PATTERNS OF NERVE STIMULATION

There is currently no single pattern of nerve stimulation that will permit accurate monitoring at all levels of neuromuscular block; some patterns are suitable for monitoring a shallow block while others are more appropriate for the assessment of a profound block. The response to a single stimulus in isolation is of little value unless a control response has been recorded before the administration of a muscle relaxant. In practice, this pattern of nerve stimulation is inappropriate if simple, tactile assessment of the force of contraction is a requirement. An interval of at least 10 seconds should be permitted between single stimuli if an effect of the previous stimulus is to be avoided during partial nondepolarizing neuromuscular block (Ali and Savarese 1980).

Tetanic stimulation

Tetanic fade is characteristic of a nondepolarizing block. A tetanus is a contraction that continues throughout repetitive stimulation. At low stimulation frequencies, the force of contraction may oscillate (unfused tetanus). If the frequency of stimulation is increased, the tetanus becomes fused, and the force of contraction increases to reach a sustained maximum of three to five times that of a single twitch response. The most commonly used stimulus frequency is 50 Hz. In the absence of neuromuscular disease or neuromuscular blocking drugs, an individual is usually able to sustain a contractile force for at least five seconds in response to 50 Hz stimulation (Stanec *et al.* 1978) This implies that sufficient acetylcholine is manufactured, mobilized and released from the motor nerve terminal to fulfil the requirements for normal, sustainable neuromuscular transmission. It must be borne in mind that repetitive nerve stimulation facilitates acetylcholine mobilization within the nerve terminal, and also that the number of acetylcholine molecules liberated is normally considerably in excess of that needed to activate all of the individual nerve fibres. Thus, if the voltage clamp technique is applied to an *in vitro* preparation, the end-plate potential is maintained even at high stimulation frequencies (Glavinovic 1979). The effect of neuromuscular block on the muscle contraction produced by tetanic nerve stimulation is shown in Fig. 16.1.

High frequency fade is generally considered to be a prejunctional phenomenon which results in a progressive reduction of the rate of release of acetylcholine by the motor nerve terminal. In clinical practice, tetanic stimulation has several disadvan-

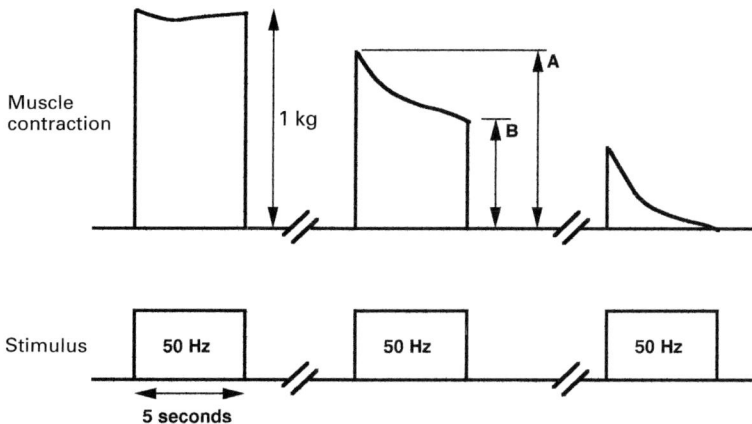

Fig. 16.1 The effect of neuromuscular blockade on the muscle contraction produced by tetanic nerve stimulation. Tetanic fade ratio = B/A. The force of muscle contraction may be up to 1 kg.

tages. A considerable interval between successive tetanic bursts must be permitted (5–6 min). Post-tetanic facilitation will influence the response to subsequent single, TOF or double burst stimulation unless there is an interval of at least two minutes when intermediate-duration relaxant drugs are used. A greater interval may be necessary during block with longer-acting drugs (Katz 1973). Using tactile assessment, tetanic fade to a 50 Hz stimulus train is detected reliably only when the tetanic fade ratio (Fig. 16.1) is 0.3 or less; it is probably no better than TOF stimulation in the clinical detection of residual block at the end of anaesthesia (Dupuis *et al.* 1990). Unfortunately, the limiting factor is the relatively poor performance of the anaesthetist's finger as a force transducer. Increasing the tetanic frequency to 100 Hz may induce fade even in the absence of a muscle relaxant (Kopman *et al.* 1982).

Train-of-four stimulation: train-of-four ratio

Train-of-four stimulation was introduced by Ali and colleagues (1970) and remains the standard method of monitoring nondepolarizing neuromuscular block. It represented a significant advance because it is not necessary to obtain a pre-relaxant control

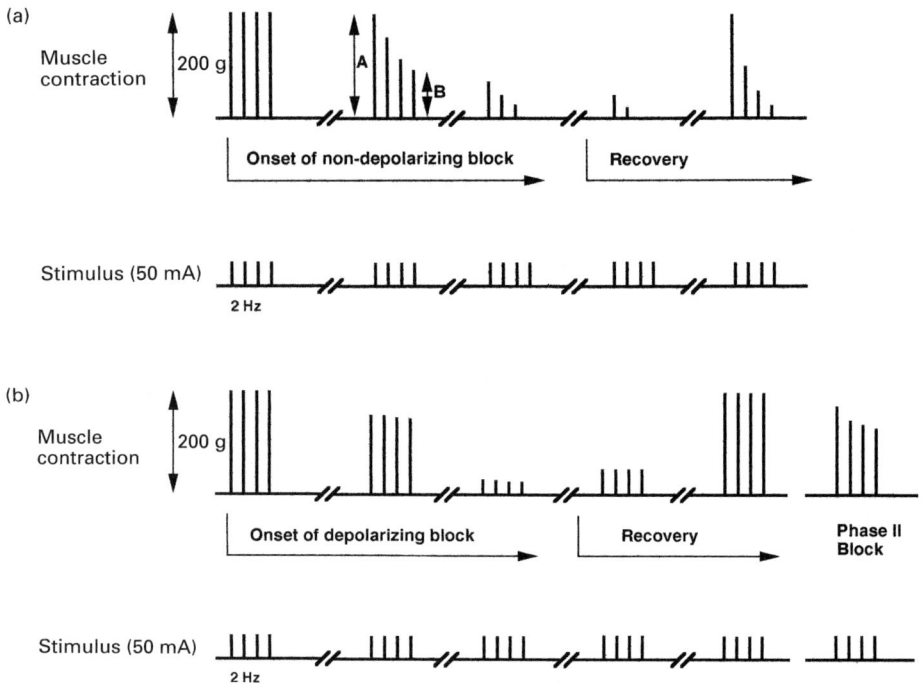

Fig. 16.2 (a) Train-of-four stimulation during the onset and offset of non-depolarizing block. Train-of-four ratio = B/A. There is usually less fade during onset than during offset. (b) Train-of-four stimulation during the onset and offset of depolarizing block. Significant fade is present only when phase II block intervenes.

value for comparison. Each train comprises four stimuli at a frequency of 2 Hz (Fig. 16.2). During nondepolarizing neuromuscular block there is progressive fade in the four responses. The TOF ratio is a comparison of the amplitude of the fourth response of the train with the amplitude of the first response of the train (Fig. 16.2). Ali and colleagues (1971*a*) demonstrated a highly significant, linear, positive association between the TOF ratio and the ratio of the first response of the train to the pre-relaxant control response. It rapidly became obvious that the TOF ratio was a more sensitive and consistent index of returning muscle power than the single twitch (Ali *et al.* 1971*b*).

Train-of-four fade is more evident during recovery from block than during onset. The extent to which the responses fade varies between muscle relaxant drugs. The magnitude of the TOF decrement has been shown to increase in the order alcuronium < atracurium < tubocurarine < gallamine (Williams *et al.* 1980). It is necessary to allow at least 10 seconds between TOF stimuli to ensure that each measurement has not been influenced by the previous train (Lee 1975).

Although TOF stimulation has become the standard method of assessing neuromuscular block, the ability of the anaesthetist to interpret the response of the muscle using simple, manual assessment of the force of contraction is severely limited. It is clearly important that any method of monitoring neuromuscular transmission should be capable of identifying the patient in whom residual block is of sufficient severity to impair spontaneous ventilation in the immediate postoperative period. It is generally accepted that, during recovery from nondepolarizing block, a TOF ratio of 0.7 corresponds with the ability to maintain adequate spontaneous ventilation (Brand *et al.* 1977). At this level of block, the ability of the anaesthetist to detect fade in the TOF responses by clinical (non-instrumental) means is extremely poor; when the ratio approached 0.7, only approximately 25% of experienced observers were able to detect any fade in the four responses using tactile assessment of the force of contraction. It was possible to consistently detect fade only when the ratio was as low as 0.3–0.4 (Viby-Mogensen *et al.* 1985).

Train-of-four stimulation: train-of-four count

As block deepens, the fourth, third, second, and first responses successively disappear and the number of measurable responses is expressed as the TOF count. Although the TOF ratio is important during reversal of block, the TOF count is a more useful simple index for monitoring neuromuscular block at the level appropriate for abdominal surgery (DeJong 1966). In general terms, during spontaneous recovery, the second, third, and fourth twitches reappear at approximately 87%, 81%, and 79% depression of the first twitch response. Thus, at the time when the second twitch becomes palpable, the force of contraction of the first twitch will have recovered to approximately 10% of its pre-relaxant control value; and when the fourth twitch first becomes apparent, relaxation will have recovered to the limits of acceptability for abdominal surgery (Ham and Redpath 1985). The relation between the extent of recovery of the first response and the TOF count varies slightly between relaxants and also appears to depend upon which inhalational agent is used (Table 16.2).

Table 16.2 The percentage block at which the TOF twitches can be expected to reappear during recovery from nondepolarizing neuromuscular block

| | Percentage block at the reappearance of twitch number: | | |
Four	Three	Two	Source
75%	80	90	1
76%	81	88	2a
76%	79	86	2b
74%	76	86	2c
93%	89	86	3

[1]Lee 1975: halothane and tubocurarine.

[2]Ham and Redpath 1985: halothane and atracurium (a), pancuronium (b), tubocurarine (c).

[3]O'Hara *et al.* 1986*a*: enflurane (atracurium, vecuronium, and tubocurarine were not significantly different in this study).

Double burst stimulation

In recent years, clinical research has been directed towards developing a sequence of stimuli that will provide the same information as the TOF, but without the need to use measuring apparatus to assess accurately the response of the muscle. Double burst stimulation (DBS) has considerable promise in achieving that goal (Engbaek *et al.* 1989). The stimulation pattern comprises two short tetanic bursts, separated by 0.75 seconds (Fig. 16.3a). The muscle response to DBS is felt as two discrete twitches. During partial nondepolarizing block, the second twitch is less forceful than the first, and a comparison of the two responses can be expressed as the double-burst ratio (Fig. 16.3b).

Double burst stimulation elicits a degree of fade that is almost identical to TOF stimulation; its advantage lies in the relative accuracy with which this fade is detectable by the palpating finger of the anaesthetist. In comparative studies DBS 3,3 revealed tactile fade in almost all cases when the TOF ratio was below 0.5, whereas TOF fade was present in only three-quarters of the estimations even when the TOF ratio had fallen below 0.4 (Drenk *et al.* 1989). DBS 3,3 represents a considerable improvement compared with the TOF ratio in routine clinical use. Although DBS was devised to improve the clinical detection of residual neuromuscular block, it has recently been suggested that it might be useful during the deeper block necessary for abdominal surgery (Braude *et al.* 1991).

Figure 16.4 shows a comparison of detectable fade between the TOF responses and the DBS responses at varying depths of neuromuscular block, demonstrating the advantages of DBS.

Changing the DBS pattern slightly so that there are two stimuli in the second burst (DBS 3,2) increases the probability that tactile fade will be present when the TOF ratio is below 0.7. Unfortunately, fade in the responses to DBS 3,2 may also be present when the TOF ratio is above 0.7 (indicating satisfactory reversal) which might lead to the unnecessary administration of neostigmine (Engbaek *et al.* 1989). No stimulation pattern is currently able to distinguish reliably between satisfactory and unsatisfactory reversal using simple tactile assessment of the force of muscular contraction.

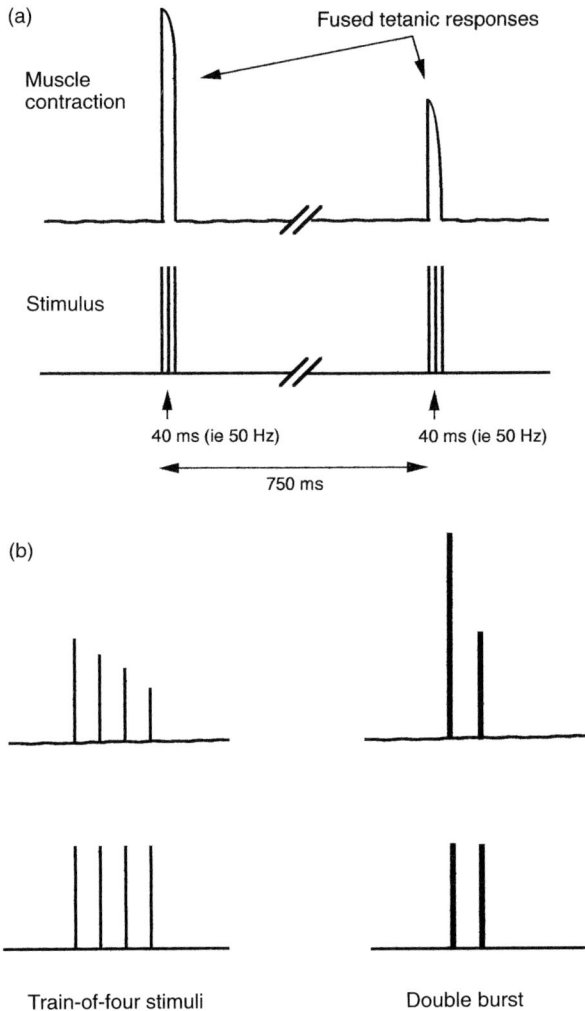

Fig. 16.3 (a) Double burst stimulation. The tetanic bursts at 50 Hz are separated by 0.75 seconds. DBS 3,3 has three stimuli in each burst; DBS 3,2 has only two stimuli in the second burst. The muscle response is detectable as two fused tetanic twitches. (b) The twitch response to DBS is considerably more forceful than the train-of-four responses although the DBS ratio is numerically close to the train-of-four ratio.

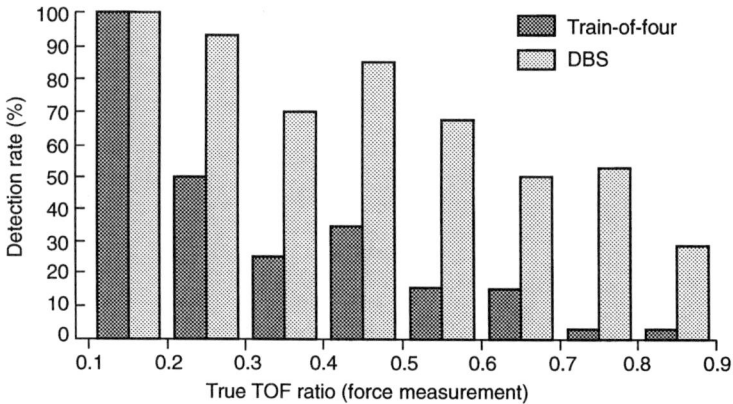

Fig. 16.4 Clinical fade is reliably detectable with train-of-four stimulation only when there is considerable neuromuscular block and the true train-of-four ratio (measured with a force transducer) is very low. During DBS stimulation, fade is detectable clinically at a lesser degree of block. DBS is a more sensitive measure of residual neuromuscular blockade at the end of anaesthesia. (After Drenk *et al.* 1989.)

Post-tetanic count

When neuromuscular block is exceptionally profound there is no muscle twitch response to any of the patterns of nerve stimulation so far discussed. It is clearly as important to have the means to quantify block of this extreme intensity as it is to measure the extent of lesser degrees of block.

For a while after a tetanic stimulus has been applied to a motor nerve, the release of acetylcholine in response to subsequent low-frequency stimulation is enhanced by post-tetanic facilitation. The phenomenon of post-tetanic facilitation may be employed in the measurement of profound block by applying a standardized tetanus followed by stimuli at a lower frequency. The responses to the low-frequency stimuli will be enhanced by post-tetanic facilitation so that they become sufficiently forceful to be measured. Post-tetanic facilitation soon wanes so that the force of the post-tetanic twitches declines to zero. The post-tetanic count (PTC) is the number of measurable twitches following a standardized tetanus (Viby-Mogensen *et al.* 1981). A tetanic burst (50 Hz for 5 s) is followed after an interval of 3 s by stimulation at 1 Hz until the responses have declined to zero (Fig. 16.5).

The PTC is able to quantify profound neuromuscular block by predicting the duration of the period during which there is no response to TOF stimulation. A low PTC is associated with a prolonged period before the first response of the TOF and, conversely, a greater PTC is associated with a shorter period.

There is a close linear relation between the time before the first response of the TOF becomes detectable and the square root of the PTC (Viby-Mogensen *et al.* 1981). This relation can be expressed as follows:

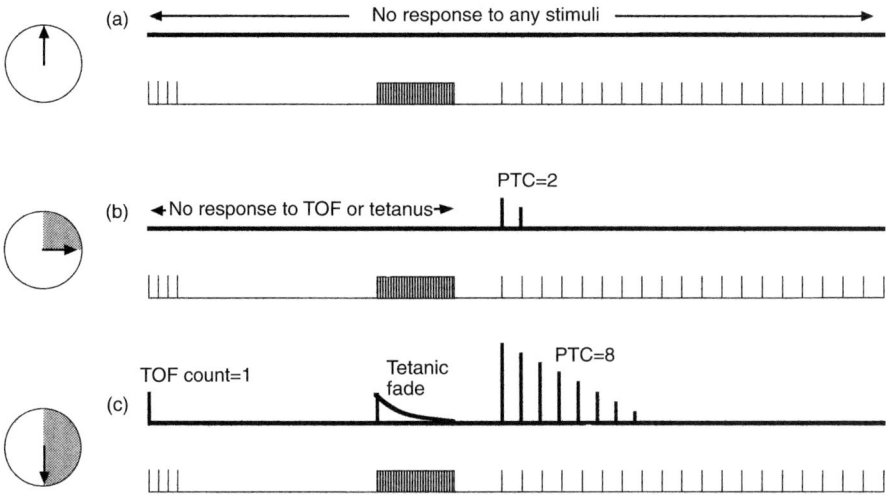

Fig. 16.5 Post-tetanic count. (a) During profound neuromuscular blockade there is no response to TOF, tetanic, or 1 Hz stimulation. (b) Neuromuscular blockade is less intense. There is still no response to TOF or tetanic stimuli but the process of post-tetanic facilitation has enhanced neuromuscular transmission so that the two post-tetanic twitches are palpable when tetanic stimulation for 5 s is followed by stimuli at 1 Hz. The post-tetanic count is 2. (c) Blockade has lessened to the extent that the first TOF twitch is palpable. There is a small, transient tetanic response and the post-tetanic count has risen to 8. The re-appearance of the first TOF twitch occurs at a PTC which is characteristic of each particular muscle relaxant drug.

$$t = a + b \, PTC.$$

Where t is the time from a given PTC to the reappearance of the first response of the TOF. In order to determine a and b, the graph has to be plotted of time to first response against square root of PTC. On this graph a is the intercept and b is the slope of the graph. These constants are characteristic for each individual muscle relaxant. Table 16.3 shows the relation between the PTC and the predicted time before the first response of the TOF reappears.

If tactile assessment is used both for the TOF and for the DBS responses, the predicted times vary little from those obtained using a force transducer (Howardy-Hansen *et al.* 1984).

Because the diaphragm is relatively insensitive to nondepolarizing agents, it has been suggested that PTC may be the stimulation pattern of choice in those situations when complete diaphragmatic paralysis is desirable. During light halothane and vecuronium anaesthesia, the re-appearance of the first TOF response is associated with a diaphragmatic response to carinal stimulation in approximately 50% of patients. This incidence is reduced to 2% when the PTC is 2 (Fernando *et al.* 1987). Reversal of this degree of block with neostigmine may be extremely prolonged. Adequate reversal of atracurium block with neostigmine from very intense block (PTC = 2) may take 30 minutes (Engbaek *et al.* 1990).

Table 16.3   The relation between the post tetanic count (PTC) and the predicted time before the first response of the TOF reappears

| | Time (min) to first response of TOF | | |
PTC	Pancuronium[1]	Atracurium[2]	Vecuronium[3]
1	35	9	16
2	25	7	14
4	20	4	10
6	12	2	6
8	5	0	4
10	0	–	2

[1]Viby-Mogensen *et al*. 1981.
[2]Bonsu *et al*. 1987.
[3]Eriksson *et al*. 1990.

Inhalational agents appear to increase the interval between the administration of the muscle relaxant drug and the appearance of the first post-tetanic twitch (i.e. PTC = 1). However, the subsequent progression through increasing numbers of post-tetanic twitches is only very slightly delayed (Bonsu *et al*. 1987). Tetanic stimulation affects acetylcholine release for a considerable time and at least 5–6 minutes should elapse between successive estimations of PTC (Viby-Mogensen *et al*. 1981).

No single mode of stimulation is suitable for monitoring all levels of neuromuscular block. Each of the methods described above is appropriate to a particular

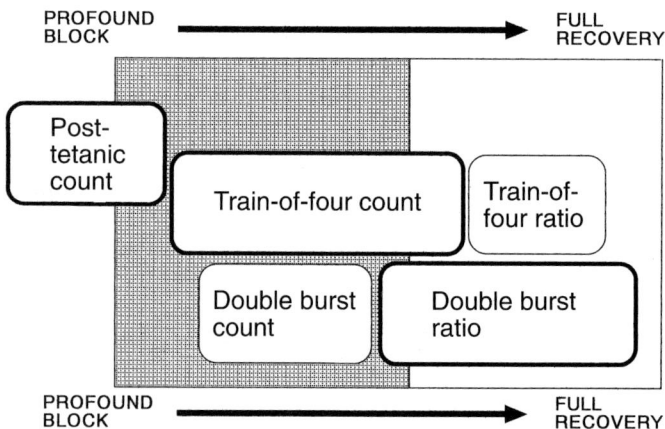

Fig. 16.6 After the intensity of neuromuscular blockade changes during a surgical procedure, the most appropriate mode of nerve stimulation also changes. As profound block wanes and eventually there is full recovery of neuromuscular function, the most appropriate pattern of stimulation changes from PTC, to TOF count, to double burst ratio. The hatched area represents 'surgical blockade'. When clinical, tactile assessment of the twitch response is used, TOF ratio is less useful than DBS ratio.

phase; from profound block to full recovery of neuromuscular transmission. Figure 16.6 indicates the usefulness of the various stimulation modes when the response is assessed by the tactile or visual methods. Single twitch and tetanic fade offer no particular advantages and it can be argued that DBS supplants the TOF ratio unless some form of instrumentation is employed to measure the response of the muscle. The most useful techniques, therefore, are PTC, TOF count, and DBS ratio which are highlighted in the figure.

NERVE STIMULATION

If a nerve is stimulated with a brief, externally applied current, the force of contraction of the muscle will depend on the number of muscle fibres reaching the threshold for contraction. A small current, for example 10–20 mA applied transcutaneously will activate only a small proportion of the motor units and will elicit a weak contraction. If the current is gradually increased, the force of contraction will increase as more muscle fibres contract until the maximum force of contraction is reached. The current required to elicit the maximum force of contraction is the maximal current and any current greater than this is termed supramaximal. It is generally accepted that a supramaximal current should be used for monitoring neuromuscular transmission so that the entire range of motor fibres is monitored. A current of at least 65 mA is usually required to produce supramaximal stimulation in all patients (Kopman and Lawson 1984). Submaximal stimulation is less painful, and it has been suggested that a current of 20–30 mA may be used for TOF monitoring with reasonable accuracy.

The quantity of electrical energy delivered to the nerve also depends on the duration of the stimulating pulse. The pulse duration should be sufficiently great to deliver adequate energy to the nerve. An excessively wide pulse which exceeds the duration of the neuromuscular refractory period may stimulate the nerve more than once. If a second nerve action potential is generated 1–2 ms after the first, the muscle will not respond because all the muscle fibres are refractory during this period. During partial neuromuscular block a proportion of muscle fibres will not have contracted in response to the first stimulus due to the presence of the neuromuscular blocking drug. When the second stimulus arrives, the release of acetylcholine by the motor nerve terminal is enhanced (prejunctional facilitation) and a greater number of muscle fibres will reach their depolarization threshold, resulting in a stronger contraction (Berry 1966). As a consequence the degree of neuromuscular block may be under-estimated. A pulse duration of 0.2 ms is commonly used both for research and for clinical monitoring.

Self-adhesive surface ECG-type electrodes are satisfactory and convenient for routine clinical monitoring. It is desirable, but not essential, first to degrease the skin site with acetone. The electrodes should be placed near to the nerve, either parallel to, or straddling it. If the electrodes are separated by more than a few centimetres, the positive electrode should be the proximal one (Berger *et al.* 1982). Needle electrodes permit more exact nerve stimulation and are less likely to be subject to high impedance that will limit the output of some low-power stimulators (Caplan *et al.* 1981). Spherical 'ball electrodes' are invariably associated with a variable, high impedance and cannot be recommended.

It is useful to make a distinction between a nerve stimulator that is appropriate to research, and one that is suitable for routine clinical use. Excessive complication should be avoided in a clinical stimulator. It is desirable to equip every location where muscle relaxant drugs are given so that all patients may be monitored. A stimulator designed for monitoring neuromuscular block should provide 1 Hz, TOF, PTC and DBS modes and be capable of delivering at least 60 mA when connected to the patient. This is at least ten times the maximum current required when a needle is used to locate a nerve for a local anaesthetic nerve-block, and if applied accidentally could damage the nerve. For this reason, dual-purpose stimulators should be treated with circumspection and stimulators capable of a high output current should be used only with surface electrodes.

METHODS OF MEASURING THE RESPONSE OF THE MUSCLE

It is useful to observe several general principles when monitoring neuromuscular transmission in the clinical setting. It is necessary to permit sufficient time to elapse between successive observations. Heat loss over time tends to reduce the response of the muscle and can be minimized by insulating the limb (Thornberry and Mazumdar 1988).

Force of contraction: force transducer

Accurate measurement of the force of contraction of a muscle can be accomplished only with a force transducer. The most commonly used technique is measurement of the force of adduction of the thumb (adductor pollicis) in response to ulnar nerve stimulation. The adductor pollicis is the only thenar muscle supplied by the ulnar nerve. Because muscles vary in their sensitivity to relaxants, it may be valuable to assess the response of a single muscle for research purposes. For routine clinical use a simple force transducer may be attached to an invasive pressure channel in the patient's vital-signs monitor which amplifies and displays the signal. Simple visual or tactile assessment of the force of contraction usually under-estimates the extent of TOF fade (see below).

For research applications, it is extremely important to stabilize the monitored arm to minimize drift due to displacement of the thumb in relation to the transducer. Measurement should be isometric, i.e. very little movement of the thumb should be permitted. A tetanic contraction can generate a force of 2 kg and the apparatus should be accurate up to this level. Starling's law applies, of course, to the adductor pollicis so that the force of contraction varies in proportion to the preload, within limits. The optimum preload for the thumb appears to be in the range 200–300 *g* (Donlon *et al.* 1979) and it is important to maintain this resting tension throughout the period of measurement. Drift may also occur when strain gauges in the transducer change their characteristics due to a heating effect. It is normal to arrange strain gauges in a Wheatstone-bridge configuration which minimizes this effect in addition to increasing sensitivity. The duration of a single muscle twitch is similar to the duration of the QRS complex of the electrocardiogram (50–100 ms) and the apparatus must have a similarly high frequency response, with sufficient damping to prevent overshoot. Stable fixation in relation to the origin of the muscle and the point of measurement is also important.

Force of contraction: visual and tactile assessment

Visual assessment of muscle contraction is possibly more closely related to estimating the acceleration of the thumb than to its force of contraction. Tactile assessment aims to emulate a force transducer. The greatest problem, which may be confusing even to experienced anaesthetists, is direct muscle stimulation. Even during profound neuromuscular block, electrical stimulation over a muscle bypasses the neuromuscular junction and may produce a twitch response. This direct response may present problems of interpretation. When the ulnar nerve is stimulated at the wrist, direct stimulation of the superficial flexors of the forearm may occur, producing spurious movement of the hand. Under these circumstances a TOF stimulus will elicit four (small) twitches of the hand during profound neuromuscular block. It may be impossible to eradicate direct muscle stimulation but it may be minimized by ensuring that the stimulating electrodes are accurately placed, avoidance of an excessive stimulus current, and positioning the positive electrode over the ulnar groove at the elbow and the negative electrode at the wrist. Visual assessment appears to be more susceptible to erroneous direct stimulation twitches than tactile assessment, and DBS appears to cause more direct stimulation than TOF stimulation for a given current and pulse duration (personal observation).

Visual or tactile measurements are inevitably less accurate than methods which use instrumentation. Using TOF stimulation, error is apparent when assessing the return of the second, third, and fourth twitches (TOF count), when assessing the TOF ratio, and when assessing the force of contraction of the first twitch in the absence of a pre-relaxant control twitch. The TOF count is underestimated by visual assessment. When a force transducer is used to measure recovery from a vecuronium block, the second twitch (T2) of the train reappears when there is 93% residual block, and the third twitch (T3) at 89% block (O'Hara *et al.* 1986*a*). If visual assessment is substituted, T2 re-appears only when residual block has recovered to 84% (measured), and T3 re-appears at 76% block. Thus the visual approach may not detect the re-appearance of a second twitch until the time when a force transducer detects two or three twitches. In addition, there is a greater variation between patients in the time taken for the twitches to re-appear using visual assessment (O'Hara *et al.* 1986*b*).

Tactile assessment improves on the accuracy of visual assessment. In the absence of a documented pre-relaxant control twitch, there is a tendency to over-estimate or under-estimate the force of contraction of the first response of the TOF

(T1) when non-instrumental techniques are used. Visual assessment makes an over-estimation in approximately 30% of measurements; the frequency can be reduced to approximately 10% if the tactile method is used (Tammisto *et al.* 1988). Although tetanic stimulation at 50 Hz is a rigorous test of neuromuscular transmission when measuring apparatus is employed, clinical assessment of tetanic fade is relatively insensitive. Tetanic fade is detected reliably by the tactile method only when the tetanic fade ratio has fallen to less than 0.3 (measured with a force transducer) (Dupuis *et al.* 1990). Thus, if simple clinical monitoring is used, tetanic stimulation appears to be no more sensitive to residual block than TOF stimulation.

Electromyography

Measurement of the electrical activity of contracting muscles has been applied to the measurement of neuromuscular transmission for many years. Churchill-Davidson and Christie (1959) used surface electrodes placed over the hypothenar eminence in a wide-ranging study of the effects of different patterns of nerve stimulation on the EMG response during neuromuscular block with several depolarizing and nondepolarizing muscle relaxants, and the effects of edrophonium and neostigmine. Subsequently, EMG apparatus has developed to the extent that electromyography is frequently more convenient than mechanomyography in the clinical setting. It is clear that these two methods measure different aspects of neuromuscular function and there is currently some debate concerning their relative merits in research and in the clinical situation. Depolarization of a single muscle fibre membrane is an all-or-none phenomenon that results from a supra-threshold endplate potential. The depolarization of an individual muscle fibre may be detected by a fine, exploring needle which is insulated except at its tip as a single fibre action potential. If a larger electrode is placed over the surface of the muscle, a compound muscle action potential (CMAP) is detected. The compound action potential comprises the vector of the summated electrical activity of the individual, single fibre potentials in the direction of the surface recording electrode. A single fibre action potential is a brief event in relation to the compound action potential but both exhibit the characteristic initial depolarization phase, followed by the repolarization phase. In the absence of a neuromuscular blocking drug, and if the stimulation is supramaximal, all the muscle fibres reach their endplate potential threshold. However, if neuromuscular transmission is impaired by the presence of a muscle relaxant drug, fewer fibres reach the threshold for generating a single fibre action potential and the amplitude of the CMAP diminishes as the number of contributing fibres declines. The amplitude of both the depolarization phase and the repolarization phase is diminished and the CMAP becomes slightly elongated (Pugh *et al.* 1987), which may reflect increased variability in the synaptic delay at the neuromuscular junction (Ekstedt and Stalberg 1969) and is related to a change in the power spectrum of the CMAP to favour lower frequencies (Harper *et al.* 1987).

Although it is possible to measure the amplitude of the CMAP on a simple storage oscilloscope, newer electromyographs designed for monitoring neuromuscular block convert the signal to a voltage by rectification and integration; an example is the Relaxograph[R]. The electrical artefact caused by the stimulus is excluded from this process electronically, and the voltage derived from the CMAP is displayed on a paper chart (Fig. 16.7). Newer equipment permits the display of the CMAP waveform at set-up which enables the user to confirm that the electrode positions are satisfactory.

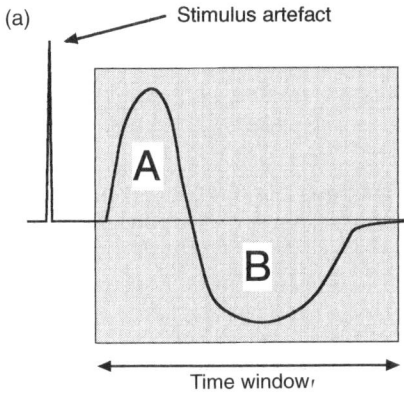

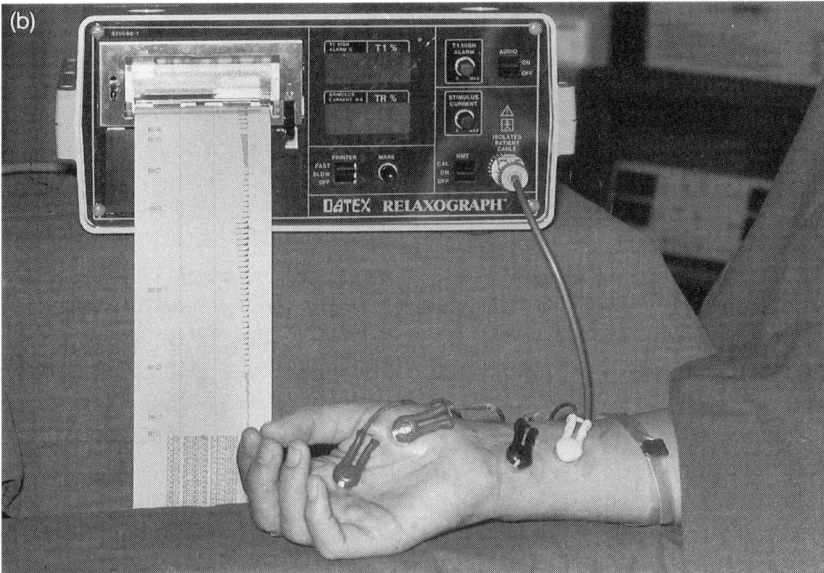

Fig. 16.7 (a) The relaxograph processes the raw EMG signal by rectification and integration so that a voltage is produced that is proportional to the areas A+B within a time window that excludes the stimulus artefact. (b) Suitable electrode positions for recording the EMG of the adductor pollicis. The recording is more stable if the hand is immobolized in a simple back-splint.

The quality of the EMG signal is crucially dependent on the care with which the recording electrodes are applied to the skin. It is important to degrease the skin with a solvent and to slightly abrade before applying the electrodes. It is often recommended that the earth electrode should be placed between the stimulating electrodes and the recording electrodes. The active recording electrode should be placed over the motor-point of the muscle where the electrical activity is maximal, and the indifferent electrode over a nearby bony point. A muscle should be chosen which gives a large EMG signal and this should be checked in the anaesthetized patient before calibrating the signal and administering a muscle relaxant. The first dorsal interosseous muscle gives a larger CMAP than the adductor pollicis. Some EMG equipment is able to operate in an uncalibrated mode in which the TOF ratio is acceptably accurate but it is not possible to compare the first response of the TOF with a pre-relaxant control value.

It is common for the EMG signal to become attenuated during a period of monitoring. The TOF ratio is unaffected but the absolute magnitude of the responses is diminished so that the first response of the TOF may not ultimately reach the pre-relaxant value when the muscle relaxant drug is no longer acting. This drift may be due to a change in the impedance characteristics of the electrode — tissue interface and it appears to have reached its maximum approximately ten minutes after the period of monitoring has begun (Meretoja and Brown 1989). It is possible that both central and peripheral effects of general anaesthesia might contribute to the initial reduction in the integrated EMG signal. However, it is unlikely that this effect is mediated via the motor nerve (Smith 1991). Drift is also less likely to occur if the monitored hand is immobilized (Kosek *et al.* 1988) with a suitable splint.

The relation between electromyographic and force measurements is complex and depends upon the nature of the neuromuscular blocking drug and the inhalational anaesthetic agent (and the nature of the reversal agent). Electromyography measures only the electrical component of neuromuscular function. EMG measurements therefore reflect events occurring at the neuromuscular junction but changes in the contractile process are not measured. Nevertheless, electromyography has the advantage that muscles not amenable to force measurement can be monitored. In the absence of a neuromuscular blocking drug, post-tetanic facilitation of the force of the twitch response can be observed but there is no corresponding increase in the amplitude of the CMAP (Botelho 1955). During voluntary contraction of a muscle, the integrated EMG increases with the force of contraction. If the initial fibre length is increased, the force of a maximal effort increases (Starling's law); however, this is not matched by a concomitant increase in the integrated EMG (Inman *et al.* 1952). These observations suggest that correlation between EMG and force measurements should be closer when stimulus frequency and preload are well controlled. The CMAP is depressed more rapidly by suxamethonium than the force of contraction and recovers more slowly. After the administration of suxamethonium, there is a characteristic, brief increase in the twitch response which is not seen in the CMAP. The force of the twitch response frequently recovers to greater than the pre-suxamethonium value for approximately ten minutes after the CMAP has recovered to 100% (Katz 1973; Shanks and Jarvis 1980). The initial increase in contractile force is associated with a change in the shape of the CMAP suggesting repetitive firing of the muscle fibres (Donati and Bevan 1984). In contrast, after the administration of a nondepolarizing neuromuscular blocking drug, the force of contraction is depressed more rapidly than the CMAP and takes longer to recover.

When comparing methods of recording it is important to measure the responses of the same muscle. When the CMAP and the force of contraction of the adductor pollicis are measured simultaneously, the relation between the two methods appears to be drug-specific, the discrepancy being considerably greater after alcuronium and tubocurarine than atracurium (Harper *et al.* 1986; Harper *et al.* 1987); the difference between the methods is less pronounced during reversal with neostigmine (Harper *et al.* 1986).

Accelerometry

The requirement for a more convenient method led to the application of accelerometry to the measurement of neuromuscular transmission during anaesthesia. This method uses Newton's second law (force = mass × acceleration) to measure the force of contraction of the thumb indirectly (Viby-Mogensen *et al.* 1988). A small acceleration transducer containing a piezoelectric ceramic wafer is taped to the pad of the thumb. When the thumb moves, a voltage is generated that is proportional to the acceleration of the transducer. Providing that the hand is positioned so that the thumb is able to move freely, accelerometric measurements of neuromuscular block appear to correlate well with mechanometric measurements (Jensen *et al.* 1988). The device is commercially available as the Accelograph[(R)], the Mini-Accelograph[(R)], and the TOF Guard[(R)] (Fig. 16.8) which have the advantage of providing automated

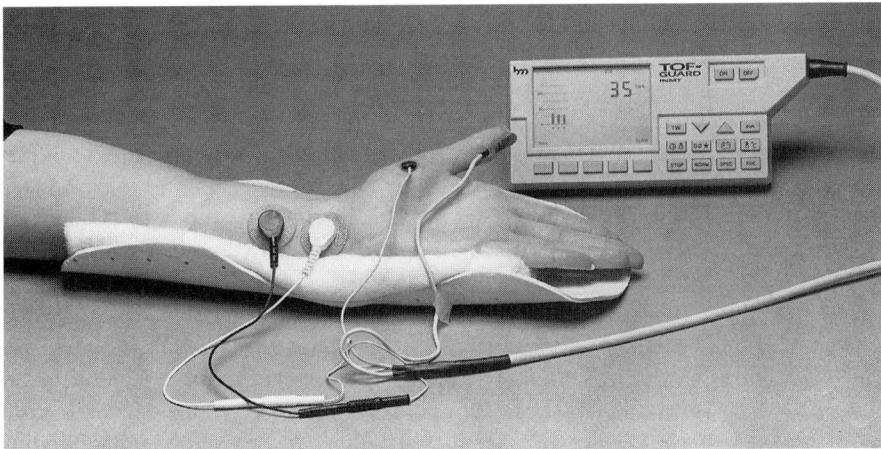

Fig. 16.8 The TOF Guard employs accelerography to detect the muscle twitch. The transducer is taped to the thumb. The temperature of the thenar eminence is measured to assist in avoiding spurious results due to excessive cooling.

measurement of the post-tetanic count, in addition to the TOF ratio. The Mini-Accelograph is designed to connect to a vital-signs monitor via an invasive pressure channel. Accelerometry appears to be unsuitable for double burst monitoring, which, in any case is more applicable to visual or tactile assessment of the muscle response. In common with all methods of monitoring, accelerometry requires a period of stabilization before consistent recordings can be made. Using accelerometry, it is common to observe a TOF ratio of greater than 1.0 in the unparalysed patient. The reason for this augmented response is obscure and development of TOF fade tends to lag behind the mechanometric TOF fade during the onset of block (personal observation). Accelerometry appears to be well suited to clinical monitoring of neuromuscular block; its place in neuromuscular research has not yet been defined.

MONITORING NEUROMUSCULAR BLOCK IN DIFFERENT MUSCLES

There is considerable variation between muscles in their sensitivity to muscle relaxants. In addition, the relation between the sensitivities of two muscles may alter if a different muscle relaxant is administered. For example, the duration of effect of pancuronium at the adductor pollicis is approximately twice that at the diaphragm. If tubocurarine is substituted, the corresponding ratio is three to one (Derrington and Hindocha 1990).

The muscles of the hand

The adductor pollicis is well suited to each of the commonly used measurement techniques, and is usually accessible during anaesthesia. Hand muscles other than the adductor pollicis may be used for electromyographic monitoring. The first dorsal interosseous muscle gives an large surface CMAP (Kalli 1990) which appears to be less vulnerable to movement artefact and to give identical results to the adductor pollicis (Harper 1988). The evoked compound muscle action potential obtained over the hypothenar eminence is also used for monitoring (Churchill-Davidson and Christie 1959). This site has the disadvantage of monitoring several dissimilar muscles, and these muscles may be more or less sensitive to muscle relaxants than the adductor pollicis. During recovery from tubocurarine, the hypothenar CMAP recovers more rapidly than the adductor pollicis CMAP (Katz 1973).

The diaphragm

The diaphragm is relatively resistant to competitive and non-competitive neuromuscular blocking drugs; it is an everyday observation that spontaneous ventilation recovers more rapidly than peripheral muscle function during the offset of neuromuscular block. Every muscle has a considerable excess of cholinoceptors at the neuromuscular junction; this represents the margin of safety. In a limb muscle, neuromuscular transmission appears normal until approximately 75% of receptors are blocked (Paton and Waud 1967). The diaphragm has a greater margin of safety than peripheral muscles and requires only half the number of unblocked receptors for neuromuscular transmission to proceed normally in laboratory studies (Waud and Waud 1972). In humans, when the adductor pollicis is 90% blocked by pancuronium, the EMG response of the diaphragm is reduced by approximately 25% (Donati *et al*. 1986).

Other factors, however, also determine the pattern of the response of a muscle to a neuromuscular blocking drug. The blood supply to the muscle is very important in determining how rapidly the drug is conveyed to the neuromuscular junction, and the richness of diaphragmatic muscle blood flow might explain the rapidity with which the diaphragm becomes paralysed after the administration of a muscle relaxant drug. After pancuronium 0.08 mg/kg, maximum block of the diaphragm occurs in approximately one minute — 30% faster than the adductor pollicis. Spontaneous recovery is also more rapid in the diaphragm. The time taken for the first response of the TOF in the diaphragm to recover is approximately half that of the adductor pollicis (Derrington and Hindocha 1990). During anaesthesia, neuromuscular transmission in the diaphragm may be measured by stimulating one phrenic nerve using ECG electrodes at the neck, and measuring the EMG response using ECG electrodes in the eighth intercostal space (costal fibres), or using an oesophageal electrode (crural fibres). The force of contraction of the diaphragm may be measured indirectly using trans-diaphragmatic pressure or inspiratory pressure. These methods of measurement are not appropriate for routine clinical monitoring.

The larynx

Satisfactory conditions for endotracheal intubation can be obtained only if the masseter muscles, the muscles of the neck, the diaphragm, and the laryngeal adductor muscles are relaxed. In common with the diaphragm, depolarizing and nondepolarizing neuromuscular block of the laryngeal adductors is more rapid in onset and offset than the adductor pollicis. Although adequate intubating conditions may exist before the adductor pollicis has become completely paralysed, ideal intubating conditions — suitable, for example, in a penetrating eye injury — may take a little longer to become established (Bencini and Newton 1984).

Facial muscles

If it is necessary to position the anaesthetized patient so that the limbs are inaccessible to neuromuscular monitoring, it may be convenient to monitor the response of the facial muscles to surface stimulation of the facial nerve. The stimulating electrodes are positioned just anterior to the tragus of the ear. The facial muscles appear to behave as 'central' muscles rather than 'peripheral' muscles. In comparison with the adductor pollicis, neuromuscular block is more rapid in both onset (Harper and Wilson 1987) and offset (Caffrey *et al*. 1986). It is important to remember that the facial muscles will underestimate the extent of neuromuscular block in comparison with the adductor pollicis so that the unwary might be tempted to give an excessive dose of relaxant.

Abdominal muscles

In view of the importance attached to the ability of the anaesthetist to manipulate abdominal muscle tone during abdominal surgery, it is unfortunate that it is difficult to monitor the degree of paralysis of these muscles. Tonic contraction of the abdominal wall muscles (abdominal wall tension) has been measured mechanically using abdominal retractors equipped with a strain-gauge force transducer. As neuromuscular block with atracurium and vecuronium was deepened, abdominal wall tension declined to a minimum before adductor pollicis block had exceeded approximately 80% depression of the control, suggesting that there is little value in maintaining profound neuromuscular block for abdominal surgery (Weber *et al.* 1985).

Muscles of the leg

Occasionally it may be more convenient to monitor the response of the muscles of the leg to nerve stimulation, for example during neurosurgery. Published work suggests that the gastrocnemius muscle is similar to the adductor pollicis in its sensitivity to muscle relaxants (Harper and Wilson 1989). In a volunteer study, the volitional strength of the soleus muscle was diminished to a lesser extent than the gastrocnemius muscle by a small dose of tubocurarine (Secher *et al.* 1982). This observation supports the hypothesis that the predominant muscle fibre type (slow or fast) is one determinant of the sensitivity of a muscle to muscle relaxants. If the posterior tibial nerve is stimulated in the popliteal fossa, a satisfactory EMG can be measured over the gastrocnemius and soleus muscles. Stimulation over the medial plantar nerve (a terminal division of the posterior tibial nerve) at the ankle elicits contraction of the short flexors of the foot and plantar flexion of the great toe (flexor hallucis brevis) which is suitable for tactile assessment by the anaesthetist.

CONCLUSION

Whenever a drug is administered to a patient, it is logical to monitor its effect. It is only by routinely monitoring neuromuscular function that the most appropriate level of block can be obtained without running the risk of post-operative problems. Care must be taken to ensure that the electrodes are carefully positioned, that the mode of stimulation is appropriate to the extent of block and that sufficient time is permitted to elapse between measurements. Neuromuscular monitoring then becomes a valuable adjunct to management whenever a neuromuscular blocking drug is given.

REFERENCES

Ali, H. H., and Savarese, J. J. (1980). Stimulus frequency and dose–response curve to *d*-tubocurarine in man. *Anesthesiology*, **52**, 36–9.

Ali, H. H., Utting, J. E., and Gray, T. C. (1970). Stimulus frequency in the detection of neuromuscular block in humans. *British Journal of Anaesthesia*, **42**, 967–77.

Ali, H. H., Utting, J. E., and Gray, T. C. (1971*a*). Quantitative assessment of residual anti-depolarizing block (part I). *British Journal of Anaesthesia*, **43**, 473–6.

Ali, H. H., Utting, J. E., and Gray, T. C. (1971*b*). Quantitative assessment of residual anti-depolarizing block (part II). *British Journal of Anaesthesia*, **43**, 478–85.

Bencini, A. and Newton, D. E. F. (1984). Rate of onset of good intubating conditions, respiratory depression and hand muscle paralysis after vecuronium. *British Journal of Anaesthesia*, **56**, 959–65.

Berger, J. J., Gravenstein, J. S., and Munson, E. S. (1982). Electrode polarity and peripheral nerve stimulation. *Anesthesiology*, **56**, 402–4.

Berry, F. R. (1966). Detection of neuromuscular block in man. *British Journal of Anaesthesia*, **38**, 929–35.

Bonsu, A. K., Viby-Mogensen, J., Fernando, P. U. E., Muchhal, K., Tamilarasan, A., and Lambourne, A. (1987). Relationship of post-tetanic count and train-of-four response during intense neuromuscular blockade caused by atracurium. *British Journal of Anaesthesia*, **59**, 1089–92.

Botelho, S. Y. (1955). Comparison of simultaneously recorded electrical and mechanical activity in myasthenia gravis patients and in partially curarized humans. *American Journal of Medicine*, **19**, 693–6.

Brand, J. B., Cullen, D. J., Wilson, N. E., and Ali, H. H. (1977).Spontaneous recovery from nondepolarizing neuromuscular blockade: correlation between clinical and evoked responses. *Anesthesia and Analgesia*, **56**, 55–8.

Braude, N., Vyvyan, H. A. L., and Jordan, M. J. (1991). Intraoperative assessment of atracurium-induced neuromuscular block using double-burst stimulation. *British Journal of Anaesthesia*, **67**, 574–8.

Caffrey, R., Warren, M. L., and Becker, K. E. (1986). Neuromuscular blockade monitoring comparing the orbicularis oculi and adductor pollicis muscles. *Anesthesiology*, **65**, 95–7.

Caplan, L. M., Satyanarayana, T., Patel, K. P., Turndorf, H., and Ramanathan, S. (1981). Assessment of neuromuscular blockade with surface electrodes. *Anesthesia and Analgesia*, **60**, 244–5.

Churchill-Davidson, H. C. and Christie, T. H. (1959). The diagnosis of neuromuscular block in man. *British Journal of Anaesthesia*, **31**, 290–301.

DeJong, R. H. (1966). Controlled relaxation. 1. Quantitation of electromyogram with abdominal relaxation. *Journal of the American Medical Association*, **197**, 393–5.

Derrington, M. C. and Hindocha, N. (1990). Comparison of neuromuscular block in the diaphragm and hand after administration of tubocurarine, pancuronium and alcuronium. *British Journal of Anaesthesia*, **64**, 294–9.

Donati, F. and Bevan, D. R (1984). Muscle electromechanical correlations during succinylcholine infusions. *Anesthesia and Analgesia*, **63**, 206.

Donati, F., Antzaka, C., and Bevan, D. R. (1986). Potency of pancuronium at the diaphragm and the adductor pollicis muscle in humans. *Anesthesiology*, **65**, 1–5.

Donlon, J. V., Savarese, J. J., and Ali, H. H. (1979). Cumulative dose–response curves for gallamine: effect of altered resting thumb tension and mode of stimulation. *Anesthesia and Analgesia*, **58**, 377–91.

Drenk, N. E., Ueda, N., Olsen, N. V., Engbaek, J., Jensen, E., Skorgaard, L. T., *et al.* (1989). Manual evaluation of residual curarization using double burst stimulation: a comparison with train-of-four. *Anesthesiology*, **70**, 578–81.

Dupuis, J. Y., Martin, R., Tessonnier, J. M., and Tetrault, J. P. (1990). Clinical assessment of the muscular response to tetanic nerve stimulation. *Canadian Journal of Anaesthesia*, **37**, 397–400.

Ekstedt, J. and Stålberg, E. (1969). The effect of non-paralytic doses of *d*-tubocurarine on individual motor end-plates in man, studied with a new electrophysiological method. *Electroencephalography and Clinical Neurophysiology*, **27**, 57–62.

Engbaek, J., Ostergaard, D., and Viby-Mogensen, J. (1989). Double burst stimulation (DBS): a new pattern of nerve stimulation to identify residual neuromuscular block. *British Journal of Anaesthesia*, **62**, 274–8.

Engbaek, J., Ostergaard, D., Skovgaard, L. T., and Viby-Mogensen, J. (1990). Reversal of intense neuromuscular blockade following infusion of atracurium. *Anesthesiology*, **72**, 803–6.

Eriksson, L., Lennmarken, C., Staun, P., and Viby-Mogensen, J. (1990). Use of post-tetanic count in assessment of a repetitive vecuronium-induced neuromuscular block. *British Journal of Anaesthesia*, **65**, 487–93.

Fernando, P. U. E., Viby-Mogensen, J., Bonsu, A. K., Tamilarasan, A., Muchhal, K. K., and Lambourne, A. (1987). Relationship between posttetanic count and response carinal stimulation during vecuronium-induced neuromuscular blockade. *Acta Anaesthesiologica Scandanavica*, **31**, 593–6.

Glavinovic, M. I. (1979). Presynaptic action of curare. *Journal of Physiology* (*London*), **290**, 499–506.

Ham, J. and Redpath, J. H. (1985). Comparative monitoring of non-depolarizing neuromuscular blockade in humans. *Anesthesia and Analgesia*, **64**, 225.

Harper, N. J. N. (1988). Comparison of the adductor pollicis and the first dorsal interosseous muscles during atracurium and vecuronium blockade: an electromyographic study. *British Journal of Anaesthesia*, **61**, 477–8.

Harper, N. J. N. and Wilson, A. (1987). Onset of atracurium-induced blockade in the muscles of the face: orbicularis oculi and adductor pollicis compared. *British Journal of Anaesthesia*, **59**, 932–3P.

Harper, N. J. N. and Wilson, A. (1989). Characteristics of atracurium block in the gastrocnemius muscle. *British Journal of Anaesthesia*, **63**, 240–1P.

Harper, N. J. N., Bradshaw, E. G., and Healy, T. E. J. (1986). Evoked electromyographic and mechanical responses of the adductor pollicis compared during the onset of neuromuscular blockade by atracurium or alcuronium, and during antagonism by neostigmine. *British Journal of Anaesthesia*, **58**, 1278–84.

Harper, N. J. N., Pugh, N. D., Healy, T. E. J., and Petts, H. V. (1987). Changes in the power spectrum of the evoked compound action potential of the adductor pollicis with the onset of neuromuscular blockade. *British Journal of Anaesthesia*, **59**, 200–5.

Harper, N. J. N., Chadwick, I. S., and Linsley, A. (1993). Suxamethonium and atracurium: sequential and simultaneous administration. *European Journal of Anaesthesiology*, **10**, 13–7.

Howardy-Hansen, P., Viby-Mogensen, J., Gottschau, A., Skovgaard, L. T., Chraemmer-Jorgensen, B., and Engbaek, J. (1984). Tactile evaluation of post tetanic count (PTC). *Anesthesiology*, **60**, 372–4.

Inman, V. T., Ralston, H. J., Saunders, J. B. deC. M., Feinstein, B., and Wright, E. W. (1952). Relation of human electromyogram to muscular tension. *Electroencephalography and Clinical Neurophysiology*, **4**, 187–94.

Jensen, E., Viby-Mogensen, J., and Bang, U. (1988). The Accelograph: a new neuromuscular transmission monitor. *Acta Anaesthesiologica Scandanavica*, **32**, 49–52.

Kalli, I. (1990). Effect of surface electrode position on the compound action potential evoked by ulnar nerve stimulation during isoflurane anaesthesia. *British Journal of Anaesthesia*, **65**, 494–9.

Katz, R. L. (1973). Electromyographic and mechanical effects of suxamethonium and tubocurarine on twitch, tetanic and post-tetanic responses. *British Journal of Anaesthesia*, **45**, 849–59.

Kopman, A. F. and Lawson, D. (1984). Milliamperage requirements for supramaximal stimulation of the ulnar nerve with surface electrodes. *Anesthesiology*, **61**, 83–5.

Kopman, A. F., Epstein, R. H. and Flashburg, M. H. (1982). Use of 100-Hertz tetanus as an index of recovery from pancuronium-induced nondepolarizing neuromuscular blockade. *Anesthesia and Analgesia*, **61**, 439–41.

Kosek, P. S., Sears, D. H., and Rubenstein, E. H. (1988). Minimizing movement-induced changes in twitch response during integrated electromyography. *Anesthesiology*, **69**, 142–3.

Lee, C. M. (1975). Train-of-4 quantitation of competitive neuromuscular block. *Anesthesia and Analgesia*, **54**, 649–53.

Meretoja, O. A. and Brown, T. C. K. (1989). Drift of the thenar EMG signal. *Anesthesiology*, **71**, A824.

O'Hara, D. A., Fragen, R. J., and Shanks, C. A. (1986*a*). Reappearance of the train-of-four after neuromuscular blockade induced with tubocurarine, vecuronium or atracurium. *British Journal of Anaesthesia*, **58**, 1296–9.

O'Hara, D. A., Fragen, R. J., and Shanks, C. A. (1986*b*). Comparison of visual and measured train-of-four recovery after vecuronium-induced neuromuscular blockade using two anaesthetic techniques. *British Journal of Anaesthesia*, **58**, 1300–2.

Paton, W. D. M., and Waud, D. R. (1967). The margin of safety of neuromuscular transmission. *Journal of Physiology*, **191**, 59–90.

Pugh, N. D., Harper, N. J. N., Healy, T. E. J., and Petts, H. V. (1987). Effects of atracurium on the latency and the duration of the negative deflection of the evoked compound action potential of the adductor pollicis. *British Journal of Anaesthesia*, **59**, 195–9.

Secher, N. H., Rube, N., and Secher, O. (1982). Effect of tubocurarine on human soleus and gastrocnemius muscles. *Acta Anaesthesiologica Scandanavica*, **26**, 231–4.

Shanks, C. A. and Jarvis, J. E. (1980). Electromyographic and mechanical twitch responses following suxamethonium administration. *Anaesthesia and Intensive Care*, **8**, 341–4.

Smith, D. C. (1991). Central enhancement of evoked electromyographic monitoring of neuromuscular function. *British Journal of Anaesthesia*, **66**, 562–5.

Stanec, A., Heyduk, J., Stanec, G., and Orkin, L. R. (1978). Tetanic fade and post-tetanic tension in the absence of neuromuscular blocking agents in anesthetized man. *Anesthesia and Analgesia*, **57**, 102–7.

Tammisto, T., Wirtavuori, K., and Linko, K. (1988). Assessment of neuromuscular block: comparison of three clinical methods and evoked electromyography. *European Journal of Anaesthesiology*, **5**, 1–8.

Thornberry, E. A. and Mazumdar B. (1988). The effect of changes in arm temperature on neuromuscular monitoring in the presence of atracurium blockade. *Anaesthesia*, **43**, 447–9.

Viby-Mogensen, J., Chraemmer-Jorgensen, B., and Ording, H. (1979). Residual curarization in the recovery room. *Anesthesiology*, **50**, 539–41.

Viby-Mogensen, J., Howardy-Hansen, P., Chraemmer-Jorgensen, B., Ording, H., Engbaek, J., and Nielsen, A. (1981). Post tetanic count (PTC): a new method of evaluating an intense nondepolarizing neuromuscular blockade. *Anesthesiology*, **55**, 458–61.

Viby-Mogensen, J., Jensen, N. H., Engbaek, J., Ording, H., Skovgaard, L. T., Stat, C., *et al.* (1985). Tactile and visual evaluation of the response to train-of-four nerve stimulation. *Anesthesiology*, **63**, 440–3.

Viby-Mogensen, J., Jensen, E., Werner, M., and Kirkegaard Nielsen, H. (1988). Measurement of acceleration: a new method of monitoring neuromuscular function. *Acta Anaesthesiologica Scandanavica*, **32**, 45–8.

Waud, B. E. and Waud, D. R. (1972). The margin of safety of neuromuscular transmission in the muscle of the diaphragm. *Anesthesiology*, **37**, 417–22.

Weber, S., Muravchick, S., DeFeo, S. P., and Rosato, E. F. (1985). Correlation of evoked twitch response to abdominal wall tension during surgery. *Anesthesiology*, **63**, A325.

Williams, N. E., Webb, S. N., and Calvey, T. N. (1980). Differential effects of myoneural blocking drugs on neuromuscular transmission. *British Journal of Anaesthesia*, **52**, 1111–4.

17

The future in neuromuscular block and its reversal

L.H.D.J. Booij

Curare was studied in animals as early as 1850 by Claude Bernard. Curarine was administered to a patient for the first time as an adjunct to anaesthesia by Läwen (1912). In 1939 Francis Sibson had attempted to treat patients with rabies with curare, and in 1857 Lewis Albert Sayre had advocated its use to relieve spasms of tetanus (Bevan *et al.* 1988).

The introduction of muscle relaxants into routine clinical anaesthesia by Griffith and Johnson (1942) has radically changed the practice of anaesthesia and increased the surgical possibilities to the benefit of all mankind. In the following year, Cullen (1943) described the benefits of curare administration during laparotomy under inhalational anaesthesia, and nowadays relaxants are part of the standard armamentarium of every anaesthestist. Operations which until 1942 could only be thought of were suddenly feasible, while the safety of anaesthesia improved markedly because lighter levels of anaesthesia with muscle relaxation were possible. Shortly after their introduction, it became apparent that muscle relaxants have side-effects, can cause adverse effects, and are potentially dangerous drugs which must be administered with extreme caution (Beecher and Todd 1954). It was also realized that numerous factors relating to the physical condition of the patient, and to the pharmacological properties of the relaxant, contributed to these problems (Foldes 1959).

The mechanism of action of the depolarizing relaxants results in a number of potentially serious side-effects, which include myalgia, potassium release, increase in intraocular, intracranial, and intragastric pressure, salivation, and a number of cardiovascular effects. From this group only suxamethonium, introduced in 1951 (Brucke *et al.* 1951) is still in clinical use because of its unique rapidity of onset and short duration of action. Decamethonium, first used in 1949, has disappeared completely. The nondepolarizing relaxants, depending upon their structure, may give rise to histamine release, cardiovascular changes, and cumulation.

In an attempt to improve on the profile of the relaxants, a large series of nondepolarizing drugs has been developed and introduced into clinical practice. These include gallamine (Bovet *et al.* 1947), alcuronium (Lund and Stovner 1962), pancuronium (Baird and Reid 1967), metocurine (originally introduced in 1948 and reintroduced in 1972) (Sobell *et al.* 1972), dioxonium (Kimenis *et al.* 1972), and fazadinium (Simpson *et al.* 1972). The pharmacodynamic profile of none or these compounds, however, has fully met all clinical requirements and because of this, Savarese and Kitz (1975) suggested the need for three types of relaxants classified according to their duration of action: short, intermediate, or long acting. Other requirements of an ideal relaxant were also defined as follows:

(1) a nondepolarizing mechanism of action;

(2) a fast onset;

(3) no cumulation;

(4) no cardiovascular side-effects;

(5) no histamine release;

(6) prompt and complete reversal with anticholinesterases;

(7) rapid elimination from the body;

(8) elimination independent of renal and/or liver function;

(9) any metabolites should be inactive.

Since those desiderata were defined, vecuronium bromide (Marshall *et al.* 1980; Crul and Booij 1980) and atracurium dibesylate (Payne and Hughes 1981; Basta *et al.* 1982) have been introduced in an attempt to satisfy the need for a non-cumulative intermediate-acting relaxant. Although they meet many of the requirements of the ideal neuromuscular blocking agent and provide more flexibility in usage, they still are not ideal. They do possess some disadvantages, e.g. vecuronium is unstable in solution and atracurium may cause histamine release, both have a rather long onset of action, and both show, like the older relaxants, a large variability in the degree of block and the time-course of action in individual patients.

There are many other reasons why there is still a need for new relaxants. Muscle relaxants seem to be responsible for up to 50% of the adverse reactions during anaesthesia (Vervloet 1985). The most frequent reactions are tachycardia, cardiovascular collapse, urticaria, and bronchospasm. Besides these factors, many relaxants depend on intact kidney and liver function for their plasma elimination, which may result in prolonged effects in patients with renal or hepatic diseases.

PATHWAYS FOR THE DEVELOPMENT OF NEW RELAXANTS

Theoretically there are several possibilities for drugs to interfere with muscle contraction. These form the potential pathways for the future development of new relaxants.

Firstly, it is possible to interfere with the generation and conduction of stimuli in the motor nerve through the administration of local anaesthetic-like agents. For this route to be applicable following systemic administration, large doses of local anaesthetic drugs are required. With the currently available drugs, a selective block of motor nerve conductivity alone cannot be anticipated but block will also be seen in other parts of the nervous system and probably even in the cardiovascular system. Tetrodotoxin, from the puffer fish and some other animals, inhibits nerve conduction through the irreversible mechanism of sodium channel block. Saxitoxin, from the Alaskan butterclam, also acts via this route. A variety of other drugs interfere with nerve conduction through an effect on potassium and calcium channels. They are not suitable for clinical use because their effect is in most cases irreversible.

Secondly, it is possible to interfere with the synthesis, mobilization, and release of acetylcholine in the motor nerve terminal. Interference with the synthesis (e.g. hemicholinium) and mobilization of acetylcholine is also likely to interfere with transmission at synapses other than the neuromuscular junction. These will result, for example, in autonomic imbalance and central nervous system effects. Vesamicol (AH5183) inhibits the uptake of acetylcholine into the vesicles thereby causing a slowly developing neuromuscular block. Vesamicol also inhibits the release of non-vesicular acetylcholine. These effects are reversed by 4-aminopyridine. A similar effect is produced by quinacrine and tetraphenylboron. These agents, however, also affect cholinergic mechanisms other than neuromuscular transmission.

It is well known that some of the nondepolarizing relaxants do block presynaptic acetylcholine receptors and thus inhibit acetylcholine release (Bowman 1980; Foldes *et al.* 1989). Block of such receptors is thought to be involved in the fade in response to train-of-four and tetanic stimulation when nondepolarizing relaxants are administered. The amount of fade produced by different nondepolarizing drugs varies, and so, presumably, does the effect on the nerve terminal (Williams *et al.* 1980). Further development of this concept of selective inhibition of acetylcholine release at the motor nerve terminal may be a feasible new pathway. Beta-bungarotoxin is a toxin that selectively blocks presynaptic acetylcholine release in an irreversible manner, and thus is not useful clinically.

Thirdly, it is possible to block the postsynaptic acetylcholine receptor, thus preventing its occupation by acetylcholine. Alpha-bungarotoxin causes selective but irreversible block of the postsynaptic receptors. Botulinum toxin and tetanus toxin do the same but also have presynaptic effects. The currently used depolarizing and nondepolarizing relaxants block the postsynaptic receptors in a reversible manner. Development of new, more selective, drugs acting only on the postsynaptic acetylcholine receptors is feasible.

The discovery that various subtypes of muscarinic and nicotinic acetylcholine receptors exist, and that they are unevenly distributed over the various muscles, may make selective block of muscles feasible. Differences in response of various muscle groups to administration of a relaxant have already been demonstrated (Caffrey *et al.* 1986; Laycock *et al.* 1988; Donati *et al.* 1990, 1991). It may thus be possible to develop relaxants that will selectively block the diaphragm or the hypopharyngeal and laryngeal muscles without significant effects on other muscles of the body.

It has recently been demonstrated that block of ion channels located near the acetylcholine receptor does result in muscle relaxation. Channel block can only occur if the channel has first been opened by an agonist (Dreyer 1982). A wide variety of substances of different chemical structure, including most agonists themselves, can block open ion channels. The degree of block is dependent upon the concentration of the substance. Channel blocking substances include steroids, barbiturates, tubocurarine, atropine, decamethonium, ethidium bromide, antibiotics, local anaesthetics, acetylcholinesterase inhibitors, and many other drugs. Many of these concepts merit further development.

The fourth and probably last possibility lies in the inhibition of excitation–contraction coupling in the muscle. Studies with one such agent, dantrolene, have shown, however, that there is lack of selectivity when high doses are used in order to obtain complete paralysis.

At present, it appears that only developments with agonists and antagonists for the postsynaptic acetylcholine receptor are regarded as feasible by the pharmaceutical industry. Thus the only new developments which are likely to occur over the next 10 years concern depolarizing or nondepolarizing relaxants.

DESIRABLE CHARACTERISTICS FOR NEW RELAXANTS

Besides the characteristics of an ideal relaxant listed above (Savarese and Kitz 1975; Booij and Crul 1983), some new ones can be formulated.

A clinically important characteristic is that new relaxants should have less variability in their effects (e.g. degree of block, or duration) when administered to an individual patient. This would make the effect of the relaxants more reliable and predictable. Because so many factors, including various diseases (Booij 1989a), contribute to this variability, it is unlikely that this will ever be obtained.

It would be ideal if block of particular muscles could be selectively obtained. For example, selective block of the hypopharyngeal and laryngeal muscles would make intubation in spontaneously breathing patients simpler. Selective paralysis of abdominal muscles would allow intra-abdominal surgery in spontaneously breathing patients under general anaesthesia. As previously noted, the development of relaxants acting selectively on particular muscles seems theoretically feasible.

A number of the older requirements have been reached in some compounds. Certain of these characteristics seem to depend on the chemical structures. While some members of the benzoisoquinolinium family are likely to cause histamine release, the steroids appear to be mainly free from such an effect. The steroids, however, seem to depend more on hepatic function for their plasma elimination than do the benzylisoquinolinium drugs. Only relaxants which are totally metabolized in plasma, extracellular fluid, or in the muscle itself, will be completely independent of renal and hepatic function.

The metabolites produced should be inactive and non-toxic. At present only suxamethonium and some previously investigated esters are metabolized by plasma cholinesterase. In a small number of patients with atypical or low plasma cholinesterase activity, a prolonged effect is observed. Hydrolysis by plasma cholinesterase therefore remains a possible solution for the development of a short-acting relaxant. The new compound mivacurium is an example of a compound which is hydrolysed by plasma cholinesterase. Atracurium is partly broken down by Hofmann elimination which is pH and temperature dependent and also partly by hydrolysis (by an atypical cholinesterase). Whether this feature can be built into other molecules remains to be investigated.

At present a fast onset of action to facilitate early endotracheal intubation of the patient is regarded as one of the most desirable features of a relaxant. Attempts have been made to shorten the onset of action by using the priming principle (Foldes 1984). The intubating conditions obtained with this technique are, however, inferior to those obtained with suxamethonium (Jones 1989). For a fast onset of action, a rapid association of the drug to the receptor is needed. For a short duration and rapid recovery a very fast dissociation and low receptor binding of the compound is needed (Paton and Waud 1962). A fast onset can also be produced by the administration of a large amount of relaxant (Lennon *et al.* 1986). This will, however, increase the duration of action for most compounds (as demonstrated with vecuronium) and may lead to an increase in the frequency of undesirable side-effects (e.g. histamine release with atracurium and vagolysis with pancuronium). Some investigators believe that it will be impossible to develop a fast onset nondepolarizer, because 75–80% of the receptors have to be blocked with a nondepolarizer before muscular relaxation becomes apparent (Waud and Waud 1975).

With depolarizers, only 20–25% of the receptors have to be occupied in order to initiate depolarization. Because hydrolysis of suxamethonium by plasma cholinesterase is fast, only a small amount of the compound will actually reach the neuromuscular junction and thus be effective. A large overdose of suxamethonium therefore has to be administered. The onset of suxamethonium, however, remains faster than any other relaxant presently available probably because the occupancy of only 20–25% of the receptors is faster than the occupancy of 75–80% of the receptors as needed with nondepolarizers. Thus with a nondepolarizing neuromuscular blocking agent, large amounts must be administered in order to secure a fast onset of action. This means that fast onset relaxants will of necessity have a low potency.

An additional, and fascinating possibility would be a gaseous relaxant. There is presently no such drug. If there were such an agent, it would depend on ventilation for its elimination, and would thus be independent of hepatic or renal function.

NEW THEORIES ON THE ONSET OF NEUROMUSCULAR BLOCK

The onset time of an individual compound clearly decreases with an increase in the dose, as has been demonstrated for atracurium (Mirakhur *et al.* 1985) and vecuronium (Feldman *et al.* 1990). Another factor which influences the onset of action is the circulation time. It is not, however, feasible to decrease circulation time to shorten the onset of relaxants.

It has been suggested that with nondepolarizing muscle relaxants a large number of molecules have to be administered in order to obtain a fast onset of action. This means that the lower the potency, the faster the onset, when equipotent doses of compounds are administered. It has been demonstrated in cats that within a series of chemically related compounds possessing the same mechanism of action and administered at equipotent dosages, the least potent compound has the fastest onset of action (Bowman et al. 1988). This has been confirmed in both dogs and rhesus monkeys (Booij, unpublished data) with the same group of steroidal relaxants. The least potent one (rocuronium) has the shortest onset of action. This principle is not only applicable to muscle relaxants, but can also be observed for other groups of drugs like amide local anaesthetics, and fentanyl analogues. According to this theory and the results of studies with a series of steroid analogues, it must be concluded that a very rapid onset, short duration of action nondepolarizing muscle relaxant can probably be synthesized. One must, however, realise that an increase in plasma concentration is only a limited possibility because this will very likely increase the incidence of side-effects. Indeed, the series of compounds with a time-course of action similar to suxamethonium which have been tested so far showed major cardiovascular side-effects.

THE CHEMICAL STRUCTURE OF MUSCLE RELAXANTS

A variety of chemical structures possess a neuromuscular blocking effect. For such an effect is it important that the compound contains cationic centres for electrostatic binding to both alpha-chain proteins of the acetylcholine receptor. It has been demonstrated that the sites of binding of the various agonists and antagonists, and thus their effects on the conformation of the receptor, are likely to be different (Wu et al. 1990). When more information on this topic becomes available it may be possible to synthesize compounds with a more specific effect on a particular part of the receptor.

Most frequently the muscle relaxants are quaternary ammonium salts; more rarely they are secondary or tertiary amines (Kharkevich 1990). For a long time it was thought that only bisquaternary compounds (pancuronium, pipecuronium, atracurium, fazadinium, metocurine, alcuronium, suxamethonium) were active. Nowadays, however, examples of monoquarternary (tubocurarine, vecuronium, rocuronium, stercuronium) and trisquarternary (gallamine) relaxants are available. Bisquaternary ammonium compounds are not necessarily more potent than mono-quaternary or trisquaternary ammonium compounds.

New compounds are being developed in several different structural families. These include the benzylisoquinolinium family (tubocurarine, atracurium, doxacurium, mivacurium, etc.), the steroid family (pancuronium, vecuronium, pipecuronium, chandonium, rocuronium, etc.), the tropanyl esters (Gyermek et al. 1990), and a group of what are described as bulky esters (dioxonium, diadonium, anatruxonium, cyclobutonium, and truxilonium) (Kharkevich 1974).

It is appropriate now to discuss the present and possible future developments in each group of relaxants. It is impossible not to glance back to the past while looking forwards.

FUTURE DEVELOPMENTS WITH DEPOLARIZING RELAXANTS

The naturally occurring agonist at the neuromuscular junction is acetylcholine. Several other substances, however, show an agonist action, and lead to depolarization of the postjunctional membrane. Amongst these are carbamylcholine, suberyldicholine, choline, decamethonium, suxamethonium, and nicotine. They have different efficacies in their ability to depolarize the postsynaptic membrane and also different affinities for the acetylcholine receptor.

It is most unlikely that new depolarizing relaxants will be developed because they will all exhibit the same side-effects that are the result of a depolarizing mechanism of action. Nevertheless there are some new observations regarding suxamethonium that may influence the opinion of anaesthesiologists on these compounds and possibly other depolarizers in the future.

It has been demonstrated that suxamethonium has a large variability in its individual effect. The duration of action seems to be inversely correlated with the plasma cholinesterase activity of the patient, even in patients with genotypically normal enzyme (Ritter *et al.* 1988). In a recent study, researchers have demonstrated that this is also true for the potency (degree of block) of suxamethonium (Van Linthout *et al.* 1992). The interindividual difference in plasma cholinesterase activity is thus one of the major factors involved in the variability in response to suxamethonium. Since plasma cholinesterase activity is decreased in a variety of situations (for instance chronic liver disease, pregnancy, some cancers, use of cytotoxic drugs, use of anticholinesterases), is it unlikely that variability in effect can be prevented. Another point to consider is that, owing to the fast hydrolysis of suxamethonium by plasma cholinesterase, only a small part of the suxamethonium injected does reach the neuromuscular junction. Such a small amount is effective because only 25–30% of the acetylcholine receptors need to be occupied. Furthermore, the number of patients who experience an extremely prolonged effect is small, and because artificial ventilation for a short period of time should be available in most recovery rooms, this, in my opinion, no longer presents an unacceptable problem.

In Russia, the depolarizing compound dioxonium has been developed. Soon after administration it changes characteristics from a depolarizing block into a stable nondepolarizing block. This last type of block can be reversed by anticholinesterases (Tammisto and Salmenpera 1980). The change of characteristics seems to depend on the dose administered: low doses (30 μg/kg) remain depolarizing in nature (Salmenpera and Tammisto 1980). In the above studies any cardiovascular or other adverse effects were not observed. A disadvantage is that there seems to be tachyphylaxis to dioxonium upon repeated administration. The change in characteristics and the observed tachyphylaxis raises the question as to whether or not this effect is comparable to the occurrence of a phase II block after administration of suxamethonium, except that it appears earlier, and at a lower dose. Whether this is also the case with the apparently nondepolarizing relaxant mivacurium, which is metabolized by plasma cholinesterase, remains to be studied. The mechanism through which a block changes its characteristics from phase I to phase II is unknown. However, certain of the characteristics of a nondepolarizing block (fade in response) are probably due to interference with presynaptic acetylcholine receptors (Bowman 1980).

In phase II block, besides a selective postsynaptic effect, there may exist a sudden presynaptic effect of the depolarizers. Whether in this case reversal of such a block is a pure presynaptic effect of the cholinesterase inhibitors is unknown. It is, however, known that anticholinesterases also have a strong presynaptic effect (Blaber and Bowman, 1963; Riker and Standaert 1966; Riker and Okamoto 1969). This may be the reason for phase II block reversal and it is clear that further research in this field is needed. If early conversion of a depolarizing block into a nondepolarizing block, as with dioxonum, is feasible, than it may be possible to develop such compounds, provided that they are free from the other adverse effects of depolarizers. This possibility has already been raised (Paton and Waud 1962).

FUTURE DEVELOPMENTS WITH NONDEPOLARIZING RELAXANTS

During the last decade intermediate- and long-acting nondepolarizing relaxants have been developed from an expanding understanding of the mechanisms of neuromuscular transmission and its block. This has greatly improved the versatility of the armamentarium of the anaesthesiologist.

Recently, two clean, long-lasting benzoisoquinolinium and steroid relaxants have been tested both in animals and in clinical trials: doxacurium (BW A938U) (Basta *et al.* 1988) and pipecuronium. These agents are devoid of cardiovascular side-effects. However, because it is possible to administer the available clean, intermediate-acting relaxants by continuous infusion for long procedures, is it doubtful that such compounds are really needed in clinical practice.

The search for a fast-onset short-acting nondepolarizer still continues. If such a compound is clean, non-cumulative, and devoid of active metabolites, then it can be administered by continuous infusion, and could be used in all procedures: short, intermediate or long.

The muscle relaxants under current investigation belong to the benzylisoquinolinium family, the aminosteroid family, the bulky esters, and the tropanyl esters. Some polypeptide toxins derived from snakes and snails have a reversible neuromuscular blocking effect. They act through a highly selective interaction with acetylcholine receptors (Olivera *et al.* 1985). Whether they will result in clinically applicable relaxants remains to be seen.

The benzylisoquinolinium family

The current clinically used relaxants tubocurarine, metocurine, and atracurium (BW 33A) belong to this group. Some other benzylisoquinolinium agents have been tested for a short duration of action in the past. Both BW 252C64 and BW 403C65 were short acting and free from cardiovascular effects in animal experiments. Important cardiovascular effects were, however, demonstrated in preliminary human studies with BW 403C65, while hypersalivation and bronchial secretion were observed with BW 252C64. Furthermore, BW 252C64 could not be reversed with anticholinesterases (Hughes 1972); this might indicate a basically depolarizing or other nonspecific mechanism of action.

BW954U has been tested in animals recently, and shown to be a potent blocker of short duration with minimal cumulative effect and reasonable cardiovascular safety (Fiamengo *et al.* 1990). It has significant prejunctional effects.

Other recent and more successful developments are mivacurium (BW B1090U) (Savarese *et al.* 1988) and doxacurium (BW A938U) (Basta *et al.* 1988).

Mivacurium (BW B1090U)

Mivacurium is a bisquaternary intermediate-acting nondepolarizing relaxant which, administered under balanced nitrous oxide–opioid anaesthesia, has an ED_{95} of 0.07–0.08 mg/kg. The onset of action is dose dependent. At one ED_{95} it is approximately 3–5 min, with a duration to 90% recovery of around 30 min, and a recovery index (25–75%) of 5–7 min (Savarese *et al.* 1988). Mivacurium is a mixture of three stereoisomers, all possessing neuromuscular blocking activity (Maehr *et al.* 1991). In children, mivacurium is less potent (Goudsouzian *et al.* 1989*a*). Inhalational anaesthetics reduce the ED_{95} by 20–30% (Caldwell *et al.* 1989). An increase in dose causes a disproportionally small increase in the duration of action, and has no effect on recovery rate. Cardiovascular effects may, however, appear. Upon rapid (but not upon slow) injection of larger bolus doses (two to three times ED_{95}), a transient decrease in arterial pressure may occur. This is accompanied by facial flush and an increase in serum histamine (Savarese *et al.* 1989). In a clinical study, a decrease in arterial pressure and cutaneous flushing were demonstrated in 30% of cases when 0.2 mg/kg of mivacurium was administered (Goldhill *et al.* 1991).

Mivacurium is metabolized by plasma cholinesterase at a rate of approximately 70–90% that of suxamethonium (Cook *et al.* 1989). The metabolites are inactive. There is an inverse relation between the plasma cholinesterase activity and the duration of action of mivacurium (Ostergaard *et al.* 1989), thus there is a prolonged effect in patients with atypical pseudocholinesterase. The compound is suitable for continuous infusion (Shanks *et al.* 1989). Mivacurium has recently been introduced into some countries.

Doxacurium (BW A938U)

Doxacurium is a bisquaternary long-acting nondepolarizer. The solution contains 0.9% benzylalcohol as a preservative. Unlike atracurium and mivacurium it does not release histamine. With an ED_{95} of 0.025–0.030 mg/kg it is the most potent relaxant available — two to three times more potent than pancuronium. At that dose it has a slow onset time of 10–13 min, a clinical duration to 25% recovery of 90–120 min, and a recovery index of 30–50 min (Basta *et al.* 1988). There is a large variability both in degree and in duration of block. Because a large part of the drug is excreted unchanged via the kidneys, the duration of action is prolonged in patients with renal failure (Cashman *et al.* 1990). Hepatic diseases appear to have no influence on the duration of action of doxacurium (Cook *et al.* 1991).

Doxacurium possesses excellent cardiovascular stability (Stoops *et al.* 1988). Inhalational anaesthetics decrease the ED_{95} by 20–40% (Katz *et al.* 1989). In children the onset of action is more rapid, the duration is shorter, and there is a need for relatively higher doses of doxacurium than in adults (Sarner *et al.* 1988; Goudsouzian *et al.* 1989*b*). The block is reversible with neostigmine. Doxacurium has recently been introduced into clinical practice.

A number of other benzylisoquinolinium drugs are still under laboratory investigation in the search for an ideal fast-onset, short-acting relaxant. In the future it is likely that we will hear more about these substances.

Steroids

A series of steroid compounds have been tested over the years (Durant *et al.* 1979; Bowman *et al.* 1988). As stated above, both onset and duration of action are inversely correlated with the potency of these compounds. Over the years a variety of steroid compounds have been tested in animals. Some have even undergone preliminary studies in humans. From this series pancuronium (Org NA96), vecuronium (Org NC45), pipecuronium, and rocuronium (Org 9426) have emerged.

Org 6368 appeared, in animal studies, to be a short-acting compound with a fast onset of action. The short-lasting effect seemed to be dependant on its rapid hepatic uptake. However, preliminary human studies did not confirm this effect (Baird 1974).

Reports on preliminary studies with steroid relaxants have appeared in the literature. It seems that it should be possible to develop a nondepolarizer with an onset time that in animal experiments is similar to that of suxamethonium.

The steroidal nondepolarizers Org 7617 and Org 9616 have a potency of one third to one tenth that of vecuronium in several animal species (Booij *et al.* 1988; Muir *et al.* 1989). In cats and monkeys, their duration of action is equivalent to that of suxamethonium, but in dogs and pigs it is slightly longer (Booij *et al.* 1988; Booij 1989*b*). Org 9616 is associated with elevations in heart rate and blood pressure, whereas Org 7617 causes hypotension by a direct vasodilator effect mediated through calcium channel block, which prevented further development (Marshall *et al.* 1988; Shanks 1988; Muir *et al.* 1989). Org 7617 is, in addition, less potent in humans than in monkeys.

Org 9991 has, in animals, a pharmacodynamic profile similar to suxamethonium. Unfortunately, however, it produces tachycardia and hypotension in a dose-dependent manner (Cason *et al.* 1990; Muir *et al.* 1991). The compound seems not to depend on renal function for its elimination (Rodrigues *et al.* 1989).

Org 8764, the desacetoxy analogue of vecuronium, showed, in contrast to vecuronium and atracurium, a more rapid onset on the vocal cords than on both tibialis muscle and diaphragm in rats (Gilly *et al.* 1988). However, it has a low potency and acts on the cardiac muscarinic receptors. This shows that non-depolarizers could be developed with a higher affinity for particular muscles.

Pipecuronium

Pipecuronium, a bisquaternary steroidal long-lasting nondepolarizing relaxant has, under balanced anaesthesia, an ED_{95} of 0.05 mg/kg, resulting in an onset time of 3–4 min, and a total duration to 90% recovery of approximately 85 min (Wierda *et al.* 1989). The pharmacodynamic profile is therefore similar to that of pancuronium (Dubois *et al.* 1991*a*). It is, however, free from cardiovascular effects (Barankay 1980). Children are slightly more sensitive to pipecuronium than adults; in infants the duration is shorter than both children and adults (Pittet *et al.* 1990). Inhalational anaesthetics do not potentiate the effect of pipecuronium. They do, however, prolong the duration of action (Pittet *et al.* 1989). Approximately 40% of the dose administered is excreted via the kidneys and thus the effect is prolonged in renal failure (Caldwell *et al.* 1987). The remainder of the drug is slowly deacetylated in the liver and then excreted in the bile.

Rocuronium (Org 9426)

Rocuronium is an intermediate-acting monoquaternary steroid nondepolarizing muscle relaxant. The compound has been extensively tested in animal experiments (Muir *et al.* 1991). It is, in contrast to vecuronium, stable in solution and has a notably fast onset of action (1.5–2 min). This makes intubation possible within 1 min after administration of a dose two times the ED_{95} (Lapreye *et al.* 1990; Foldes *et al.* 1991). The ED_{95} is approximately 0.3–0.4 mg/kg with a duration of action similar to vecuronium (Booij and Knape 1991). Inhalational anaesthetics potentiate the effects of rocuronium (Quil *et al.* 1991; Dubois *et al.* 1991*b*). There are no cardiovascular side-effects nor is there any sign of histamine release (Davis *et al.* 1991) following the administration of rocuronium. Its plasma clearance is mainly through liver uptake and biliary excretion (Khuenl-Brady *et al.* 1990), so renal failure does not influence the time-course of action in humans (Szenohradszky *et al.* 1991). Rocuronium has recently been introduced in some countries.

Aza-steroid compounds

Chandonium (HS-310) is a steroid relaxant developed in India. Pharmacological studies with these aza-steroid compounds have been performed in Glasgow. In cats chandonium had a rapid onset and short duration of action, but was accompanied by cardiovascular effects due to vagolysis and cardiac noradrenalin re-uptake block, which resulted in tachycardia (Gandiha *et al.* 1975). Preliminary studies in humans led to the same conclusions (Booij and Agoston 1976, unpublished observations) which stopped its development. Human studies with the compound were subsequently performed in India (Suri 1984) and these also showed that chandonium produces a marked increase in heart rate and blood pressure.

HS-342 is an analogue that in animals causes a fast-onset and short-lasting neuromuscular block. It also, however, possesses a strong vagolytic and autonomic ganglion blocking effect (Marshall *et al.* 1973). This compound has not been tested in humans.

It is doubtful whether either of these two compounds will ever reach the Western market.

RGH 4201 (Duador) is the 3-alpha isomer of chandonium. It was, like pipecuronium, developed in Hungary. Its pharmacodynamic profile is similar to that of vecuronium; in humans the ED_{90} is 0.4 mg/kg, which has an onset time to maximal effect of 6.4 min, a duration to 25% recovery of 28.4 min and a recovery index of 51.9 min (Fitzal *et al.* 1982). The compound is in clinical use in some eastern European countries.

Ester-type nondepolarizing relaxants

In 1973, some short-acting esters were tested in animal experiments (D-188, JJ-142, and HH-85) (Savarese *et al.* 1973, 1975). The presence of vagolytic cardiovascular effects, however, prevented their further development. Intermediate-acting esters were also tested (BW985U, BW785U, BW444U) (Savarese and Wastila 1979*a, b*; Wastila and Savarese 1979). These are all hydrolysed by plasma cholinesterase into inactive products. Some of the compounds underwent preliminary testing in humans, and were longer acting than expected (Savarese *et al.* 1980, 1981). Because most of the compounds have anticholinesterase effects themselves, the ability to reverse such compounds with anticholinesterases might be impaired. Most of them showed histamine release (Savarese *et al.* 1980) with cardiovascular effects, and some exhibited tachyphylaxis (Rosow *et al.* 1980; Basta *et al.* 1981), all of which are good reasons why they were not developed further.

In Russia, a number of bulky ester compounds have been developed and are in clinical use: anatruxonium, cyclobutonium, truxilonium, and diadonium (Kharkevich 1974). Diadonium has been tested in animals in the USA. The resulting neuromuscular block was rapid in onset and had a short duration, but was accompanied by moderate hypotension and mydriasis. In guinea-pigs and monkeys the block was reversible by neostigmine. In mice, rats and also in humans, however, this was not the case (Foldes *et al.* 1989*b*).

Tropanyl ester compounds

G1-64

G1-64 is a tropanyl ester derivative with neuromuscular blocking activity. In animals it has a short onset (shorter than atracurium or vecuronium) and a relatively short duration of action (comparable to vecuronium and atracurium). In the cat it is slightly more vagolytic than pancuronium (Gyermek *et al.* 1990). Human studies have not yet been undertaken with tropanyl esters.

CURRENT STATUS AND POSSIBLE DEVELOPMENTS WITH ANTAGONISTS

The ability to reverse the effect of the muscle relaxants is one of the basic requirements for muscular relaxation. At present only the anticholinesterases neostigmine, pyridostigmine, and edrophonium are clinically used for this purpose. In the past has it been demonstrated that the benzhydryl piperazines, especially BW 52.212, antagonize both suxamethonium and the nondepolarizers (Ellis *et al.* 1953). Another compound, BW49-204, was effective against the depolarizer decamethonium, (VanDam *et al.* 1953). No further studies have been performed with these compounds, which may be effective reversing agents.

Anticholinesterases

Acetylcholinesterase plays an important role in neuromuscular transmission by eliminating the acetylcholine molecules from the cleft through hydrolysis. Only 50% of the acetylcholine molecules liberated from the nerve terminal reach the postsynaptic receptors, the remainder being hydrolysed during the passage across the junctional cleft. Such agents do also have a presynaptic effect and it is believed that the reversing agents also act through this mechanism. Presynaptic effects lead to repetitive firing and increased acetylcholine release. All these factors contribute to the reversing activity (Riker and Okamoto 1969).

Toxic cholinesterase inhibition leads to severe spastic paralysis through accumulation of acetylcholine. Cholinesterase inhibitors may also block the ionic endplate channels, especially at high doses, leading to increase in paralysis. Cholinesterase inhibitors are also used clinically to increase the acetylcholine concentration in patients with myasthenia gravis. For the reversal of nondepolarizing neuromuscular block, neostigmine and pyridostigmine are usually used.

Clinical investigations have demonstrated that edrophonium, administered in adequate high doses, is also a reliable reversal agent, especially for the intermediate-acting nondepolarizers. It has been demonstrated that too small a dose of neostigmine leads to residual paralysis (Viby-Mogensen *et al.* 1979) and that too large a dose leads to neostigmine-induced neuromuscular block (Goldhill *et al.* 1989). An antagonist should thus be titrated under close monitoring of neuromuscular function. The amount of reversing agent that has to be administered depends upon the type of anaesthetic administered, the type of relaxant used and the degree of spontaneous recovery of neuromuscular block. If the neuromuscular block is profound, then recovery may be prolonged, no matter what dose of neostigmine is administered (Caldwell *et al.* 1986). In renal failure the effect of neostigmine and pyridostigime is prolonged.

L.H.D.J. Booij

In view of the fact that cholinesterase inhibitors have many unwanted side-effects it has been tempting to develop reversal agents which possess a different mechanism of action.

Aminopyridines

4-Aminopyridine and its analogues increase presynaptic acetylcholine release, which increases the competition with nondepolarizing relaxants for the postjunctional acetylcholine receptors. They are therefore drugs that can potentially be used for reversal of a neuromuscular block. Because 4-aminopyridine is a tertiary amine, it crosses the blood–brain barrier, and causes central nervous system effects. In clinical studies, 4-aminopyridine had a relatively weak effect which, in the doses used, only partly reversed the non-depolarizing block. It was, however, able to reverse an antibiotic-induced block (Booij *et al.* 1978). Furthermore it does potentiate the effect of the anticholinesterases (Miller *et al.* 1978, 1979).

2,4-diaminopyridine and 3,4-diaminopyridine are more potent and more polar compounds. They thus cross the blood–brain barrier to a lesser extent, and have more specific peripheral effects (Biessels *et al.* 1984). These compounds and some of their analogues are currently being investigated.

Acetamino pyridine-*N*-oxide is another more polar derivative, which is also more potent than 4-aminopyridine (Amaki *et al.* 1980).

Germine mono-acetate

Germine mono-acetate is able to antagonize both a depolarizing and a non-depolarizing neuromuscular block. The mechanism seems to be a direct effect o the muscle fibre (Brennan *et al.* 1971). Although its efficacy has been demonstrated in animal studies (Detwiller 1972; Hyashi *et al.* 1973), the compound has not been routinely used in clinical practice. In cats it reversed muscle relaxation from dantrolene (Lee *et al.* 1980).

REFERENCES

Amaki, Y., Kobayashi, K., and Kibayashi, C. (1980). *In vitro* neuromuscular effect of acetaminopyridine-*N*-oxide. *Anesthesiology*, **53**, S283.
Baird, W. L. M. (1974). Initial studies in man with a new myoneural blocking agent (Org 6368). *British Journal of Anaesthesia*, **46**, 658–61.
Baird, W. L. M., and Reid, A. M. (1967). The neuromuscular blocking properties of a new steroid compound, pancuronium bromide. *British Journal of Anaesthesia*, **39**, 775–80.
Barankay, A. (1980). Circulatory effects of pipecuronium bromide during anaesthesia of patients with severe valvular and schaemic heart disease. *Drug Research*, **30**, 386–9.
Basta, S. J., Moss, J., Savarese, J. J., Ali, H. H., Sunder, N., Gionfriddo, M. *et al.* (1981). Cardiovascular effects of BW444U: correlation with plasma histamine levels. *Anesthesiology*, **55**, A198.

Basta, S. J., Ali, H. H., Savarese, J. J., Sunder, N., Gionfriddo, M., Cloutier, G. (1982). Clinical pharmacology of atracurium besylate (BW 33A): A new non-depolarizing muscle relaxant. *Anesthesia and Analgesia*, **61**, 723–9.

Basta, S. J., Savarese, J. J., Ali, H. H., Embree, P. B., Schwartz, A. F., Rudd, G. D., *et al.* (1988). Clinical pharmacology of doxacurium chloride. *Anesthesiology*, **69**, 478–86.

Beecher, H. K. and Todd, D. P. (1954). A study of the deaths associated with anesthesia and surgery. *Annals of Surgery*, **140**, 2–34.

Bevan, D. R., Bevan, J. C., and Donati, F. (1988). The arrival of curare in Montreal. In *Muscle relaxants in clinical anesthesia*. (ed. D. R. Bevan, J. C. Bevan, and F. Donati), pp. 1–12. Year Book Medical Publishers, Chicago.

Biessels, P. T. M., Agoston, S., and Horn, A. S. (1984). Comparison of the pharmacological actions of some new 4-aminopyridine derivatives. *European Journal of Pharmacology*, **106**, 319–25.

Blaber, L. C. and Bowman, W. C. (1963). Studies on the repetitive discharge evoked in ulnar nerve and skeletal muscle after injection of anticholinesterase drugs. *British Journal of Pharmacology*, **20**, 326–44.

Booij, L. H. D. J. (1989a). Muscle relaxants and medical status of the patient. *Current Opinion in Anaesthesiology*, **2**, 488–92.

Booij, L. H. D. J. (1989b). The development of new steroidal non-depolarizing neuromuscular blocking agents. *Acta Anaesthesiologica Scandinavica*, **33**, (Suppl 91), 101–3.

Booij, L. H. D. J. and Crul, J. F. (1983). A comparison of vecuronium with the hypothetical ideal neuromuscular blocking drug. In *Clinical experiences with Norcuron* (Org NC45, vecuronium bromide), (ed. S. Agoston), pp. 3–8. Excerpta Medica, Amsterdam.

Booij, L. H. D. J. and Knape, J. T. A. (1991). The neuromuscular blocking effect of Org 9426. *Anaesthesia*, **46**, 341–3.

Booij, L. H. D. J., Miller, R. D., and Crul, J. F. (1978). Neostigmine and 4-aminopyridine antagonism of lincomycin-pancuronium neuromuscular blockade in man. *Anesthesia and Analgesia*, **57**, 316–21.

Booij, L. H. D. J., Crul, J. F., and van der Pol, F. (1988). Cardiovascular and neuromuscular blocking effects of four new muscle relaxants in anaesthetized Beagle dogs. *European Journal of Anaesthesiology*, **6**, 70.

Booij, L. H. D. J., Marshall, I. G., Crul, J. F., and Muir, A. W. Pharmacology of four steroidal muscle relaxants. In *Abstracts, 9th World Congress of Anaesthesiologists*, Washington, pp. A0533.

Bovet, D., Depoierre, F., and Lestrange, Y. (1947). Proprietes curarisantes des ethers phenoliques a onctions ammonium quarternaires. *Comptes Rendus Hebdomadaires des Scéances de l'Academie des Sciences*, **225**, 74–6.

Bowman, W. C. (1980). Prejunctional and postjunctional cholinoceptors at the neuromuscular junction. *Anaesthesia and Analgesia*, **59**, 935–43.

Bowman, W. C., Rodger, I. W., Houston, J., Marshall, R. J., and McIndewar, I. (1988). Structure–action relationships among some deacetoxy analogues of pancuronium and vecuronium in the anesthetized cat. *Anesthesiology*, **69**, 57–61.

Brennan, J. L., Jones, S. F., and McLeod, J. G. (1971). Effect of germine acetates on neuromuscular transmission. *Journal of Neurological Sciences*, **13**, 321–31.

Brucke, H., Ginzel, K. H., and Klupp, H. (1951). Bis-cholinester von Dicarbonsäuren als Muskelrelaxantien in der Narkose. *Wiener Klinische Wochenschrift*, **63**, 464–6.

Caffrey, R. R., Warren, M. L., and Becker, K. E. (1986). Neuromuscular blockade monitoring comparing the orbicularis oculi and adductor pollicis muscles. *Anesthesiology*, **65**, 95–7.

Caldwell, J. E., Robertson, E. N., and Baird, W. L. M. (1986). Antagonism of profound neuromuscular blockade induced by vecuronium or atracurium. *British Journal of Anaesthesia*, **58**, 1285–9.

Caldwell, J. E., Canfell, P. C., Castagnoli, K. P., Lynam, D. P., Fahey, M. R., Fisher, D. M., *et al.* (1987). The influence of renal failure on the pharmacokinetics and duration of action of pipecuronium bromide. *Anesthesiology*, **67**, A612.

Caldwell, J. E., Kitts, J. B., Heier, T., Fahey, M. R., Lynam, D. P., and Miller, R. D. (1989). The dose–response relationship of mivacurium chloride in humans during nitrous oxide–fentanyl or nitrous oxide–enflurane anaesthesia. *Anesthesiology*, **70**, 31–5.

Cashman, J. N., Luke, J., and Jones, R. M. (1990). Neuromuscular block with doxacurium (BE A938U) in patients with normal or absent renal function. *British Journal of Anaesthesia*, **64**, 186–92.

Cason, B., Baker, D. G., Hickey, R. F., Miller, R. D., and Agoston, S. (1990). Cardiovascular and neuromuscular effects of three steroidal neuromuscular blocking drugs in dogs (Org 9616, Org 9426 and Org 9991). *Anesthesia and Analgesia*, **70**, 382–8.

Cook, D. R., Stiller, R. L., Weakly, J. N., Chakravorti, S., Brandom, B. W., and Welch, R. M. (1989). *In vitro* metabolism of mivacurium (BW1090U) and succinylcholine. *Anesthesia and Analgesia*, **68**, 452–6.

Cook, D. R., Freeman, J. A., Lai, A. A., Robertson, K. A., Kang, Y., Stiller, R. L., *et al.* (1991). Pharmacokinetics and pharmacodynamics of doxacurium in normal patients and those with hepatic or renal failure. *Anesthesia and Analgesia*, **72**, 145–50.

Crul, J. F. and Booij, L. H. D. J. (1980). First clinical experiences with Org NC45. *British Journal of Anaesthesia*, **52**, S49–52.

Cullen, S. C. (1943). The use of curare for the improvement of abdominal muscle relaxation during inhalation anesthesia. *Surgery*, **14**, 261–6.

Davis, G. K., Sziam, F., Lowdon, J. D., and Levy, J. H. (1991). Evaluation of histamine release following Org 9426 administration using a new radioimmunoassay. *Anesthesiology*, **75**, A818.

Detwiller, P. B. (1972). The effects of germine-3-acetate on neuromuscular transmission. *Journal of Pharmacology and Experimental Therapeutics*. **180**, 244–54.

Donati, F., Meistelman, C., and Plaud, B. (1990). Vecuronium neuromuscular blockade at the diaphragm, the orbicularis oculi and adductor policis muscles. *Anesthesiology*, **73**, 870–5.

Donati, F., Meistelman, C., and Plaud, B. (1991). Vecuronium neuromuscular blockade at the adductor muscles of the larynx and the adductor pollicis. *Anesthesiology*, **74**, 833–7.

Dreyer, F. (1982). Acetylcholine receptor. *British Journal of Anaesthesia*, **54**, 115–30.

Dubois, M. Y., Fleming, N. W., and Lea, D. E. (1991*a*). Effects of succinylcholine on the pharmacodynamics of pipecuronium and pancuronium. *Anesthesia and Analgesia*, **72**, 364–8.

Dubois, M., Kataria, B., Lea, D., and Lapeyre, G. (1991*b*). Neuromuscular effects of Org 9426 in humans during general anesthesia with and without enflurane. *Anesthesia and Analgesia*, **72**, S57.

Durant, N. N., Marshall, I. G., Savage, D. S., Nelson, D. J., Sleigh, T., and Carlyle, I. C. (1979). The neuromuscular and autonomic blocking activities of pancuronium, Org NC45, and other pancuronium analogues, in the cat. *Journal of Pharmacy and Pharmacology*, **31**, 831–6.

Ellis, C. H., Wnuck, A. L., and de Beer, E. J. (1953). Succinylcholine Antagonists. *Federation Proceedings*, **1**, 12–39.

Feldman, S., Fauvel, N., and Harrop-Griffiths, W. (1990). The onset of neuromuscular blockade. In *Neuromuscular blocking agents: past, present and future*, (ed. W. C. Bowman, P. A. F. Denissen, and S. Feldman), pp. 44–51. Excerpta Medica, Amsterdam.

Fiamengo, S. A., Savarese, J. J., Chiscolm, D., Lien, C., and Wastila, W. B. (1990). Pharmacology of BW954U. *Anesthesiology*, **73**, A863.

Fitzal, S., Ilias, W., Kalina, K., Schwarz, S., Foldes, F. F., and Steinbereithner, K. (1982). Neuromuskulare Effekte von Duador einem neuen kurz wirksamen nicht depolarisierenden Muskelrelaxans. *Anaesthesist*, **31**, 674–9.

Foldes, F. F. (1959). Factors which alter the effects of muscle relaxants. *Anesthesiology*, **20**, 464–504.

Foldes, F. F. (1984). Rapid tracheal intubation with non-depolarizing neuromuscular blocking drugs: the priming principle. *British Journal of Anaesthesia*, **56**, 663.

Foldes, F. F., Chaudhry, I. A., Kinjo, M., and Nagashima, H. (1989*a*). Inhibition of mobilization of acetylcholine. *Anesthesiology*, **71**, 218–23.

Foldes, F. F., Chaudhry, I. A., Barakat, T., Flores, C. A., Kinjo, M., Bikhazi, G. B., *et al.* (1989*b*). Species variation in the site and mechanism of the neuromuscular effects of diadonium in rodents. *Anesthesia and Analgesia*, **68**, 638–44.

Foldes, F. F., Nagashima, H., Nguyen, H. D., Schiller, W. S., Mason, M. M., and Ohta, Y. (1991). The neuromuscular effects of Org 9426 in patients receiving balanced anesthesia. *Anesthesiology*, **75**, 191–5.

Gandiha, A., Marshall, I. G., Paul, D., Rodger, I. W., Scott, W., and Singh, H. (1975). Some actions of chandonium iodide, a new short-acting muscle relaxant, in anesthetized cats and on isolated muscle preparations. *Clinical and Experimental Pharmacology and Physiology*, **2**, 150–70.

Gilly, H., Hirtschl, M. M., and Steinbereithner, K. (1988). Pharmacodynamics of Org 8764, atracurium and vecuronium: a comparison of vocal cord, diaphragm and tibial muscle relaxation. *Anesthesiology*, **69**, A481.

Goldhill, D. R., Wainright, A. P., Stuart, C. S., and Flynn, P. J. (1989). Neostigmine after spontaneous recovery from neuromuscular blockade. Effect on depth of blockade monitored with train-of-four and tetanic stimuli. *Anaesthesia*, **44**, 293–9.

Goldhill, D. R., Whitehead, J. P., Emmott, R. S., Griffith, A. P., Bracey, B. J., and Flynn, P. J. (1991). Neuromuscular and clinical effects of mivacurium chloride in healthy adult patients during nitrous oxide–enflurane anaesthesia. *British Journal of Anesthesia*, **67**, 289–95.

Goudsouzian, N. G., Alifirmoff, J. K., Eberly, C., Smeets, R., Griswold, J., Miller, V., *et al.* (1989*a*). Neuromuscular and cardiovascular effects of mivacurium in children. *Anesthesiology*, **70**, 237–42.

Goudsouzian, N. G., Alifimoff, J. K., Liu, L. M. P., Foster, V. J., McNulty, B. F., and Savarese, J. J. (1989*b*). Neuromuscular and cardiovascular effects of doxacurium in children anaesthetized with halothane. *British Journal of Anaesthesia*, **62**, 263–8.

Griffith, H. R. and Johnson, G. E. (1942). The use of curare in general anesthesia. *Anesthesiology*, **3**, 418–20.

Gyermek, L., Nguyen, N., and Lee, C. (1990). G1-64, a new, rapidly acting nondepolarizing neuromuscular blocking agent. *Anesthesiology*, **73**, A862.

Hughes, R. (1972). Evaluation of the neuromuscular blocking properties and side-effects of the two new isoquinolinium bisquarternary compounds (BW 252C64 and BW 403C65). *British Journal of Anaesthesia*, **44**, 27–42.

Hyashi, H., Yonemura, K., and Slimoji, K. (1973). Antagonism of neuromuscular block by germine mono acetate. *Anesthesiology*, **38**, 145–52.

Jones, R. M. (1989). The priming principle how does it work and should we be using it? *British Journal of Anaesthesia*, **63**, 1–3.

Katz, J. A., Fragen, R. J., Shanks, C. A., Dunn, K., McNulty, B., and Rudd, G. D. (1989). Dose–response relationships of doxacurium chloride in humans during anesthesia with nitrous oxide and fentanyl, enflurane, isoflurane, or halothane. *Anesthesiology*, **70**, 432–6.

Kharkevich, D. A. (1974). New curare-like agents. *Journal of Pharmacy and Pharmacology*, **26**, 153–65.

Kharkevich, D. A. (1990). Chemical structures of neuromuscular blocking agents. In *Muscle relaxants: Monographs in anaesthesiology*, Vol. 19, (ed. S.Agoston S and W. C. Bowman), pp. 59–86. Elsevier Science Publishers, Amsterdam.

Khuenl-Brady, K., Castagnoli, K. P., Canfell, C., Caldwell, J. E., Agoston, S., and Miller, R. D. (1990). The neuromuscular blocking effect and pharmacokinetics of Org 9426 and Org 9616 in the cat. *Anesthesiology*, **72**, 669–74.

Kimenis, A., Klusha, V. E., and Ginters, Y. A. (1972). Pharmacology of dioxonium, a new myorelaxant. *Farmakologiya i toxicologiya*, **35**, 172.

Lapreye, G., Dubois, M., Lea, D., Kataria, B., and Tram, D. (1990). Effects of 3 intubating doses of Org 9426 in humans. *Anesthesiology*, **73**, A906.

Läwen A. (1912). Über die Verbindung Lokalanästhesie mit der Narkose, über hohe Extraduralanesthesie und epidurale Injektionen anästhesierender Lösungen bei tabetischen Magenkrisen. *Beiträge zur Klinischen Chirurgie*, **80**, 168–9.

Laycock, J. R. D., Donati, F., Smith, C. E., and Bevan, D. R. (1988). Potency of atracurium and vecuronium at the diaphragm and the adductor pollicis muscle. *British Journal of Anaesthesia*, **61**, 286–91.

Lee, C., Au, E., Durant, N. N., and Katz, R. L. (1980). Germine monoacetate counteracts dantrolene sodium. *Anesthesiology*, **3**, S278.

Lennon, R. L., Olson, R. A., and Gronert, G. A. (1986). Atracurium or vecuronium for rapid sequence endotracheal intubation. *Anesthesiology*, **64**, 510–3.

Lund, I. and Stovner, J. (1962). Experimental and clinical experiences with a new muscle relaxant RO 4-3816, diallyl-nortoxiferine. *Acta Anaesthesiologica Scandinavica* **62**, 85–97.

Maehr, R. B., Belmont, M. R., Wray, D. L., Savarese, J. J., and Wastila, W. B. (1991). Autonomic and neuromuscular effects of mivacurium and isomers in cats. *Anesthesiology*, **75**, A772.

Marshall, I. G., Paul, D., and Singh, H. (1973). The neuromuscular and other blocking actions of 4,17a-diomethyl-4,17*a*-diaza-d-homo-5*a*-androstane dimethiodide (HS-342) in the anaesthetized cat. *European Journal of Pharmacology*, **22**, 129–34.

Marshall, I. G., Agoston, S., Booij, L. H. D. J., Durant, N. N., and Foldes, F. F. (1980). Pharmacology of Org NC45 compared with other nondepolarizing neuromuscular blocking drugs. *British Journal of Anasthesia*, **52**, 11–9S.

Marshall, R. J., Muir, A. W., Booij, L., Crul, J., and Marshall, I. G. (1988). The cardiovascular effects of four new non-depolarising neuromuscular blocking drugs in rat, cats, dogs, pigs and monkeys. *World Congress of Anaesthesiologists*, **2**, A034.

Miller, R. D., Denissen, P. A. F., van der Pol, F., Agoston, S., Booij, L. H. D. J., and Crul, J. F. (1978). Potentiation of neostigmine and pyridostigmine by 4-aminopyridine in the rat. *Journal of Pharmacy and Pharmacology*, **30**, 699–702.

Miller, R. D., Booij, L. H. D. J., Agoston, S., and Crul, J. F. (1979). 4-aminopyridine potentiates neostigmine and pyridostigmine in man. *Anesthesiology*, **50**, 416–20.

Mirakhur, R. K., Lavery, G. G., Clarke, R. S. J., Gibson, F. M., and McAtees, E. (1985). Atracurium in clinical anaesthesia: effect of dosage on onset, duration and conditions for tracheal intubation. *Anaesthesia*, **40**, 801–5.

Muir, A. W., Houston, J., Marshall, R. J., Bowman, W. C., and Marshall, I. G. (1989). A comparison of the neuromuscular blocking and autonomic effects of two new short-acting muscle relaxants with those of succinylcholine in the anesthetized cat and pig. *Anesthesiology*, **70**, 533–40.

Muir, A. W., Anderson, K., Marshall, R. J., Booij, L. H. D. J., Crul, J. F., Bowman, W. C., Marshall, I. G. (1991). The effects of a 16-*N*-homopiperidino analogue of vecuronium on neuromuscular transmission in anaesthetized cats, pigs, dogs and monkeys, and in isolated preparations. *Acta Anaesthesiologica Scandinavica*, **35**, 85–90.

Olivera, B. M., Gray, W. K., and Zeikus, R. (1985). Peptide neurotoxins from fish-hunting cone snails. *Science*, **230**, 1338–43.

Ostergaard, D., Jensen, F. S., Jensen, E., and Viby-Mogensen, J. (1989). Influence of plasma cholinesterase activity on recovery from mivacurium-induced neuromuscular blockade. *Acta Anaesthesiologica Scandinavica*, **33** (suppl 91), 165.

Paton, W. D. M. and Waud, D. R. (1962). Drug–receptor interactions at the neuromuscular junction. In *Curare and curare-like agents* (ed. A. V. S. DeReuck), pp. 34–47. Churchill, London.

Payne, J. P. and Hughes, R. (1981). Evaluation of atracurium in anaesthetized man. *British Journal of Anaesthesia*, **53**, 45–54.

Pittet, J. F., Taasonyi, E., Morel, D. R., Gemperle, G., Richter, M., and Rouge, J. C. (1989). Pipecuronium-induced neuromuscular blockade during nitrous oxide–fentanyl, isoflurane, and halothane anesthesia in adults and children. *Anesthesiology*, **71**, 210–13.

Pittet, J. F., Taasonyi, E., Morel, D. R., Gemperle, G., and Rouge, J. C. (1990). Neuromuscular effect of pipecuronium bromide in infants and children during nitrous oxide-alfentanil anesthesia. *Anesthesiology*, **72**, 432–5.

Quil, T. J., Begin, M., Glass, P. S. A., Ginsberg, B., and Gorback, M. S. (1991). Clinical responses to Org 9426 during isoflurane anesthesia. *Anesthesia and Analgesia*, **72**, 203–6.

Riker, W. F. and Okamoto, M. O. (1969). Pharmacology of motor nerve terminals. *Annual Review of Pharmacology*, **9**, 173–208.

Riker, W. F. and Standaert, F. G. (1966). The action of facilitatory drugs and acetylcholine on neuromuscular transmission. *Annals of New York Academy of Sciences*, **135**, 163–76.

Ritter, D. M., Rettke, S. R., Ilstrup, D. M., and Burritt, M. F. (1988). Effect of plasma cholinesterase activity on the duration of action of succinylcholine in patients with genotypically normal enzyme. *Anesthesia and Analgesia*, **67**, 1123–6.

Rodrigues, R. C., Kyubg, C., Caldwell, E., Sharma, M., Canfell, P. C., and Miller, R. D. (1989). Pharmacokinetics and the neuromuscular blocking effects of Org 991 in the cat. *Anesthesiology*, **71**, A775.

Rosow, C. E., Basta, S. J., Savarese, J. J., Ali, H. H., Kniffen, K. J., and Moss, J. (1980). BW785U: correlation of cardiovascular effects with increases in plasma histamine. *Anesthesiology*, **53**, S271.

Salmenpera, M. and Tammisto, T. (1980). The use of dioxonium as a neuromuscular blocking agent. *Acta Anaesthesia Scandinavica*, **24**, 395–8.

Sarner, J. B., Brandom, B. W., Cook, D. R., Dong, M. L., Horn, M. C., Woelfel, S. K., *et al.* (1988). Clinical pharmacology of doxacurium chloride (BW 938U) in children. *Anesthesia and Analgesia*, **67**, 303–6.

Savarese, J. J. and Kitz, R. J. (1975). Does clinical anesthesia need new neuromuscular blocking drugs? *Anesthesiology*, **42**, 236–9.

Savarese, J. J. and Wastila, W. B. (1979*a*). Pharmacology of BW985U: A short acting nondepolarizing neuromuscular blocking agent. *Anesthesiology*, **51**, S277.

Savarese, J. J. and Wastila, W. B. (1979*b*). BW444U: an intermediate-duration nondepolarizing blocking agent with significant lack of cardiovascular and autonomic effect. *Anesthesiology*, **51**, S279.

Savarese, J. J., Ginsberg, S., Lee, C. M., and Kitz, R. J. (1973). The pharmacology of new short-acting nondepolarizing ester neuromuscular blocking agents: clinical implications. *Anesthesia and Analgesia*, **52**, 982–8.

Savarese, J. J., Antoniom, R. P., and Ginsberg, S. (1975). Potential clinical uses of short-acting nondepolarizing neuromuscular-blocking agents as predicted from animal experiments. *Anesthesia and Analgesia*, **54**, 669–78.

Savarese, J. J., Ali, H. H., Basta, S. J., Ramsey, F. M., Rosow, C. E., Lebowitz, P. W., *et al.* (1980). Clinical neuromuscular pharmacology of BW785U, an ultra-short-acting nondepolarizing ester neuromuscular blocking agent. *Anesthesiology*, **53**, S274.

Savarese, J. J., Basta, S. J., Ali, H. H., Sunder, N., Gionfriddo, M., Goudsouzian, N. G., *et al.* (1981). Clinical neuromuscular pharmacology of BW444U. *Anesthesiology*, **55**, A197.

Savarese, J. J., Ali, H. H., Basta, S. J., Embree, P. B., Scott, R. P. F., Sunder, N., *et al.* (1988). The clinical neuromuscular pharmacology of mivacurium chloride (BW 1090U). *Anesthesiology*, **68**, 723–32.

Savarese, J. J., Ali, H. H., Basta, S. J., Scott, R. P. F., Embree, P. B., Wastila, W. B. *et al.* (1989). The cardiovascular effects of mivacurium chloride (BW B1090U) in patients receiving nitrous oxide–opiate–barbiturate anesthesia. *Anesthesiology*, **70**, 386–94.

Shanks, C. A. (1988). What's new in skeletal muscle relaxants and their antagonists? *Anesthesiology Clinics of North America*, **6**, 335–55.

Shanks, C. A., Fragen, R. J., Pemberton, D., Katz, J. A., and Rizner, M. E. (1989). Mivacurium induced neuromuscular blockade following single bolus doses and with continuous infusion during either balanced or enflurane anesthesia. *Anesthesiology*, **71**, 362–6.

Simpson, B. R., Savege, T. M., and Foley, E. T. (1972). An azobisarylimidazo-pyridinium derivative: A rapidly acting non-depolarizing muscle-relaxant. *Lancet*, **i**, 516–9.

Sobell, H. M., Sakore, T. D., and Tavale, S. S. (1972). Stereochemistry of curare alkaloid: 0,01, *N*-trimethyl-*d*-tubocurarine. *Proceedings of the National Academy of Sciences of the USA*, **69**, 2212–5.

Stoops, C. M., Curtis, C. A., Kovach, D. A., McCammon, R. L., Stoelting, R. K., Warren, T. M., *et al.* (1988). Hemodynamic effects of doxacurium chldoride in patients receiving oxygen sufentanil anesthesia for coronary arterey bypass grafting or valve replacement. *Anesthesiology*, **69**, 365–70.

Suri, Y. V. (1984). Chandonium iodide–new non-depolarizing muscle relaxant. In *Anesthesiology clinical pharmacology*, (ed. Y. V. Suri and D. Singh), pp. 28–35. Vani Educational Books, New Dehli.

Szenohradszky, J., Segredo, V., Caldwell, J. E., Sharma, M., Gruenke, L. D., and Miller, R. D. (1991). Pharmacokinetics, onset and duration of action of Org 9426 in humans: normal vs. absent renal function. *Anesthesia and Analgesia*, **72**, S290.

Tammisto, T. and Salmenpera, M. (1980). Neuromuscular blocking properties of dioxonium. *Acta Anesthesiologica Scandinavica* **24**, 439–43.

VanDam, L. D., Safar, P., and Dumke, P. R. (1953). A new antagonist to syncurine. *Anesthesia and Analgesia*, **32**, 113–22.

Van Linthout, L. E. H., Van Egmond, J., De Boo, T., Lerou, J. G. C., Wevers, R. A., and Booij, L. H. D. J. (1992). Factors affecting the magnitude and time course of neuromuscular block produced by suxamethonium. *British Journal of Anaesthesia* **69**, 29–35.

Vervloet, D. (1985). Allergy to muscle relaxants and related compounds. *Clinical Allergy*, **15**, 501–8.

Viby-Mogensen, J., Jorgensen, B. C., and Ording, H. (1979). Residual curarization in the recovery room. *Anesthesiology*, **50**, 539–41.

Wastila, W. B. and Savarese, J. J. (1979). Autonomic/neuromuscular dose-ratios and hemo-dynamic effects of BW785U), a short-acting nondepolarizing ester neuromuscular block-ing agent. *Anesthesiology*, **51**, S278.

Waud, B. E. and Waud, D. R. (1975). Physiology and pharmacology of neuromuscular blocking agents. In *Muscle relaxants. Monographs in anaesthesiology*, Vol. 3, (ed. R. L. Katz), pp. 1–58. North Holland, Amsterdam.

Wierda, J. M. K. H., Richardson, F. J., and Agoston, S. (1989). Dose response relation and time course of action of pipecuronium bromide in humans anesthetized with nitrous oxide and isoflurane, halothane, or droperidol/fentanyl. *Anesthesia and Analgesia*, **69**, 208–13.

Williams, N. E., Webb, S. N., and Calvey, T. N. (1980). Differential effects of myoneural blocking drugs on neuromuscular transmission. *British Journal of Anaesthesia*, **52**, 1111–4.

Wu, C. S. C., Sun, X. H., and Yang, J. T. (1990). Confirmation of acetylcholine receptor in the presence of agonists and antagonists. *Journal of Protein Chemistry*, **9**, 119–26.

18

Neuromuscular blocking agents in specific clinical situations

B. J. Pollard

The majority of patients are medically fit apart from the pathological process which has precipitated the admission for surgery. There is little reason to believe that the response of the patient to the neuromuscular blocking agent will not be exactly as predicted. There are a number of situations, however, where special precautions apply, or an abnormal response should be expected. Certain of these situations have been noted already in other sections. It is the purpose of this chapter to bring all of these together such that they can be more easily considered.

RENAL DISEASE

The kidneys represent the principal site for the removal of waste products, drugs, and their metabolities. The muscle relaxant drugs are all highly ionized and are therefore water soluble and would be expected to be freely filtered at the glomerulus. They will remain ionized at the pH of the glomerular filtrate and thus not be reabsorbed, but excreted in the urine. Those which undergo metabolic breakdown produce water-soluble compounds which are also excreted principally via the kidneys.

Protein binding does not greatly affect the renal elimination of the neuromuscular blocking agents because they are only about 20–50% protein bound. At least half of the relaxant molecules are therefore in the unbound form dissolved in plasma and freely filterable in the kidney (Hunter 1991).

The kidneys are not the only pathway for elimination of certain neuromuscular blocking agents. Many have more than one pathway of elimination and such agents would be suitable for use in patients with renal insufficiency. Renal failure is probably the principal cause of a prolongation of action of a number of the neuromuscular blocking agents, and this effect has been reported in several papers (Feldman and Levi 1963; Riordon and Gilbertson 1971; Morgan and Lumley 1975).

Established texts in the specialty show that caution used to be advised in all cases when a neuromuscular blocking agent was used in the presence of impaired renal function in view of the risk of recurarization. The delayed elimination of the neuromuscular blocking agent was thought to allow the reappearance of the block as the effect of the antagonist waned (Miller and Cullan 1976). It has, however, been shown that the anticholinesterases also rely upon the kidney to some extent for their elimination. Their duration of action is therefore also prolonged in renal failure, making recurarization unlikely (Cronnelly *et al.* 1979, 1980; Morris *et al.* 1981).

Alcuronium

There is very little information on the use of alcuronium in patients with renal failure. It has been used safely in patients with renal insufficiency but cannot be recommended. It is almost exclusively renally excreted and several reports exist of a prolonged duration of action in the presence of renal failure (Hofer *et al.* 1969; Raaflaub and Frey 1972; Cozanitis and Haapanen 1979; Smith *et al.* 1987). Alcuronium would seem, therefore, to be best avoided in patients with renal insufficiency.

Tubocurarine

There are a number of studies and reports which have examined the influence of renal failure on the action of tubocurarine. Most conclude that the duration of action is prolonged but there is not universal agreement about the extent of the prolongation (Hunter *et al.* 1984). Miller and Cullen (1976) reported that the elimination half-life of tubocurarine was increased from 232 minutes in normal patients to 330 minutes in renal failure patients. Riordon and Gilbertson (1971) described a patient with renal failure who exhibited a prolongation of action of tubocurarine, while Churchill-Davidson *et al.* (1967) found there to be no change in the duration of action in renal failure. Tubocurarine is a suitable drug, therefore, for patients with renal failure, provided that care is taken with its use.

Metocurine

Metocurine is more dependent upon renal excretion than is tubocurarine, despite their structural similarity. Its elimination half-life in patients with renal failure is longer than in patients with normal renal function (Meijer *et al.* 1979; Brotherton and Matteo 1981). Metocurine is therefore not a wise choice for use in the patient with renal failure.

Gallamine

Gallamine is metabolized to such a small extent that it relies almost exclusively on the kidney for its elimination and therefore for the termination of its effect (Feldman and Levi 1963; Agoston *et al.* 1978). Theoretically, its action would be expected to be prolonged almost indefinitely in the patient with absent renal function, although in practice, an increase in terminal half-life of about six times has been described (Ramzan *et al.* 1982). Gallamine may be removed from the plasma by either peritoneal dialysis (Lowenstein *et al.* 1970) or haemodialysis (Singer *et al.* 1971). Gallamine is generally regarded as being contraindicated in patients with impaired renal function.

Pancuronium

Pancuronium has been used in patients with impaired renal function without any apparent problems. A prolongation of the duration of action was, however, reported by d'Hollander *et al.* (1978) and by Miller *et al.* (1973). The elimination half-life is increased, due probably to a reduction in clearance to about half that of normal patients (McCloud *et al.* 1976; Buzello and Ruthven-Murray 1976; Somogyi *et al.* 1977*a*).

Atracurium

Atracurium is probably the most studied relaxant in renal failure patients. The studies have all demonstrated that there is no significant difference between the pharmacodynamics and pharmacokinetics of atracurium in renal failure when compared to patients with intact renal function (Hunter *et al.* 1982; Fahey *et al.* 1984; Lebrault *et al.* 1984; de Bros *et al.* 1986; Mongin-Long *et al.* 1986). The notable feature of atracurium which is responsible for these observations, and which sets it apart from all of the other neuromuscular blocking agents, is its spontaneous degradation (by the Hofmann elimination reaction) in the body to metabolites which are devoid of neuromuscular blocking activity.

There is one metabolite of atracurium, laudanosine, which can cause cerebral excitation in laboratory animals. In view of the fact that laudanosine is renally excreted, this metabolite has the potential to accumulate in renal failure and much debate has centred around the possibility of significant adverse effects resulting from the accumulation of laudanosine in renal failure. No adverse effects have, however, been conclusively attributed to laudanosine. The highest plasma concentration recorded so far was in excess of 8 μg/ml (Gwinnutt *et al.* 1989) and this was not associated with any adverse effects. The jury must therefore remain out on this issue, at least for the time being. Atracurium is presently regarded as the muscle relaxant of choice in the patient with compromised renal function.

Vecuronium

Vecuronium is renally excreted as the parent compound and is also fairly rapidly metabolized. It is actively taken up by various tissues of the body, which results in a large apparent volume of distribution. Although the effect of renal failure on vecuronium is only small, a gradual increase in duration of action is seen with repeated doses. This accumulation is presumably the result of the gradual saturation of peripheral storage sites (Bevan *et al.* 1984). Single doses of vecuronium or the use of a small number of incremental bolus doses for shorter duration surgery is safe in the anephric patient, although an increase in the duration of action of even a single dose can be detected in renal failure (Meistelman *et al.* 1983). Prolonged neuromuscular block may, however, result from the use of larger doses or from an infusion in a patient with severely impaired renal function (Slater *et al.* 1988; Segredo *et al.* 1990).

The possibility has been raised that the prolonged duration of action under these circumstances is the result of the accumulation of the 3-desacetyl metabolite rather than the parent compound (Segredo *et al.* 1990). Vecuronium would appear, therefore, to be a suitable drug for use in patients with renal failure for short duration procedures, provided that care is taken and neuromuscular transmission is monitored.

Mivacurium

Mivacurium is broken down in the blood by plasmacholinesterase to substances which are devoid of neuromuscular activity (Cook *et al.* 1989). The destruction of mivacurium will therefore be affected by any factor which interferes with either the activity or the quantity of plasma cholinesterase, including congenital atypical cholinesterase variants and anticholinesterase agents. One might, therefore, expect it not to be affected by renal impairment. The duration of action of mivacurium has, however, been shown to be slightly prolonged in the anephric patient (Phillips and Hunter 1992). The likely reason is the small decrease in plasma cholinesterase activity which is a common finding in renal failure. It would appear therefore that mivacurium is safe to use in renal failure patients, although a small prolongation of effect may be observed.

Pipecuronium

This long-acting relaxant is eliminated substantially unchanged by the kidney. A prolongation of effect might therefore be expected in renal failure and has indeed been observed (Caldwell *et al.* 1988, 1989).

Doxacurium

The elimination half-life of doxacurium is approximately 86 minutes (Dresner *et al.* 1990) and this is markedly increased in patients with renal disease (Cook *et al.* 1991). Cashman *et al.* (1990) found the time to 25% recovery of twitch height to be approximately doubled in the presence of renal failure.

Rocuronium

The majority of a dose of rocuronium is excreted into the bile and thus eliminated through the gut. It appears that less than 10% is secreted in the urine in the cat (Khunl-Brady *et al.* 1990) and only about 30% is excreted in the urine in the human

(Wierda *et al.* 1991). One might therefore expect that the duration of action of rocuronium would not be significantly altered in patients with renal failure and this has been borne out in practice. Rocuronium therefore seems to be a suitable relaxant to use in the renal failure patient. It is interesting to note that there is a close structural similarity between rocuronium and vecuronium, yet one appears to be suitable for use in renal failure and the other requires caution.

Suxamethonium

Suxamethonium may be used safely in the patient with renal failure, provided that its capacity to increase the plasma potassium is remembered. Patients with impaired renal function frequently have a raised plasma potassium and this should be checked by appropriate biochemical screening before surgery. The elimination of suxamethonium is the result of its hydrolysis by plasma cholinesterase and should therefore be principally independent of kidney function. It is not uncommon to observe a small reduction in plasma cholinesterase in renal failure patients (Phillips and Hunter 1992) which may led to a minor prolongation of the duration of action of suxamethonium. This is unlikely to be of clinical significance.

It appears, therefore, that at present the drug of choice for anaesthesia in patients with renal failure is atracurium. It is possible, however, that mivacurium and rocuronium may also achieve a place in the management of these patients in the future. It is wise always to monitor neuromuscular function in patients with renal failure whenever a neuromuscular blocking agent is used, whichever one is chosen.

LIVER DISEASE

The liver plays a central role in the metabolism and elimination of many drugs. The muscle relaxants, being water soluble polar compounds, do not usually require hepatic metabolism for their inactivation and removal. Liver metabolism does, however, take place with a number of the relaxants and if this impaired, then the duration of action of the relaxant may be prolonged. Some relaxants are actively taken up by the liver and decreased hepatic uptake will affect activity. Those relaxants which are excreted into the bile will have their plasma clearance reduced in the presence of cholestasis. Plasma volume and plasma proteins may also be changed and the pharmacokinetics of many of the relaxants will be altered in hepatic failure.

Tubocurarine

Resistance to tubocurarine has been reported in patients with liver failure (Dundee and Gray 1953; El-Hakim and Baraka 1963). The likely explanation would seem to be due to a change in the volume of distribution. The duration of action of tubocurarine is increased in patients with cholestasis, probably reflecting the pathway of excretion in the bile.

Pancuronium

Patients with chronic liver disease are resistant to pancuronium. There is an increase in elimination half-life associated with a decrease in plasma clearance and an increase in the volume of distribution (Nana *et al.* 1972; Ward *et al.* 1975; Duvaldestin *et al.* 1978*a*; Westra *et al.* 1981*a*). The liver uptake of pancuronium is reduced (Westra *et al.* 1981*b*) which results in a prolongation of the block, and if cholestasis is present the duration of action is also increased (Somogyi *et al.* 1977*b*). It is probable that the resistance due to pancuronium is not caused by an alteration in protein binding (Duvaldestin and Henzel 1982).

Vecuronium

Vecuronium is actively taken up by the liver (Upton *et al.* 1982; Bencini *et al.* 1985, 1986), which to some extent accounts for its brevity of action (Sohn *et al.* 1986). In view of this, any liver disorder which impairs the ability to take up vecuronium will lead to a significant prolongation of its action (Lebrault *et al.* 1985). The duration of action is also increased by cholestasis (Lebrault *et al.* 1986).

Atracurium

Atracurium appears to be the relaxant which is least affected by liver disease (Ward and Neill 1983; Cook *et al.* 1984; Gyasi and Naguib 1985). The pharmacokinetics, including elimination half-life, are unaffected by liver disease.

Suxamethonium

Plasma cholinesterase is synthesized in the liver. A decrease in the concentration of plasma cholinesterase in patients with liver disease would therefore be expected, which would result in an decrease in the rate of breakdown of suxamethonium and hence a prolongation of its action. In practice plasma cholinesterase is present in great excess and any effect on the rate of metabolism of suxamethonium is only small (McArdle 1940; Bowen 1960).

The newer relaxants

There is little information available on the effect of liver disease on the actions of pipecuronium, doxacurium, mivacurium, and rocuronium. The liver is important for the elimination of pipecuronium in the pig, so the action of pipecuronium is significantly prolonged in that animal. It is unlikely that this effect occurs in humans. Cook *et al.* (1991) suggested that the duration of action of doxacurium would be likely to be prolonged in patients with liver disease. Mivacurium relies upon plasma cholinesterase for its breakdown. Plasma cholinesterase is manufactured in the liver, and it would therefore seem highly probable that the duration of action of mivacurium would be longer in patients with liver failure. It is known that the liver is important in the termination of effect and metabolism of rocuronium. It would therefore be surprising if the duration of action of rocuronium was not extended in liver disease and this has indeed been demonstrated (Magorian *et al.* 1991).

MYOTONIAS

This group of muscle disorders includes myotonia dystrophica, myotonia congenita, and paramyotonia congenita. They are inherited conditions and present a number of problems for the anaesthetist, including cardiac abnormalities and an abnormal sensitivity to respiratory depressants. There are also abnormal responses to certain neuromuscular blocking agents.

The response to the nondepolarizing neuromuscular blocking agents is normal (Mitchell *et al.* 1978; Boheimer *et al.* 1985). A neuromuscular blocking agent will not, however, have any affect on a pre-existing myotonic spasm because such spasms are the result of a phenomenon distal to the neuromuscular junction. The response to anticholinesterases is unpredictable. A neuromuscular block may be inadequately reversed (Aldridge 1985) or the anticholinesterase itself may precipitate a myotonic episode (Buzello *et al.* 1982). It may therefore be advisable to use one of the shorter acting muscle relaxants and to await spontaneous recovery (Nightingale *et al.* 1985; Stirt *et al.* 1985). It is possible that mivacurium may be useful in these cases.

The response to suxamethonium is unpredictable. Suxamethonium is likely to precipitate a myotonic episode leading to severe tonic spasms (Talmage and McKechnie 1959; Kaufman 1960; Paterson 1962; Cody 1968; Aldridge 1985). These can last for several hours and may be very difficult to treat. A further dose of muscle relaxant will have no effect because the contractures are generated beyond the neuromuscular junction. In the meantime, the contractures will be unpleasant to the patient and may also be hazardous because respiration will be impaired. It is generally accepted that suxamethonium is contraindicated in patients with myotonia.

MALIGNANT HYPERPYREXIA

This is an inherited disorder of calcium flux in muscle fibres. The incidence in the general population is low, although it may appear to be surprisingly high in certain discrete areas due to the presence of affected families. It is of importance to anaesthetists because a number of the drugs used in anaesthesia are potent trigger agents. Once an episode has been triggered it may be very difficult to abort and has potentially serious consequences.

The nondepolarizing neuromuscular blocking agents appear to be safe. No hyperthermic crisis has ever been conclusively attributed to a nondepolarizing agent. The depolarizing agent suxamethonium is, however, probably the most potent triggering agent known. Suxamethonium therefore is absolutely contraindicated in known or suspected cases of malignant hyperpyrexia. The anticholinesterases should also be avoided in these patients and it is therefore wise to use one of the shorter-acting nondepolarizing neuromuscular blocking agents, e.g. mivacurium, and await spontaneous recovery.

MYASTHENIA

Myasthenia gravis is a disorder of the neuromuscular system. It usually presents in the second or third decade of life and affects females more often than males. There is a second smaller peak in incidence around about the sixth decade, when both sexes are equally affected. The aetiology is still not fully understood, but there appears to be an autoimmune component characterized by antibodies to the acetylcholine receptor at the neuromuscular junction (Bender *et al.* 1975; Drachman *et al.* 1976). Up to 80% of patients have abnormalities of the thymus gland and removal of that gland frequently improves symptoms.

The onset of myasthenia gravis is usually marked by a slowly developing weakness and fatigue, often affecting the ocular and pharyngeal muscles first. The symptoms and signs bear a close resemblance to what is seen in the patient who is partially paralysed with a subclinical dose of a nondepolarizing neuromuscular blocking agent. Relief of the symptoms is brought about by the administration of an anticholinesterase. It would therefore not be surprising to find an increased sensitivity to nondepolarizing neuromuscular blocking agents in patients with myasthenia gravis. Patients with myasthenia gravis are often also receiving therapy with steroids and immunosuppressants and drug interactions must also be considered (see Chapter 12).

In view of the increased sensitivity to nondepolarizing neuromuscular blocking agents, a much reduced dose is required. Both pancuronium (Blitt *et al.* 1975) and tubocurarine (Lake 1978) have been used successfully in low dosage. It is, however, advantageous to use a neuromuscular blocking agent with a short duration of action and which has negligible potential for accumulation or prolongation of effect. The two intermediate-acting agents atracurium and vecuronium have therefore become popular. Vecuronium has been reported to be a suitable agent (Hunter *et al.* 1985) although it has been noted that there may be delayed recovery (Buzello *et al.* 1986). Atracurium has received more attention and it is generally accepted at present that atracurium is the drug of choice given in reduced doses (Bell *et al.* 1984; Baraka and Dajani 1984; MacDonald *et al.* 1984; Ward and Wright 1984; Vacanti *et al.* 1985; Ramsey and Smith 1985; Pollard *et al.* 1989). Whichever drug is used it is important to monitor the neuromuscular block in myasthenic patients.

At the termination of surgery the administration of an anticholinesterase should antagonize the remaining action of the neuromuscular blocking agent and increase muscle power again. A short period of post-operative controlled ventilation is occasionally required.

It is interesting to speculate upon the possible use of the two newer nondepolarizing agents, mivacurium and rocuronium. The profile of rocuronium is very similar to that of vecuronium, except for its more rapid onset. It is likely, therefore, that it would behave in a similar fashion to vecuronium in the myasthenic patient. Mivacurium is the shortest acting nondepolarizing available at present and might therefore be expected to be of value in the myasthenic patient. It does, however, rely upon plasma cholinesterase for its metabolism, the activity of which will be reduced by the anticholinesterase agent present to treat the myasthenic symptoms. It is possible that the duration of action of mivacurium might be less easy to predict, although this has not so far been tested.

The myasthenic syndrome (Eaton–Lambert syndrome) has certain similarities to myasthenia gravis in being a disorder of the neuromuscular junction with weakness as a feature. In the myasthenic syndrome, however, exercise often reduces weakness rather than accentuating it and anticholinesterases generally have little effect. It is a disorder of the prejunctional region rather than of the postjunctional receptors. These patients are extremely sensitive to neuromuscular blocking agents. There is one report of 5 mg of tubocurarine lasting for 24 hours (Wise 1962) and it would seem wise to avoid neuromuscular blocking agents altogether in these patients if possible.

MUSCULAR DYSTROPHY

This heading includes a group of related neurological disorders which have a genetic basis. Muscular weakness and wasting are common findings. The patient's responses to the nondepolarizing neuromuscular blocking agents are generally unremarkable. A normal response can be expected (Cobham and Davies 1964; Richards 1972). The response to suxamethonium may, however, produce serious problems. Hypokalaemia, cardiac arrhythmias, muscular rigidity, rhabdomyolysis, myoglobinuria, and renal failure may result from the administration of suxamethonium and it should therefore be avoided (Genever 1971; Scay et al. 1978; Linter et al. 1982; Milne and Rosales 1982).

BURNS

Patients who suffer from burns or scalds demonstrate an abnormal response to neuromuscular blocking agents. The response to nondepolarizing agents is quite different from that to depolarizers. It would appear likely that these responses are the result of a change in the distribution of acetylcholine receptors together with an overall decrease in their sensitivity.

The nondepolarizing neuromuscular blocking agents

Burns patients exhibit an increased resistance to nondepolarizing agents. The more extensive the burn, the greater is this resistance and this has been demonstrated for tubocurarine (Martyn et al. 1980), pancuronium (Martyn et al. 1986), metocurine

(Martyn *et al.* 1982*a*, 1983), and atracurium (Dwersteg *et al.* 1986; Mills *et al.* 1986). The extent of this resistance can be considerable.

The effect begins approximately six days after the burn or scald and reaches a maximum between about two and six weeks. It then begins to decline but may still be present over a year later (Dwersteg *et al.* 1986; Martyn *et al.* 1982*a*). At its peak, doses of between 2.5 and 12 times normal may be required.

It is likely that this increased resistance is not the direct result of one mechanism. There is an alteration in protein binding which may result in a decrease in unbound drug in the plasma (Paifsky 1980; Leibel *et al.* 1981), although this would not be enough to account for the whole of the alteration in drug response. Alterations in pharmacokinetics may also be another factor in the equation (Martyn *et al.* 1982*b*). The most significant factor is probably secondary to an increase in the number of extrajunctional receptors combined with a decrease in the sensitivity of all acetylcholine receptors.

Suxamethonium

The depolarizing neuromuscular blocking agents will produce satisfactory relaxation in patients with burns. Their use is inadvisable, however, because the rise in plasma potassium which follows their administration is accentuated markedly (Tolmine *et al.* 1967). This acute increase in plasma potassium is related to the extent of the burn and will almost certainly be of such an extent that serious cardiac arrythmias will result. It is likely that the mechanism underlying the acute hyperkalaemia following the administration of a depolarizing agent to burns patients is also due to the extrajunctional spread of acetylcholine receptors (Gronert 1980).

OBSTETRICS

There is presently a trend away from general anaesthesia and towards spinal and epidural analgesia in obstetric practice. There will always, however, be a requirement for general anaesthesia in obstetrics, and there are a number of important considerations for which the reader is referred to any major textbook. It is appropriate to consider some aspects of this topic here, because a relaxant-intubation technique is necessary the majority of the time. A rapid sequence induction technique is required and so suxamethonium is the drug of choice at present for intubation. It will then be necessary to administer a nondepolarizing agent to continue the block in many cases. It must be remembered that magnesium sulphate and phenytoin are commonly used in obstetrics for the management of pre-eclampsia. Both of these interact quite markedly with the neuromuscular blocking agents (see Chapter 12).

Suxamethonium

The onset characteristics are identical to those individuals who are not pregnant. The duration of action may, however, be prolonged in some patients under certain conditions. Suxamethonium does not appear to have any direct effect on uterine muscle (Wiqvist and Wahlin 1962). It is interesting to note that the frequency of post-operative muscle pains following suxamethonium is less in pregnant patients than in the general population (Bryson and Ormstøn 1962; Crawford 1971; Datta *et al.* 1977).

There is a general decrease in the level of plasma cholinesterase during pregnancy such that activity has fallen to approximately 75% of normal by the second trimester. It may fall further in the immediate post-partum period before returning to normal by about two months post-partum (Hazel and Monier 1971; Leighton *et al.* 1986; Blitt *et al.* 1977). Plasma cholinesterase is, however, normally present in such great excess that the small reduction in the rate of breakdown of suxamethonium is not usually clinically detectable. Leighton *et al.* (1986) did observe a prolongation of recovery time in post-partum patients which they attributed partly to a reduction in the extra-cellular fluid volume as well as to the reduction in activity of plasma cholinesterase.

Suxamethonium carries two charged quaternary nitrogen centres and so would not be expected to cross biological membranes. There is good evidence, however, to show that it is capable of crossing the placenta (Krisselgaard and Moya 1961). This is of no significance if the neonate has genotypically normal plasma cholinesterase even though cholinesterase activity in the neonate is only about half of that in the adult. There is also unlikely to be any problem if mother, neonate or both are heterozygous for atypical plasma cholinesterase. If either is homozygous, then the neonate should exhibit no neuromuscular deficit. If both are homozygous, then both will remain paralysed for a prolonged time after delivery (Baraka *et al.* 1975).

The nondepolarizing agents

The nondepolarizing agents have been used in obstetric anaesthesia since their introduction and they have probably all been used at some time. Despite all being highly ionized polar molecules, they do cross the placenta to a greater or lesser extent and can be detected in the fetal circulation very shortly after their administration to the mother (Pittinger and Morris 1955; Duvaldestin *et al.* 1978*b*; Ho *et al.* 1981; Demetriou *et al.* 1982). The neonate is, however, unaffected by the usual clinical doses which cause full paralysis in the mother.

Tubocurarine, metocurine, alcuronium, and gallamine are not used to any great extent in obstetric anaesthesia, due principally to their unwanted side-effects rather than any problem specific to the pregnant mother or neonate. Pancuronium is safe and has proved to be popular. The intermediate-acting agents atracurium and vecuronium are also very popular, probably because of their greater cardiovascular stability.

NEUROANAESTHESIA

There are very few specific situations in neuroanaesthesia where a muscle relaxant is necessary for assisting surgical access. A neuromuscular blocking agent is commonly used however, for example, because the operations are lengthy, because tracheal intubation is necessary to secure the airway, and because coughing on a tracheal tube must be avoided. Although in many cases the choice of neuromuscular blocking agent is not important, there are a number of situations in neuroanaesthesia where it is of profound importance.

The patient with raised intracranial pressure is one such situation. It is clearly important to avoid any actions which might further increase the intracranial pressure, for example, hypercarbia, hypertension, and compression of the neck veins. The administration of an intubating dose of suxamethonium will also produce a rise in intracranial pressure (Halldin and Wahlin 1959) and this agent should therefore be avoided if possible. The rise in intracranial pressure is probably secondary to a rise in intra-abdominal pressure caused by the muscle fasciculations, which is transmitted to the central veins and thence to the cerebral venous system. It might also be related in part to an increase in brain activation due to an increased input from muscle proprioception feedback at the time of the fasciculations (Lanier *et al.* 1986).

In patients with a raised intracranial pressure, most anaesthetists would avoid suxamethonium and rely upon the use of a generous dose of a nondepolarizing agent. Pancuronium, vecuronium, and atracurium are presently popular in this respect. A problem arises when the patient requires a rapid sequence induction technique (which should include suxamethonium) in order to secure the airway as rapidly as possible. The other risks to the life of the patient must then be balanced against the risks of a potential rise in intracranial pressure and this can only be done by consideration of the circumstances of each individual patient. Precurarization with a small dose of a nondepolarizer will blunt the rise in intracranial pressure but will not completely prevent it (Minton *et al.* 1986).

The patient who has suffered a head injury must also be carefully assessed before a neuromuscular blocking agent is administered. The intracranial pressure may be raised, and so the considerations above will apply. The cervical spine must also be assessed. Great care must be taken when administering a neuromuscular blocking agent to a patient with an unstable cervical spine. The subsequent loss of muscle tone may allow the head to be moved into a potentially dangerous position with very serious long-term consequences. An awake fibreoptic intubation technique may be appropriate together with external fixation of the neck before a relaxant is considered.

The potential for drug interactions must also be remembered in neurosurgical patients. Many patients receive treatment with anticonvulsants or calcium antagonists and members of these families of drugs are known to modify the action of a neuromuscular blocking agent (Chapter 12). The technique of anaesthesia during neurosurgery includes moderate hyperventilation. Changes in acid–base balance also affect a neuromuscular block (Chapter 12).

CARDIOTHORACIC ANAESTHESIA

Good cardiostability is clearly of paramount importance in the choice of drugs for use in patients who are undergoing anaesthesia for cardiac surgery. The use of tubocurarine is commonly associated with hypotension and so it is not generally regarded as suitable for cardiac anaesthesia. The same problems may occur with metocurine and alcuronium, although to a lesser extent and these agents are also not used often. Pancuronium is popular because of its tendency to maintain the blood pressure and increase the heart rate. This effect balances the potential bradycardia which is a feature of high-dose narcotic techniques. Atracurium and vecuronium have become popular due to their stable cardiovascular profiles, although it is necessary to be on guard for a bradycardia which is a not uncommon occurrence with these drugs in the presence of high-dose narcotics. The relatively short duration of action of atracurium and vecuronium necessitates their administration by continuous infusion for best effect. The newer longer-acting nondepolarizing agents pipecuronium and doxacurium possess excellent cardiovascular stability and may prove to be more suitable for these long procedures. It is rarely necessary to perform a rapid sequence induction in these patients, but should suxamethonium be required there is no contraindication to its use.

When cardiopulmonary bypass is required, the haemodynamic changes which take place markedly affect a neuromuscular block (d'Hollander *et al.* 1983*a*). When the bypass circuit is connected into the patient's circulation, a sudden dilution of the blood volume takes place. The plasma concentration of the neuromuscular blocking agent will suddenly fall, with a rapid recovery of neuromuscular function. This can be prevented by adding a supplementary dose of neuromuscular blocker to the pump prime. Following the initial effect of haemodilution, there is a subsequent increase in the level of block. This is the result of an increase in the plasma concentration of neuromuscular blocking agent. This increase appears to be due to a reduction in the volume of distribution secondary to the reduction in blood flow to certain vital organs which actively take up these drugs, e.g. lungs and liver. A simultaneous reduction in renal blood flow will also reduce urinary elimination. Once stable on bypass, hypothermia may be required. An enhancement of the action of the neuromuscular blocking agents is seen as the temperature falls, reversing as rewarming occurs. Although this effect of hypothermia has been shown to be true for all of the neuromuscular blocking agents (Futter *et al.* 1983; Buzello *et al.* 1987; d'Hollander *et al.* 1983*a*), it is more marked for both atracurium and vecuronium (Flynn *et al.* 1984; Buzello *et al.* 1985).

AGE

When a drug effect is described, the implication is usually that the drug is being administered to adults unless otherwise qualified. Patients at either limit of age may, however, behave differently from adults. The response of the paediatric population are considered in Chapter 15. This section concerns the older age group.

With advancing age, a number of changes take place. There is a slow deterioration in function of most vital organs, the liver, kidneys, and neuromuscular junctions being most relevant to the actions of the neuromuscular blocking agents. Total body water also falls. This is accompanied by an overall increase in total body fat and reduction in lean body mass. The volume of distribution (real or apparent) for many of the neuromuscular blocking agents correspondingly falls. These changes have been observed and recorded for many of the neuromuscular blocking agents.

The reduced clearance, increased elimination half-life and reduction in distribution volume have been demonstrated to a certain extent for alcuronium (Stephens *et al.* 1984), tubocurarine (Matteo *et al.* 1985), metocurine (Matteo *et al.* 1985), pancuronium (Duvaldestin *et al.* 1982), and vecuronium (d'Hollander *et al.* 1982). The duration of action of each of these may therefore be expected to be prolonged in the elderly patient, although not always to such an extent that it is clinically important. A number of studies have created disagreements with respect to these general guidelines. Somogyi (1980), reported that the pharmacokinetics of pancuronium were unchanged in the older age groups and Rupp *et al.* (1983) reached a similar conclusion with respect to vecuronium. The only neuromuscular blocking agent which has consistently been reported to be unaffected by age is atracurium (d'Hollander *et al.* 1983*b*).

NEUROLOGICAL DISORDERS

There are a number of neurological disorders which may affect the responses to neuromuscular blocking agents and which have not been covered elsewhere. These conditions include motor paralysis as a result of intracranial pathology or poliomyelitis, cerebrovascular accident, disuse atrophy from immobilization, Parkinson's disease, and a number of other less common neurological conditions. Whether the origin is principally an upper motor neurone lesion, a lower motor neurone lesion, or a combination of the two, there are certain common factors.

The important consideration with respect to the neuromuscular blocking agents in these conditions is the response to suxamethonium. There are a number of reports of exaggerated side-effects with potentially serious consequences. Hyperkalaemia with associated serious cardiac arrythmias has been described following the use of suxamethonium in hemiplegic and paraplegic patients (Cooperman *et al.* 1970; Tobey 1970; Smith and Grenvik 1970; Stone *et al.* 1970). The principal at-risk time appears to be from about six days to six months, although outside this time window care should also be exercised. A similar hyperkalaemic response to suxamethonium may also be seen in patients with poliomyelitis (Beach *et al.* 1971), Parkinson's disease (Gravlee 1980), denervation (John *et al.* 1976), peripheral neuropathies (Gronert *et al.* 1973; Fergusson *et al.* 1981), and Friedreich's ataxia (Kume *et al.* 1976; Bell *et al.* 1986). Muscle contractures may also be seen in certain of these patients. The abnormal responses to depolarizing agents are probably secondary to the spread of acetylcholine receptors away from the junctional region (Dreyer and Peper 1974; Gronert and Theye 1975; Snider and Harris 1979). It is interesting to note that this effect may not be confined to the affected limb(s) (Waud *et al.* 1985; Shayevitz and Matteo 1985).

The responses to nondepolarizing agents may be variable. Hemiplegic patients demonstrate resistance to the nondepolarizing agents (Graham 1980; Moorthy and Hilgenberg 1980; Shayevitz and Matteo 1985), as do patients with an immobilized limb (Gronert 1981; Gronert et al. 1984). It is interesting to note that the contralateral limb will also demonstrate resistance despite being normally mobile or unaffected (Iwasaki et al. 1985; Shayevitz and Matteo 1985; Waud et al. 1985). Patients with degenerative diseases of the anterior horn cells of the spinal cord — e.g. poliomyelitis and amyotrophic lateral sclerosis — are not resistant, but sensitive to nondepolarizing agents (Rosenbaum et al. 1971; Brown and Charlton, 1975).

When a neuromuscular blocking agent is required in patients with any neurological disorder, it is wise to avoid the use of suxamethonium in view of the potential for serious exaggerated side-effects. A link between some neurological or muscular disorders and malignant hyperthermia has been suggested and it is also wise to avoid suxamethonium for this reason. The responses to nondepolarizing agents may be unpredictable and so the use of one of the intermediate- or shorter-acting agents is advisable. It is also recommended to monitor neuromuscular block in these patients, bearing in mind that such monitoring should be undertaken in a 'normal' limb if possible.

REFERENCES

Agoston, S., Vermeer, G. A., and Kersten-Kleef, U. W. (1978). A preliminary investigation of the renal and hepatic elimination of gallamine triethiodide in man. *British Journal of Anaesthesia*, **50**, 345–51.

Aldridge, L. M. (1985). Anaesthetic problems in myotonic dystrophy: a case report and review of the Aberdeen experience comprising 48 general anaesthetics in a further 16 patients. *British Journal of Anaesthesia*, **57**, 1119–30.

Baraka, A. and Dajani, A. (1984). Atracurium in myasthenics undergoing thymectomy. *Anesthesia and Analgesia*, **63**, 1127–30.

Baraka, A., Haroun, S., Bassilli, M., and Abu-Haider, G. (1975). Response of the newborn to succinylcholine injection in homozygotic atypical mothers. *Anesthesiology*, **43**, 115–6.

Beach, T. P., Stone, W. A., and Hamelberg, W. (1971). Circulatory collapse following succinylcholine: Report of a patient with diffuse lower motor neurone disease. *Anesthesia and Analgesia*, **50**, 431–7.

Bell, C. M., Florence, A. M., Hunter, J. M., Jones, R. S., and Utting, J. E. (1984). Atracurium in the myasthenic patient. *Anaesthesia*, **39**, 961–8.

Bell, C. F., Kelly, J. M., and Jones, R. S. (1986). Anaesthesia for Friedreich's ataxia: Case report and review of the literature. *Anaesthesia*, **41**, 296–301.

Bencini, A. F., Houwertjes, M. C., and Agoston, S. (1985). Effects of hepatic uptake of vecuronium bromide and its putative metabolites and their neuromuscular blocking actions in the cat. *British Journal of Anaesthesia*, **57**, 789–95.

Bencini, A. F., Scaf, A. H. J., Sohn, Y. J., Kersten, U. W., and Agoston, S. (1986). Hepatobiliary disposition of vecuronium bromide in man. *British Journal of Anaesthesia*, **58**, 988–95.

Bender, A. N., Ringel, S. P., Engel, W. K., Daniels, M. P., and Vogel, Z. (1975). Myasthenia gravis: A serum factor blocking acetylcholine receptors of the human neuromuscular junction. *Lancet*, **i**, 607–9.

Bevan, D. R., Donati, F., and Gyasi, H. (1984). Vecuronium in renal failure. *Canadian Anaesthetists' Society Journal*, **31**, 491–6.

Blitt, C. D., Wright, W. A., and Peat, J. (1975). Pancuronium and the patient with myasthenia gravis. *Anesthesiology*, **42**, 624–6.

Blitt, C. D., Petty, W. C., Alberternst, E. E., and Wright, B. J. (1977). Correlation of plasma cholinesterase activity and duration of action of succinylcholine during pregnancy. *Anesthesia and Analgesia*, **56**, 78–83.

Boheimer, N., Harris, J. W., and Ward, S. (1985). Neuromuscular block in dystrophica myotonica. *Anaesthesia*, **40**, 872–4.

Bowen, R. A. (1960). Anaesthesia in operations for the relief of portal hypertension. *Anaesthesia*, **15**, 3–10.

Brotherton, W. P. and Matteo, R. S. (1981). Pharmacokinetics and pharmocodynamics of metocurine in humans with and without renal failure. *Anesthesiology*, **55**, 272–6.

Brown, J. C. and Charlton, J. E. (1975). Study of sensitivity to curare in certain neurological disorders using a regional technique. *Journal of Neurology Neurosurgery and Psychiatry*, **38**, 34–54.

Bryson, T. H. L. and Ormston, T. O. G. (1962). Muscle pains following the use of suxamethonium in caesarian section. *British Journal of Anaesthesia*, **34**, 476–80.

Buzello, W., Kreig, N., and Schlickewei, A. (1982). Hazards of neostigmine in patients with neuromuscular disorders. *British Journal of Anaesthesia*, **54**, 529–34.

Buzello, W., and Ruthven-Murray, J. (1976). Der Konzentrationsverlauf von Pancuronium im serum anurischer Patienten. *Anaesthesist*, **25**, 440–3.

Buzello, W., Schluermann, D., Schindler, M., and Spillner, G. (1985). Hypothermic cardiopulmonary bypass and neuromuscular blockade by pancuronium and vecuronium. *Anesthesiology*, **62**, 201–4.

Buzello, W., Noeldge, G., Kreig, N., and Brobmann, G. F. (1986). Vecuronium for muscular relaxation in patients with myasthenia gravis. *Anesthesiology*, **64**, 507–9.

Buzello, W., Schluermann, D., Pollmaecher, T., and Spillner, G. (1987). Unequal effects of cardiopulmonary bypass-induced hypothermia on neuromuscular blockade from constant infusion of alcuronium, *d*-tubocurarine, pancuronium and vecuronium. *Anesthesiology*, **66**, 842–6.

Caldwell, J. E., Castagnoli, K. P., Canfell, P. C., Fahey, M. R., Lynam, D. P., Fisher, D. M., and Miller, R. D. (1988). Pipecuronium and pancuronium: comparison of pharmacokinetics and duration of action. *British Journal of Anaesthesia*, **61**, 693–7.

Caldwell, J. E., Canfell, P. C., Castagnoli, K. P., Lynam, D. P., Fahey, M. R., Fisher, D. M., and Miller, R. D. (1989). The influence of renal failure on the pharmacokinetics and duration of action of pipecuronium bromide in patients anesthetized with halothane and nitrous oxide. *Anesthesiology*, **70**, 7–12.

Cashman, J. N., Luke, J. J., and Jones, R. M. (1990). Neuromuscular block with doxacurium (BWA938U) in patients with normal or absent renal function. *British Journal of Anaesthesia*, **64**, 186–92.

Churchill-Davidson, H. C., Way, W. L., and de Jong, R. H. (1967). The muscle relaxants and renal excretion. *Anesthesiology*, **28**, 540.

Cobham, I. G. and Davies, H. S. (1964). Anesthesia for muscular dystrophy patients. *Anesthesia and Analgesia*, **43**, 22–9.

Cody, J. R. (1968). Muscle rigidity following administration of succinylcholine. *Anesthesiology*, **29**, 159–60.

Cook, D. R., Brandom, B. W., Stiller, R. L., Woelfer, S., Lair, A., and Slater, J. (1984). Pharmacokinetics of atracurium in normal and liver failure patients. *Anesthesiology*, **61**, A433.

Cook, D. R., Stiller, R. L., Weakly, J. N., Chakravorti, S., Brandom, B. W., and Welch, R. M. (1989). *In vitro* metabolism of mivacurium chloride (BW1090U) and succinylcholine. *Anesthesia and Analgesia*, **68**, 425–6.

Cook, D. R., Freeman, J. A., Lai, A. A., Robertson, K. A., Kang, Y., Stiller, R. L., *et al.* (1991). Pharmacokinetics and pharmacodynamics of doxacurium in normal patients and in those with hepatic or renal failure. *Anesthesia and Analgesia*, **72**, 145–50.

Cooperman, L. H., Strobel, G. E., and Kennell, E. M. (1970). Massive hyperkalaemia after administration of succinylcholine. *Anaethesiology*, **32**, 161–4.

Cozanitis, D. and Haapanen, E. (1979). Studies on muscle relaxants during haemodialysis. *Acta Anaesthesiologica Scandinavica*, **23**, 225–34.

Crawford, J. S. (1971). Suxamethonium muscle pains and pregnancy. *British Journal of Anaesthesia*, **43**, 677–80.

Cronelly, R., Stanski, D. R., and Miller, R. D. (1979). Renal function and the pharmacokinetics of neostigmine in anesthetized man. *Anesthesiology*, **51**, 222–6.

Cronelly, R., Stanski, D. R., Miller, R. D., and Sheiner, L. B. (1980). Pyridostigmine kinetics with and without renal function. *Clinical Pharmacology and Therapeutics*, **28**, 78–81.

d'Hollander, A. A., Camu, F. and Sanders, M. (1978). Comparative evaluation of neuromuscular blockade after pancuronium administration in patients with and without renal failure. *Acta Anaesthesiologica Scandinavica*, **22**, 21–6.

d'Hollander, A. A., Massaux, F., Nevelsteen, M., and Agoston, S. (1982). Age dependant dose–response relationships of ORG NC45 in anaesthetized patients. *British Journal of Anaesthesia*, **54**, 653–7.

d'Hollander, A. A., Duvaldestin, P., Henzel, D., Nevelsteen, M., and Bomblet, J. P. (1983*a*). Variations in pancuronium requirement, plasma concentration and urinary excretion induced by cardiopulmonary bypass and hypothermia. *Anesthesiology*, **58**, 505–9.

d'Hollander, A. A., Luyckx, C., Barvais, L., and de Ville, A. (1983*b*). Clinical evaluation of atracurium besylate requirement for a stable muscle relaxation during surgery: lack of age-related effects. *Anesthesiology*, **59**, 237–40.

Datta, S., Crocker, J. S., and Alper, M. H. (1977). Muscle pain following administration of suxamethonium to pregnant and non-pregnant patients undergoing laparoscopic tubal ligation. *British Journal of Anaesthesia*, **49**, 625–8.

de Bros, F., Lai, A., Scott, R. P. F., de Bros, J., Batson, G., Goudsouzian, N., Ali, H. H., Cosimi, A. B., and Savarese, J. J. (1986). Pharmacokinetics and pharmacodynamics of atracurium during isoflurane anesthesia in normal and anephric patients. *Anesthesia and Analgesia*, **65**, 743–6.

Demetriou, M., Depoix, J. P., Diakite, B., Fromentin, M., and Duvaldestin, P. (1982). Placental transfer of Org NC45 in women undergoing caesarian section. *British Journal of Anaesthesia*, **54**, 643–5.

Drachman, D. B., Kao, I., Pestronk, A., and Toyka, K. V. (1976). Myasthenia gravis as a receptor disorder. *Annals of the New York Academy of Sciences*, **274**, 226–34.

Dresner, D. L., Basta, S. J., Ali, H. H., Schwartz, A. F., Embree, P. B., Wargin, W. A., *et al.* (1990). Pharmacokinetics and pharmacodynamics of doxacurium in young and elderly patients during isoflurane anesthesia. *Anesthesia and Analgesia*, **71**, 498–502.

Dreyer, F. and Peper, K. (1974). The spread of acetylcholine sensitivity afeter denervation of frog skeletal muscle fibres. *Pflugers Archiv*, **348**, 287–92.

Dundee, J. W. and Gray, T. C. (1953). Resistance to *d*-tubocurarine chloride in the presence of liver damage. *Lancet*, **ii**, 16–8.

Duvaldestin, P. and Henzel, D. (1982). Binding of tubocurarine, fazadinium, pancuronium and ORG NC45 to serum protein in normal man and in patients with cirrhosis. *British Journal of Anaesthesia*, **54**, 513–6.

Duvaldestin, P., Agoston, S., Henzel, D., Kersten, U. W., and Desmonts, J. M. (1978*a*). Pancuronium pharmacokinetics in patients with liver cirrhosis. *British Journal of Anaesthesia*, **50**, 1131–6.

Duvaldestin, P., Demetriou, M., Henzel, D. and Desmonts, J. M. (1978*b*). The placental transfer of pancuronium and its pharmacokinetics during caesarian section. *Acta Anaesthesiologica Scandinavica*, **22**, 327–33.

Duvaldestin, P., Saada, J., Berger, J. L., d'Hollander, A. A. and Desmonts, J. M. (1982). Pharmacokinetics, pharmacodynamics and dose–response relationships of pancuronium in control and elderly subjects. *Anesthesiology*, **56**, 36–40.

Dwersteg, J. F., Pavlin, E. G., and Heinbach, D. M. (1986). Patients with burns are resistant to atracurium. *Anesthesiology*, **65**, 517–20.

El Hakim, M. and Baraka, A. (1963). *d*-Tubocurarine in liver disease. *Kasr-El-Aini Journal of Surgery*, **4**, 99–101.

Fahey, M. R., Rupp, S. M., Fisher, D. M., Miller, R. D., Sharma M., Canfell, C., *et al.* (1984). The pharmacokinetics and pharmacodynamics of atracurium in patients with and without renal failure. *Anesthesiology*, **61**, 699–702.

Feldman, S. A. and Levi, J. A. (1963). Prolonged paresis following gallamine. *British Journal of Anaesthesia*, **35**, 804–6.

Fergusson, R. J., Wright, D. J., Willey, R. F., Crompton, G. K., and Grant, I. W. (1981). Suxamethonium is dangerous in polyneuropathy. *British Medical Journal*, **282**, 298–9.

Flynn, P. J., Hughes, R., and Walton, B. (1984). Use of atracurium in cardiac surgery involving cardiopulmonary bypass with induced hypothermia. *British Journal of Anaesthesia*, **56**, 967–72.

Futter, M. E., Whalley, D. G., Wynands, J. E., and Bevan, D. R. (1983). Pancuronium requirements during hypothermic cardiopulmonary bypass in man. *Anaesthesia and Intensive Care*, **11**, 216–9.

Genever, E. E. (1971). Suxamethonium-induced cardiac arrest in unsuspected pseudohypertrophic muscular dystrophy. *British Journal of Anaesthesia*, **43**, 984–6.

Graham, D. H. (1980). Monitoring neuromuscular block may be unreliable in patients with upper motor neurone lesions. *Anesthesiology*, **52**, 74–5.

Gravlee, G. P. (1980). Succinylcholine induced hyperkalaemia in a patient with Parkinson's disease. *Anesthesia and Analgesia*, **59**, 444–6.

Gronert, G. A. (1980). A possible mechanism of succinylcholine induced hyperkalaemia. *Anesthesiology*, **53**, 356.

Gronert, G. A. (1981). Disuse atrophy with resistance to pancuronium. *Anesthesiology*, **55**, 547–9.

Gronert, G. A. and Theye, R. A. (1975). Pathophysiology of hyperkalaemia induced by succinylchlorine. *Anesthesiology*, **43**, 89–99.

Gronert, G. A., Lambert, E. H., and Theye, R. A. (1973). The response of denervated muscle to succinylcholine. *Anesthesiology*, **39**, 13–22.

Gronert, G. A., Matteo, R. S., and Perkins, S. (1984). Canine gastrocnemius disuse atrophy: Resistance to paralysis by dimethyltubocurarine. *Journal of Applied Physiology*, **57**, 1502–6.

Gwinnutt, C. L., Eddleston, J. M., Edwards, D., and Pollard, B. J. (1989). Concentrations of atracurium and laudanosine in cerebrospinal fluid and plasma in 3 intensive care patients. *British Journal of Anaesthesia*, **65**, 829–32.

Gyasi, H. K. and Naguib, M. (1985). Atracurium and severe hepatic disease: A case report. *Canadian Anaesthetists' Society Journal*, **32**, 161–4.

Halldin, M. and Wahlin, H. (1959) Effect of succinylcholine on intraspinal fluid pressure. *Acta Anaesthesiologica Scandinavica*, **38**, 155–61.

Hazel, B. and Monier, D. (1971) Human serum cholinesterase: variations during pregnancy and postpartum. *Canadian Anaesthetists' Society Journal*, **18**, 272–7.

Ho, P. C., Stephens, I. D., and Triggs, E. J. (1981). Caesarian section and placental transfer of alcuronium. *Anaesthesia and Intensive Care*, **9**, 113–9.

Hofer, R., Krenn, J., Pfeiffer, G., and Steinbereithner, K. (1969). Untersuchungenzer ausscheidung von Diallyl-nor-Toxiferin bei nierentransplantation. *Anaesthesist*, **18**, 304–8.

Hunter, J. M., Jones, R. S., and Utting, J. E. (1982). Use of atracurium in patients with no renal function. *British Journal of Anaesthesia*, **54**, 1251–8.

Hunter, J. M. (1991). Resistance to non-depolarizing neuromuscular blocking agents. *British Journal of Anaesthesia*, **67**, 511–4.

Hunter, J. M., Bell, C. F., Florence, A. M., Jones, R. S., and Utting, J. E. (1985). Vecuronium in the myasthenic patient. *Anaesthesia*, **40**, 848–53.

Hunter, J. M., and Jones, R. S., and Utting, J. E. (1984). Comparison of vecuronium, atracurium and tubocurarine in normal patients and in patients with no renal function. *British Journal of Anaesthesia*, **56**, 941–51.

Iwasaki, H., Namiki, A., Omote, K., Omote, T., and Takahashi, T. (1985). Response differences of paretic and healthy extremities to pancuronium and neostigmine in hemiplegic patients. *Anesthesia and Analgesia*, **64**, 864–6.

John, D. A., Tobey, R. E., Homer, L. D., and Rice, C. L., (1976). Onset of succinlycholine induced hyperkalaemia following denervation. *Anesthesiology*, **45**, 294–8.

Kaufman, L. (1960). Anaesthesia in dystrophica myotonica. *Proceedings of the Royal Society of Medicine*, **53**, 183–5.

Khunl-Brady, K., Castagnoli, K. P., Canfell, P. C., Caldwell, J. E., Agoston, S., and Miller, R. D. (1990). The neuromuscular blocking effects and pharmacokinetics of Org 9426 and Org 9616 in the cat. *Anesthesiology*, **72**, 669–74.

Krisselgaard, N. and Moya, F. (1961). Investigation of placental thresholds of succinylcholine. *Anesthesiology*, **22**, 7–10.

Kume, M., Sin, T., and Oyama, T. (1976). Anesthetic experience with a patient with Freidrich's ataxia: A case report. *Japanese Journal of Anesthesiology*, **25**, 877–80.

Lake, C. L. (1978). Curare sensitivity in steroid treated myasthenia gravis: A case report. *Anesthesia and Analgesia*, **57**, 132–4.

Lanier, W. L., Milde, J. H., and Michenfelder, J. D. (1986). Cerebral stimulation following succinylcholine in dogs. *Anesthesiology*, **64**, 551–9.

Lebrault, C., Lavaud, E., Strumza, P., Nebout, T., and Duvaldestin, P. (1984). Effet myorelaxant de l'atracurium chez les patients insuffisants renaux chroniques. *Annales Francais Anesthesie et Reanimation*

Lebrault, C., Berger, J. L., d'Hollander, A. A., Gomeni, R., Henzel, D., and Duvaldestine, P. (1985). Pharmacokinetics and pharmacodynamics of vecuronium (ORG NC45) in patients with cirrhosis. *Anesthesiology*, **62**, 601–5.

Lebrault, C., Duvaldestin, P., Henzel, D., Chauvin, M., and Guesnon, P. (1986). Pharmacokinetics and pharmacodynamics of vecuronium in patients with cholestasis. *British Journal of Anaesthesia*, **58**, 983–7.

Leighton, B. L., Cheek, T. G., Gross, J. B., Apfelbaum, J. L., Shantz, B. B., Gutsche, B. B., and Rosenberg, H. (1986). Succinylcholine pharmacodynamics in peripartum patients. *Anesthesiology*, **64**, 202–5.

Linter, S. P. K., Thomas, P. R., Withington, P. S., and Hall, G. M. (1982). Suxamethonium associated hypertonicity and cardiac arrest in suspected pseudohypertrophic muscular dystrophy. *British Journal of Anaesthesia*, **54**, 1331–2.

Leibel, W. S., Martyn, J. A. J., Szyfelbein, S. K., and Miller, K. W. (1981). Elevated plasma binding cannot account for burn related *d*-tubocurarine hyposensitivity. *Anesthesiology*, **54**, 378–82.

Lowenstein, E., Goldfine, C., and Flacke, W. E. (1970). Adminstration of gallamine in the presence of renal failure — reversal of neuromuscular blockade by peritoneal dialysis. *Anesthesiology*, **33**, 556–8.

Macdonald, A. M., Keen, R. I., and Pugh, N. D. (1984). Myasthenia gravis and atracurium. *British Journal of Anaesthesia*, **56**, 651–4.

Magorian, T., Wood, P., Caldwell, J. E., Szenohradszky, J. Segredo, V., Sharma, H., *et al.* (1991). Pharmacokinetics, onset and duration of action of rocuronium in humans: normal vs hepatic dysfunction. *Anesthesiology*, **75**, A1069.

Martyn, J. A. J., Szyfelbein, S. K., Ali, H. H., Matteo, R. S., and Savarese, J. J. (1980). Increased *d*-tubocurarine requirement following major thermal injury. *Anesthesiology*, **52**, 352–5.

Martyn, J. A. J., Matteo, R. S., Szyfelbein, S. K., and Kaplan, R. F. (1982*a*). Unprecedented resistance to neuromuscular blocking effects of metocurine with persistance after complete recovery in a burned patient. *Anesthesia and Analgesia*, **61**, 614–7.

Martyn, J. A. J., Matteo, R. S., Greenblatt, D. J., Lebowitz, P. W., and Savarese, J. J. (1982*b*). Pharmacokinetics of *d*-tubocurarine in patients with thermal injury. *Anesthesia and Analgesia*, **61**, 241–6.

Martyn, J. A. J., Goudsouzian, N. G., Matteo, R. S., Liu, L. M., Szyfelbein, S. K., and Kaplan, R. F. (1983), Metocurine requirements and plasma concentrations in burned paediatric patients. *British Journal of Anaesthesia*, **55**, 263–8.

Martyn, J. A. J., Goldhill, D. R., and Goudsouzian, N. G. (1986). Clinical pharmacology of muscle relaxants in patients with burns. *Journal of Clinical Pharmacology*, **26**, 680–5.

Matteo, R. S., Backus, W. W., McDaniel, D. D., Brotherton, W. P., Abraham, R., and Diaz, J. (1985). Pharmacokinetics and pharmacodynamics of *d*-tubocurarine in the elderly. *Anesthesia and Analgesia*, **64**, 23–9.

McArdle, R. (1940). The serum cholinesterase in jaundice and diseases of the liver. *Quarterly Journal of Medicine*, **9**, 107–27.

McCloud, K., Watson, M. J., and Rawlins, M. D. (1976). Pharmacokinetics of pancuronium in patients with normal and impaired renal function. *British Journal of Anaesthesia*, **48**, 341–5.

Meijer, D. K. F., Weitering, J. G., Vermeer, A., and Scaf, A. H. J. (1979). Comparative pharmacokinetics of *d*-tubocurarine and metocurine in man. *Anesthesiology*, **51**, 402–7.

Meistelman, C., Lienhart, D., Leveque, C., Bitker, M. O., Pigot, B., and Viars, P. (1983). Pharmacology of vecuronium in patients with end stage renal failure. *Anesthesiology*, **59**, A293.

Miler, R. D. and Cullen, D. J. (1976). Renal failure and postoperative respiratory failure: Recurarization? *British Journal of Anaesthesia*, **48**, 253–6.

Miller, R. D., Stephens, W. C. and Way, W. L. (1973). The effect of renal failure and hyperkalaemia on the duration of pancuronium neuromuscular blockade in man. *Anesthesia and Analgesia*, **52**, 661– 6.

Miller, R. D., Matteo, R. D., Bennet, L. Z., and Sohn, Y. J. (1977). The pharmacokinetics of *d*-tubocurarine in man with and without renal failure. *Journal of Pharmacology and Esperimental Therapeutics*, **202**, 1–7.

Mills, A., Schriefer, T., and Martyn, J. A. J. (1986). Electromyographic studies of patients with thermal injury. *Anesthesiology*, **65**, A294.

Milne, B. and Rosales, J. K. (1982). Anaesthetic considerations in patients with muscular dystrophy undergoing spinal fusion and Harrington rod insertion. *Canadian Anaesthetists Society Journal*, **29**, 250–4.

Minton, M. D., Grosslight, K., Stirt, J. A., and Bedford, R. F. (1986). Increases in intracranial pressure from succinylcholine: Prevention by prior nondepolarizing blockade. *Anesthesiology*, **65**, 165–9.

Mitchell, M. M., Ali, H. H., and Savarese, J. J. (1978). Myotonia and neuromuscular blocking agents. *Anesthesiology*, **49**, 44–8.

Moorthy, S. S. and Hilgenberg, J. C. (1980). Resistance to nondepolarizing muscle relaxants in paretic upper extremities of patients with residual hemiplegia. *Anesthesia and Analgesia*, **59**, 624–7.

Morgan, M. and Lumley, J. (1975). Anaesthetic considerations in chronic renal failure. *Anaesthesia and Intensive Care*, **3**, 218–25.

Mongin-Long, D., Chabrol, B., Baude, C., Ville, D., Renaudie, M., Dubernaud, J. M., and Moskovtchenko, J. F. (1986). Atracurium in patients with renal failure. *British Journal of Anaesthesia*, **58**, 44S.

Morris, R. B., Cronnelly, R., and Miller, R. D. (1981). Pharmacokinetics of edrophonium in anephric and renal transplant patients. *British Journal of Anaesthesia*, **53**, 131–4.

Nana, A., Cardan, E., and Leitersdorfer, T. (1972). Pancuronium bromide: Its use in asthmatics and patients with liver disease. *Anaesthesia*, **27**, 154–8.

Nightingale, P., Healy, T. E. J., and McGuinness, K. (1985). Dystrophica myotonica and atracurium. *British Journal of Anaesthesia*, **57**, 1131–5.

Paterson, I. S. (1962). Generalised myotonia following suxamethonium. *British Journal of Anaesthesia*, **34**, 340–2.

Phillips. B. J., and Hunter, J. M. (1992). Use of mivacurium chloride by constant infusion in the anephric patient. *British Journal of Anaesthesia*, **68**, 492–8.

Piafsky, K. M. (1980). Disease induced changes in plasma binding of basic drugs. *Clinics in Pharmacokinetics*, **5**, 246–62.

Pittinger, C. B. and Morris, L. E. (1955). Observations of the placental transmission of gallamine triethiodide (Flaxedil), succinylcholine chloride (Anectine) and decamethonium bromide (Syncurine) in dogs. *Anesthesia and Analgesia*, **34**, 107–11.

Pollard, B. J., Harper, N. J. N., and Doran, B. R. H. (1989). Use of continuous prolonged administration of atracurium in the ITU management of a patient with myasthenia gravis. *British Journal of Anaesthesia*, **62**, 95–7.

Raaflaub, J. and Frey, P. (1972). Zur Pharmacokinetik von Diallylnortoxiferin beim Menschen. *Arzneimittel Forschung*, **22**, 73–8.

Ramsey, F. M. and Smith, G. D. (1985). Clinical use of atracurim in myasthenia gravis: A case report. *Canadian Anaesthetists Society Journal*, **32**, 642–5.

Ramzan, M. I., Shanks, C. A., and Triggs, E. J. (1981). Gallamine disposition in surgical patients with chronic renal failure. *British Journal of Clinical Pharmacology*, **12**, 141–7.

Riordan, D. D. and Gilbertson, A. A. (1971). Prolonged curarization in a patient with renal failure. *British Journal of Anaesthesia*, **43**, 506–8.

Richards, W. C. (1972). Anaesthesia and serum creatinine phosphokinase levels in patients with Duchenne's pseudohypertrophic muscular dystrophy *Anaesthesia and Intensive Care*, **1**, 150–3.

Rosenbaum, K. J., Neigh, J. L., and Stobell, G. E. (1971). Sensitivity to non-depolarizing muscle relaxants in amyotrophic lateral sclerosis. *Anesthesiology*, **35**, 638–41.

Rupp, S. M., Fisher, D. M., Miller, R. D., and Castagnoli, K. (1983). Pharmacokinetics and pharmacodynamics of vecuronium in the elderly. *Anesthesiology*, **59**, A270.

Scay, A. R., Ziter, F. A., and Thompson, J. A. (1978). Cardiac arrest during induction of anaesthesia in Duchenne muscular dystrophy. *Journal of Pediatrics*, **93**, 88–90.

Segredo, V., Matthay, M. A., Sharma, M. L., Gruenke, C. D., Caldnutt, J. E., and Miller, R. D. (1990). Prolonged neuromuscular blockade after long-term administration of vecuronium in two critically ill patients. *Anesthesiology*, **72**, 566–70.

Slater, R. M., Pollard, B. J., and Doran, B. R. H. (1988). Prolonged neuromuscular blockade with vecuronium in renal failure. *Anaesthesia*, **43**, 250–1.

Shayevitz, J. R. and Matteo, R. S. (1985). Decreased sensitivity to metocurine in patients with upper motor neurone disease. *Anesthesia and Analgesia*, **64**, 767–72.

Singer, M. M., Dutton, R., and Way, W. L. (1971). Untoward results of gallamine administration during bilateral nephrectomy: treatment with haemodialysis. *British Journal of Anaesthesia*, **53**, 404–5.

Smith, R. B. and Grenvik, A. (1970). Cardiac arrest following succinlycholine in patients with central nervous system injuries. *Anesthesiology*, **33**, 558–60.

Smith, C. L., Hunter, J. M., and Jones, R. S. (1987). Prolonged paralysis following an infusion of alcuronium in a patient with renal dysfunction. *Anaesthesia*, **42**, 522–5.

Snider, W. D. and Harris, G. L. (1979). A physiological correlates of disuse-induced sprouting at the neuromuscular junction. *Nature*, **281**, 69–71.

Sohn, Y. J., Bencini, A. F., Scaf, A. H. J., Kersten, U. W., and Agoston, S. (1986). Comparative pharmacokinetics and dynamics of vecuronium and pancuronium in anesthetized patients. *Anesthesia and Analgesia*, **65**, 233–9.

Somogyi, A. A. (1980). Pancuronium plasma clearance and age. *British Journal of Anaesthesia*, **52**, 360.

Somogyi, A. A., Shanks, C. A., and Triggs, E. J. (1977a). The effect of renal failure on the disposition and neuromuscular blocking action of pancuronium bromide. *European Journal of Clinical Pharmacology*, **12**, 23–29.

Somogyi, A. A., Shanks, C. A., and Triggs, E. J. (1977b). Disposition kinetics of pancuronium bromide in patients with total biliary obstruction. *British Journal of Anaesthesia*, **49**, 1103–8.

Stephens, I. D., Ho, P. C., Holloway, A. M., Bourne, D. W., and Triggs, E. J. (1984). Pharmacokinetics of alcuronium in elderly patients undergoing total hip replacement or aortic reconstructive surgery. *British Journal of Anaesthesia*, **56**, 465–71.

Stirt, J. A., Stone, D. J., Weinberg, G., Wilson, D. F., Sterreck, C. S., and Sussman, M. D. (1975). Atracurium in a child with myotonic dystrophy. *Anesthesia and Analgesia*, **64**, 369–70.

Stone, W. A., Beach, T. P., and Hamelberg, G. W. (1970). Succinylcholine: Danger in the spinal cord injured patient. *Anesthesiology*, **32**, 168–9.

Talmage, E. A. and McKechnie, F. B. (1959). Anesthetic management of patients with myotonia dystrophica. *Anesthesiology*, **20**, 717–9.

Tobey, R. E. (1970). Paraplegia, succinylcholine and cardiac arrest. *Anesthesiology*, **32**, 359–64.

Tolmine, J. D., Joyce, T. H., and Mitchell, G. D. (1967). Succinylcholine danger in the burned patient. *Anesthesiology*, **28**, 467 70.

Upton, R. A., Nguyen, T. L., Miller, R. D., and Castagnoli, N., Jr (1982). Renal and biliary elimination of vecuronium (ORG NC45) and pancuronium in rats. *Anesthesia and Analgesia*, **61**, 313–6.

Vacanti, C. A., Ali, H. H., Schweiss, J. F., and Scott, R. P. F. (1985). The response of myasthenia gravis to atracurium. *Anesthesiology*, **62**, 692–4.

Ward, M. E., Adu-Gyamfi, Y., and Strunin, L. (1975). Althesin and pancuronium in chronic liver disease. *British Journal of Anaesthesia*, **47**, 1199–204.

Ward, S. and Wright, D. J. (1984) Neuromuscular blockade in myasthenia gravis with atracurium besylate. *Anaesthesia*, **39**, 51–3.

Ward, S. and Neill, E. A. M. (1983). Pharmacokinetics of atracurium in acute hepatic failure (with acute renal failure). *British Journal of Anaesthesia*, **55**, 1169–72.

Waud, B. E., Amaki, Y. and Waud, D. R. (1985). Disuse and *d*-tubocurarine-induced sensitivity in isolated muscles. *Anesthesia and Analgesia*, **64**, 1178–82.

Westra, P., Vermeer, G. A., de Lange, A. R., Scaf, A. H., Meijer, D. K., and Wesseling, H. (1981*a*). Hepatic and renal disposition of pancuronium and gallamine in patients with extrahepatic cholestasis. *British Journal of Anaesthesia*, **53**, 331–8.

Westra, P, Keulemans, G. T. P., Houwertjes, M. C., Hardonk, M. J., and Meijer, D. K. (1981*b*). Mechanism underlying the prolonged duration of action of muscle relaxants caused by extrahepatic cholestasis. *British Journal of Anaesthesia*, **53**, 217–26.

Wierda, J. M. K. H., Kersten-Kleef, U. W., Lambalk, L. M., Kloppenburg, W. D., and Agoston, S. (1991). The pharmacodynamics and pharmacokinetics of Org 9426, a new nondepolarizing neuromuscular blocking agent in patients anaesthetized with nitrous oxide and halothane. *Canadian Journal of Anaesthesia*, **38**, 430–5.

Wiqvist, N. and Wahlin, A. (1962). Effect of succinlycholine on uterine motility. *Acta Anaesthesiologica Scandinavica*, **6**, 71–5.

Wise, R. P. (1962). A myasthenic syndrome complicating bronchial carcinoma. *Anaesthesia*, **17**, 488–504.

19

Species differences in response to relaxants

R. S. Jones

During the search for any new muscle relaxant, the compounds are tested in a variety of species of animals. It is often at this stage that different responses in the variety of species are noted, particularly in relation to the duration of action and the cardiovascular effects of any particular compound.

The use of relaxants was first described in animals. A century or more ago, they were used for killing several species for food. The great advantage of the technique was that no residues were present in the carcass which could be toxic to the people who ate the animals. In addition, muscle relaxants were also administered to animals as an aid to the study of their anatomy.

The first recorded administration of curare to animals was by Sir Benjamin Brody, and he was also the first person to demonstrate that artificial respiration could maintain life in the curarized animal (Holmes 1898).

The first recorded person to bring curare to Europe from South America was Charles Waterton (1825). He performed the famous experiment on an ass following his return to England. The ass could be kept alive for four hours, until the effects of the drug wore off, by regularly inflating the lungs with bellows inserted into a tracheal incision. The animal survived and grew fat and lively thereafter. Youatt (1838), who had obtained supplies of the crude curare from Waterton, described attempts to treat rabies in dogs. The following year (Youatt 1839) he described the use of the drug in the treatment of tetanus in a horse.

In 1850 Claude Bernard in his classic experiments showed that curare acted by paralysing the myoneural junction (Bernard 1851). He sounded a warning at that time which is still as important today as it was then. This was in relation to the use of paralysis as a substitute for adequate anaesthesia:

Within the motionless body behind the staring eye, with all the appearance of death–feeling and intelligence persist in all their force. Can we conceive of a suffering more horrible than that of intelligence present after the succumbing one by one of all the organs which are destined to find themselves imprisoned alive within a cadaver? (Smithcors. 1971).

Griffith and Johnson (1942) are credited with the first description of the use of curare to produce relaxation during surgery in humans. Gray and Halton (1946) administered the drug in human anaesthesia in Liverpool in 1943. It was not until eight years later, however, that the first clinical attempts to use curare in the form of the pure preparation (Introcostrin) in dogs were described by Pickett (1951).

There were three reasons why the results were unimpressive. Firstly, the preparation was crude; secondly, it was not appreciated that the compound caused histamine release in dogs; and thirdly the dogs were allowed to breathe spontaneously. The first report of the use of the muscle relaxant suxamethonium accompanied by intermittent positive pressure ventilation in dogs was by Hall (1952). Two years later, the concept of balanced anaesthesia was discussed and the use of the nondepolarizing muscle relaxant gallamine together with intermittent positive ventilation was described (Hall and Weaver 1954).

PHARMACOLOGY OF THE MUSCLE RELAXANT DRUGS

Depolarizing muscle relaxants

For the purposes of this discussion suxamethonium and decamethonium can be taken together. It was shown that both drugs interrupted neuromuscular transmission in humans by long-lasting depolarization. Stimulation associated with fasciculation preceded the onset of the block and action potential records showed that these effects were the result of repetitive firing of the muscle fibres. Anticholinesterase drugs were ineffective in reversing the block and tubocurarine administration reduced the action of both drugs (Zaimis and Head 1976). It was, however, somewhat fortuitous that the early workers had chosen the cat as their experimental animal, as it is the species which most closely resembles man in its response to depolarizing muscle relaxants.

It was also demonstrated that the administration of these drugs would cause a release of potassium from muscle which was sufficient to produce a rise in the plasma potassium concentration. This was shown in humans (Mazze et al. 1969), cats (Paton 1956), and dogs (Stevenson 1960a). Stevenson (1960b) also demonstrated that the rise in serum potassium was not abolished by adrenalectomy, ganglionic block, adrenolytic drugs, or high epidural block and was therefore likely to be due to potassium release from muscle.

It is interesting to reflect that whereas the overall response to the nondepolarizing muscle relaxants is similar throughout the mammalian species, this is not true for the depolarizing drugs. It was demonstrated by Bovet et al. (1951) that decamethonium block in the rabbit could be antagonized by eserine. Jarcho et al. (1951) showed that, in normally innervated rat muscle, decamethonium appeared to act in some ways like acetylcholine, in others, like curare. Similar findings were reported in the dog by Philippot and Dallemagne (1952). It was later shown that, in the monkey, dog, rabbit, and hare (Zaimis 1953) and guinea-pig (Hall and Parkes 1953), the depolarizing relaxants initially exhibit a depolarizing action but during the blocking process their action changes into that resembling a substance competing with acetylcholine. This was first referred to as a 'dual' block by Zaimis (1953). Bowman (1962) also demonstrated dual block in the ferret.

The concept of the dual block demonstrated by Zaimis (1953) arose during her study of the effects of tridecamethonium in chicks. Tubocurarine produces a flaccid paralysis in birds, and the depolarizing drugs produce a contracture characterized by extension of the limbs and retraction of the head. When tridecamethonium was administered, however, a completely different situation was observed. Initially a slow contracture appeared, then, whilst the legs were extended, the head drooped forward in paralysis. This paralysis then extended to the leg muscles and the whole bird became flaccid. This would suggest that tridecamethonium produced an initial depolarization but changed during the blocking process to a competitive inhibitor. The effect of the drug on the tibialis muscle of the cat was similar to that in the monkey, dog, and hare tibialis caused by suxamethonium and decamethonium. Thus it appeared that the muscles of different species have differing responses and that the action of the quaternary molecules is determined by their structure and by the properties of the muscles on which they act.

Rat skeletal muscle has been shown to be particularly insensitive to depolarization by suxamethonium and decamethonium (Derkx *et al.* 1971). They also demonstrated that endplate depolarization is not the cause of the interruption of neuromuscular transmission. In addition they demonstrated that, whilst neostigmine will potentiate the action of suxamethonium in the dog, it antagonizes the block in the rat. Iveson *et al.* (1969) suggested that suxamethonium block in rats is due only to competition with acetylcholine and has none of the normal characteristics of a depolarization block. Similar results were obtained with decamethonium by Humphrey (1973).

It was also shown that a single drug may produce different types of neuromuscular block in different skeletal muscles of a particular animal. In the cat, the red muscles, as exemplified by the soleus, are slow-contracting and the white muscles, as exemplified by the tibialis, are fast-contracting. In the tibialis decamethonium produces a typical depolarization, while the soleus block has all the characteristics of a dual block. In the intact dog while recording mechanical responses of the fore limb to ulnar nerve stimulation, Cullen and Jones (1980*a*) noted the development of phase II (dual) block and tachyphylaxis to suxamethonium. There did not appear, however, to be any connection between the development of tachyphylaxis and dual block in the dog. They demonstrated that when a dose of 0.3 mg/kg of suxamethonium was administered intravenously to a dog dual block began to develop after a single dose but was not fully developed until the third or fourth dose. With the onset of the dual block a more prolonged return of neuromuscular activity could be expected, but when it was fully developed it could be reversed by anticholinesterase drugs.

It had already been shown in earlier experiments that when neostigmine was administered prior to the administration of suxamethonium the duration of suxamethonium block was increased by 100 per cent (Jones *et al.* 1980).

Avian muscle would appear to respond differently from mammalian muscle to the administration of muscle relaxants. Whereas tubocurarine produces a flaccid paralysis in chicks and adult fowl, decamethonium and suxamethonium produce a rigid extension of the limbs and retraction of the head in a similar manner to acetylcholine. If the dose is small an abrupt recovery will occur but if it is large the bird dies in contracture and never shows a flaccid paralysis. It was suggested by Buttle and Zaimis (1949) that avian muscle might be used to differentiate a true curare-like action from that of drugs which produce a prolonged depolarization. This 'chicktest' is still used in pharmocology.

There are extremely wide differences between species of domestic animals in their sensitivity and hence their response to suxamethonium. Horses, cats, and pigs are relatively resistant but dogs, sheep, and cattle are paralysed by relatively small doses. Suxamethonium is hydrolysed by cholinesterase in a similar manner to acetylcholine and it is suggested that this hydrolysis is responsible for recovery from the effects of the drug (Hall and Clarke 1991).

The pseudocholinesterase concentration in the serum of the horse and pig is about half that in the human. The pseudocholinesterase concentration in dog serum is about one quarter that in the human but the level of true cholinesterase in the red blood cells is only about one-seventh of the human level. It is suggested that the correlation between the higher sensitivity and the lower true cholinesterase is likely to influence the duration of suxamethonium apnoea in the dog. When the serum level of pseudocholinesterase was raised it produced a marked resistance to suxamethonium (Hall *et al.* 1953). In view of this information, attempts have been made to correlate the sensitivity of an animal to suxamethonium with the concentration of blood cholinesterase. The use of a test involving the ability of plasma cholinesterase to hydrolyse butyrylthiocholine, which is used to predict suxamethonium sensitivity in humans, has been shown to be of no practical use in animals (Hansson 1957*a*). It would appear that the affinities of cholinesterase for different substrates vary between species, and whereas the hydrolysis of the various substrates parallels that of suxamethonium in humans this is not the case in other animal species. Therefore it is essential to use only suxamethonium as the substrate for assay. Whilst the atypical forms of pseudocholinesterase and its inheritance has been well documented in humans, their significance and inheritance has not been studied in animals.

The dose of suxamethonium which is used in horses tends to vary with the state of anaesthesia. In the anaesthetized horse a dose of 100 μg/kg is used to produce paralysis for up to five minutes (Jones 1991). When the drug was used in the conscious horse for casting, however, a dose of 150 μg/kg was suggested (Hansson 1957*b*). This latter practice is now considered to be totally inhumane and is not recommeded. In cattle and sheep, a much lower dose of 20 μg/kg is recommended. In pigs, a much larger dose of 2 mg/kg is required. In dogs 300 μg/kg and in cats 1.5 mg/kg are the recommended doses (Jones 1991). This relatively small dose in the dog will, however, produce apnoea for some 25–30 minutes (Jones *et al.* 1978).

Non-depolarizing muscle relaxants

In general, the response to nondepolarizing muscle relaxants is much more uniform in mammalian species than that to the depolarizing drugs. The potency of the other drugs has been compared with that of tubocurarine (Maclagan 1976). The potency does not vary significantly between species. In the cat, dog, and human both alcuronium and pancuronium are much more potent than tubocurarine.

There is considerable species variation in the duration of action of these drugs. Tubocurarine and gallamine have a comparable duration of action in the cat, dog, and human. It would, however, appear that the steroid-based neuromuscular blocking drugs have a relatively short duration of action in cat and dog (5–10 min) when compared with human and monkey (30 min) (Maclagan 1976). It has long been considered that the cat closely resembled the human in its sensitivity and response to muscle relaxant drugs (Paton and Zaimis 1952). There would appear to be an exception to this rule in that the steroid relaxants behave differently in the two species. It has been demonstrated that dipyrandium has a short duration of action, comparable with that of suxamethonium, when administered to cats, rabbits, and chickens. In the rhesus monkey, however, the duration of action was similar to that of tubocurarine (Biggs *et al.* 1964). In the human this drug was found to have a duration of action similar to that of tubocurarine (Mushin and Mapleson 1964).

More recently it has been demonstrated that there is a considerable species variation between the time-course of action and the potencies of the two steroid relaxants pancuronium and vecuronium. The drugs appear to be of similar potency, with a greater potency in the dog and somewhat less in rats, cats, and Rhesus monkeys. The onset of action of vecuronium is slightly more rapid and its duration of action and recovery time are substantially slower than that of pancuronium (Marshall *et al.* 1980). It would appear that the dose and the duration of action in the dog and cat are similar to that in humans (Feldman and Liban 1987; Jones 1991).

When atracurium was administered to cats, dogs, and Rhesus monkeys, the time-course of the block was similar for all three species. The drug was, however, more potent in dogs than in either cats or monkeys (Hughes and Chapple 1981). Prediction based on the potency and time-course of the block in the three animal species proved accurate for anaesthetized man (Payne and Hughes 1981).

Tubocurarine

Whilst this drug was shown to release histamine in the human as early as 1945 (Whitacre and Fischer 1945) this has not been considered a contraindication to its use. It was, however, demonstrated by Pickett (1951) that the drug had histamine-releasing properties which produced profound cardiovascular effects which preclude its use in this species. This was confirmed by Smith *et al.* (1970) who demonstrated that a fall in cardiac output and heart rate occurred in anaesthetized dogs, which was associated with hypotension. It was also demonstrated that the lung compliance decreased when tubocurarine was administered to the pentobarbitone-anaesthetized dog (Safar and Bachman 1956). Similar cardiovascular effects have also been demonstrated in cats by McCullough *et al.* (1970). However, tubocurarine has minimal cardiovascular effects in horses (Klein 1987) and in pigs (Hall 1971).

There appear to be a significant difference in the dosage of tubocurarine between species. Initial doses of 300 μg/kg have been suggested in the horse, 400 μg/kg in the pig, 60 μg/kg in cattle, and 40 μg/kg in sheep, with increments of one-quarter to one-sixth of the original dose (Jones 1991).

Gallamine

This was the first synthetic nondepolarizing muscle relaxant to be available for clinical use in humans and animals. The administration of the drug will produce tachycardia and slight hypertension in dogs and pigs due to its vagal blocking action (Hall 1971). In the halothane-anaesthetized horse, the drug appears to have very little effect on the cardiovascular system (Klein 1981).

There also appear to be differences in doses between domestic species. In horses, pigs, cats, and dogs the usual dose is 1 mg/kg followed by increments of one-fifth of the original dose. In cattle 500 μg/kg is recommended as an initial dose followed by one fifth of that dose as an increment (Jones 1991).

Alcuronium

This is another synthetic muscle relaxant which has only been used to any real extent in horses and dogs. It would appear that the horse is somewhat more sensitive than the dog to this drug. The recommended dose for the horse is 50 μg/kg and for the dog 100 μg/kg followed by increments of one fifth of the original dose (Jones 1991).

Pancuronium

This is a steroid derivative which has no hormonal activity. It has been used widely in veterinary anaesthesia, particularly in small animals. There appear to be considerable species variation in response to pancuronium under clinical conditions. In the horse an initial dose of 120–180 μg/kg has been recommended by Hildebrand (1990). Recommended doses for other domestic species are available (Jones 1991). These are 40 μg/kg in cattle 25 μg/kg in sheep and goats, 60 μg/kg in dogs, 100 μg/kg in pigs, and 80 μg/kg in cats. Incremental doses of one-quarter to one-fifth of the original dose are appropriate for continuing the neuromuscular block. As pancuronium is cumulative, it is essential that monitoring of the neuromuscular block should be carried out.

Atracurium

Whilst atracurium has been shown to produce symptoms associated with the release of histamine in humans this does not appear to be a feature of its administration to other species. As dogs seem to be extremely susceptible to compounds which release histamine the use of tubocurarine is precluded in this species. Hence it was decided to investigate the cardiovascular effects of a relatively large dose (0.6 μg/kg) of atracurium in the dog. No signs of hypertension or any other untoward effects were observed (Jones *et al.* 1983). Apart from the horse, in which a dose of 150 μg/kg is recommended, the majority of other species which have been studied require a dose of 500 μg/kg to produce neuromuscular block. Incremental doses of 40 per cent of the original dose are recommended (Jones 1991).

Vecuronium

As this drug has only recently become available for use in veterinary anaesthesia, there is a relative dearth of information on its use in many species. With the exception of sheep, in which a dose of 40 μg/kg is recommended, the recommended dose in most other species is 100 μg/kg. Incremental doses of 20 per cent of the original dose are suitable (Jones 1991).

FACTORS AFFECTING RESPONSES TO MUSCLE RELAXANTS

There are a variety of factors such as age, other drugs, pH, and neuromuscular disease, which may affect an animal's response to neuromuscular blocking drugs. These have been reviewed by both Klein (1987) and Hall and Clarke (1991). There are very few differences between species. The subject has been reviewed in the human by Ali and Savarese (1976). One or two aspects of this subject are of importance and will be discussed here.

Animals with a relatively small body weight are particularly susceptible to the effects of hypothermia. Reducing the temperature of the tibialis anterior muscle of the cat reduced the block produced by tubocurarine (Bigland *et al.* 1958). The same workers also demonstrated the opposite effect in that the magnitude and duration of a depolarizing block was increased by a reduction in temperature.

It is well recognized that age has an effect on the response to muscle relaxants. The muscles of young cats are very sensitive to tubocurarine and insensitive to depolarizing drugs (Maclagan and Vrbova 1966). The sensitivity to depolarizing drugs increases with age until maturity (Mann and Salafsky 1970). Young animals appear to be less sensitive to the newer nondepolarizing drugs vecuronium and atracurium.

Human patients with myasthenia gravis are very sensitive to nondepolarizing muscle relaxants (Foldes 1975). This is also the situation in the dog. However, both atracurium and vecuronium can be used in dogs in doses of one-tenth to one-fifth of that normally recommended (Jones and Sharp 1985; Jones *et al.* 1988).

Myotonia congenita has been described in dogs, horses, and goats (Blood and Radostits 1989). It has been shown in the horse that such animals are extremely sensitive to suxamethonium (Jones and Ritchie 1965). It has also been demonstrated that neostigmine does not produce spasms in halothane-anaesthetized horses with myotonia (Klein 1987).

The effect of acid–base balance changes on the action of muscle relaxants has been shown to be somewhat complex and the reports tend to be conflicting (Hughes 1970). It has also been reported that when vecuronium was administered to cats, the magnitude of the effect varied with the muscle type. The soleus and the diaphragm were affected more than the tibialis (Funk *et al.* 1980).

MONITORING OF NEUROMUSCULAR BLOCK

Whilst pharmacologists have isolated single muscles or groups of muscles in a variety of species and recorded their response to nerve stimulation for a number of years, the use of monitoring techniques in intact animals is relatively recent.

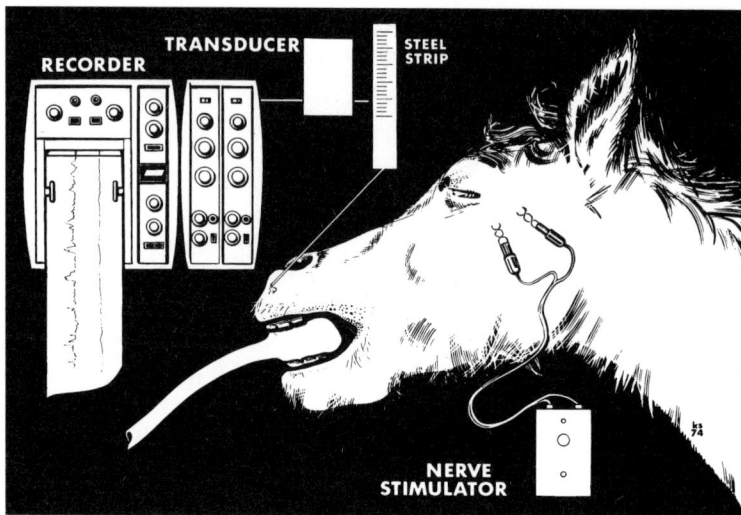

Fig. 19.1 A representation of the head of the horse and the equipment for recording neuro-muscular block in the anaesthetized horse. (Reprinted from Jones, R. S. and Prentice, D. E. (1976) with permission of the editors of the *British Veterinary Journal*.)

One of the earliest reports was by Bowen (1969), who described an experimental technique for assessing the twitch response of the hind-limb of the dog and the cow to peroneal nerve stimulation, and the response of the upper lip and nose of the horse to stimulation of the superior buccal branch of the facial nerve. He used a stimulus frequency of 0.5 Hz in the dog and 0.2 Hz in cattle and horses, and employed single stimuli.

A similar technique was adapted for use in the horse under conditions of clinical anaesthesia by Jones and Prentice (1976). They used a single stimulus at a frequency of 0.2 Hz and a tetanus of 50 Hz for 10 seconds (Fig. 19.1).

A comparison of the effects of various muscle relaxant drugs, and the use of the response of the upper lip and of the hind limb have been discussed by Klein (1987). The sites of stimulation are shown on the hind limb (Fig. 19.2) and on the face (Fig. 19.3). The use of the train-of-four technique was first described by Ali *et al.* (1971) in humans. There is little correlation in sheep and horses between the responses to stimulation of the facial nerve and of the peroneal nerve. In the dog a technique for recording both the evoked electrical and mechanical activity in response to ulnar nerve at stimulation was described by Heckmann *et al.* (1977). They demonstrated that the electrical and mechanical responses are similar and tend to show close correlation when muscle relaxant drugs were administered. The train-of-four techniques has been adapted for use in the dog and applied to both the facial nerve and the ulnar nerve in the intact dog (Cullen and Jones 1980*b*). Recordings from the foreleg showed the presence of train-of-four fade until complete neuromuscular block had been established. Simultaneous recordings from the

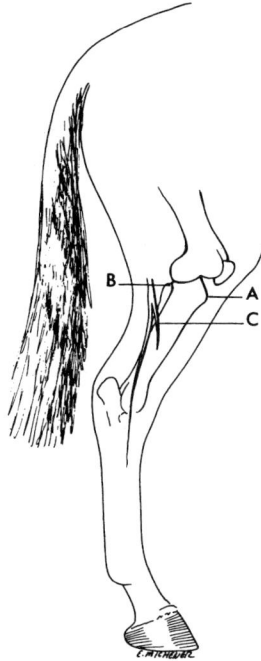

Fig. 19.2 Subcutaneous location of the peroneal nerve of the horse. A, tibial tuberosity; B, head of fibula; C, motor branch of peroneal nerve to digital exterior muscles, which can be palpated as it crosses the shaft of the fibula. (Reprinted with permision from Klein, L. V. (1981).)

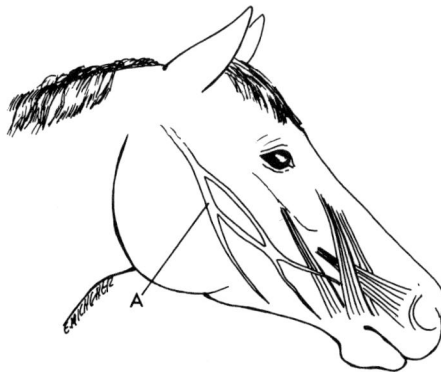

Fig. 19.3 Subcutaneous location of the facial nerve of the horse. The active electrode should be placed approximately at the level of the lateral canthus of the eye A to avoid direct muscle stimulation. (Reprinted with permission from Klein, L. V. (1981).)

nose demonstrated the development of train-of-four fade in the early stages but as the block developed all four twitch heights became equal. This phenomenon occurred with both suxamethonium and nondepolarizing muscle relaxants.

USE OF MUSCLE RELAXANTS IN CLINICAL VETERINARY ANAESTHESIA

The use of muscle relaxants in clinical anaesthesia in animals has been described by Klein (1987) and more specifically in cats and dogs by Hall (1982).

In cats they are used to facilitate endotracheal intubation, bronchoscopy and oesophagoscopy. In addition they are used to assist in the institution and maintenance of intermittent positive pressure ventilation.

In dogs there are similar indications to the cat, although muscle relaxants are not usually necessary or required for endotracheal intubation. In the dog, however, these drugs have wider indications on the provision of muscle relaxation for a spectrum of surgical procedures including laparotomies and a variety of orthopaedic procedures.

Whilst the number of general anaesthetics administered to pigs is relatively few, muscle relaxants are used for endotracheal intubation and for a number of surgical procedures, particularly in the experimental animal. In cattle, sheep, and goats the indications for the use of muscle relaxants are few. It is probably only in the experimental situation for certain procedures — for example, thoracotomy — that these agents are used.

The indications for the use of muscle relaxants in horses are more numerous and have been discussed by Hildebrand (1990). Suxamethonium was often administered following the administration of thiopentone for the induction of anaesthesia, in order to provide better control of the fall from the upright to the recumbent position and facilitate endotracheal intubation. This technique of induction of anaesthesia has, however, been superseded by a number of improved techniques such as xylazine — ketamine. The indications for the use of these drugs in horses are similar to those in the dog. It is, however, essential that proper facilities are available for intermittent positive pressure ventilation and the monitoring of the neuromuscular block.

Reversal of neuromuscular block in domestic animals has been discussed by Jones (1988). In general, either neostigmine or edrophonium are used, preceded by either atropine or glycopyrrolate. In the horse, however, if atropine is administered with neostigmine, which is essential with this drug in this species, a number of undesirable side-effects are observed. It has been suggested that edrophonium can be used alone, and hence the use of anticholinesterases be avoided in this species (Hildebrand 1990).

REFERENCES

Ali, H. H., Utting, J. E., and Gray, T. C. (1971). Quantitative assessment of residual anti-depolarising block. *British Journal of Anaesthesia*, **43**, 473–7.

Bernard, C. (1851). Leçon sur les effets des substances toxiques et medicamenteuses. *Compte Rendue de la Sociétié Biologique du Paris*, **2**, 195–206.

Biggs, R. S., Davis, M., and Wien, R. (1964). Muscle relaxant properties of a steroid quaternary ammonium salt. *Experientia*, **20**, 119–21.

Bigland, B., Goetzee, B., Maclagan, J., and Zaimis, E. (1958). The effect of lowered muscle temperature or the action of neuromuscular blocking drugs. *Journal of Physiology (London)*, **141**, 425–34.

Blood, D. C. and Radostits, O. M. (1989). *Veterinary medicine* (7th edn). Baillière Tindall, London.

Bovet, D., Bovet-Nitti, F., Guarino, S., Longo, S., and Fusco, R. (1951). Recherches sur les poisons curarisants de synthèse. *Archives International Pharmacodynamics*, **88**, 1–50.

Bowen, J. M. (1969). Monitoring neuromuscular function in intact animals. *American Journal of Veterinary Research*, **30**, 857–9.

Bowman, W. C. (1962). Mechanisms of neuromuscular blockade. In *Progress in medicinal chemistry*, (ed. G. B. West and G. P. E. Ellis) Vol. 2, pp. 88–131. Butterworth, London.

Buttle, G. A. M. and Zaimis, E. (1949). The action of decamethonium iodide in birds. *Journal of Pharmacy and Pharmacology*, **1**, 991–2.

Cullen, L. K. and Jones, R. S. (1980*a*). Recording of train of four evoked muscle responses from the nose and foreleg in the intact dog. *Research in Veterinary Science*, **29**, 277–80.

Cullen, L. K. and Jones, R. S. (1980*b*). The nature of suxamethonium neuromuscular block in the dog assessed by train of four stimulation. *Research in Veterinary Science*, **29**, 281–8.

Derkx, F. H. M., Bonta, I. L., and Lagendijk, A. (1971). Species-dependent effect of neuromuscular blocking agents. *European Journal of Pharmacology*, **16**, 105–8.

Feldman, S. A. and Liban, J. B. (1987). Vecuronium — a variable dose technique. *Anaesthesia*, **42**, 199–201.

Foldes, F. F. (1975). Myasthenia gravis. In *Muscle relaxants* (ed. R. L. Katz), pp. 345–93. Elsevier, New York.

Funk, D. I., Crul, J. F., and van der Pol, F. M. (1980). Effects of changes in acid–base balance on neuromuscular blockade produced by ORG-NC 45. *Acta Anaesthesiologica Scandinavica*, **24**, 119–24.

Gray, T. C. and Halton, J. (1946). A milestone in anaesthesia? (*d*-tubocurarine chloride). *Proceedings of the Royal Society of Medicine*, **34**, 400–6.

Griffith, H. R. and Johnson, G. E. (1942). The use of curare in general anaesthesia. *Anesthesiology*, **3**, 418–20.

Hall, L. W. (1952). A report on the clinical use of bis (beta-dimethylaminoethyl)-succinate bisethiodide (Brevedil E, M and B 2210) during anaesthesia in the dog. *Veterinary Record*, **64**, 491–3.

Hall, L. W. (1971). In *Wright's veterinary anaesthesia and analgesia* (7th edn), p. 19. Balliere Tindall, London.

Hall, L. W. (1982). Relaxant drugs in small animal anaesthesia. *Proceedings of the Association of Veterinary Anaesthetists*, **10**, (Supplement), 144–55.

Hall, L. W. and Clarke, K. W. (1991). In *Veterinary anaesthesia* (9th edn), pp. 113–35. Baillière Tindall, London.

Hall, L. W. and Weaver, B. M. Q. (1954). Some notes on balanced anaesthesia for the dog and cat. *Veterinary Record*, **66**, 289–93.

Hall, R. A. and Parkes, M. W. (1953). The effect of drugs upon neuromuscular transmission in the guinea pig. *Journal of Physiology*, **122**, 1274–81.

Hall, L. W., Lehman H., and Silk, E. (1953). Response in dogs to relaxants derived from succinic acid and choline. *British Medical Journal*, **i**, 134–6.

Hansson, C. H. (1957a). Blood cholinesterase activity in relation to tolerance for succinylcholine. *Acta Pharmacologica et Toxicologica Scandinavica*, **14**, 6–10.

Hansson, C. H. (1957b). Observations on casting horses and cows with succinylcholine. *Nordisk veterinaermedicin*, **9**, 753–62.

Heckmann R., Jones, R. S., and Wuersch, W. (1977). A method for recording electrical and mechanical activity of muscle in the dog. *Research in Veterinary Science*, **23**, 1–6.

Hildebrand, S. (1990). Neuromuscular blocking agents in equine anaesthesia. In *The veterinary clinics of North America — Large animal practice*, Vol. 6, No. 3, pp. 597–606. Saunders, London.

Holmes, T. (1898). *Brody*. Fisher Unwin, London.

Hughes, R. (1970). The influence of changes in acid–base balance on neuromuscular blockade in cats. *British Journal of Anaesthesia*, **42**, 658–68.

Hughes, R. and Chapple, D. J. (1981). The pharmacology of atracurium: a new competitive neuromuscular blocking agent. *British Journal of Anaesthesia*, **53**, 31–44.

Humphrey, P. P. A. (1973). Depolarization and neuromuscular block in the rat. *British Journal of Pharmacology*, **48**, 636–7P.

Iveson, T. D., Ford, R., and Loveday, C. (1969). The neuromuscular blocking action of suxamethonium in the anaesthetised rat. *Archives International Pharmacodynamics*, **181**, 283–6.

Jarcho, L. W., Berman, B., Eyzaguirre, C., and Lilienthal, J. L. (1951). Curarization of denervated muscle. *Annals of the New York Academy of Sciences*, **54**, 337–46.

Jones, R. S. (1988). Reversal of neuromuscular blockade: a review. *Journal of the Association of Veterinary Anaesthetists*, **15**, 80–8.

Jones, R. S. (1991). Drugs modifying neuromuscular transmission. In *The veterinary formulary* (ed. Y. Debut). The Pharmaceutical Press, London.

Jones, R. S. and Prentice, D. E. (1976). A technique for the investigation of the action of drugs on the neuromuscular junction in the intact horse. *British Veterinary Journal*, **132**, 226–30.

Jones, R. S. and Ritchie, H. E. (1965). The effects of suxamethonium in a case of myotonia in a horse. *British Journal of Anaesthesia*, **37**, 142.

Jones, R. S. and Sharp, N. J. H. (1985). The use of the muscle relaxant atracurium in a myasthenic dog. *Veterinary Record*, **117**, 500–1.

Jones, R. S., Heckmann, R., and Wuersch, W. (1978). Observations on the duration of action of suxamethonium in the dog. *British Veterinary Journal*, **134**, 521–3.

Jones, R. S., Heckmann, R., and Wuersch, W. (1980). The effect of neostigmine on the duration of action of suxamenthonium in the dog. *British Veterinary Journal*, **136**, 71–3.

Jones, R. S., Hunter, J. M., and Utting, J. E. (1983). Neuromuscular blocking action of atracurium in the dog and its reversal by neostigmine. *Research in Veterinary Science*, **34**, 173–76.

Jones, R. S., Brown, A., and Watkins, P. E. (1988). The use of the muscle relaxant vecuronium in a myasthenic dog. *Veterinary Record*, **122**, 611.

Klein, L. V. (1981). Neuromuscular blocking agents in equine anaesthesia. In *The veterinary clinics of North America — Large animal practice*, Vol. 3, No. 1, pp. 135–62. Saunders, London.

Klein, L. V. (1987). Neuromuscular blocking agents. In *Principles and practice of veterinary anaesthesia* (ed. C. E. Short) pp. 134–53. Williams and Wilkins, Baltimore.

Maclagan, J. (1976). Competitive neuromuscular blocking drugs. In *Neuromuscular junction*, (ed. E. Zaimist), pp. 421–86. Springer-Verlag, Berlin.

Maclagan, J. and Vrbova, G. (1966). The importance of peripheral changes in determining the sensitivity of striated muscle to depolarising drugs. *Journal of Physiology (London)*, **184**, 618–30.

Mann, W. S. and Salafsky, B. (1970). Development of the differential response to succinyl-choline in the fast and slow twitched skeletal muscle of the kitten. *Journal of Physiology (London)*, **210**, 581–92.

Marshall, I. G., Agoston, S., Booij, L. H. D. J., Durant, N. H., and Foldes, F. F. (1980). Pharmacology of ORG NC 45 compared with other non-depolarising neuromuscular blocking drugs. *British Journal of Anaesthesia*, **52**, 11–95.

Mazze, R. E., Escue, H. M., and Houston, J. B. (1969). Hyperkalaemia and cardiovascular collapse following administration of succinylcholine to the traumatised patient. *Anesthesiology*, **31**, 540–7.

McCullough, L. S., Reier, C. E., Delaunois, A. L., Gardier, R. W., and Hamelberg, W. (1970). The effects of *d*-tubocurarine on spontaneous postganglionic sympathetic activity and histamine release. *Anesthesiology*, **33**, 328–34.

Mushin, W. W. and Mapleson, W. W. (1964). Relaxant action in man of dipyrandium chloride (M & B 9105A). *British Journal of Anaesthesia*, **36**, 761–8.

Paton, W. D. M. (1956). Mode of action of neuromuscular blocking agents. *British Journal of Anaesthesia*, **28**, 470–80.

Payne, J. P. and Hughes, R. (1981). Evaluation of atracurium in anaesthetised man. *British Journal of Anaesthesia*, **53**, 45–54.

Paton, W. D. M. and Zaimis, E. (1952). The methonium compounds. *Pharmacological Reviews*, **4**, 219–53.

Philippot, E. and Dallemagne, M. J. (1952). Les inhibiteurs de la transmission neuro-musculaires étudiés chez le chien. *Experientia*, **8**, 273–4.

Pickett, D. (1951). Curare in canine surgery. *Journal of the American Veterinary Medical Association*, **119**, 346–53.

Safar, P. and Bachman, L. (1956). Compliance of the lungs and thorax in dogs under the influence of muscle relaxants. *Anesthesiology*, **17**, 334–46.

Smith, G., Proctor, D. W. and Spence, A. A. (1970). A comparison of some cardiovascular effects of tubocurarine and pancuronium in dogs. *British Journal of Anaesthesia*, **42**, 923–27.

Smithcors, J. F. (1971). History of veterinary anaesthesia. In *Textbook of veterinary anesthesia* (ed. L. R. Soma), pp. 14–15. Williams and Wilkins, Baltimore.

Stevenson, D. E. (1960a). A review of some side-effects of muscle relaxants in small animals. *Journal of Small Animal Practice*, **1**, 77–83.

Stevenson, D. E. (1960b). Changes in the blood electrolytes of anaesthetized dogs caused by suxamethonium. *British Journal of Anaesthesia*, **32**, 364–71.

Waterton, C. (1825). *Wanderings in South America*. Longman, Green, Brown, and Longman.

Whitacre, R. J. and Fischer, A. J. (1945). Clinical observations on the use of curare in anesthesia. *Anesthesiology*, **6**, 124–30.

Youatt, W. (1838). Animal pathology lecture XXII, Rabies. *Veterinarian*, **11**, 457–66.

Youatt, W. (1839). Tetanus v wourali. *Veterinarian*, **12**, 633–8.

Zaimis, E. (1953). Motor end-plate differences as a determining factor in the mode of action of neuromuscular blocking substances. *Journal of Physiology*, **122**, 238–51.

Zaimis, E. and Head, S. (1976). Depolarizing neuromuscular blocking drug. In *Neuromuscular junction* (ed. E. Zaimis), pp. 365–414. Springer-Verlag, Berlin.

20

Use patterns in different countries

François Donati and Claude Meistelman

The choice of muscle relaxant made by the clinician is based on many factors, many of which have very little to do with the scientific merits of the drug. The type of practice, personal experience, and training of the individual anaesthetist influences the choice of drug. Within a hospital or clinic, the selection of muscle relaxants is affected by the preferences of the anaesthetists taken as a group, tradition, efficiency of surgeons, organization of recovery rooms, and availability of the various products through pharmacy. These choices are, in turn, influenced by outside forces, such as the prestige and personal opinions of experts at the local and national level, the marketing strategies of the various pharmaceutical firms, and the approval (or lack of it) by the national regulatory boards.

Thus, use patterns vary from one anaesthetist to the next, and from one hospital to the next. Furthermore, there are hardly any published data about muscle relaxant use at the local or national level, so generalizations must be avoided. However, when comparing various countries, different patterns emerge. These patterns should not be regarded as rules implemented by influential academic anaesthetists in the various locations, but rather as different answers by different people to the same problems. In practice, the answer depends on the perception of what the reality is. Beyond the facts, which are difficult to tabulate, it is most interesting to find out how anaesthetists of different countries have come up with different solutions to the same problems, such as the relaxant for intubation, maintenance of relaxation, and management of recovery.

AVAILABILITY AND USE OF RELAXANTS AND REVERSAL AGENTS

The drugs available vary slightly from country to country in the industrialized world. Some are not used, because they have been replaced by more attractive alternatives. Gallamine is an example (Table 20.1). Most countries now have only one short-acting drug (suxamethonium), two intermediate-acting drugs (atracurium and vecuronium), and a variable selection of long-acting drugs. The new, long-acting drug doxacurium was, at the time of writing, only available in the USA. Pipecuronium has been marketed only recently in the West and is restricted to a few

Table 20.1 Neuromuscular relaxant availability in four countries

	UK	France	USA	Canada
Suxamethonium	++	++	++	++
d-Tubocurarine	++	0	++	++
Pancuronium	++	++	++	++
Metocurine	0	0	+	+
Gallamine	+	+	+	+
Alcuronium	++	+	0	0
Atracurium	++	++	++	++
Vecuronium	++	++	++	++
Doxacurium*	0	0	+	0
Pipecuronium*	0	0	+	0
Mivacurium*	+	0	+	0

0, not available; +, available, but rarely used; ++, used.
* Recent introduction into clinical use in those countries marked.

countries, such as the USA and France. Mivacurium, the shortest-acting nondepolarizing drug available to date, has recently been released in the UK and the USA.

Other drugs are available in the eastern European countries and the former USSR. For example, pipecuronium was developed in Hungary before 1980 and the first clinical trials were carried out in Hungary and the USSR (Agoston and Richardson 1985). It has been used in eastern Europe for more than a decade. Tercuronium, whose duration of action is comparable to that of pancuronium, was introduced into clinical practice in the USSR in the late 1970s (Danilov 1986). The recent political changes in these countries will probably lead to more uniformity with the West, although cost might be a problem in the East. Financial considerations are even more important in Third World countries, where resources in personnel, drugs, and equipment are extremely scarce.

The reversal drugs edrophonium, neostigmine, and pyridostigmine are available in most industrialized countries. However, their use is quite variable. The drug 4-aminopyridine was developed in Bulgaria and was the subject of several clinical trials in The Netherlands (Agoston *et al.* 1985). Its use is probably limited to eastern European countries.

Published data on relaxant agents used in different countries are difficult to obtain. Information on the sales of these various products was not available to the authors, and would reflect the use outside the operating room and the amount wasted. A recent article was published on the relative contribution of neuromuscular relaxants to the anaesthesia literature (Shanks 1992). During the decade 1980–90, the number of articles on atracurium and vecuronium increased, and those on older relaxants decreased. In 1989–90, of the 267 articles published on muscle relaxants in the English language literature, atracurium and vecuronium were each mentioned in approximately one-quarter of the titles (64 and 66, respectively). Since 1988, articles on pipecuronium, doxacurium, and mivacurium have

Table 20.2 Drug used for intubation in published articles, June–December 1991

Country	Succinylcholine Precur.	Alone	Atracurium	Vecuronium	Pancuronium	Alcuronium
United Kingdom	1	1	3	4	0	1
Scandinavia	1	1	2	1	2	1
Rest of Europe	3	1	0	3	1	0
Total Europe	5	3	5	8	3	2
USA	1	5	2	6	2	0
Canada	1	0	0	3	1	0
Total North America	2	5	2	9	3	0
Rest of World	1	2	1	2	0	0
Total	8	10	8	19	6	2

been published. Suxamethonium appears to generate a constant level of interest. It was the subject of 60 publications in 1980–90. This distribution does not necessarily reflect the use of the various drugs, but the interests of the investigators and the needs of the research sponsors.

Another approach is to examine the choice made by investigators who published clinical articles on topics other than neuromuscular blockade. For the last six months of 1991, six English language journals were surveyed: *Acta Anaesthesiologica Scandinavica, Anaesthesia, Anesthesia and Analgesia, Anesthesiology, British Journal of Anaesthesia, and Canadian Journal of Anaesthesia.* Articles involving general anaesthesia for adults or children, scheduled for surgical procedures other than cardiac, neurosurgical or obstetrical, were retained. Articles on the pharmacology of muscle relaxants were not included. Suxamethonium was used in 34% of cases, and

Table 20.3 Drug used for maintenance in published articles, June–December 1991

Country	Atracurium	Vecuronium	Pancuronium	Alcuronium	Metocurine
United Kingdom	4	5	0	3	0
Scandinavia	2	2	2	1	0
Rest of Europe	0	4	2	1	0
Total Europe	6	11	4	5	0
USA	3	7	2	0	1
Canada	1	4	1	0	0
Total North America	4	11	3	0	1
Rest of World	2	2	0	0	0
Total	12	24	7	5	1

Table 20.4 Reversal drugs in published articles, June–December 1991

Country	Neostigmine	Edrophonium	Pyridostigmine
United Kingdom	4	0	0
Scandinavia	4	0	0
Rest of Europe	0	0	1
Total Europe	8	0	1
USA	0	2	0
Canada	0	1	0
Total North America	0	3	0
Rest of World	0	0	0
Total	8	3	1

there was no obvious geographical pattern (Table 20.2). Atracurium or vecuronium was chosen in 51% of studies, without any definite trend. For maintenance of relaxation, atracurium or vecuronium was used in 73% of cases (Table 20.3). Pancuronium, and alcuronium outside North America, were the most popular long-acting drugs. Among reversal agents, neostigmine was preferred in Europe, and edrophonium in North America, but the numbers were small, because most investigators did not specify which drug they used for reversal (Table 20.4). Although this probably indicates the use pattern in academic centres only, it appears that intermediate-acting agents are very popular, but suxamethonium is still used relatively frequently.

EFFECTS IN DIFFERENT COUNTRIES

In 1969, Katz *et al.* reported the results of a study which had been triggered by the clinical impression that clinicians used more relaxants in the UK than in the USA. They reported that the maximum blockade produced by *d*-tubocurarine, 0.1 mg/kg, and its duration of action were greater in New York (75% and 31 min, respectively), than in London (43% and 14 min). The same sort of findings were reported for succinylcholine 1 mg/kg. Duration to 90% recovery was 9.1 min in London and 14.6 min in New York. Genetic differences play a role in the sensitivity to, and elimination of, many drugs, but this was probably not the explanation for the differences between London and New York, as the study was conducted in a predominantly white population.

The Katz *et al.* (1969) study was conducted before the modern techniques of monitoring became widespread, and before the concept of dose–response relationships had gained wide acceptance in anaesthesia. The study was also limited to two locations, and the stimulation pattern (one impulse every 3–4 s) might appear inappropriate to the present-day reader. However, the investigation was conducted with the same methodology at both sites, and the background anaesthetic was the same.

Comparison of data obtained in different locations must be made with caution, because many factors may affect the measurement of potency and duration of neuromuscular relaxants. The demographic characteristics (age, sex, weight) of the population studied must be similar, the background anaesthetic the same, and the measurement technique rigorously identical. For example, allowing the train-of-four response to stabilize for five more minutes before injecting the drug can alter measured onset time dramatically (Curran *et al.* 1987). Nevertheless, there seems to be a tendency for dose–responses of neuromuscular relaxants obtained in Europe to be shifted to the right compared with those in North America (Fig. 20.1). For example, Fiset *et al.* (1991) surveyed the literature and reported that measurements of the ED_{50} for vecuronium tended to be lower in North America (mean 23 μg/kg) than in Europe (mean 31 μg/kg). Interestingly, the lowest figures originated from studies conducted in California (15–17 μg/kg).

Recently, a comparative study was undertaken simultaneously in Montreal and Paris (Fiset *et al.* 1991). Vecuronium dose–response relationships were obtained in both locations in an adult population with a thiopentone–N_2O–narcotic anaesthetic. The Paris dose–response curve was shifted to the right by an average of 30% with respect to that in Montreal, the ED_{50}s being 26 and 33 μg/kg, respectively (Fig. 20.1). Furthermore, the same data were essentially unchanged (26 and 36 μg/kg),

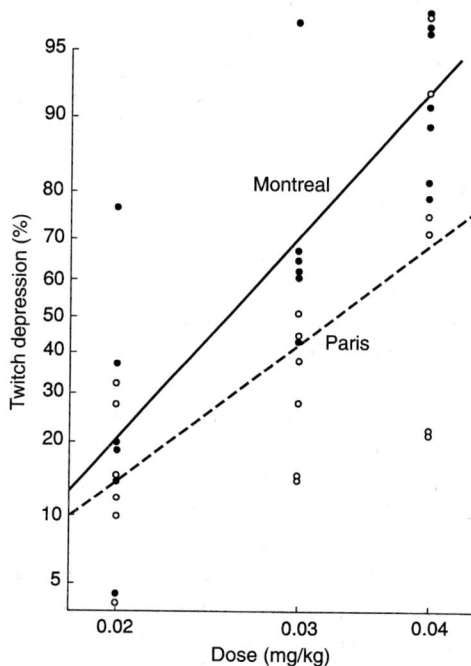

Fig. 20.1 Dose–response relationships for vecuronium in Montreal and Paris. (From Fiset *et al.* 1991.)

when expressed per kilogram ideal body weight, suggesting that the lower ED_{50} in Montreal patients was not related to differences in body habitus.

Unfortunately, it is impossible to determine whether these differences reported above apply to all of Europe and North America. In addition, there are no data available for other parts of the world. Although the differences measured between the USA and the UK and between Canada and France were less than the variability normally seen between individuals, it appears that geographical location of anaesthetic practice might determine the average requirement for muscle relaxants. Thus, local experience with relaxant dose requirement is essential in 'fine tuning' one's clinical practice.

Genetic factors play a major role in the metabolism of suxamethonium. Absent or abnormal plasma cholinesterase in certain individuals is associated with prolonged blockade. The incidence of this defect does not appear to vary among populations. However, to obtain meaningful comparison between countries, a large number of properly randomized individuals need to be tested, because of the low incidence of the phenomenon. No such large scale study has been undertaken.

No such comparative data have been obtained for reversal agents. Such a study would be even more difficult to perform than for the muscle relaxant drugs, because the number of factors to standardize is greater for a reversal study. These include relaxant given, background anaesthetic, spontaneous recovery at reversal, dose of reversal drug, and anticholinergic given. Finally, it should be remembered that data on the potency of relaxants in different countries is, at present, extremely fragmentary. The populations studied (eastern North America and western Europe) do not necessarily lie at opposite ends of the potency spectrum, and even greater differences might be found in genetically different populations. In other words, potency differences worldwide are likely to exceed the 30% observed between Montreal and Paris.

CONCERNS AND SOLUTIONS

Suxamethonium versus nondepolarizing drugs

The availability of the intermediate-acting drugs vecuronium and atracurium since the early to mid-1980s has undoubtedly decreased the use of suxamethonium. Yet, there are two undisputed advantages to suxamethonium: a rapid onset and short duration. Thus, its use decreases the probability of aspiration of gastric contents and allows an escape route if the intubation and ventilation are difficult or impossible. Consequently, the use of suxamethonium depends, at least in part, on the perceived risk of difficult intubation and aspiration of gastric contents. Most practitioners in multi-ethnic areas have the impression that tracheal intubation is noticeably more difficult in individuals of certain ethnic communities, but it is difficult to confirm such anecdotal experience. Nevertheless, the use of suxamethonium is affected not by the real, but by the perceived, risk of difficult intubation, and this in turn may be modified by the experience and skill of the anaesthetist, which in turn depends on training and type of practice, both of which are different in various countries.

Other influences also play a role. For example, the use of suxamethonium has decreased significantly in France over the past few years, and a large part of this decline is attributed to the apparently high incidence of anaphylactic reactions. Awareness of this phenomenon has been influenced greatly by the work of a referral centre, located in Nancy, where appropriate testing of patients having suspected anaphylactic reactions during anaesthesia is performed. The centre quoted an incidence of one anaphylactic reaction per 1500 anaesthetics (Laxenaire and Moneret-Vautrin 1985), suxamethonium being incriminated most often as the triggering agent. Since suxamethonium is not administered in all cases, incidence of anaphylaxis to suxamethonium could be even greater than 1:1500. If this was the approximate incidence worldwide, each practitioner would encounter the problem every year or two, with cases every month in busy centres. Although the number of reports of anaphylaxis to suxamethonium worldwide is greater than for any other drug used in anaesthesia, the incidence of anaphylaxis is probably much less than 1:1500 in most of the world. A prospective survey conducted in France between 1978 and 1982 revealed 26 anaphylactoid shocks at induction in 198 103 anaesthetics, or one in 7619, and the role of suxamethonium was not specified (Tiret *et al.* 1986). The reasons for the apparently large incidence of anaphylactic reactions in France are not known, but this undoubtedly affects the use of suxamethonium. Interestingly, the number of reactions attributed to other muscle relaxants reported to the Nancy laboratory has increased since 1980 (Laxenaire and Moneret-Vautrin 1990).

Intermediate versus long-acting

The choice of nondepolarizing relaxant depends on the surgical procedure to be performed and its duration. There are wide variations in the duration required for a given procedure, even when surgeons of the same hospital are compared. Thus, it is not surprising to find different use patterns for relaxant drugs. However, considerations other than duration are important. One such consideration is cost. Atracurium and vecuronium are more expensive than the older nondepolarizing relaxants, and the cost differential is even more striking for maintenance of relaxation for long procedures.

The intermediate-acting drugs, however, are used frequently worldwide for surgical procedures exceeding one hour in duration. Their rapid recovery rate makes their use more flexible and reversal is easier. Many studies from Scandinavia (Viby-Mogensen *et al.* 1979; Anderson *et al.* 1988), Australia (Beemer and Rozental 1986), Canada (Bevan *et al.* 1988), and the USA (Brull *et al.* 1991) have all confirmed the high (20–40%) incidence of residual curarization in the recovery room after administration of long-acting relaxants. The incidence was reduced to practically zero with atracurium or vecuronium.

Use of monitoring

The use of a nerve stimulator has increased in the last few years, but it is the authors' impression that a large proportion of general anaesthetics with neuromuscular blockade are given without monitoring. There are no published data on the clinical use of neuromuscular monitoring. It appears, however, that the use of nerve stimulators in hospitals where training takes place is of crucial importance, because the use of stimulators tends to spread to centres where former trainees practice.

Use of reversal agents

The routine use of reversal agents is widespread in certain countries, especially in the Anglo-Saxon world. This does not seem to be the case in certain countries of continental Europe. For example, in a survey of nearly 200 000 anaesthetics in France, reversal agents were given to only 4.9% of patients (Hatton *et al.* 1983), and the study covered the period 1978–1982, before the introduction of atracurium and vecuronium. Perhaps as a result of this survey, the use of reversal agents has definitely increased in France, probably to 50% of cases. Although it appears that anticholinesterase drugs were under-used in the French survey, the availability of atracurium, vecuronium, and eventually mivacurium, probably decreases the need for reversal. In fact, many patients probably do not need reversal, but the problem is to identify which patients do need it. Routine neuromuscular monitoring can be unreliable in the detection of residual blockade (Viby-Mogensen *et al.* 1985).

CONCLUSION

The basic principles of securing the airway and attaining full neuromuscular recovery at the end of a surgical procedure are adhered to worldwide. There is, however, considerable variation in the ways to achieve these goals. There are also differences in the availability of relaxant drugs between countries, and even pharmacological variations between geographical locations. Thus, it is important for the individual clinician to be familiar with the local experience with the agents available.

REFERENCES

Agoston, S., Langrehr, D., and Newton D. E. F. (1985). Pharmacology and possible clinical applications of 4-aminopyridine. In *Muscle relaxants: Basic and clinical aspects*, (ed. R. L. Katz) pp. 285–293. Grune and Station, Orlando.

Agoston, S. and Richardson, F. J. (1985). Pipecuronium bromide (Arduan) — a new long-acting non-depolarizing neuromuscular blocking drug. *Clinics in Anaesthesiology*, **3**, 361–9.

Anderson, B. N., Madsen, J. V., Schurizek, B. A., and Juhl, B. (1988). Residual curarisation: a comparative study of atracurium and pancuronium. *Acta Anaesthesioligica Scandinavica*, **32**, 79–81.

Beemer, G. H. and Rozental, P. (1986). Postoperative neuromuscular function. *Anaesthesia Intensive Care*, **14**, 41–5.

Bevan, D. R., Smith, C. E., and Donati, F. (1988). Postoperative neuromuscular blockade: a comparison between atracurium, vecuronium and pancuronium. *Anesthesiology*, **69**, 272–6.

Brull, S. J., Ehrenwerth, J., Connerly, N. R., and Silverman, D. G. (1991). Assessment of residual curarization using low-current stimulation. *Canadian Journal of Anaesthesia*, **38**, 164–8.

Curran, M. J., Donati, F., and Bevan, D. R. (1987). Onset and recovery of atracurium and suxamethonium-induced neuromuscular blockade with simultaneous train-of-four and single twitch stimulation. *British Journal of Anaesthesia*, **59**, 989–94.

Danilov, A. F. (1986). Tercuronium. In *New neuromuscular blocking agents: Handbook of experimental pharmacology*, Vol. 79, (ed. D. A. Kharkevich), 485–497. Springer-Verlag, Berlin.

Fiset, P., Donati, F, Balendran, P., Meistelman, C., Lira, E., and Bevan, D. R. (1991). Vecuronium is more potent in Montreal than in Paris. *Canadian Journal of Anaesthesia*, **38**, 717–21.

Hatton, F., Tiret, L., Maujoi, L., N'Doye, P., Vourc'h, G., Desmonts, J. M., *et al.* (1983). Enquête epidémiologique sur les anesthésies. *Annales Français Anesthesie Réanimation*, **5**, 333–65.

Katz, R. L., Norman, J., Seed, R. F., and Conrad, L. (1969). A comparison of the effects of suxamethonium and tubocurarine in patients in London and New York. *British Journal of Anaesthesia*, **41**, 1041–7.

Laxenaire, M. C. and Moneret-Vautrin, D. A. (1985). The French experience of anaphylactoid reactions. *International Anesthesiology Clinics*, **23**, 145–60.

Laxenaire, M. C. and Moneret-Vautrin, D. A. (1990). *Le risque Allergique en Anesthésie-Réanimation*. Masson, Paris.

Shanks, C. A. (1992). Neuromuscular contributions in eight anaesthesia journals. *Canadian Journal of Anaesthesia*, **39**, 66–8.

Tiret, L., Desmonts, J. M., Hatton, F., and Vourc'h, G. (1986). Complications associated with anaesthesia — a prospective survey in France. *Canadian Anaesthetists' Society Journal*, **33**, 336–44.

Viby-Mogensen, J., Jensen, N. H., Engbaek, J., Ording, H., Skovgaard, L. T., and Chraemmer-Jorgensen, B. (1985). Tactile and visual evaluation of the response to train-of-four nerve stimulation. *Anesthesiology*, **63**, 440–3.

Viby-Mogensen, J., Jorgensen, B. C., and Ording, H. (1979). Residual curarization in the recovery room. *Anesthesiology*, **50**, 539–41.

The action of relaxants on different muscles of the body

Claude Meistelman and François Donati

The main goals of muscular relaxation during induction of anaesthesia are the paralysis of the vocal cords and jaw muscles to facilitate tracheal intubation and the relaxation of the respiratory muscles, particularly the diaphragm, to ensure controlled ventilation. Paralysis of the abdominal muscles and the diaphragm is often required intraoperatively, particularly during abdominal surgery. During recovery of neuromuscular block, restoration of complete skeletal muscular strength is essential to ensure adequate spontaneous ventilation and the patency of the upper airway (jaw muscles, intrinsic muscles of the tongue) (Pavlin *et al.* 1989).

For practical reasons it is almost impossible to monitor the response of the respiratory or abdominal muscles during anaesthesia. Stimulation of the ulnar nerve and monitoring of the adductor pollicis has been used for many years to determine the time-course and intensity of neuromuscular block. The underlying assumption is that relaxation of the adductor pollicis is a reliable reflection of the intensity of paralysis in other muscles. One must, however, recognize that large discrepancies exist in the sensitivity of the neuromuscular junctions of the body to the effects of neuromuscular relaxants. Paton and Zaimis (1951) demonstrated that respiratory muscles were more resistant to curare than other muscles. In humans, several studies have reported some discrepancies between the level of peripheral paralysis and respiratory depression or intubating conditions (Norman *et al.* 1980; Bencini and Newton 1984; Carnie *et al.* 1986). It has been demonstrated more recently that the time-course of neuromuscular block in various skeletal muscles was different from that in the adductor pollicis and discrepancies could exist in onset time, duration of action, and intensity of paralysis (Donati *et al.* 1986; Chauvin *et al.* 1987; Pansart *et al.* 1987; Smith *et al.* 1989*a*, *b*; Donati *et al.* 1991*a*; Meistelman *et al.* 1991). Therefore the understanding and knowledge of the relationship between neuromuscular function at the monitored muscle and the other muscles are important in the interpretation of monitoring.

RESPIRATORY MUSCLES

In awake volunteers, minute volume and end-tidal pCO_2 are little affected, if at all, by doses of tubocurarine which abolish grip strength almost completely (Gal and Smith 1976; Gal and Goldberg 1980, 1981; Rosenbaum *et al.* 1983; Pavlin *et al.* 1989). After the injection of tubocurarine 0.2 mg/kg, for example, grip strength is only 3% of control, but tidal volume is normal. Vital capacity, inspiratory capacity, respiratory and expiratory pressures, and maximum voluntary ventilation are decreased to 40–60% of their normal, unparalysed values (Gal and Smith 1976; Gal and Goldberg 1980) (Fig. 21.1). Still, these values are considerably greater than indices of peripheral muscle function. A dose of 0.1 mg/kg of tubocurarine induced a maximum decrease of the vital capacity of 12% whereas the grip strength was decreased by 77%. Similar effects were found with depolarizing muscle relaxants (suxamethonium, decamethonium), but to a lesser extent. A similar decrease of grip strength decreased vital capacity by 51 and 37%, respectively (Foldes *et al.* 1961). Similar results were obtained by Williams and Bourke (1985) for suxamethonium.

It is tempting to suggest that patients need only partial peripheral muscle recovery to have an adequate respiratory function, because normal gas exchange can be maintained. In fact, it is necessary to ensure return of full respiratory reserve because a decrease in vital capacity impairs the ability to cough (Arora and Gal 1981). A small number of studies sought to determine the smallest train-of-four ratio at the adductor pollicis which is associated with normal vital capacity. This level is approximately 0.7 (Ali *et al.* 1975; Dupuis *et al.* 1990). However, these studies were performed on

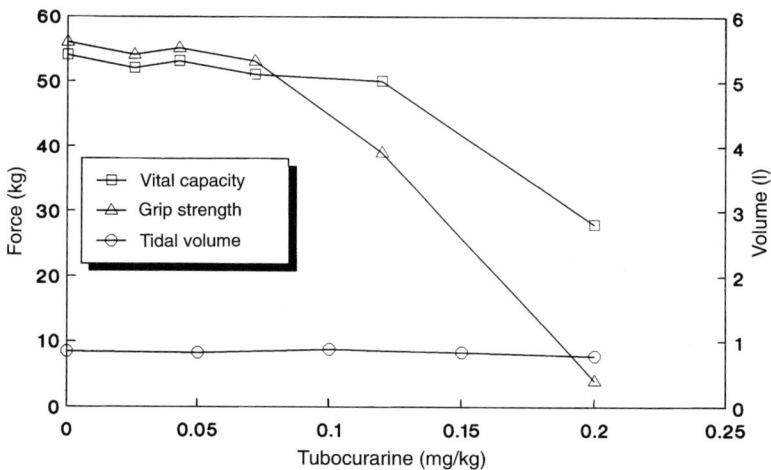

Fig. 21.1 Effect of tubocurarine in awake volunteer. At doses which abolish hand grip almost completely, tidal volume is normal, and vital capacity and inspiratory capacity are depressed 40–50%. (From Gal and Smith 1976; Gal and Goldberg 1980.)

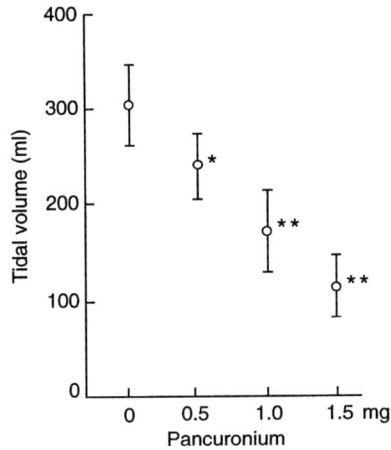

Fig. 21.2 Tidal volume versus dose of pancuronium injected to adult patients under anesthesia. Small doses (0.5 mg, equivalent to approximately 0.05 mg/kg tubocurarine) depress tidal volume. By contrast, higher doses 0.2 mg/kg tubocurarine do not affect tidal volume in awake humans (see Fig. 21.1). From Nishino *et al.* 1988.)

a small number of subjects, and it is highly probable that some individuals might not regain full respiratory function until the train-of-four ratio is greater than 0.7.

In anaesthetized patients, the respiratory system appears to be more sensitive to the effects of neuromuscular relaxants than in awake subjects. Wymore and Eisele (1978) measured inspiratory force during quiet breathing under halothane anaesthesia and found that a 50% decrease required a mean dose of 0.129 mg/kg of *d*-tubocurarine. This is in contrast to the lack of effects produced in quiet breathing by as much as 0.2 mg/kg in awake subjects. More convincingly, respiratory rate is decreased in anaesthetized animals (Oliven *et al.* 1984) and humans (Nishino *et al.* 1988) when given neuromuscular blocking agents. Respiratory rate increases in awake individuals (Rigg *et al.* 1970; Gal and Smith 1976). Furthermore, small doses of pancuronium (0.5–1.5 mg), which would not be expected to alter tidal volume in awake subjects, depress tidal volume and minute ventilation in enflurane-anaesthetized patients (Nishino *et al.* 1988) (Fig. 21.2). This effect cannot be due to diaphragmatic block (see below), even if potentiation by enflurane is accounted for. A possible explanation is interference with the control of breathing via an effect of small doses of neuromuscular blockers on muscle spindles (Oliven *et al.* 1984). Whatever the mechanism, anaesthetized patients should be regarded as extremely sensitive to neuromuscular relaxants, even given in small doses.

Diaphragm

With the development of nerve stimulation in association with electromyographic recording of the diaphragmatic activity or measurement of transdiaphragmatic pres-

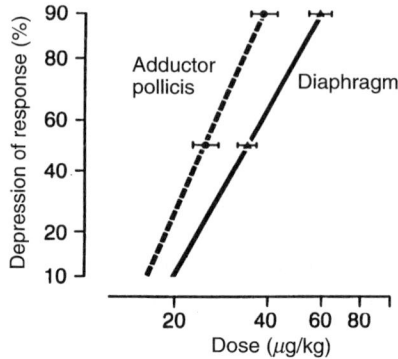

Fig. 21.3 Cumulative dose–response relationship for vecuronium at the adductor pollicis and the diaphragm. (From Laycock *et al.* 1988*b*.)

sure, the assessment and the comparison of neuromuscular block, both at the diaphragm and the peripheral muscles, have been made possible. The advantage of this technique is that the diaphragm can be separated from other respiratory muscles. Three types of data can be obtained: dose–response curve, onset characteristics and recovery characteristics. The cumulative dose–response curve for the diaphragm is shifted to the right compared with that of the adductor pollicis for pancuronium (Donati *et al.* 1986), atracurium (Laycock *et al.* 1988*b*), and vecuronium (Laycock *et al.* 1988b; Lebreault *et al.* 1989) (Fig. 21.3). The dose of pancuronium associated with 50% depression of response of the diaphragm to the first stimulation in the train of four (ED_{50}) is twice that of the adductor pollicis (Donati *et al.* 1986). The ED_{50} ratios are 1.56 for atracurium and 1.47 for vecuronium, suggesting that both atracurium and vecuronium exhibit a similar degree of sparing at the diaphragm (Laycock *et al.* 1988*b*). Thus complete paralysis of the diaphragm is not expected with a dose of relaxant that barely blocks the adductor pollicis. Laycock *et al.* (1988*a*) have compared the potency of pancuronium at both muscles in children and demonstrated that the ratio of diaphragm to adductor pollicis ED_{50} varied between 1.64 and 1.75 in children compared with 2.14 in adults. Smith *et al.* (1988) demonstrated that the diaphragm-sparing effect of suxmethonium was comparable to that previously reported for nondepolarizing muscle relaxants.

These data suggest that the diaphragm requires a greater concentration of neuromuscular blocking agent than the adductor pollicis for a similar degree of block. Theoretically, these differences could be attributed to differences in type of receptors, number of receptors, amount of neurotransmitter released with each stimulus, or quantity of acetylcholinesterase. Lu (1970) has compared the affinity of muscle relaxants for the acetylcholine receptors of the isolated diaphragm, latissimus dorsi, and serratus anterior muscles in guinea-pig. He found that the concentration required for a certain percentage occupancy (say 50%) was the same for all three muscles. However the concentration of relaxant required for any degree of block was greater at the diaphragm. Similar results were obtained by Waud and Waud (1972) in cats, who found that, following tubocurarine administration, neuromuscular transmission occurs when approximately 18% of the receptors are free at the diaphragm, whereas 29% free receptors are required at the tibialis muscle. This indicates that the diaphragm does not necessarily have a different acetylcholine receptor, but may have a higher receptor density, higher acetylcholine release, or smaller acetylcholinesterase activity. Sterz *et al.* (1983) determined the dose–response relationship of motor endplates in mammalian fast and slow muscles by performing quantitative iontophoresis, and demonstrated that differences in the density of ionic channels could exist between muscles. 'Fast-twitch muscles' such as the omohyoideus or the extensor digitorum muscle have a similar density of channel whereas in the soleus muscle, a 'slow-twitch muscle', the channel density is half of that of the former two. The lack of significant difference in the Hill coefficient or slope off dose–response curve suggests that postjunctional receptors are similar at both fast and slow muscles. This lower density of acetylcholine receptors in slow muscle could explain, at least in part, the lower margin of safety for neuromuscular transmission compared with fast muscle.

Surprisingly, the onset of neuromuscular block is significantly more rapid at the diaphragm than at the adductor pollicis despite the resistance of the diaphragm to muscle relaxants in humans. This was observed with paralysing doses of atracurium (Pansart *et al.* 1987; Derrington and Hindocha 1988), vecuronium 0.1 mg/kg (Chauvin *et al.* 1987; Derrington and Hindocha 1988), pancuronium, tubocurarine, alcuronium (Derrington and Hindocha 1990), and suxamethonium (Pansart *et al.* 1987). The onset of neuromuscular block is influenced by several factors among which the access to muscle plays an important role. Goat *et al.* (1976) demonstrated that the onset time of gallamine neuromuscular block was shortened by increasing blood flow to muscle. The diaphragm receives a larger blood flow than limb

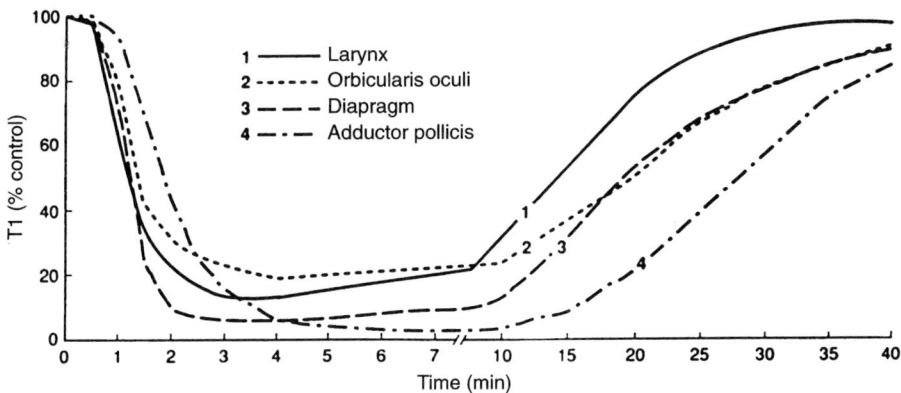

Fig. 21.4 Onset and recovery of neuromuscular blockade after injection of vecuronium 0.07 mg/kg at four muscles. (Data from Donati *et al.* 1990, 1991.)

skeletal muscles, because of its main role for breathing and its proximity to the aorta (Rochester and Briscoe 1979). It follows that the diaphragmatic muscle tends to be paralysed more rapidly than more peripheral, less perfused muscles, such as the adductor pollicis (Donati 1988). When subparalysing doses of relaxants are given, time to maximum block is shorter at the diaphragm. For vecuronium 0.04 mg/kg, onset time is 2.9 min for the diaphragm and 6.6 min for the adductor pollicis (Donati *et al.* 1990). Maximum block (77 and 83%, respectively) is, however, similar at both muscles. (Fig. 21.4). This seems to contradict the concept that the diaphragm is resistant to the effects of relaxants. The apparent paradox is resolved if one considers that plasma concentrations decrease rapidly after a bolus dose. Thus, they are greater when the diaphragm is blocked maximally than when the adductor pollicis is (Fig. 21.5). In pharmacokinetic–dynamic terms, the diaphragm has a greater concentration for 50% block (CP50) (Walker *et al.* 1987; Debaene *et al.* 1990), and a faster transfer rate constant (ke_0) (Walker *et al.* 1987).

Distinct ultrastructural differences exist at the neuromuscular junction according to the type of myofibre (Padykula and Gauthier 1970). Some authors have raised the hypothesis that these differences could influence the rate of access of neuromuscular blocking drug to the neuromuscular junction, although this has never been confirmed.

Because the diaphragm recovers at higher plasma concentrations, recovery from diaphragmatic block occurs sooner than does adductor pollicis recovery. With vecuronium 0.1 mg/kg, the twitch height at the diaphragm returned to 25% of control value after 27 min compared with 41 min at the adductor pollicis. Complete twitch height recovery was achieved after 49 min for the diaphragm and 74 min for the adductor pollicis (Chauvin *et al.* 1987). Similar findings were obtained with atracurium, and when the diaphragm had completely recovered the twitch height of the adductor pollicis was still 50% with either vecuronium or atracurium. Recovery

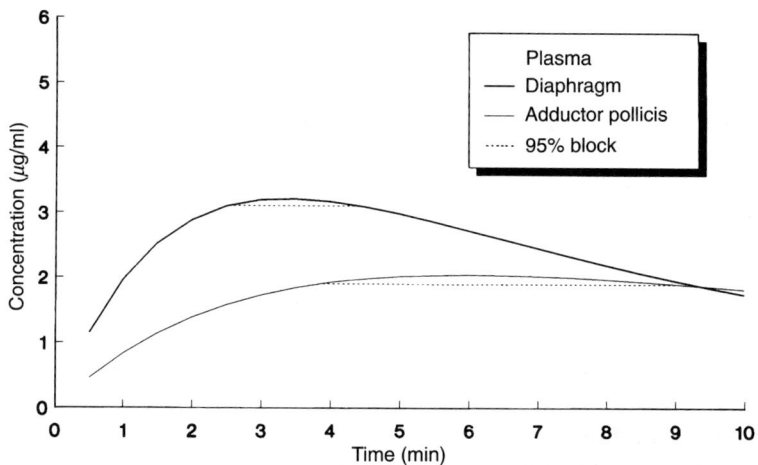

Fig. 21.5 Predicted muscle relaxant concentration time-course both in plasma and in the effect compartment at both diaphragm and adductor pollicis.

was also faster at the diaphragm with tubocurarine, pancuronium, and alcuronium (Derrington and Hindocha 1990). After suxamethonium administration, the diaphragm also started to recover from paralysis sooner than the adductor pollicis, full recovery occurring 2 min later at the adductor pollicis than at the diaphragm (Pansart *et al.* 1987). Recovery is much slower than onset and the concentration gradient between neuromuscular junction and plasma is small (pseudo-equilibrium state). It is likely that the concentrations of muscle relaxant are the same at both muscles. Thus, blood flow plays a minor role in recovery from block. Neuromuscular effect follows declining plasma concentrations. For example, CP_{50} for the diaphragm and the adductor pollicis were 122 and 74 ng/ml, respectively, suggesting the lower sensitivity of the diaphragm to muscle relaxants (Debaene *et al.* 1990).

Other respiratory muscles

No data have been obtained using single twitch or train-of-four stimulation of a nerve supplying intercostal, abdominal or accessory muscles of respiration. Indirect data in awake subjects, however, suggest that these muscles are less resistant to nondepolarizing drugs than is the diaphragm. Spontaneous EMG during partial paralysis was greater for the diaphragm than for other muscles of respiration (De Troyer *et al.* 1980). Inspiratory pressures are affected less by tubocurarine than expiratory pressures (Johansen *et al.* 1964; Arora and Gal 1981), and the diaphragm is an inspiratory muscle.

UPPER AIRWAY

There is indirect evidence that the muscles of the upper airway are particularly sensitive to the effects of relaxants. In many studies involving awake subjects, many individuals needed to have their airway maintained by the investigator at levels of paralysis associated with only a modest decrease in vital capacity. De Troyer *et al.* (1980) attributed the decrease in maximal minute ventilation produced with partial paralysis to increases in upper airway resistance. Pavlin *et al.* (1989) reported that total airway obstruction was achieved with a dose of tubocurarine which produced an inspiratory pressure of 45 cm H_2O, i.e. as much as 50% of control. Small doses of pancuronium (0.02 mg/kg) depress the swallowing reflex to a greater extent than the strength of peripheral muscles (Isono *et al.* 1991) (Fig. 21.6). This indicates that muscles involved with maintenance of airway patency are more sensitive to relaxants than other respiratory muscles and possibly peripheral muscles. Thus following administration of small doses of nondepolarizing muscle relaxants, such as used during the priming technique, there is a risk of aspirating gastric content by paralysis of upper airway muscles.

Although it is generally agreed that the upper airway is kept patent through an active mechanism (Brouillette and Tach 1979), the roles of the masseter, geniohyoid, genioglossus, pharyngeal muscles, and laryngeal adductors are not known.

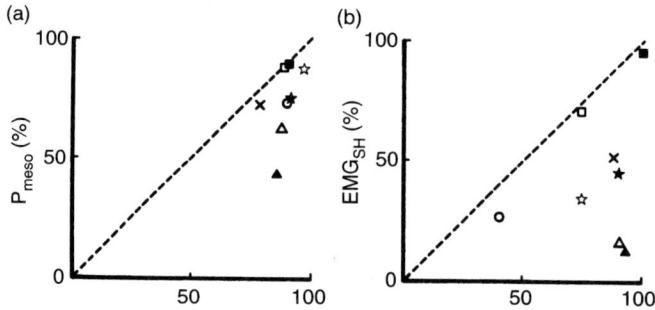

Fig. 21.6 (a) Mesopharyngeal pressure (P_{meso}) versus hand grip strength. (b) Electromyographic activity of hypopharynx (EMG_{sh}) versus train-of-four ratio at hypothenar eminence. (Data from in volunteers receiving pancuronium 0.02 mg/kg. Indices of pharyngeal function are depressed more than peripheral muscle function.) (From Isono *et al.* 1991.)

Of those, the masseter has been studied most extensively because it is relatively easy to investigate.

Masseter

In cats the masseter has been found to be more sensitive than respiratory or limb muscles to tubocurarine, pancuronium or pipecuronium (Kharkevich and Fisenko 1981). The cumulative dose–response curve for pancuronium is shifted to the left compared with the adductor pollicis, i.e. the masseter is approximately 15% more sensitive to the drug (Smith *et al.* 1989*a*). The neuromuscular blocking effects of suxamethonium are approximately the same for both muscles in adults (Smith *et al.* 1989*b*), and more profound at the masseter in children (Plumley *et al.* 1990). Onset of action is more rapid at the masseter, for all drugs tested, and both in adults and children (Smith *et al.* 1989*a*; Plumley *et al.* 1990; Saddler *et al.* 1990*a, b*). These data indicate that jaw relaxation, which is required for adequate intubating conditions, can be obtained rapidly with small doses of neuromuscular blocking drugs. Recovery of the masseter and possibly other upper airway muscles is probably, however, slower than other respiratory muscles such as the diaphragm.

The masseter has an unusual response to suxamethonium. A significant reduction in mouth opening and an increase in jaw stiffness occurs at a time when full relaxation of the limb muscles is obtained (Van der Spek *et al.* 1987). This reduction in mouth opening is observed within 60 seconds after loss of twitch at hand muscles and cessation of fasciculations (Van der Spek *et al.* 1990). The increase in masseter tone may be greater than 500 *g* (Leary and Ellis 1990), usually occurs within one minute, returns to normal within one to two minutes after suxamethonium administration (Plumley *et al.* 1990) (Fig. 21.7), and is usually overcome easily by the laryngoscopist. It is now accepted, however, that the normal response of the masseter to suxamethonium is an increase in jaw stiffness which is maximal at the time of muscle fasciculations, is transient, and is not accompanied by other signs of hyper-

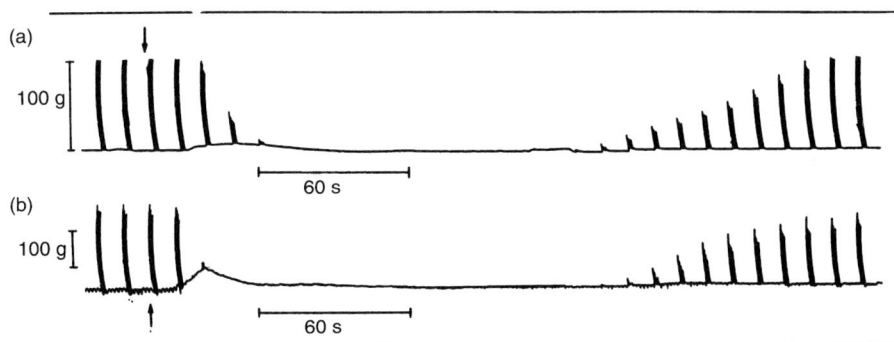

Fig. 21.7 Response of adductor pollicis (a) and masseter (b) to suxamethonium given at the arrow in a normal child. Neuromuscular blockade occurs sooner at the masseter. However, there is an increase in tone (baseline shifts upwards) at the masseter which persists even after evoked twitch height is abolished completely. A similar increase in tone, but of smaller magnitude, is also observed at the adductor pollicis. (From Saddler *et al.* 1990.)

metabolism (Saddler 1991). The adductor pollicis also shows an increase in tension after suxamethonium, but of much less magnitude (Plumley *et al.* 1990). This phenomenon is not observed after nondepolarizing agents (Van der Spek 1990).

The mechanism of action for this effect remains speculative; the increase in tone might be present even in the presence of total neuromuscular block at the masseter. The ineffectiveness of subparalysing doses of tubocurarine in preventing tension increases suggests that this effect of suxamethonium is not presynaptic. A paralysing dose of atracurium, however, abolished the effect entirely (Smith *et al.* 1990), suggesting that nicotinic acetylcholine receptors — either junctional or extrajunctional — are involved. A direct action on muscle is unlikely as atracurium, which acts at the neuromuscular junction, blocks this increase in tone. It had been suggested that masseter spasm might be an extreme case of the apparently normal dose-related increase in resting tension (Brandom 1990). Nevertheless patients who are at increased risk for masseter spasm or masseter muscle rigidity, such as children with strabismus, do not show a significantly different increase in masseter tone from normal children (Saddler *et al.* 1990*b*).

For many years, the phenomenon called masseter spasm (Donlon *et al.* 1978), suxamethonium spasm (Ellis and Halsall 1984), masseter muscle rigidity (Rosenberg and Fletcher 1986), or trismus (Rosenberg 1987) has been felt to be an unusual sign presaging malignant hyperthermia (MH). Because this is a subjective diagnosis, reported instances are very variable. Retrospective studies in the USA have suggested an incidence of 1 in 800 (Schwartz *et al.* 1984) whereas incidence has been described as 1 in 12 000 in Denmark (Ording 1985). Jaw stiffness may be an early sign of MH, but is not specific for it (Hackl *et al.* 1990). Therefore, both Van der Spek *et al.* (1990) and Saddler (1991) have suggested that, after appearance of a jaw stiffness, signs of hypermetabolism (increased core temperature, increased end-tidal core temperature, metabolic and respiratory acidosis) should be sought before a diagnosis of

MH is contemplated. Expressing the opposite opinion, Allen and Rosenberg (1990) have recommended discontinuation of anaesthesia, unless the procedure is urgent, because of the inability to predict outcome after an increased jaw stiffness.

Laryngeal muscles

It has been known for several years that the effects of a neuromuscular blocking drug could differ at the laryngeal and peripheral muscles (Baer 1984), and that discrepancies could exist between tracheal intubating conditions and the intensity of peripheral paralysis. Carnie *et al.* (1986) demonstrated that after injection of suxamethonium, intubation could be attempted before the response to the train of four at the adductor pollicis is abolished.

The assessment of the effects of muscle relaxants at the laryngeal muscles has been made possible by stimulation of the recurrent laryngeal nerve in association with measurements of contraction of laryngeal adductor muscles (Donati *et al.* 1991*b*). All of the intrinsic laryngeal muscles controlling movements of vocal folds induce vocal cord adduction except the cricothyroid, which is a tensor of the vocal cords, and the posterior cricoarytenoid muscle which causes vocal cord abduction (Snell and Katz 1988; Bartlett 1989). Stimulation at the notch of the thyroid cartilage causes a selective stimulation of adductor muscles because this site of stimulation is close to the anterior branches of the recurrent laryngeal nerve which supply these muscles (Steinberg *et al.* 1986).

Laryngeal adductor muscles are more resistant to nondepolarizing muscle relaxants than is the adductor pollicis. The ED_{90} of vecuronium is 46 μg/kg at the adductor pollicis and 80 μg/kg at the vocal cords (Donati *et al.* 1991*a*). The same sparing effect on the laryngeal muscles has been also described with rocuronium (Org 9426) in humans, and the ED_{50} ratio is 1.52 (Plaud *et al.* 1991). Therefore complete paralysis of vocal cords requires doses greater than those which block the adductor pollicis. No information is available on the margin of safety of the laryngeal muscles. This resistance might, however, be explained by histological and physiological differences between laryngeal and peripheral muscles, e.g. the adductor pollicis. The laryngeal adductor muscles, particularly the thyroarytenoid muscle have fast contraction times (Sanders *et al.* 1987), whereas the adductor pollicis is made up mostly of slow fibres (Johnson *et al.* 1973) and exhibits slow contraction time. Experimental data in the cat and in the pig have shown that nondepolarizing muscle relaxants tend to produce a larger block at fast-twitch than slow-twitch muscles (Sutherland *et al.* 1983; Muir and Marshall 1987; Muir *et al.* 1989). Furthermore Secher *et al.* (1982) demonstrated that there was a relationship between the percentage of slow-twitch fibres and the degree of curarization in humans. These differences in sensitivity of different muscles might be due to the larger number of acetylcholine receptors in fast-twitch fibres (Sterz *et al.* 1983). Recovery from neuromuscular block at the vocal cords occurs sooner than adductor pollicis (Fig. 21.4). Following administration of twice the ED_{95}, recovery of the vocal cords to 90% of control value occurred in approximately in 23 minutes whereas similar recovery at the adductor pollicis took 40 minutes for both vecuronium and atracurium (Donati *et al.* 1991*a*; Plaud *et al.* 1991). This was probably due to the sparing effects of nondepolarizing muscle relaxants on fast-contracting muscles, an effect previously observed at the diaphragm. Onset of neuromuscular block is faster at the vocal cords than at the adductor pollicis. Following approximately twice the ED_{95}, maximum block of the laryngeal adductor muscles occurred 3.3 min and 1.3 min after vecuronium and rocuronium administration, respectively, whereas the adductor pollicis was blocked in 5.7 min and 2.4 min, respectively (Donati *et al.* 1991*a*; Plaud *et al.* 1991) (Fig. 21.4). These findings, already reported for the diaphragm, are probably due to the greater vascularity and the proximity to the central circulation of the laryngeal muscles, compared to peripheral muscles.

Unlike nondepolarizing muscle relaxants, suxamethonium produces a more profound block at the vocal cords than at the adductor pollicis. After 0.25 mg/kg, block of the first twitch is 66% of control at the vocal cords and 45% at the adductor pollicis. With 0.5 mg/kg, maximum block is slightly greater at the vocal cords (93%) than at the adductor pollicis (84%) (Meistelman *et al.* 1991) (Fig. 21.8). This sparing effect on the adductor pollicis might also be related to the different sensitivities of different fibre types and muscle relaxants. Experimental data in cats (Sutherland *et al.* 1983; Choi *et al.* 1984) and pigs (Muir and Marshall 1987) suggest that, unlike nondepolarizing blockers, suxamethonium is more effective in blocking the fast-contracting tibialis than the slow-contracting soleus. Suxamethonium produces more rapid vocal cord neuromuscular block than the adductor pollicis. With 0.5 mg/kg, time to maximum neuromuscular block was 0.9 min at the vocal cords and 1.7 min at the adductor pollicis, with the onset at the laryngeal muscles occurring during fasciculations of peripheral muscles. Therefore rapid onset of action and some selectivity for laryngeal adductor muscles make this drug particularly suitable for tracheal intubation.

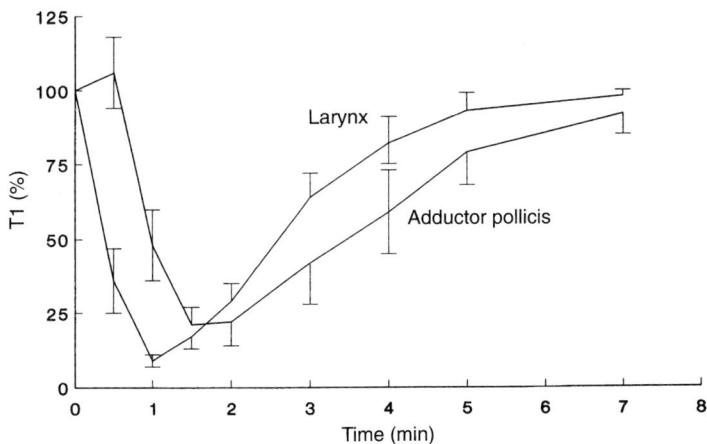

Fig. 21.8 Effect of suxamethonium 0.5 mg/kg on adductor muscles of the larynx and adductor pollicis. (From Meistelman *et al.* 1991.)

ORBICULARIS OCULI MUSCLE

Initial studies had demonstrated that the orbicularis oculi was relatively resistant to the effects of muscle relaxants and recovered more rapidly than did the adductor pollicis (Stiffel *et al.* 1980; Caffrey *et al.* 1986). The onset and the intensity of paralysis at the orbicularis oculi and the diaphragm are very close during vecuronium-induced neuromuscular block (Donati *et al.* 1990) (Fig. 21.4). Since the sensitivity of the orbicularis oculi to a neuromuscular blocking drug is probably less than that of other muscles, its paralysis probably indicates complete block of almost all muscles whose relaxation is required for good intubating conditions. Following a bolus of atracurium (0.5 mg/kg), the onset of neuromuscular block at the orbicularis oculi (145 s) and at the vocal cords (132 s) do not differ significantly, both being blocked faster than the adductor pollicis (242 s) (Ungureanu *et al.* 1993). Thus, monitoring the orbicularis oculi by stimulating the facial nerve may be valuable for assessing the onset of neuromuscular block at the respiratory muscles and the vocal cords. It also might be a better indicator of deep neuromuscular block than the adductor pollicis, and be useful for maintenance of profound block. Recovery characteristics of the orbicularis oculi are similar to those of the diaphragm.

The facial nerve also supplies the orbicularis ori. With both vecuronium and atracurium, it was demonstrated that this muscle recovered more rapidly than the hand muscles (Sharpe *et al.* 1991). It must, however, be stressed than the sensitivity and time-course are not necessarily the same as the orbicularis oculi.

PERIPHERAL MUSCLES

Many superficial nerves supplying one or more muscles can be used for monitoring purposes. In clinical anaesthesia and in research, monitoring of the adductor pollicis following ulnar nerve stimulation is a standard procedure for monitoring of neuromuscular block. The ulnar nerve supplies several other hand muscles (hypothenar muscles, interosseous muscles) (Rosenberg and Greenhow 1978), but their response to muscle relaxants could differ slightly from the adductor pollicis. The muscles of the hypothenar eminence, including the abductor digiti minimi, are more resistant to nondepolarizing muscle relaxants than the adductor pollicis (Katz 1973; Kopman 1985; Dupuis *et al.* 1990) (Fig. 21.9). A train-of-four ratio of 0.9 at the hypothenar muscles has approximately the same significance as a train of four of 0.7 at the adductor pollicis muscle. Following administration of a nondepolarizing muscle relaxant, the time-course and intensity of neuromuscular block at the first dorsal interosseous muscle of the hand are the same as those at the adductor pollicis (Harper 1988; Kopman 1988). Because the electromyographic signal recorded over the first dorsal interosseous has a large amplitude (Kalli 1990) and the response is similar to that of the adductor

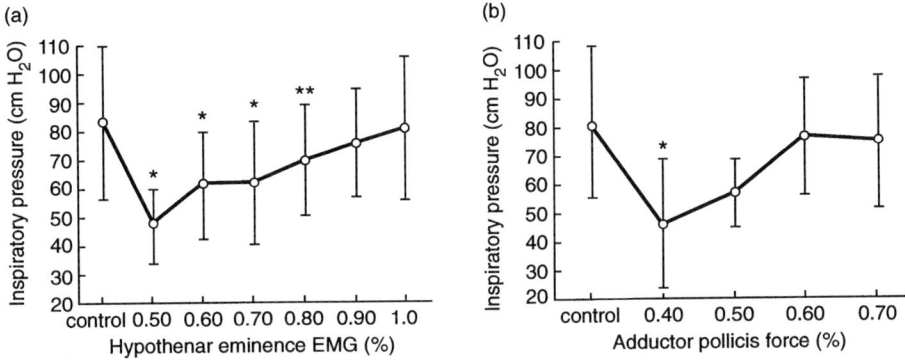

Fig. 21.9 Relationship of inspiratory force to hypothenar eminence EMG (a) or adductor pollicis force (b) in volunteers given vecuronium. Return of normal inspiratory force occurs at a higher level at the former than the latter, because the hypothenar eminence is more resistant to vecuronium than the adductor pollicis is. (From Dupuis *et al.* 1990.)

pollicis, it has been suggested than it could be a site of choice for the electromyographic monitoring. Stimulation of the ulnar nerve at the elbow also induces contraction of the flexor carpi ulnaris and flexor digitorum profundus muscles. The sensitivity of these muscles may, however, be different from that of the adductor pollicis.

Stimulation of the posterior tibial nerve induces contraction of the flexor hallucis brevis and large toe plantar flexion. Its use has been suggested when the hand muscles were not accessible. Onset and recovery from nondepolarizing block do not appear different from that at the adductor pollicis (Sopher *et al.* 1988).

IMPLICATIONS FOR MONITORING

For many years the monitoring of neuromuscular transmission has almost only used the adductor pollicis because of its ease of use and the invaluable information it may give. During induction of anaesthesia the adductor pollicis has been used widely to determine the optimal time to intubation, but discrepancies have been described between tracheal intubating conditions and the intensity of peripheral paralysis (Bencini and Newton 1984; Carnie *et al.* 1986). This may be explained by differences in onset time and intensity of neuromuscular block between the respiratory and the upper airway muscles and the adductor pollicis. The onset of paralysis at the orbicularis oculi approaches that of the diaphragm (Donati *et al.* 1990) and the laryngeal adductor muscles (Ungureanu *et al.* 1993). Monitoring of the orbicularis oculi may therefore be useful to determine onset of paralysis at muscles whose relaxation is required for good intubating conditions. Since the sensitivity of the orbicularis oculi to muscle relaxants is a good reflection of diaphragmatic and laryngeal adductor muscles block, paralysis of the orbicularis oculi probably indicates complete block of the respiratory muscles.

During surgery when an intense neuromuscular block is required, disappearance of the train of four at the adductor pollicis does not eliminate the possibility of hiccups, cough, and extrusion of abdominal contents. The use of the post-tetanic count (PTC) technique may allow the evaluation of the very intense block (Viby-Mogensen *et al*. 1981, Viby-Mogensen 1982), although it cannot be repeated more often than every five minutes as facilitation of subsequent responses may occur. Monitoring of the orbicularis oculi, using train-of-four stimuli, appears to be preferable to the use of PTC at the adductor pollicis because the response of the orbicularis oculi is a good reflection of diaphragmatic paralysis. When profound block is not required, monitoring of the adductor pollicis using train-of-four is sufficient and allows easier antagonism of relaxation at the end of surgery.

Although the orbicularis oculi may be valuable for monitoring the onset of relaxation and for maintenance of a profound block, the adductor pollicis is probably preferable for the management of recovery because it is a sensitive muscle (Donati *et al*. 1990). When the adductor pollicis has almost completely recovered it can be assumed that no residual paralysis exists at either the diaphragmatic muscle or the laryngeal adductor muscles. It is, however, important that monitoring of the adductor pollicis be used in association with clinical tests of recovery such as the patient's ability to lift the head for five seconds, to protrude the tongue or to swallow, because in the latter, muscles of the upper airway are very sensitive to muscle relaxants.

CONCLUSION

Neuromuscular relaxants are usually thought of as working at the neuromuscular junction. In fact their sites of action are the neuromuscular junction of many muscles, which all have different sensitivities to these drugs and their time-course of effect. These differences have important implications for the safe conduct of relaxation and for monitoring.

Data regarding intensity and time-course of muscle relaxation has been obtained for only a few muscles and only a few neuromuscular blocking drugs have been tested. However, it is not necessary to have information about all muscles. It is probably only sufficient to know the behaviour of extreme cases: the most resistant and the most sensitive, and the ones with the fastest and the slowest onsets. Current evidence suggest that the laryngeal adductor muscles are the most resistant muscles to nondepolarizing block, and upper airway musculature and the adductor pollicis are among the most sensitive. On the other hand, peripheral muscles have slower onsets than centrally located muscles.

Thus, it is suggested that the site of monitoring should be adapted to the requirements for paralysis. A fast-onset, resistant muscle such as the orbicularis oculi appears best suited to tracheal intubation and maintenance of profound relaxation, whereas a slow-onset, sensitive muscle such as the adductor pollicis would appear ideal for the monitoring of less intense levels of paralysis and for recovery.

REFERENCES

Ali, H. H., Wilson, R. S., Savarese, J. J., and Kitz, R. J. (1975). The effect of tubocurarine on indirectly elicited train-of-four muscle response and respiratory measurements in humans. *British Journal of Anaesthesia*, **47**, 570–4.

Allen, G. C. and Rosenberg, H. (1990). Malignant hyperthermia susceptibility in adult patients with masseter muscle rigidity. *Canadian Journal of Anaesthesia*, **37**, 31–5.

Arora, N. S. and Gal, T. J. (1981). Cough dynamics during progressive expiratory muscle weakness in healthy curarized subjects. *Journal of Applied Physiology*, **51**, 494–8.

Baer, G. A. (1984). Laryngeal muscle recovery after suxamethonium. *Anaesthesia*, **39**, 143–6.

Bartlett, D. (1989). Respiratory functions of the larynx. *Physiological Reviews*, **69**, 33–57.

Bencini, A. and Newton, D. E. F. (1984). Rate of onset of good intubating conditions, respiratory depression and hand muscles paralysis after vecuronium. *British Journal of Anaesthesia*, **56**, 959–65.

Brandom, B. W. (1990). Atracurium and succinylcholine on the masseter muscle. *Canadian Journal of Anaesthesia*, **37**, 7–11.

Brouilette, R. T. and Tach, B. T. (1979). A neuromuscular mechanism maintaining extrathoracic airway patency. *Journal of Applied Physiology*, **46**, 772–9.

Caffrey, R. R., Warren, M. L., and Becker, K. E. (1986). Neuromuscular blockade monitoring comparing the orbicularis oculi and adductor pollicis muscles. *Anesthesiology*, **65**, 95–7.

Carnie, J. C., Street, M. K., and Kumar, B. (1986). Emergency intubation of the trachea facilitated by suxamethonium. *British Journal of Anaesthesia*, **58**, 498–501.

Chauvin, M., Lebrault, C., and Duvaldestin, P. (1987). The neuromuscular blocking effect of vecuronium on the human diaphragm. *Anesthesia and Analgesia*, **66**, 117–22.

Choi, W. W., Gergis, S. D., and Sokoll, M. D. (1984). Effects of succinylcholine chloride on the response of fast and slow muscle in the cat. *Acta Anaesthesiologica Scandinavica*, **28**, 516–20.

Debaene, B., Guesde, R., Clergue, F., and Lienhart, A. (1990). Plasma concentration–response relationship of pancuronium for the diaphragm and the adductor pollicis in anesthetized man. *Anesthesiology*, **73**, A887.

De Troyer, A., Bastenier, J., and Delhez, L. (1980). Function of respiratory muscles during partial curarization in humans. *Journal of Applied Physiology*, **49**, 1049–56.

Derrington, M. C. and Hindocha, N. (1988). Comparison of neuromuscular block in the diaphragm and hand. *British Journal of Anaesthesia*, **61**, 279–85.

Derrington, M. C. and Hindocha, N. (1990). Comparison of neuromuscular block in the diaphragm and hand after administration of tubocurarine, pancuronium and alcuronium. *British Journal of Anaesthesia*, **64**, 294–9.

Donati, F. (1988). Onset of action of relaxants. *Canadian Journal of Anaesthesia*, **35**, S52–8.

Donati, F., Antzaka, C., and Bevan, D. R. (1986). Potency of pancuronium at the diaphragm and the adductor pollicis in humans. *Anesthesiology*, **65**, 1–5.

Donati, F., Meistelman, C., and Plaud, B. (1990). Vecuronium neuromuscular blockade at the diaphragm, the orbicularis oculi and adductor pollicis muscles. *Anesthesiology*, **73**, 870–75.

Donati, F., Meistelman, C., and Plaud, B. (1991*a*). Vecuronium neuromuscular blockade at the adductor muscles of the larynx and adductor pollicis. *Anesthesiology*, **74**, 833–7.

Donati, F., Plaud, B., and Meistelman, C. (1991*b*). A method to measure elicited contraction of laryngeal adductor muscles during anesthesia. *Anesthesiology*, **74**, 827–32.

Donlon, J. W., Newfield P., Sreter, F., and Ryan, J. F. (1978). Implications of masseter spasm after succinylcholine. *Anesthesiology*, **49**, 298–301.

Dupuis, J. Y., Martin, R., and Tetrault, J. P. (1990). Clinical, electrical and mechanical correlations during recovery from neuromuscular blockade with vecuronium. *Canadian Journal of Anaesthesia*, **37**, 192–6.

Ellis, F. R. and Halsall P. J. (1984). Suxamethonium spasm. A differential diagnostic conundrum. *British Journal of Anaesthesia*, **56**, 381–4.

Foldes, F. F., Monte, A. P., Brunn, H. M., and Wolfson, B. (1961). Studies with muscle relaxants in anaesthetized subjects. *Anesthesiology*, **22**, 230–6.

Gal, T. J. and Goldberg, S. K. (1980). Diaphragmatic function in healthy subjects during partial curarization. *Journal of Applied Physiology*, **48**, 921–6.

Gal, T. J. and Goldberg, S. K. (1981). Relationship between respiratory muscle strength and vital capacity during partial curarization in awake subjects. *Anesthesiology*, **34**, 141–7.

Gal, T. J. and Smith, T. C. (1976). Partial paralysis with *d*-tubocurarine and the ventilatory response to CO_2. *Anesthesiology*, **45**, 22–28.

Goat, V. A., Yeung, M. L., Blakeney, C., and Feldman, S. A. (1976). The effect of blood flow upon the activity of gallamine triethiodide. *British Journal of Anaesthesia*, **48**, 69–73.

Hackl, W., Mauritz, W., Schemper, M., Winkler, M., Sporn, P., and Steinbereithner, K. (1990). Prediction of malignant hyperthermia susceptibility: statistical evaluation of clinical signs. *British Journal of Anaesthesia*, **64**, 425–9.

Harper, N. J. N. (1988). Comparison of the adductor pollicis and the first dorsal interosseous muscles during atracurium and vecuronium blockade: an electromyographic study. *British Journal of Anaesthesia*, **61**, 477–8.

Isono, S., Ide, T., Kochi, T., Mizuguchi, T., and Nishino, T. (1991). Effects of partial paralysis on the swallowing reflex in conscious humans. *Anesthesiology*, **75**, 980–4.

Johansen, S. H., Jorgensen, M., and Molbech, S. (1964). Effect of tubocurarine on respiratory and nonrespiratory muscle power in man. *Journal of Applied Physiology*, **19**, 990–4.

Johnson, M. A., Polgar, J., Weightman, D., and Appleton, D. (1973). Data on the distribution of fibre types in thirty six human muscles: an autopsy study. *Journal of the Neurological Sciences*, **18**, 111–29.

Kalli, L. (1990). Effect of surface electrode position on the compound action potential evoked by ulnar nerve stimulation during isoflurane anaesthesia. *British Journal of Anaesthesia*, **64**, 494–9.

Katz, R. L. (1973). Electromyographic and mechanical effects of suxamethonium and tubocurarine on twitch, tetanic and post-tetanic responses. *British Journal of Anaesthesia*, **45**, 849–59.

Kharkevich, D. A. and Fisenko, V. P. (1981). The effects of neuromuscular blocking agents on the acetylcholine receptors of different skeletal muscles. *Archives Internationales de Pharmacodynamie et de Thérapie*, **251**, 255–69.

Kopman, A. F. (1985). The relationship of evoked electromyographic and mechanical responses following atracurium in humans. *Anesthesiology*, **63**, 208–11.

Kopman, A. F. (1988). The dose–effect relationship of metocurine: the integrated electromyogram of the first dorsal interosseous muscle and the mechanomyogram of the adductor pollicis compared. *Anesthesiology*, **68**, 604–7.

Laycock, J. R. D., Baxter, M. K., Bevan, J. C., Sangwan, S., Donati, F., and Bevan, D. R. (1988*a*). The potency of pancuronium at the adductor pollicis and diaphragm in infants and children. *Anesthesiology*, **68**, 908–11.

Laycock, J. R. D., Donati, F., Smith, C. E., and Bevan, D. R. (1988*b*). Potency of atracurium and vecuronium at the diaphragm and the adductor pollicis muscle. *British Journal of Anaesthesia*, **61**, 286–91.

Leary, N. P. and Ellis, F. R. (1990). Masseteric muscle spasm as a normal response to suxamethonium. *British Journal of Anaesthesia*, **64**, 488–92.

Lebrault, C., Chauvin, M., Guirimand, F., and Duvaldestin, P. (1989). Relative potency of vecuronium on the diaphragm and the adductor pollicis. *British Journal of Anaesthesia*, **63**, 389–92.

Lu, T. C. (1970). Affinity of curare-like compounds and their potency in blocking neuromuscular transmission. *Journal of Pharmacology and Experimental Therapeutics*, **174**, 560–6.

Meistelman, C., Plaud, B., and Donati, F. (1991). Neuromuscular effects of succinylcholine on the vocal cords and adductor pollicis muscles. *Anesthesia and Analgesia*, **73**, 278–82.

Muir, A. W. and Marshall, R. J. (1987). Comparative neuromuscular blocking effects of vecuronium, pancuronium, ORG 6368 and suxamethonium in the anaesthetized domestic pig. *British Journal of Anaesthesia*, **59**, 622–9.

Muir, A. W., Houston, J., Green, K. L., Marshall, R. J., Bowman, W. C., and Marshall, I. G. (1989). Effects of a new neuromuscular blocking agent (ORG 9426) in anaesthetized cats and pigs and in isolated nerve–muscle preparations. *British Journal of Anaesthesia*, **63**, 400–10.

Nishino, T., Yokokawa, N., Hiraga, K., Honda, Y., and Mizuguchi, T. (1988). Breathing patterns of anesthetized humans during pancuronium-induced partial paralysis. *Journal of Applied Physiology*, **64**, 78–83.

Norman, J., Read, D., and du Boulay, M. (1980). Hand and respiratory paralysis by Org NC45 in man. *British Journal of Anaesthesia*, **52**, 956P.

Oliven, A., Deal E. C., Jr, Kelsen, S. G., and Cherniak, N. S. (1984). Respiratory response to partial paralysis in anaesthetized dogs. *Journal of Applied Physiology*, **56**, 1583–8.

Ording, H. (1985). Incidence of malignant hyperthermia in Denmark. *Anesthesia and Analgesia*, **64**, 700–4.

Padykula, H. A. and Gauthier, G. F. (1970). The ultrastructure of the neuromuscular junctions of mammalian red, white and intermediate skeletal muscle fibers. *Journal of Cell Biology*, **46**, 27–41.

Pansart, J. L., Chauvin, M., Lebrault, C., Gauneau, P., and Duvaldestin, P. (1987). Effect of an intubating dose of succinylcholine and atracurium on the diaphragm and the adductor pollicis muscle in humans. *Anesthesiology*, **67**, 326–30.

Paton, W. D. M., and Zaimis, E. J. (1951). The action of *d*-tubocurarine and of decamethonium on respiratory and other muscles in the cat. *Journal of Physiology* (*London*), **112**, 311–31.

Pavlin, E. G., Holle, R. H., and Schoene, R. B. (1989). Recovery of airway protection compared with ventilation after paralysis with curare. *Anesthesiology*, **70**, 381–5.

Plaud, B., Meistelman, C., and Donati, F. (1991). Organon 9426 neuromuscular blockade at the adductor pollicis of the larynx and adductor pollicis in man. *Anesthesiology*, **75**, A784.

Plumley, M. H., Bevan, J. C., Saddler, J. M., Donati, F., and Bevan, D. R. (1990). Dose-related effects of succinylcholine on the adductor pollicis and masseter muscles in children. *Canadian Journal of Anaesthesia*, **37**, 15–20.

Rigg, J. R. A., Engel, L. A., and Ritchie, B. C. (1970). The ventilatory response to carbon dioxide during partial paralysis with tubocurarine. *British Journal of Anaesthesia*, **42**, 105–8.

Rochester, D. F. and Briscoe, A. M. (1979). Metabolism of working diaphragm. *American Review of Respiratory Disease*, **119**, 101–6.

Rosenbaum, S. H., Askanazi, J., Hyman, A. I., and Kinney, J. M. (1983). Breathing patterns during curare-induced muscle weakness. *Anesthesia and Analgesia*, **62**, 809–14.

Rosenberg, H. (1987). Trismus is not trivial. *Anesthesiology*, **67**, 453–5.

Rosenberg, H. and Fletcher, J. E. (1986). Masseter muscle rigidity and malignant hyperthermia susceptibility. *Anesthesia and Analgesia*, **65**, 161–4.

Rosenberg, H. and Greenhow, D. E. (1978). Peripheral nerve stimulator performance: the influence of output, polarity and electrode placement. *Canadian Anaesthetic Society Journal*, **25**, 424–6.

Saddler, J. M. (1991). Jaw stiffness — an ill understood condition. *British Journal of Anaesthesia*, **67**, 515–6.

Saddler, J. M., Bevan, J. C., Plumley, M. H., Donati, F., and Bevan, D. R. (1990*a*). Potency of atracurium on masseter and adductor pollicis muscles in children. *Canadian Journal of Anaesthesia*, **37**, 26–30.

Saddler, J. M., Bevan, J. C., Plumley, M. H., Polomeno, R. C., Donati, F., and Bevan, D. R. (1990*b*). Jaw muscle tension after succinylcholine in children under going strabismus surgery. *Canadian Journal of Anaesthesia*, **37**, 21–5.

Sanders, I, Aviv, J., Kraus, W. M., Racenstein, M. M., and Biller, H. F. (1987). Transcutaneous electrical stimulation of the recurrent laryngeal nerve in monkeys. *Annals of Otology, Rhinology and Laryngology*, **96**, 38–42.

Schwartz, L., Rockoff, M. A., and Koka, B. V. (1984). Masseter spasm with anesthesia: incidence and implications. *Anesthesiology*, **61**, 772–5.

Secher, N. H., Rube, N., and Secher, O. (1982). Effect of tubocurarine on human soleus and gastrocnemius muscle. *Acta Anaesthesiologica Scandinavica*, **26**, 231–4.

Sharpe, M. D., Moote, C. A., Lam, A. M., and Manninen, P. H. (1991). Comparison of integrated evoked EMG between the hypothenar and facial muscle groups following atracurium and vecuronium administration. *Canadian Journal of Anaesthesia*, **38**, 318–23.

Smith, C. E., Donati, F., and Bevan, D. R. (1988). Potency of succinylcholine at the diaphragm and at the adductor pollicis muscle. *Anesthesia and Analgesia*, **67**, 625–30.

Smith, C. E., Donati, F., and Bevan, D. R. (1989*a*). Differential effects of pancuronium on masseter and adductor pollicis muscles in humans. *Anesthesiology*, **71**, 57–61.

Smith, C. E., Donati, F., and Bevan, D. R. (1989*b*). Effects of succinylcholine at the masseter and adductor pollicis muscles in adults. *Anesthesia and Analgesia*, **69**, 158–62.

Smith, C. E., Saddler, J. M., Bevan, J. C., Donati, F., and Bevan, D. R. (1990). Pretreatment with non-depolarizing neuromuscular blocking agents and suxamethonium-induced increase in resting jaw tension in children. *British Journal of Anaesthesia*, **64**, 577–81.

Snell, R. S. and Katz, J. (1988). *Clinical Anatomy for Anesthesiologists*, pp. 21–28. Appleton and Lange, Norwalk.

Sopher, M. J., Sears, D. H., and Walts, L. F. (1988). Neuromuscular function monitoring comparing the flexor hallucis brevis and adductor pollicis muscles. *Anesthesiology*, **69**, 129–31.

Steinberg, J. L., Khane, G. J., Fernandes, M. C., and Nel, J. P. (1986). Anatomy of the recurrent laryngeal nerve: a redescription. *Journal of Laryngology and Otology*, **100**, 919–27.

Sterz, R., Pagala, M., and Peper, K. (1983). Postjunctional characteristics of the endplates in mammalian fast and slow muscles. *Pflugers Archiv*, **398**, 48–54.

Stiffel, P., Hameroff, S. R., Blitt, C. D., and Cork, R. C. (1980). Variability in assessment of neuromuscular blockade. *Anesthesiology*, **52**, 436–7.

Sutherland, G. A., Squire, I. B., Gibb, A. J., and Marshall, I. G. (1983). Neuromuscular blocking and autonomic effects of vecuronium and atracurium in the anaesthetized cat. *British Journal of Anaesthesia*, **55**, 1119–26.

Ungureanu, D., Meistelman, C., Frossard, J., and Donati, F. (1993). The orbicularis oculi and adductor pollicis muscles as monitors of atracurium blockade of laryngeal muscles. *Anesthesia and Analgesia*, **77**, 775–9.

Van der Spek A. F. L., Fang W. B., Ashton-Miller, J. A., Stohler, C. S., Carlson, D. S., and Schork, M. A. (1987). The effects of succinylcholine on mouth opening. *Anesthesiology*, **67**, 459–65.

Van der Spek, A. F. L., Reynolds, P. I., Fang, W. B., Ashton Miller, J. A., Stohler, C. S., and Schork, M. A. (1990). Changes in resistance to mouth opening induced by depolarizing and non-depolarizing neuromuscular relaxants. *British Journal of Anaesthesia*, **64**, 21–27.

Viby-Mogensen, J. (1982). Clinical assessment of neuromuscular transmission. *British Journal of Anaesthesia*, **54**, 209–23.

Viby-Mogensen, J., Howardy-Hansen, P., Chraemer-Jorgensen, B., Ording, H., Engbaek, J., and Nielsen, A. (1981). Post tetanic count (PTC): a new method of evaluating an intense nondepolarizing neuromuscular blockade. *Anesthesiology*, **55**, 458–61.

Walker, J. S., Shanks, C. A., Borton, C., and Brown, K. F. (1987). Alcuronium pharmacodynamics in dogs: effect–concentration relationship in the diaphragmatic and limb muscles. *Journal of Pharmacy and Pharmacology*, **39**, 614–20.

Waud, B. E. and Waud, D. R. (1972). The margin of safety of neuromuscular transmission in the muscle of the diaphragm. *Anesthesiology*, **37**, 417–22.

Williams, J. P. and Bourke, D. L. (1985). Effects of succinylcholine on respiratory and non-respiratory muscle strength in humans. *Anesthesiology*, **63**, 299–303.

Wymore, M. L. and Eisele, J. H. (1978). Differential effects of *d*-tubocurarine on inspiratory and two peripheral muscles in anesthetized man. *Anesthesiology*, **48**, 360–2.

Index